KV-537-357

The International Handbook of Medical Science

SECOND EDITION

The International Handbook of Medical Science

SECOND EDITION

EDITED BY
DAVID HORROBIN
ALEXANDER GUNN

A daily reference book for medical practice

MTP
Medical and Technical Publishing Co. Ltd.
Oxford Lancaster

Published in UK by MTP, Medical and Technical Publishing Co. Ltd., Seacourt Tower, Oxford and St Leonard's House, Lancaster.

SBN 852 00038 3

Printed in UK

Editorial

The International Handbook of Medical Science is designed to provide a practical and intelligent source of daily reference for medical practice. The first edition proved particularly successful and we were most appreciative of the many letters and comments we received.

The second edition is a development of the first. The two major sections on drugs in current use and on the therapy of common diseases have been up-dated and much new information has been included. A discussion on the use of drugs in pregnancy is also included. In addition, however, there are a considerable number of completely new features. The reference section in particular has been considerably expanded and now covers such important subjects as drug addiction, alcoholism, modern contraceptive practice and electrocardiography.

It has been decided to reduce the number of articles on recent advances in medical science but instead to choose for coverage a limited number of subject areas with particular current interest to a wide readership.

We hope that this second edition, with its many innovations, proves to be a worthwhile development of the first. The aim of the volume remains the same: to provide in an intelligent and constructive way much of the information that is needed in medical practice but which it is often difficult and time-consuming to obtain.

David Horrobin, Professor of Medical Physiology, Nairobi Medical School, Kenya. Late Fellow in Physiology, Magdalen College, Oxford.

Alexander Gunn, Director of Health Services, University of Reading.

March 1972

Contents

Section A

Recent Advances in Medical Science

Sir Macfarlane Burnet presents a detailed account of current developments and contemporary research into immunological response to cancer. Possible applications at the clinical level are described.

Recent Advances in the Study of Cancer Immunity

by

Sir Macfarlane Burnet

University of Melbourne

At the present time there is a high level of interest both by immunologists and by surgeons in the topic of cancer immunity. This is based on the findings from a wide range of malignant disease, both clinical and experimental, that immune responses can occur against the patient's or animal's own primary (autochthonous) tumour. Responses are not always demonstrable and even when they are there is often little evidence that their presence can inhibit tumour growth. Nevertheless there are strong reasons to think that the process which I called immunological surveillance some years ago is constantly in action to inhibit at least a proportion of initiated neoplasms and that in the absence of an immune response there would be strikingly larger numbers of tumours and a shift of their incidence to lower ages. In principle at least there are potentialities for the application of immunological methods in the therapy of some forms of cancer.

The basic experimental findings

In 1953 Foley [1] observed that when fibrosarcomas were induced in mice by injection intramuscularly of methyl-cholanthrene (MCA) the tumours could be transferred to other mice of the same pure line (syngeneic) strain and that if a tumour was excised after a period of growth the animal was significantly resistant to inoculation with cells of the same tumour. It showed, however, no resistance to the cells of a similar tumour induced by the same dose of MCA in another mouse of the same strain. This type of experiment has been widely used in mice, rats and guinea pigs and the broad pattern of the results can be succinctly stated as follows.

Within a pure line strain tumours induced either as fibrosarcomas after intramuscular inoculation or as hepatomas after feeding or intraperitoneal injection of a carcinogen show varying degrees of immunogenicity, and of malignancy as judged by the latent period before a standard sized tumour develops. Some of the tumours produced are not demonstrably immunogenic, but when an immune response occurs it is specific to the strain of tumour. It seems likely that there is some limit to the number of new antigenic specificities which can be manifested by such tumours, but there is as yet no record of two identically patterned tumours being produced in different animals. The immunity is of the cell-mediated type involving cells of the T-system and is analogous to homograft immunity. With guinea pig tumours it has been shown directly to be associated with typical delayed hypersensitivity. In some instances no immunity can be shown while a tumour is actually growing or for a few days after its removal. After a week or two immunity becomes evident by the failure of a standardized inoculum of tumour cells to give rise to a visible tumour.

A wholly different result is obtained when tumours are produced in suitable laboratory rodents by the standard oncogenic viruses, polyoma and SV40. If polyoma virus is inoculated into new-born mice or hamsters, multiple tumours in various organs are produced, predominantly in the salivary glands of mice and in the kidneys of hamsters. Inoculated into adult mice the virus produces no tumours. When, however, a typical tumour has been produced in a mouse inoculated neonatally it can be transplanted serially in mice of syngeneic strain. In the process of passage the virus disappears, i.e. its presence as virus – technically as virions – is not necessary to the continued malignant character of the cells.

By quite straightforward experiments it can be shown that the virus-free tumour has developed two or more new antigens, the most important of which from our point of view is the TSTA (tumour-specific transplantation antigen). These antigens are common to all polyoma-induced tumours and are assumed to result from the incorporation of part of the virus DNA in the chromosomes of the malignant cell. The simplest way to demonstrate TSTA is to transplant polyoma tumour cells, induced and transferred in strain A, into a genetically different B strain of mice. After an initial 'take' the tumour is destroyed by a typical homograft reaction since it carries the foreign histocompatibility antigen A. In the process, however, host B develops immunity against TSTA and when subsequently tested with cells of polyoma raised in B no tumour results. It is also found that when an adult mouse of strain A is inoculated with cell-free polyoma virus of any source it becomes resistant to later inoculation with polyoma cells from an A mouse.

This is important because it indicates that in the adult, initially non-immune mouse the virus 'transforms' cells so that they develop the characteristic TSTA and produce small foci of potentially malignant cells. A rapid immune response against TSTA, however, ensures that the foci are destroyed before they become evident. In the neonatal mouse the capacity to respond immunologically is very poorly developed and the tumours enlarge. By the time immune competence should be attained sufficient TSTA is being produced by the tumour to paralyse the immune response. The animal is now tolerant to all the new antigens of the tumour and it grows unhindered.

Similar phenomena are shown with SV40 virus and tumours, but the new antigens induced are quite distinct from those of polyoma. Very recently it is being reported that more detailed experiments indicate that some of these virus-induced tumours may show other new antigens in addition to the major ones for which the virus is responsible.

Clinical evidence for the importance of cancer immunity

No direct experimental study remotely resembling what can be done in pure line mice is possible with human cancer and evidence for the existence and significance of immunity against malignant cells must be obtained by rather indirect and statistical methods. In general it is limited to observations on the frequency of spontaneous malignant disease in defined populations and serological or other *in vitro* evidence of immune response in an individual to his own tumour. It is, however, highly significant that a tiny proportion of established histologically-diagnosed cancers retrogress spontaneously, and on a larger scale there seem to be more recoveries after standard treatment than would be expected if every surviving cancer cell could re-initiate a malignant process. There are several features about these findings which suggest that immune responses are concerned.

If the process of immunological surveillance is of any importance we should expect to find an excess of tumours in persons whose immunological system was grossly deficient or paralysed by immuno-suppressive drugs. This is in fact the case. All the major immuno-deficiency syndromes which with adequate treatment can allow the affected infant to survive for more than a few years show a disconcertingly high incidence of malignant disease with lympho-reticular neoplasms conspicuously frequent. Even more striking has been the experience of patients who have received a transplanted kidney and survived over a year. The most recent figures I have found (Schenck and Penn [2]) record 52 primary malignant tumours in about 5,000 renal transplants, and suggest that their own experience in Denver covering eight years, with 11 tumours in 184 cases, indicates that the real incidence must be considerably higher than the 1 per cent indicated by the global figures. Of the 52 tumours there were 18 superficial carcinomas of skin, lip or cervix and 10 epithelial tumours of viscera. There were 22 lymphomatous tumours, including reticulum cell sarcoma, of which 11 involved the brain. All these figures are very much higher than the expected incidence in the relatively young subjects concerned. The average age of mesenchymal tumour patients was 30 and of those with epithelial tumours 37 years. The incidence of miscellaneous epithelial tumours is also well above the expected level, but experienced investigators, e.g. Richard Doll, feel that there may be reasons for not taking some of these figures at their face value. No one, however, has the slightest doubt that both in genetically immuno-deficient children and in patients maintained for a year or more on immuno-suppressive drugs lymphomas and related tumours are far more frequent than in normal people. The simplest interpretation is that immunological surveillance is of special importance in relation to incipient malignancies of lymphoid cells.

Spontaneous cure in relation to cancer immunity

It is convenient to combine the discussion of spontaneous cure of cancer with evidence for immune responses in man. The main evidence that spontaneous cure is an immunological process depends on the fact that it is just those cancers most frequently showing retrogression which show the best evidence for an immune response by conventional techniques. Everson and Cole [3] found acceptable evidence of spontaneous regression of cancer in 176 individuals. Four tumour types were responsible for 98 of those cases – hypernephroma 31, neuroblastoma 29, malignant melanoma 19, chorioncarcinoma 19. In 1966 Burkitt's lymphoma had only recently been described and it is not mentioned in Everson and Cole's study. This is the well known tumour widely prevalent in the malarious areas of tropical Africa and now known to occur in other parts of the world. Since then every aspect of Burkitt's lymphoma has been intensively studied and it is almost certain that if early diagnosis and follow-up studies were adequate a considerable proportion of spontaneous cures would be observed. David and Burkitt [4], for instance, reported long-term remission and probable cure of four patients treated with hexamine in 1961. There is also the well known ease with which a substantial proportion can be cured with cytotoxic drugs such as cyclophosphamide. Burkitt lymphoma will therefore be added to the other four types of tumour for further discussion.

For some reason little immunological work has been done with hypernephromas, but there is an extensive literature about each of the others. Malignant melanoma has probably been the most widely studied. Antibody in patients' serum has been demonstrated by fluorescent methods and by cytotoxicity for autologous tumour cells (Lewis *et al.*, [5]). Antigens extracted from the autologous tumour gave reactions of cutaneous hypersensitivity in patients with localised disease but not in those where the tumour had generalised (Fass *et al.*, [6]). Cell-mediated immunity was shown by Hellström *et al.* [7], by using patients' lymphocytes against autologous tumour cells and assessing colony inhibition.

The bad reputation of malignant melanoma is clear enough evidence that these various immune responses are rarely effective in eliminating the tumour. On general grounds one would expect that cell-mediated (T) immunity would be the important controlling factor and the cutaneous hypersensitivity tests of Fass *et al.* suggested that as long as this was demonstrable the tumour remained localised. The circulating antibody studied by Lewis *et al.* behaved in much the same fashion and in some cases antibody present when first tested disappeared as the disease progressed. They distinguished two types of antigen by the type of fluorescence shown on target tumour cells. One was highly specific, being shown only with autologous tumour and serum; the antigen was restricted to the cell surface. The second antigen-antibody reaction showed almost complete cross reaction between different patients and the antigen was present in the cytoplasm. Cross reaction was also seen in the Hellströms' experiments with a colony-inhibition technique, but there is a suggestion in some of their protocols that autologous cells were somewhat more susceptible than allogeneic ones.

Burkitt lymphoma results are difficult to interpret owing to the frequent association of the herpes-like EB virus with tumour cells. If we forget about this and consider the tumour simply as a clone of malignant cells with a new antigen, the results described by Fass *et al.* [8] are of special interest. Thirteen patients with Burkitt lymphoma were skin-tested with autologous cell extract before and after treatment with cyclophosphamide. The results fell into three groups. One case only was positive before treatment and remained so after effective treatment. Seven cases negative before became positive after treatment; all responded satisfactorily to the drug. Finally, five cases were negative both before and after cyclophosphamide; four of these relapsed. The suggestion is strong that an effective T-type response is necessary to 'finish the job' after treatment with a cytotoxic drug.

Chorioncarcinoma is unique amongst malignant tumours in being composed of cells derived from the foetus and therefore genetically distinct from the patient. On general grounds, therefore, one would expect that the presence of alien (paternal) antigens on the tumour cells would result in their rapid immunologically-based rejection. It is evident, however, that a chorioncarcinoma has a similar lack of antigenicity to that shown by trophoblast cells from which it is derived. This has been ascribed to the presence of a sialic-acid compound, presumably a glyco-protein, on the cell surface. The resistance to immune response is, however, not absolute and again the frequent satisfactory outcome with cytotoxic drugs makes it likely that immune processes play a part once most of the malignant cells have been destroyed.

Finally, a few words may be said about neuroblastoma, a common tumour of infants and children, well known to be particularly amenable to surgical treatment. If histological study of the adrenal is made as a routine in autopsies of children under 3 months of age, many more neuroblastoma foci are found than would be the case if all developed into clinically evident tumours. Beckwith and Perrin [9] found the incidence was approximately 10,000 times that of the clinically evident tumour. Although it has been suggested that the failure of such foci to develop results from the maturation of the neuroblastoma to a benign ganglioma, it seems more likely from Hellström's work on cell-mediated immunity in patients with such tumours that immunological surveillance is responsible for their disappearance.

The nature of tumour-specific antigens

There is no doubt that a tumour may carry antigens not present in the normal tissues of the individual in which it has arisen. The origin of such antigens is, however, controversial and there are several possibilities which for the most part are not mutually exclusive. There are three groups of tumour in which the situation seems to be reasonably clear.

(1) Most carcinomas of the human colon produce a tumour-specific antigen which appears to be identical with a foetal protein normally present in various parts of the gastrointestinal tract.

The other two are the experimentally-induced tumours already mentioned in the introductory section.

(2) Tumours produced by chemical carcinogens which show a wide range of individual antigens and a spectrum of immunogenicity ranging from high to nil.

(3) The virus-specific tumour antigens induced by some of the oncogenic viruses.

Before considering human tumours from this point of view it is worth discussing some of the theoretical possibilities as to how these antigens arise. If such discussion is not to be interminably qualified, certain conditions must be accepted for the time being as if they were axiomatic.

(1) A tumour is a clonal proliferation initiated from a single cell which has undergone an inheritable change expressible as a somatic mutation and not interfering with the viability of the cell line.

(2) Somatic mutation in the broad sense becomes clinically demonstrable only when it results in a proliferative advantage to the altered cell and its descendants.

(3) Every somatic cell carries the genetic potentialities of the whole organism to which it belongs, including potentialities normally expressible only at particular stages of embryogenesis and development.

With this background something may first be said about the possible origin of somatic mutations. I should like to introduce a suggestion here, initiated so far as I am concerned by Professor Richard Doll, in discussing informally the curious regularity of the age-specific incidence of cancer by which (with some 'fiddling' in a few cases) it takes the form of a straight line when plotted logarithmically on both axes. Almost the only necessary conditions for such behaviour are that rare and random circumstances should act with equal likelihood *over the relevant period* to produce some continuing and cumulative effect. Doll showed that most of the apparent exceptions could be brought into line by making some reasonable assumptions about the period over which the mutagenic [carcinogenic] agent was operative.

When the rule holds effectively over the whole of life one must assume that the mutagenic influence is always acting and we can postulate thermal agitation or background ionising radiation from cosmic rays or terrestrial radioactivity. The deviations of lung cancer age-incidence can be rationalised by considering the experience of cohorts of contemporaries in relation to the changing history of cigarette smoking. The remarkably steep straight line for prostatic cancer can be brought down to the standard slope of 4–5 by assuming that the mutagen concerned is active only from the age of 35 onward.

This approach fits neatly with some suggestions on the nature of carcinogenesis that I have recently elaborated (Burnet, [10, 11]). They are based on the very generalised hypothesis that a wide variety of 'non-biological' molecules, i.e. substance for which there is no evolved mechanism capable of handling them effectively in the body, may find opportunity to enter the genetic compartment of the cell and damage information-carrying DNA while still leaving the cell viable. Such damage must necessarily be minimal if the mutated cell is to survive and have descendants. It will be based on *chemically* definable changes but informationally the changes are likely to be as random as those of any spontaneous mutation. Where experimental oncogenic viruses are concerned, the intrusion into the nuclear mechanism will in general be at random but complicated by the possibility of viral nucleic acid being fused into the cell genome.

The origin of new antigens which can provide a basis for immunological surveillance or perhaps future immunotherapy of cancer can now be formulated:

(1) By definition any informationally random episode, if it is to induce a cell to initiate a malignant clone, must so modify the cell that it and its descendants have an inheritable proliferative advantage over its unmutated congeners. Usually this will be associated with a cell surface change – loss of contact inhibition for example – presumably involving both the function and detailed structure of one or more genetically coded receptors in the cell membrane. Similar random changes may also involve other cell membrane proteins not directly concerned with malignant character.

If the damage is to structural genes, change expressed in the cell membrane proteins will be in amino-acid sequence. Depending on circumstances, these may or may not modify function or confer autoimmunogenicity on the protein. Either may happen without the other.

(2) Foreign intrusion into the genome is at least equally likely to cause inheritable disturbance in non-structural operational aspects of the genetic system of the cell. In the book already referred to I have discussed at length the variety of 'inappropriate' components that can be produced by cancer cells (Burnet, [10]). It appears that once a malig-

nant clone is initiated there is either some secondary loss of integration of nuclear function or an increased vulnerability to casual mutagens. Every somatic cell exposed to an appropriate degree of random damage will be capable in principle of sometimes (even if the likelihood is almost infinitely rare) producing any protein that any cell – embryonic, foetal or adult – of the organism can make. If the protein in question is a highly active pituitary hormone it will have an immediately evident clinical effect if the clone producing it expands to more than minimal size. If it is a tissue-specific 'inaccessible' antigen to which normal immune tolerance is not provoked, severe autoimmune disease may be initiated. There are steadily increasing numbers of clinical reports of conditions that can probably be ascribed to such processes.

(3) Finally we come to a matter of great current significance: the appearance with some regularity in tumours of colon and rectum of a foetal antigen normally produced by cells ancestral to the intestinal epithelium. It would be by no means unlikely that most active cancers should produce proteins characteristic of foetal cells of the particular system concerned. The special interest of cancers of the lower bowel may be due merely to the fact that the antigen CEA (carcino-embryonic antigen) can readily be detected in the circulating blood. If the embryonic antigen had disappeared well before birth, the body is unlikely to have any intrinsic tolerance and there will be possibilities that antibodies may be produced against it or clones of T-immunocytes of appropriate specificity develop.

The manifestations (clinical and laboratory) of immune response in malignant disease

It is only too clear that any immune response to clinical malignant disease is usually ineffective and there is plainly scepticism in many quarters as to whether immunological surveillance is 'really' of any human significance. Nevertheless I can also sense that with the established facts of specific tumour antigens and of effective immune responses in a number of experimental situations there is an even wider optimism that some form of immunotherapy for at least a proportion of cancers will be developed. If this is to happen it must be by an understanding and exploitation of the types of immune responses to malignant cells which can be studied in the laboratory.

It is probably desirable first to recapitulate for readers not familiar with recent ideas in immunology the modern division of immune responses into two systems. The T-system is so called because the cells concerned, T-immunocytes, are thymus-dependent in the sense that they or their progenitors were differentiated from stem cell to lymphocytes carrying antibody-type receptors in the thymus. The cells of the T-system are concerned with cell-mediated immunity and synthesise no more antibody than is needed to maintain their specific immune receptor patches on the cell surface. They are responsible for delayed hypersensitivity reactions and various types of contact sensitivity in the skin, for the rejection of skin and organ grafts and probably for some or most forms of autoimmune disease. They are deeply concerned in both the production of symptoms and the development of immunity with most virus diseases and with chronic mycobacterial or fungal diseases.

The second system, B, takes its initial from the fact that in birds the immunocytes concerned are developed in the Bursa of Fabricius, a lymphoid organ opening off the cloaca. There is nothing equivalent in mammals and immunologists are divided as to whether the immunocytes with the corresponding functions are differentiated in the 'gut-associated lymphoid tissue' – tonsil, appendix, Peyer's patches, etc. – or in the bone marrow. The trend is toward the latter so that B can stand for bursa or bone marrow. On stimulation by antigen, B-immunocytes are transformed into plasma cells which are essentially factories producing large amounts of antibody of the same specificity as was characteristic of the ancestral immunocyte. A proportion of stimulated B-immunocytes proliferate to produce 'memory cells' from which further crops of plasma cells can be derived if the antigen is re-encountered on some subsequent occasion. All types of antibody producers fall into this series.

The disease, congenital sex-linked agammaglobulinaemia, represents a complete failure of the B-system to develop and its symptoms provide a guide to the functions of antibody in the body. The most important is protection against acute bacterial infection. In sharp contrast to the older view that all immunity was due to antibody, the modern tendency is to regard most of the other functions of antibody as relatively minor adjuvants to the functioning of the T-system. Perhaps the most important action is to 'mop up' any excess of antigen that may enter the body before it can stimulate immunocytes either to proliferate as T-cells or to produce more antibody-producing plasma cells. This negative feedback is obviously valuable in an acute infection to ensure that the whole immune system is not swung into action against the antigens of the pathogen responsible, but where for any reason the cell-mediated T response is inadequate, antibody of the same type may weaken it further. This is of special importance in relation to cancer immunity. It was disconcerting when it was found about 20 years ago that by immunising animals with some types of tumour extracts they became *more* susceptible to the tumour in question, i.e. a tumour could be produced by a smaller inoculum of cells. The same type of 'enhancement' could be produced by passive transfer of serum from an immunised animal. It is accepted as resulting from attachment of antibody to antigen of the tumour cell either free in body fluids or on the tumour cell surface. This both renders the antigen less capable of stimulating the appropriate T-immunocytes to proliferate and at the same time protects the target cells from their cytotoxic action. This enhancing effect of antibody is not always demonstrable. In some experimental systems cytotoxic antibody can be produced and shown to be capable of preventing inoculated cancer cells from growing to a tumour.

All the evidence, however, points to the prime importance of the T-system in cancer immunity. The removal of an incipient cancer focus, whether arising spontaneously or following experimental injection, is a function of lymphocytes of the T-system wholly analogous to the rejection of a transplanted organ or skin graft from another individual. There are some differences of opinion about the details of the process, but the following sequence seems to be the most likely.

The tumour cell surfaces liberate into the tissue fluid small amounts of their TSTAs which by definition are foreign to the body. These are transported either directly or carried on the surface of lymphocytes or monocytes passing through or by the tumour by the lymph flow to the regional lymph nodes. There antigen finds opportunity sooner or later to meet a T-immunocyte whose receptor has an antibody-like relationship to the tumour antigen. The immunocyte proliferates and soon there is a growing population of such cells tuned to react with the tumour cells. In due course some reach the site of the tumour nidus. Contact results in immobilisation of the immunocyte with liberation of a range of more or less actively damaging and stimulating products from its substance. By processes which need not be elaborated, other lymphocytes as well as specific immunocytes are attracted to the spot, both tumour cells and the associated capillaries are damaged, and if all goes well the tumour is eliminated.

Possible applications at the clinical level

So far there has been little clinical application of the steadily increasing fund of knowledge about cancer immunity. Some real possibilities are, however, beginning to emerge, which may be briefly enumerated.

Diagnosis: The most important development here has been the recognition that most patients with carcinoma of the colon and some with other abdominal malignancies show serologically demonstrable amount of a carcinoembryonic antigen (CEA) in the blood. This is the first useful 'blood test' for a specific type of cancer and we can expect active development of its use in screening for unsuspected abdominal malignancy and in detecting post-operative recurrences. There are already hints that foetal antigens may also be present in other types of tumour and active research on their clinical detection either as circulating antigen or from the appearance of an antibody can be expected. The advantage of these foetal antigens is that they are likely to be of the same tissue-specific pattern in all the human tumours in which they are present. Recent work by the Hellströms and their colleagues in Seattle suggests that tissue-specific, presumably foetal, antigens can be demonstrated by testing patients' lymphocytes for colony-inhibiting capacity against cell cultures of tumour. All this work is at the present time in the category of research, the techniques are elaborate and there is obvious scope for misinterpretation. It will be of much interest to see whether and when such techniques will become suitable for routine use in the handling of cancer patients.

Prognosis: Pathologists have regarded the intensity of lymphocyte and plasma cell infiltration at the margin of the malignant tissue in surgically removed tumours as a partial guide to prognosis. A heavy infiltration was favourable, absence of any cellular response very unfavourable. Should tests for antibody or cell-mediated responses develop to the practical level they will clearly be of value for prognosis as well as diagnosis.

Immunotherapy: It is hard to conceive that this will ever be more than an accessory to surgical removal. An actively growing tumour may be (1) non-antigenic, (2) producing enough antigen to maintain a state of immunological paralysis, or (3) under cell-mediated immunological attack but with sufficient intrinsic proliferative vigour to keep on growing. If a tumour is non-antigenic, clearly nothing can be done to treat it immunologically. In either of the other classes, however, removal of the primary tumour may give an opportunity for existing immune capacity to complete the elimination of any remaining tumour cells. Further help in this direction is possible in principle if an effective immunising antigen of the same specificity as the tumour was available. This is likely to be dependent on proof that the known or still to be discovered 'tumour-foetal' antigens can in fact stimulate an effective cytotoxic response. If the really relevant tumour antigens are specific for each individual tumour, there can be no serious prospect of specific immunotherapy.

Non-specific improvement of the body's own T-system responses remains something of a will-o'-the-wisp. It is easy enough to make a bodily function *less* efficient, by immunosuppressive drugs for example, but almost impossible to improve the effectiveness of anything so elaborate and controlled as the immune system. Attempts to do so with bacterial endotoxins, pertussis vaccine or BCG have been made and doubtless new suggestions will come forward for test in the future. One would guess that their efficacy is likely to remain forever non-proven.

References

1. Foley, E. J., Antigenic properties of methylcholanthrene-induced tumours in mice of the strain of origin. *Cancer Res.* (1953), **13**, 835.
2. Schenck, S. A., and Penn, I., De novo brain tumours in renal transplant recipients. *Lancet* (1971), **1**, 983.
3. Everson, T. C., and Cole, W. H., *Spontaneous Regression of Cancer* (1966), Philadelphia.
4. David, J., and Burkitt, D., Burkitt's lymphoma: remissions following seemingly non-specific therapy. *Brit. med. J.* (1968), **4**, 288.
5. Lewis, M. C., Ikonopisov, R. L., Nairn, R. C., Phillips, T. M., Fairley, C. H., Bodenham, D. C., and Alexander, P., Tumour-specific antibodies in human malignant melanoma and their relationship to the extent of the disease. *Brit. med. J.* (1969), **3**, 547.
6. Fass, L., Herberman, R. B., Ziegler, J. L., and Kiryabwire, J. W. M., Cutaneous hypersensitivity reactions to autologous extracts of malignant melanoma cells. *Lancet* (1969), **1**, 116.
7. Hellström, I., Hellström, K. E., Sjögren, H. O., and Warner, G. A., Demonstration of cell-mediated immunity to human neoplasms of various histological types. *Int. J. Cancer* (1971), **7**, 1.
8. Fass, L., Herberman, R. B., and Ziegler, J., Delayed cutaneous hypersensitivity reactions to autologous extracts of Burkitt-lymphoma cells. *New Engl. J. Med.* (1970), **282**, 776.
9. Beckwith, J. B., and Perrin, E. V., In situ neuroblastomas: a contribution to the natural history of neural crest tumors. *Amer. J. Path.* (1963), **43**, 1089.
10. Burnet, F. M., *Immunological Surveillance* (1970), Pergamon Australia, Sydney.
11. Burnet, F. M., *Transplantation Reviews*, (1971), 7, 3.

Current research directed towards an understanding of the biological significance of prostaglandins in a wide range of tissues is discussed in depth. Particular emphasis is placed on the potential applications in the field of fertility control, namely the development of a "once-a-month" contraceptive pill.

Recent Advances in Prostaglandin Research

by
Sultan M. M. Karim,
Professor of Pharmacology and Therapeutics, Makerere University Medical School, Kampala, Uganda
and
Donald Macintosh,
Senior Lecturer in Pharmacology, Department of Pharmacology and Therapeutics, Makerere University Medical School, Kampala, Uganda

Prostaglandin research has been the most stimulating feature of biomedical investigation in the past decade. Interest developed at a time of expanding knowledge of hormonal and neurohormonal behaviour and research work received a tremendous impetus in the early 1960s with the elucidation in Sweden of the chemical structure of prostaglandins followed by the independent discovery in Holland, Sweden and the USA of biosynthetic pathways, that of the Upjohn Compnay, USA providing a large supply of material for investigation.

Several detailed reviews on the subject have been published notably those of Bergström *et al.* [1] and Horton [2]. This article deals mainly with results of research indicating a probable physiological or pathophysiological role for prostaglandins, their established and potential therapeutic value.

In 1930 Kurzrok and Lieb published the first account of the actions of human seminal fluid on the uterus (Kurzrok and Lieb, [3]). They observed that uteri from women with a history of successful pregnancies were stimulated by semen whereas the activity of those from women with complete sterility or sterility of long duration was inhibited. The presence of spermatozoa was not essential for these responses. On the basis of these results, Kurzrok and Lieb classified uteri as receptive or rejective and seminal fluid as depressant or stimulant. Their investigations had been prompted by Kurzrok's observations that, in the course of every attempt to treat human sterility by artificial insemination, seminal fluid was often promptly expelled from the uterine cavity even when the patient was maintained in the extreme Trendelenberg position. Similar quantities of Ringer's solution on the other hand were successfully retained.

The findings of Kurzrok and Lieb were subsequently confirmed and extended by Goldblatt and von Euler (Goldblatt, [4] von Euler, [5]). Considering that the active principle involved originated from the prostate gland, von Euler named it prostaglandin. Goldblatt suggested that more than one active compound was present in seminal fluid and that they might be of physiological significance. He was unable however, to demonstrate their presence in extracts from adenomatous prostates.

It is now known that there are 14 structurally related compounds in the human body some of which stimulate the human uterus, others possessing activity on non-uterine tissue. These are collectively known as the prostaglandins, more simply designated PGs.

Structure synthesis and release

Prostaglandins are a series of cyclic oxygenated C_{20} fatty acids whose basic skeleton is that of prostanoic acid, a hypothetical compound (Figure 1). Their chemical structure was elucidated by Bergström and co-workers in the early 1960s (for references see Bergström and Samuelsson, [6]). Under present nomenclature they are grouped into four types – E, F, A and B. There are 14 naturally occurring prostaglandins. These are PGE_1, PGE_2, PGE_3, $PGF_{1\alpha}$, $PGF_{2\alpha}$, $PGF_{3\alpha}$, PGA_1, PGA_2, PGB_1, PGB_2, and 19-OHA_1, 19-OHA_2, 19-OHB_1 and 19-OHB_2 (Figure 2). Compounds of the E and F series are termed the primary prostaglandins. There are three unsaturated fatty acid precursors of prostaglandins, viz.: 8, 11, 14-Eicosatetraenoic acid (di-homo-y-linoleic acid), 5, 8, 11, 14-Eicosatetraenoic acid (arachidonic acid) and 5, 8, 11, 14, 17-Eicosapentaneoic acid.

Di-homo-y-lineoleic acid is derived from the essential fatty acid linolenic acid. Natural synthesis of prostaglandins is from this compound and arachidonic acid under the control of a microsomal synthetase system (prostaglandin synthetase). The pathways are outlined in Figure 3.

Distribution, synthesis and release

Prostaglandins are widely distributed in mammalian tissues although with considerable qualitative and species variation. Their possible

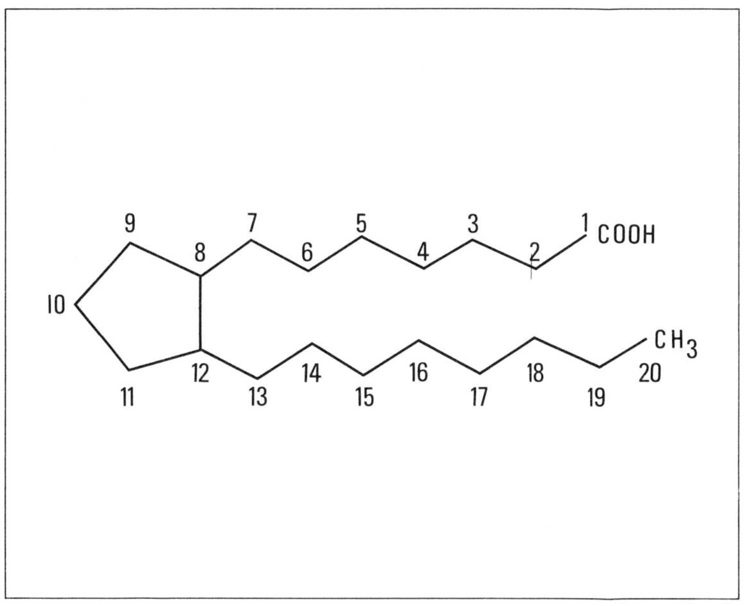

Fig. 1. The Structure of 'prostanoic acid'

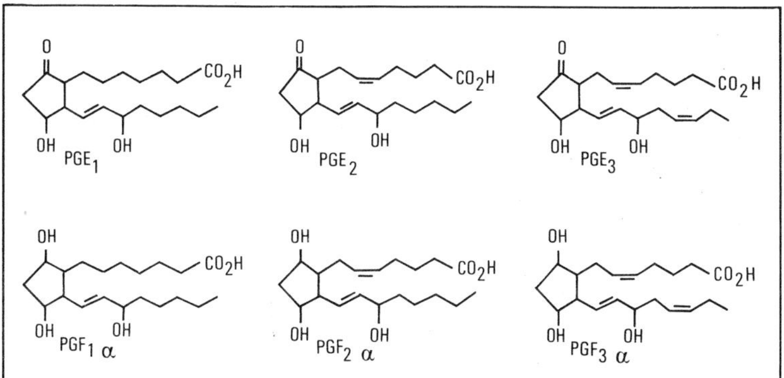

PGE$_1$ PGE$_2$ PGE$_3$

PGF$_{1\alpha}$ PGF$_{2\alpha}$ PGF$_{3\alpha}$

Fig. 2. Chemical Structures of 14 naturally occurring prostaglandins.

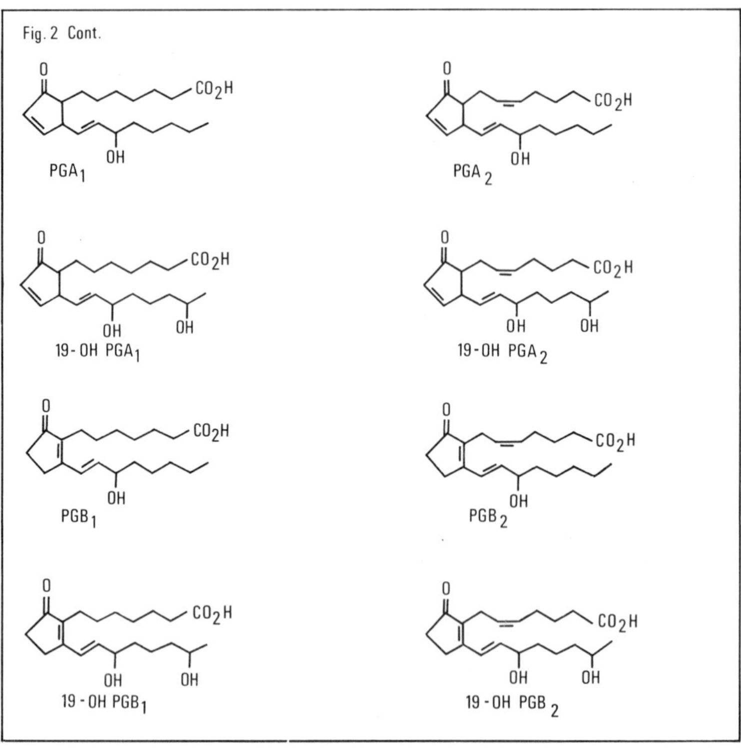

Figure 2 (Continued). Chemical structures of 14 naturally occurring prostaglandins.

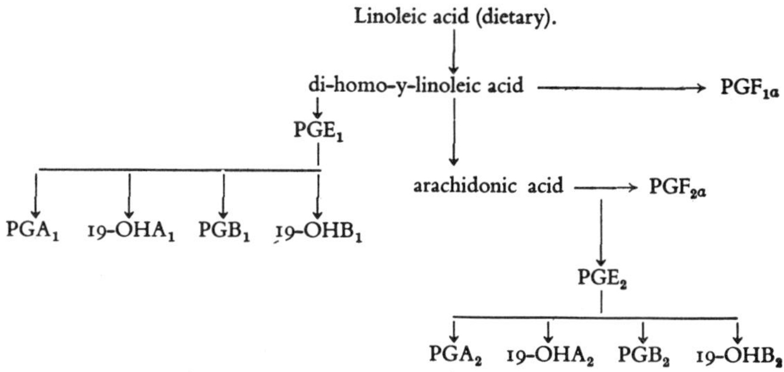

Figure 3. Outline of prostaglandin biosynthesis from linoleic acid.

occurrence in non-mammalian tissues and in plants is being investigated. Their presence and concentration in a number of human and animal tissues have been estimated by a highly sensitive biological assay technique (Bergström, Carlson and Weeks, [1]) by g.l.c. and mass spectrometry. The data are presented in Table 1.

Biosynthesis and release of prostaglandins from tissues occur so readily in response to a variety of stimuli, physiological and pathological that it would appear that any distortion of the cell membrane is an adequate trigger mechanism. Prostaglandins are stored in minute quantities and the ease with which biosynthesis is stimulated means that PG concentration values reported for many tissues do not accurately reflect the true endogenous concentration. Experimentally enhanced release may indicate accelerated biosynthesis rather than activation of release mechanisms.

The prostaglandin synthesising enzyme system is highly active in intact tissue but dependent upon the amount of substrate (precursor) available. There is good evidence that for increased biosynthesis phospholipase A, present in the cell membrane, is the essential regulating factor. By clearing precursor acids from tissue phospholipids this enzyme could provide additional substrate for conversion into prostaglandins.

Cardiovascular and renal systems

The effects of prostaglandins on the cardiovascular system vary according to species, compound used, the route of administration and where the intravenous route is employed, to single injection or infusion and rate of infusion.

Prostaglandins E (PGE_1, PGE_2 and PGE_3) consistently lower arterial

Table 1 Occurrence of prostaglandins in some human tissues

Source	Prostaglandins
Semen	E_1, E_2, E_3, $F_{1\alpha}$, $F_{2\alpha}$, A_1, A_2, B_1, B_2, 19 hydroxy A_1, 19 hydroxy A_2, 19 hydroxy B_1 19 hydroxy B_2
Menstrual fluid } Endometrium }	E_2, $F_{2\alpha}$
Lung	$F_{2\alpha}$
Lung	E_2, $F_{2\alpha}$
Umbilical and placental blood vessels, amniotic fluid, decidua	E_1, E_2, $F_{1\alpha}$, $F_{2\alpha}$
Maternal venous blood during labour	E_2, $F_{2\alpha}$
Thymus	E_1
Thyroid	E_2, $F_{2\alpha}$
Vagus nerve	E_2, $F_{2\alpha}$
Cervical sympathetic nerve	E_2, $F_{2\alpha}$
Bronchi	E_2, $F_{2\alpha}$
Cardiac muscle	E_2
Stomach mucosa	E_2

For the occurrence of prostaglandins in other human tissues and animal tissues see Bergström, Carlson and Weeks [1]; Euler and Eliasson [1]; Karim, Sandler and Williams (1967).
Modified from Karim (1971a), 'Prostaglandins and Reproduction' in *The Scientific Basis of Obstetrics and Gynaecology*, Ch. 12, P. 319. Ed. R. R. Macdonald, J. A. Churchill, London, 1971.

blood pressure in a wide range of laboratory animals including the dog, monkey and baboon, PGE_1 being the most potent. The evidence indicates a direct effect on peripheral arteries and arterioles supported by portal venoconstriction, the lowered peripheral resistance producing an increase in cardiac output. There is no evidence in favour of a cholinergic mechanism, histamine release, α-receptor blockade, or β-receptor stimulation. Prostaglandins E appear to exert physiological antagonism against noradrenaline, angiotensin and vasopressin. In intact laboratory animals, anaesthetised and non-anaesthetised, the hypotensive effect of PGE_1 is accompanied by an increase in heart rate, which in dogs is prevented by pre-treatment with reserpine, pronethalol and ganglion blocking agents. The vasodilating effect is not altered. This chronotropic action of PGE_1 would appear to be due to a reflex increase in sympathetic activity as a result of lowered systemic arterial pressure. Further studies in dogs have produced evidence that PGE_1 increases directly myocardial contractility, cardiac output and coronary artery blood flow (for references see Karim and Somers, [7]).

Several studies in man have shown that the intravenous infusion of PGE_1 produces tachycardia, fall in systemic and diastolic blood pressures, facial flushing, abdominal pain, severe pulsating headache and venous erythema at the site of infusion. During the simultaneous infusion of PGE_1 with noradrenaline, the pressor effect is less than that of noradrenaline illustrating the physiological antagonism referred to above.

The cardiovascular effects of F prostaglandins are more complex. Prostaglandins $F_{1\alpha}$ and $F_{2\alpha}$ are depressor in the cat (probably by dilating skeletal muscle vessels) and rabbit, pressor in the rat, dog and man. In the spinal chick they are also pressor but in the anaesthetised chick they may give pressor, depressor or biphasic responses. Prostaglandin $F_{2\alpha}$ is more active than $PGF_{1\alpha}$ in lowering rabbit blood pressor but much less active than PGE_2 in lowering cat blood pressure. No observations have yet been published on the cardiovascular effects of $PGF_{3\alpha}$.

The pressor effect of $F_{2\alpha}$ in man is seen with rapid single intravenous injections of 500 mg. However, infusions of up to 200 μg/minute over several hours, given to stimulate the uterus in early pregnancy, have not produced any effects on the cardiovascular system.

The pressor effect of $PGF_{2\alpha}$ in the rat and dog is considered to be due mainly to selective peripheral venoconstriction causing an increase in right arterial pressure and an increase in cardiac output. It is not known whether this mechanism operates in man.

The selective venoconstricting action of $PGF_{2\alpha}$ may be of physiological significance in reproduction. Prostaglandin $F_{2\alpha}$ is known to be present in uterine tissue and on release may reduce blood flow in the common utero-ovarian vein with resultant luteolysis and menstrual-like bleeding.

Prostaglandin $F_{1\alpha}$ in low concentrations (50 ng/ml) increases the contractile force of the perfused rat heart without altering the heart rate or coronary flow. In anaesthetised dogs neither prostaglandin $F_{1\alpha}$ or $F_{2\alpha}$ given by intracoronary infusion have any effect on myocardial contractility, blood flow or cardiac rate.

The A series of prostaglandins are potent hypotensive agents in the rat and dog, the effect in the latter being mainly due to marked peripheral vasodilation. In the dog, PGA compounds increase cardiac rate and output (as do the PGE compounds) partly by a direct inotropic effect and partly through increased sympathetic activity from the lowered arterial pressure.

The results of a few studies of the effects of PGA_1 infusion in patients with essential hypertension have been published. There was significant reduction in systolic and diastolic blood pressure levels (chiefly systolic). Post infusion hypertension was noted to be common and sometimes, the hypertensive effect was preceded by an increase in urinary flow and urinary $Na+$ and $K+$ levels.

A natriuretic effect of PGA_1 by infusion has also been noted in hyponatraemic, cirrhotic and anephric patients, this being most marked in cirrhosis with ascites.

The cardiovascular effects of PGA_2, now known to be the main constituent of renal medullin, have been studied in a 25 year old hypertensive subject using a single intravenous injection and continuous intravenous infusion. Systolic and diastolic blood pressure levels fell followed by reflex tachycardia and increased cardiac output with a fall in the total peripheral resistance. Using the single injection technique the hypotensive effect began 18 seconds after injection, was maximal at 23 seconds and had disappeared at 32 seconds. With the infusion a marked diuresis was recorded.

These studies indicate possible roles for prostaglandins in the regulation of blood pressure and renal function, and they may prove to be of therapeutic value in the treatment of hypertension and fluid retention.

The alimentary tract

Prostaglandins E_1, E_2, $F_{1\alpha}$ and $F_{2\alpha}$ occur in the alimentary tract. The presence of A and B prostaglandins has not so far been demonstrated. The precise localisation, mechanisms of storage and release of E and F compounds are not known but in the human stomach, where PGE_2 is the chief prostaglandin component, the source is the mucosa. Studies in muscle strips from the small and large bowel of animals and man have shown that on longitudinal muscle, E and F compounds induce contraction; on circular muscle E compounds produce relaxation or diminish the stimulant effect of acetylcholine and carbamylcholine, whereas F compounds produce contraction. The experimental evidence indicates a direct action on muscle cells although on longitudinal muscle a stimulant effect through the intrinsic cholinergic nerve supply may also be involved (for references see Bennett, [8]).

In humans the intravenous infusion of PGE_1 caused abdominal pain (Bergström *et al.*, [9]) and the intravenous infusion of $PGF_{2\alpha}$ (50 μg/minute) for therapeutic abortion frequently caused diarrhoea and occasionally vomiting (Karim and Filshie, [10]). Infusion of PGE_2 at 5μg/minute for the same purpose did not produce diarrhoea. Prostaglandins E_1, E_2 and $F_{2\alpha}$ administered orally caused diarrhoea (Misiewicz *et al.*, [11]; Karim, [12]). The diarrhoea has been described as normally formed faeces in clear fluid so that apart from a stimulant effect of prostaglandins on alimentary tract smooth muscle impairment of electrolyte absorption through the mucosa with consequent fluid retention in the lumen appear to be involved.

It has been suggested that the profuse diarrhoea associated with cholera may be due to release of prostaglandins from the intestinal wall by cholera endotoxin. An effective inhibition of prostaglandin synthesis or an antagonist could prove to be a significant advance in the treatment of this disease.

Antisecretory activities of E and F prostaglandins have been shown in the rat and the dog (for references see Bennett and Fleshler, [13]). Prostaglandin E_1 and E_2 decreased gastric acid secretion in response to food, pentagastrin and histamine. In rats, the release of histamine into gastric juice was not affected. Prostaglandin $F_{2\alpha}$ in dogs had no effect on histamine-induced acid secretion.

There is little information on the effects of prostaglandins on human gastric secretion, only one study having been published to date (Horton *et al.*, [14]). These authors found that PGE_1 administered orally did not affect the acid secretion response to pentagastrin. The effects of PGE_2 are not yet known.

Further animal investigations suggest that the antisecretory effects of prostaglandins are direct but there may be an indirect supporting action via reduction in gastric mucosal blood flow systemically or locally induced. Strong evidence for a direct action is that on the isolated gastric mucosa of the bullfrog, PGE_1 inhibits the secretory activity of histamine and gastrin (Way and Durbin, [15]).

Respiratory tract

Experiments *in vitro* show that E prostaglandins are bronchodilator while the F series are bronchoconstrictor (Sweatman and Collier, [16]).

Prostaglandins E_2 and $F_{2\alpha}$ are both present in human lung but their roles in lung function and in asthma are unknown.

Isolated human bronchial smooth muscle is relaxed by prostaglandin E_1 (Sweatman and Collier, [16]). When given intravenously to anaesthetised guinea-pigs, prostaglandin E_1 and isoprenaline show similar bronchodilator activity but when administered by aerosol the activity of prostaglandin E_1 is much greater (Large *et al.*, [17]). Since propanolol did not antagonise the effect, β-receptor stimulation is probably not involved.

In a clinical study in normal subjects and asthmatics the effect of prostaglandin E_1 was compared with that of isoprenaline and a placebo administered by metered aerosols (Cuthbert, [18]). In six normal subjects prostaglandin E_1 (free acid) did not alter the forced expiratory volume in one second (FEV_1) but caused upper respiratory tract irritation which was reduced in incidence and intensity when the triethanolamine salt was used. In five asthmatic subjects with reversible airway obstruction, prostaglandin E_1 (triethanolamine salt) in doses of 2·75–27·5 μg produced an increase in FEV_1 of 20–40 per cent lasting for 15–35 minutes. The increase in FEV_1 from prostaglandin E_1 (triethanolamine salt) in doses of 55 μg was comparable to that of 550 μg isoprenaline both in intensity and duration although the isoprenaline effect appeared sooner. Although none of the asthmatics in the trial experienced respiratory tract irritation, one asthmatic outside the trial did so with a progressive fall in FEV_1 followed by bronchospasm. This was considered to be secondary to the local irritant effect of prostaglandin and was reversed by isoprenaline inhalation.

Small scale clinical studies have also been carried out with prostaglandin E_2 as the triethanolamine salt. In four normal subjects the FEV_1 was unchanged as with the prostaglandin E_1 preparation, but in two asthmatic subjects FEV_1 increased by 40 per cent. and the bronchodilating effect lasted for 40–60 minutes.

These results indicate that E prostaglandins may have therapeutic application in asthma although more extensive investigation is required to establish this and their relative merits. It is possible that prostaglandin analogues of greater therapeutic advantage will be found.

Fat and carbohydrate metabolism

The formation of fatty acids from triglyceride and re-esterification back to triglyceride is a continuous process. Fatty acids pass into plasma as free fatty acids together with glycerol which is also derived from triglyceride. The mobilisation of free fatty acids from triglyceride is a complex process involving a number of hormonal, nervous and nutritional regulating factors.

In experimental preparations, PGE_1 has been shown to be a highly potent inhibitor of basal lipolysis and to depress the lipolytic effect of catecholamines, glucagon, ACTH, TSH, arginine-vasopressin, sympathetic nerve stimulation and exposure to cold. By contrast, PGE_1 promotes lipolysis in dogs and man when injected intravenously in amounts too small to affect hormonal lipolytic activity. This action is considered to be mediated through the sympathetic nervous system since it is antagonised by ganglion blocking drugs. (For references see Horton, [2]).

The mechanism of the antilipolytic effect of PGE_1 which is similar in some respects to that of insulin, is not clear. Catecholamines, ACTH and glucagon induce lipolysis by activating the adenyl cyclase enzyme system which catalyses the formation of cyclic AMP (cyclic 3′5′-adenosine monophosphate) from ATP. Cyclic AMP then activates the lipase system essential for triglyceride breakdown and is itself inactivated by phosphodiesterase. Inhibition of lipolysis by PGE_1 may therefore result from an inhibitory action on adenyl cyclase or cyclic AMP or from a stimulant effect on phosphodiesterase. At present inhibition of adenyl cyclase appears to be the most likely although the nature of the enzyme inhibition is obscure.

In summary, PGE_1 given by intravenous injection has two effects on fat metabolism. In low doses lipolysis is stimulated through sympathetic nervous system activity (possibly related lowering of blood pressure) but in high doses lipolysis is inhibited.

Apart from the lipolytic effect of PGE_1, this compound possesses some insulin-like activity on glucose metabolism. Glucose uptake and oxidation and triglyceride synthesis from glucose and acetate are stimulated by PGE_1 in isolated rat adipose tissue; administered intraperitoneally to intact rats, PGE_1 stimulates the incorporation of glucose into diaphragmatic and epididymal fat glycogen. In dogs and man intravenous infusion of PGE_1 lowers blood glucose levels. (Haessler and Crawford, [19]; Vaughan, [20]).

Whether these effects of PGE_1 on glucose metabolism are direct or secondary to decreased lipolysis is not established.

Studies on the effects of other prostaglandins are fewer. Prostaglandins E_2 and E_3 given by single intravenous injection in dogs reduced the lipolytic effect of noradrenaline; $PGF_{1\alpha}$ had no effect, and PGA_1

either had no effect or promoted lipolysis. In man, the intravenous infusion of PGE_2 for 30 minutes in doses of 0·056–0·32 μg/kg/minute had a lipolytic effect whereas the effects of prostaglandins A_1, $F_{1\alpha}$, $F_{1\beta}$ and $F_{2\alpha}$ in the same dosage were equivocal (for references see Bergström, Carlson and Weeks, [1]).

Prostaglandins would therefore appear to be implicated in intermediary metabolism but the nature of the involvement and interrelationships with hormones remain to be elucidated. An optimistic speculation would be that PGE_1 or a synthetic analogue may prove to be useful in the treatment of diabetes mellitus.

Prostaglandins and blood coagulation

Prostaglandin E_1 when added to platelet rich plasma *in vitro*, markedly inhibits platelet aggregation induced by ADP, thrombin, collagen, noradrenaline and serotonin. Prostaglandin W-homo, E_1, a synthetic prostaglandin, has a similar action but is several times more potent. Other prostaglandins with similar platelet inhibiting activity include PGE_2, A_1, A_2, $F_{1\alpha}$, $F_{2\alpha}$, B_1 and B_2. All these compounds are several times less active than PGE_1.

In vivo however, intravenous infusions of PGE_1 or PGE_2 at rate of 5–10 μg/minute do not influence platelet aggregation. The effects of higher rates of infusion on platelet function cannot be assessed because of the marked cardiovascular changes produced by PGE compounds. The possible reason for the lack of platelet inhibiting action of prostaglandins *in vivo* could be their very rapid inactivation in the body. These compounds therefore, are not of practical value in the treatment or prevention of thrombosis and atherosclerosis. Perhaps, a search for a prostaglandin analogue with selective action on platelet aggregation and with a longer life in the body would be a fruitful line for future investigations (for references see Mody, [21]).

Reproduction

Although prostaglandins have a wide range of pharmacological actions the first recognised property of this group of compound was its ability to stimulate isolated strips of human uterus. This has been demonstrated for semen, extracts of seminal fluid and for some individual pure prostaglandins (Bygdeman, [22]). Further interest in the action of prostaglandins on the uterus was stimulated by suggestions that these compounds may be involved in some natural reproductive processes. Thus Pickles and his collaborators (see Pickles, [23]), demonstrated the presence of prostaglandins in human menstrual fluid and in the disintegrating endometrium. Prostaglandin-like activity was also encountered in circulating blood only during menstruation. Pickles suggested that prostaglandins could be the menstrual stimulant. The studies of Karim and collaborators has provided evidence for the participation of prostaglandins in spontaneous abortion and in term labour. They have shown that certain prostaglandins appear in the amniotic fluid and in maternal circulation only during spontaneous abortion and labour (see Karim, [24]).

The role of uterine contractions in menstruation, spontaneous abortion and labour is well recognised. The uterine smooth muscle stimulating property of prostaglandins has been utilised for several clinical purposes in obstetrics and gynaecology. These include induction of labour, termination of early pregnancy and as post-implantation contraceptives.

Induction of labour

Several clinical trials for the induction of labour with prostaglandins have been reported. In most of these studies prostaglandins E_2 or $F_{2\alpha}$ have been given by intravenous infusions although other routes have been employed. First reports of the use of prostaglandins for the induction of labour came from Uganda in 1968 (see Karim, [24]). Karim and associates established the regime of slow infusion of dilute solutions of prostaglandins. They showed that with 0·5 μg/minute PGE_2 or 5·0 μg/minute $PGF_{2\alpha}$ it was possible to stimulate term uterus to produce labour-like contractions and induce labour. Subsequently these findings have been confirmed by many investigators although some have found it necessary to use higher rates of infusion.

Side effects reported when prostaglandins are infused for stimulating the term uterus include occasional nausea and vomiting, headache and mild superficial thrombophlebitis at the infusion site when PGE_2 is used. The only side effect of some concern is increase in the tone of the uterus with prostaglandin infusion. This, however, occurs only when higher rates of infusions are employed. There appears to be only a four-fold difference in the infusion rates required within patients at term. Thus it is possible to stimulate the uterus in term patients within the dose range of 0·5 to 2·0 μg/minute PGE_2 or 5 to 20 μg/minute $PGF_{2\alpha}$. Attempts have been made by some investigators to give prostaglandins by the titration method, i.e. doubling the dose at a fixed interval until optimum uterine stimulation is achieved. Such a method, although useful when oxytocin is employed, is not suitable for prostaglandins and produces unphysiological effects on the uterus.

Prostaglandins given by mouth are effective in stimulating the term uterus. Prostaglandins E_2 in a dose of 0·5–2·0 mg or $PGF_{2\alpha}$ 5–20 mg given orally produce labour-like contractions lasting for 2–3 hours with each dose. It has been shown that with repeated oral doses of these two prostaglandins every 2 hours it is possible to induce labour (see Karim, [24], for references).

Other methods of giving prostaglandins include intravaginal and intra-amniotic administration.

Three clinical trials comparing prostaglandins with oxytocin for the induction of labour have so far been reported. The results of such trials has depended upon the doses of drugs used and the criteria selected for successful induction. In two of these trials prostaglandin E_2 has been shown to be superior to oxytocin for the induction of labour and in one, no difference between the two drugs was encountered. (See Karim, [24].)

Intrauterine foetal death and hydatidiform mole

Retention of the products of conception following intrauterine foetal death can occur at any stage of pregnancy. Although with this condition spontaneous expulsion of the contents of the uterus eventually follows in the majority of cases, the disadvantages of such a delay are many. These include inconvenience, mental distress, abeyance of reproductive functions and restriction of full activity. It also exposes the patient to the risk of hypofibrinogenaemia. The available methods for terminating pregnancy in cases of foetal death are not entirely satisfactory. Surgical intervention in the presence of macerated products of conception is always attended by a high risk of infection, haemorrhage and trauma. A high concentration of oxytocin infusion has been shown to be effective in cases of intrauterine foetal death. However, in some cases the induction-delivery interval has been several days and side effects such as cutaneous vasoconstriction and hypertension have been reported.

Successful treatment of intrauterine foetal death with prostaglandins has been recently reported. With gestation below 28 weeks intravenous infusion of 2·5–5·0 μg/minute PGE_2 or 25–50 μg/minute $PGF_{2\alpha}$ is employed. Above 28 weeks PGE_2 infusion of 0·5–2·0 μg/minute or $PGF_{2\alpha}$ 5–20 μg/minute is employed. In the vast majority of cases expulsion of the products of conception is achieved within 12–14 hours with no side effects (see Karim, [24], for references).

Treatment of molar pregnancy is often problematical. Current practice employs high concentrations of oxytocin infusion but the results are not always satisfactory. Uterine haemorrhage can be a major problem, occurring spontaneously or during the treatment. Once again intravenous infusion of 5 μg/minute PGE_2 or 50 μg/minute $PGF_{2\alpha}$ have been reported to be effective in evacuating the hydatidiform mole, within 12 hours with minimal side effects (see Karim, [11], for references).

Abortion

The practice of abortion dates back to the origin of the human race. Over the centuries a large number of chemical compounds and plant extracts have been used for illegal abortion. In spite of this however, medical science has not produced a drug that will effectively and safely cause an abortion. At present several methods for therapeutic termination of pregnancy are in use. Before the 12th week of gestation, pregnancy is usually terminated surgically by dilatation of the cervix followed by either curettage or vacuum aspiration. In recent years with the use of thin catheters attached to suction apparatus, it has become possible to empty the uterus of its contents during this early period without dilatation of the cervix. After 12 weeks abortion is most commonly carried out by hysterotomy. Replacement of part of the amniotic fluid by hypertonic saline and glucose is also effective for second trimester pregnancy termination but the method has certain serious disadvantages and some fatalities have been reported.

Unlike oxytocin, certain prostaglandins have been shown to be able to stimulate the uterus in early pregnancy. The first study demonstrating the efficacy of prostaglandins $F_{2\alpha}$ was reported by Karim and Filshie in January, 1970 (see Karim, [24]) and aroused a great deal of interest. With 50 μg/minute continuous infusion of this compound pregnancy was successfully terminated in 14 out of 15 women within 24 hours. The same authors showed that prostaglandin E_2 is approximately 10 times more potent than $PGF_{2\alpha}$ in its uterine stimulant action and reported successful termination of pregnancy in eight women with 5 μg/minute infusion. The gestation age in the above studies varied between nine and 22 weeks.

Since the publication of the first report, several clinical trials using prostaglandins E_2 or $F_{2\alpha}$ given by continuous intravenous infusion have been reported. Because of the different rates and duration of infusion employed in different trials the results are not strictly comparable. However, some useful information regarding the efficacy and side effects has been obtained from these studies. This is summarised below.

(1) There is very little doubt that with further work prostaglandins can be developed as efficient and safe abortifacients.

(2) The abortifacient action of prostaglandins is dependent on their uterine stimulant action, with resultant cervical dilatation and expulsion of the products of conception. Since the two prostaglandins – PGE_2 and $PGF_{2\alpha}$ – employed for this purpose are very rapidly inactivated in the body, in order to maintain optimum uterine contractions, the infusion has to be continued until abortion takes place. Several investigators have reported local erythematous reaction at the site of venepuncture resulting from long term prostaglandin infusion. This may limit the use of prostaglandins given by intravenous route. However, several other routes of administering prostaglandins are being developed to overcome the above disadvantages.

(3) The side effects encountered with the use of prostaglandins seem to be related to the dose administered. With 50 μg/minute $PGF_{2\alpha}$ or 5 μg/minute PGE_2 which have been found to be sufficient for adequate uterine stimulation, the side effects commonly encountered are diarrhoea, nausea and vomiting. The incidence of diarrhoea is approximately 50 per cent. with $PGF_{2\alpha}$ and only 5–10 per cent. with PGE_2. Nausea and vomiting occur in about 25 per cent. of the women receiving prostaglandins but they respond to symptomatic treatment. In some studies reported from North America, $PGF_{2\alpha}$ has been infused up to 200 μg/minute and PGE_2 up to 20 μg/minute in order to evaluate drug tolerance. With such rates of infusion side effects such as pyrexia, vasovagal symptoms have been reported.

(4) When prostaglandins E_2 and $F_{2\alpha}$ are used for the termination of pregnancy a certain proportion of abortions are incomplete, requiring subsequent curettage. The incidence of retained placenta is higher in the first trimester than in the second trimester. Because of the available safe alternative method of terminating first trimester pregnancy, i.e. vacuum aspiration, prostaglandins do not seem to offer any advantage over the surgical method terminating first trimester pregnancy.

Direct instillation of either prostaglandins E_2 or $F_{2\alpha}$ into the uterus (between foetal membranes and uterine wall) has been shown to be effective for the termination of pregnancy in first and second trimester. Because of the local action, the dose required is much smaller than with intravenous administration. As a result the incidence of side effects is considerably reduced. In order to maintain effective uterine activity prostaglandins have to be administered by this route every 1–2 hours until abortion takes place.

Prostaglandins administered by the intravaginal route have also been shown to be effective in terminating pregnancy in the first two trimesters with minimal side effects. The drug has to be administered every 2–3 hours to maintain good uterine activity. It is possible that with a slow-release formulation abortion can be achieved with an appropriate single intravaginal dose.

The presence of prostaglandins E_2 and $F_{2\alpha}$ in amniotic fluid during spontaneous abortion and labour has led to the suggestion they are involved in the physiology of uterine contractions. Recently it has been shown that with single injection of 5 mg PGE_2 or 25 mg $PGF_{2\alpha}$ into the amniotic sac it is possible to produce an abortion. Because of the inaccessibility of the amniotic sac before the 12th week of pregnancy the use of the intra-amniotic route for terminating pregnancy can be applied to second trimester cases only. The procedure shows promise of a simple and safe method of dealing with such cases (see Karim, [24]).

Central nervous system

Prostaglandins may be implicated in the regulation of body temperature. Although detailed observations in the human have not been published there are occasional reports of the development of fever in women receiving high doses of PGE_2 and $PGF_{2\alpha}$ by intravenous infusion for therapeutic abortion (for references see Karim, [24]).

Suggestive evidence comes from experimental work in cats (Milton and Wendlandt, [25]). Injection of PGE_1 into the third ventricle produced an immediate and marked pyrexial effect accompanied by violent shivering and piloerection, which was neither prevented or reversed by the antipyretic agent 4-acetamidophenol. Prostaglandin $F_{2\alpha}$ had no pyrexial effect; prostaglandins A_1 and $F_{1\alpha}$ had a slight but inconstant effect which in contrast to that of PGE_1 was prevented by 4-acetamidophenol. Previously PGE_2 had also been shown to possess pyrexial activity though less than that of PGE_1.

Milton and Wenblandt found that the threshold pyrexial dose of PGE_1 was lower than that of 5-hydroxytryptamine (5–HT). In view of the fact that 5–HT is known to release PGE_1 from neural tissue (Ramwell, Shaw and Jessup, [26]) the pyrexial effect of 5–HT may be mediated through cerebral release of PGE_1. Mention has already been made of the possibility that antipyretic analgesic drugs may owe their antipyretic activity to an inhibition of synthesis or release of PGE_1.

Prostaglandins have been identified in the brain and spinal cord of several animal species and appear to be normal constituents of cerebrospinal fluid; their release from the surface of the brain and spinal cord occurs spontaneously and on nerve stimulation (for references see Horton, [2]). A great deal of experimental work has been carried out to test the possibility that prostaglandins might function as central transmitters. Studies in a number of animal species particularly the cat, have shown that E and F compounds have well marked effects on cerebral function and on the spinal cord (for references see Horton, [2]). For example, the injection of prostaglandins E_1, E_2 and E_3 into the lateral ventricle of the cat produce stupor and catatonia. Prostaglandin $F_{2\alpha}$ had no such effect and PGE_1 given intravenously produced only slight sedation. The potent depressor effect of the E compounds cannot be considered as being compatible with transmitter function since there was a latent period of 20–30 minutes and the effect lasted for several hours.

Prostaglandins E_2 and $F_{2\alpha}$ potentiate crossed exterior reflexes in the spinal cat (Horton and Main, [27]). This effect of PGE_1 is on the spinal cord and mediated through increased excitability of α-motoneurones, though whether directly or indirectly is not known.

In spite of the accumulation of a very large amount of experimental data, central transmitter function for prostaglandins is at present purely speculative.

PROSTAGLANDINS IN PATHOLOGICAL CONDITIONS

Tumours

The association between the clinical behaviour of certain tumours and the production of pharmacologically active substances by these tumours is now well established. For example, catecholamines secreted by phaechromocytoma are known to be responsible for episodes of hypertension and 5-hydroxytryptamine and kinins for the symptoms collectively known as carcinoid syndromes. It is also beginning to be appreciated that not one but several chemically different pharmacologically active substances may be produced by the same tumour. Since the discovery of prostaglandins, these substances have been shown to be present in different types of tumours including those deriving from fore-gut, neural crest tumours and medullary carcinoma of the thyroid (Table 2). Because of the wide range of pharamacological actions of prostaglandins attempts have been made to relate their presence in tumours and clinical symptoms associated with such tumours. No definite links have been established yet. However, the presence of prostaglandins in the medullary carcinoma of the thyroid and in circulating blood is of particular interest. An association between medullary carcinoma of the thyroid and diarrhoea has been reported by Williams who has produced evidence that the link between them is humoral.

Table 2 Prostaglandin occurrence in human tumour tissues

Tumour	Diarrhoea	Prostaglandin
Ganglioneuroma	Yes	E_2 $F_{2\alpha}$
Neuroblastome	No	E_2 $F_{2\alpha}$
Phaechromocytoma	No	E_2 $F_{2\alpha}$
Bronchial carcinoid	Yes	E_2 $F_{2\alpha}$
Carcinoma of the bronchus	No	E_2 $F_{2\alpha}$
Islet cell tumour (α)	Yes	E_2 $F_{2\alpha}$
Islet cell tumour (β)	No	No PG detected
Medullary carcinoma of thyroid	Yes	E_2 $F_{2\alpha}$
Kaposi sarcoma	Yes	E_2 $F_{2\alpha}$

Data from: Sandler *et al.* [28].

In man, abdominal cramps have been described when prostaglandin E_1 is infused. Diarrhoea is associated with oral and intravenous administration of PGE and PGF compounds. Prostaglandin secretion by tumour therefore still remains a possible cause of the diarrhoea associated with medullary carcinoma of the thyroid. Gastrin secretion is accepted as the cause of the diarrhoea, in most cases of α-cell islet tumours but in a small group such cases with diarrhoea there is no detectable gastrin in the tumour and no hyperchlorhydria. Prostaglandins have been shown to be present in one case of α-islet cell tumour with associated diarrhoea and therefore remains a mediator of this symptom.

Patients with Kaposi's Sarcoma also develop gastrointestinal symptoms such as abdominal pain and diarrhoea. Tumour tissues and blood from these patients contain high concentrations of prostaglandins (see Sandler, Karim and Williams [28].

It should however, be mentioned that phaechromocytoma tumours also contain high concentrations of prostaglandins without associated diarrhoea. Perhaps the catecholamines secreted by such tumours antagonise the diarrhoea producing effect of prostaglandins.

Cholera

Diarrhoea and vomiting are the prominent features associated with cholera. There is also a high incidence of spontaneous abortion in women who contract cholera during pregnancy. Since administration of prostaglandins produces watery diarrhoea (as in cholera) and also stimulates the human uterus it is conceivable that some of the clinical symptoms associated with cholera are mediated through prostaglandins release. So far no information on the blood levels of prostaglandins in choleraic patients is available. There is also evidence that the diarrhoea in the above two situations is due largely to an effect on intestinal electrolytes rather than on motility. In the dog intra-arterial injections of PGE_1 and PGA_1 into the mesenteric artery results in a long lasting secretion into the lumen.

Inflammation

Increased permeability of skin blood vessels of the rat by prostaglandin E_1 and A_1 has been demonstrated (Kaley and Weiner, [29]. Prostaglandin E_1 was approximately equal in potency to bradykinin and superior to histamine and serotonin. Prostaglandin A_1 was less potent than the foregoing but superior to 0·9 per cent. saline and the prostaglandin solvent alone. Prostaglandin $F_{2\alpha}$ on the other hand showed either no increase in vascular permeability or local vasoconstriction. Pre-treatment with the anti-histaminic mepyramine maleate (Anthisan) given intravenously or intradermally completely suppressed the histamine-induced increase in vascular permeability and moderately suppressed that of PGE_1 bradykinin and serotonin. On rat skin depleted of histamine and serotonin by compound 48/80 the permeability increasing effects of histamine, serotonin, bradykinin and PGE_1 were all reduced, but that of PGE_1 was least affected. Systemic pre-treatment with two serotonin antagonists (BOL-148 and UMK-491) affected only the permeability-increasing activity of serotonin.

The same workers using an *in vitro* micropore filter technique found that PGE_1 in low concentrations induced a slight degree of polymorphonuclear leucocyte migration, very much less than that obtained with activated serum but significantly greater than that from the control solution and the prostaglandin vehicle. Prostaglandins A_1 and $F_{2\alpha}$ had no such chemotactic effect in concentrations 10–100 times higher. None of the prostaglandins were found to possess chemotactic activity on mononuclear cells.

Whether the vascular changes seen are a direct effect of prostaglandins or part direct and part indirect through rupture and degranulation of most cells with liberation of vasoactive compounds has not yet been established.

The experimental work together with the widespread distribution of prostaglandins in mammalian tissues and their release from damaged tissues, suggest that these compounds are involved in the inflammatory response together with other vasoactive substances such as histamine, serotonin and bradykinin. In addition, there is some evidence indicating that polymorphonuclear leucocytes themselves may contribute to the prostaglandin effect by releasing prostaglandins during phagocytosis thereby augmenting increased vascular permeability and leucocyte migration at sites of tissue damage.

Prostaglandins may also be involved in inflammation of immunological origin since antigen releases prostaglandin E_1 and F compounds from the sensitised guinea-pig lung and activation of complement seems to be associated with the development of prostaglandin-like activity.

Recently a mixture of prostaglandins E_1, E_2, $F_{1\alpha}$ and $F_{2\alpha}$ has been obtained from the interstitial fluid of the skin patients with allergic contact eczema (Greaves *et al.*, [30]); in contrast the interstitial fluid from normal skin contained little or no prostaglandin activity. A fatty acid compound possessing prostaglandin-like activity has also been obtained from skin with delayed inflammation induced by ultra-violet light.

Although these findings cannot be interpreted as definitive evidence in man for the role of prostaglandins as mediators of the inflammatory response they point the way for the investigation of prostaglandin antagonists or inhibitors of prostaglandin synthesis as locally applied anti-inflammatory preparations, as a much-needed alternative to steroids.

Alterations in vascular permeability by prostaglandins are also seen in the eye of some species (see below).

The eye

The rabbit eye responds to mechanical or chemical irritation with prolonged miosis, vasodilation, increased capillary permeability reflected in an increase in protein content of aqueous humour and a prolonged rise in intraocular pressure; these changes are associated with the release into aqueous humour of a compound with spasmogenic and vasodilating activities termed 'irin' (Ambache, [31]). Prostaglandins E_2 and $F_{2\alpha}$ have been identified as components of rabbit and cat irin (Ambache and Brummer, [32]). Prostaglandins E_1 and E_2 injected into the anterior chamber (intracameral injection) of the rabbit eye produce a considerable rise in intraocular pressure and miosis; $PGF_{1\alpha}$ has no such effects and $PGF_{2\alpha}$ causes miosis but no rise in intraocular pressure (Waitzman and King, [33]).

Further studies in rabbits with prostaglandins E_1, E_2, $F_{1\alpha}$, $F_{2\alpha}$ and A_1 showed a large and sustained rise in intraocular pressure accompanied frequently, but not always, by miosis with all compounds except for $PGF_{1\alpha}$ where the rise was slight (Beitch and Eakins, [34]). The rise in pressure was associated with vascular congestion of the iris. The intracameral injection of PGE_1 and PGE_2 increased the protein content of the aqueous humour denoting an increased permeability of the blood/aqueous humour barrier by these compounds. This effect was related to the size of the increase in intraocular pressure.

In the cat, prostaglandins antagonise atropine-induced mydriasis and in the rabbit and cat prostaglandin induced miosis and rise in intraocular pressure are overcome by isoprenaline and noradrenaline but not by phenoxybenzamine or propanolol. Prostaglandins appear therefore to have a direct effect on iris smooth muscle of these species showing physiological antagonism towards isoprenaline and noradrenaline. Apart from the involvement of prostaglandins in the response of the rabbit eye to irritation, these compounds may also be concerned with regulation of activity of iris smooth muscle and possibly with aqueous humour production and flow.

There are no detailed reports of the ocular effects of locally or systemically administered prostaglandins in man, but in a series of women receiving prostaglandins by intrauterine injection for therapeutic abortion, no effects on intraocular pressure were observed (Embrey and Hillier, [35]).

Not only may prostaglandins participate in the inflammatory reaction, suppression of their formation may explain the action of analgesic drugs of the antipyretic anti-inflammatory group. Vane has shown that indomethacin, sodium acetylsalicylate and sodium salicylate all inhibited the synthesis of PGE_2 and $PGF_{2\alpha}$ (Vane, [36]). No inhibitory activity was found with the solvent media. Indomethacin was found to be the most active, being over twenty times more potent than sodium salicylate on a weight basis and almost fifty times more potent on a molar basis. Sodium salicylate was a weak inhibitor of prostaglandin synthesis, an interesting finding in view of the fact that in standard tests for anti-inflammatory and antipyretic activity it has approximately the same potency as sodium acetylsalicylate. A possible explanation for this is that sodium salicylate is a better inhibitor of prostaglandin synthesis from di-homo-y-linolenic acid than from arachidonic acid. Hydrocortisone showed weak inhibition of synthesis of prostaglandin E_2 and $F_{2\alpha}$.

Prostaglandins E_1, E_2 and $F_{2\alpha}$ induce fever in cats when injected into the third ventricle; tissue release of these compounds may be the basis of fever and inhibition of their synthesis may be the mode of antipyretic action of aspirin-like drugs.

Peripheral analgesic activity is related to anti-inflammatory activity but depression of prostaglandin synthesis may also account for the relief of headache of non-inflammatory origin by aspirin.

Vane has also put forward the interesting suggestion that prostaglandins may exert a normal protective effect on gastric mucosa and that interference with their synthesis may facilitate the development of mucosal erosions known to occur with salicylate therapy.

CONCLUSION

The ubiquity of prostaglandins in mammalian tissues, the ease with which they are released and their tissue effects, often obtained with nanogram quantities point to their function as regulators of many physiological and some pathological processes. It may be that prostaglandins are essential for the metabolic activity of all cells and might participate in nucleoprotein synthesis. The volume of accumulated data is equalled by the volume of speculation and concrete conclusions as to their precise biological significance cannot at present be drawn.

None the less, knowledge of some physiological effects of prostaglandins has found valuable clinical application in obstetrics. In several centres prostaglandins E_2 and $F_{2\alpha}$ are routinely employed for the termination of second trimester pregnancy and for the induction of labour.

Potential applications of prostaglandins in other clinical areas have been indicated but at the present time their greatest promise is in the field of fertility control. Population increase without a concomitant increase in food production is a problem facing many countries. The failures with and hazards attending the use of contraceptive procedures currently available are well known; prostaglandins may offer a safe and highly effective means of contraception through their ability to induce menstrual bleeding, administration being required only once a month.

References

1. Bergström, S., Carlson, L. A., and Weeks, J. R., The prostaglandins: A family of biologically active lipids. *Pharmacological reviews* (1968), **20,** 1–48.
2. Horton, E. W., Hypotheses on physiological roles of prostaglandins. *Physiol. Rev.* (1969), **49,** 122–161.
3. Kurzrok, R., and Lieb, C. C., Biochemical studies of human semen. II. The action of semen on the human uterus. *Proc. Soc. Exp. Biol. Med.* (1930), **28,** 268–272.
4. Goldblatt, M. W., A depressor substance in seminal fluid. *J. Soc. Chem. Ind., Lond.* (1933), **52,** 1056–1057.
5. Euler, U. S. von., Zur Kenntnis der pharmakologischen Wirkungen von Nativsekreten und Extrackten männlicher accessorischer Geschlechtsdrüsen. Naunyn-Schmiedebergs Arch. *Exp. Path. Pharmak.* (1934), **175,** 78–84.
6. Bergström, S., and Samuelsson, B. Prostaglandins. *Ann. Rev. Biochem.* (1965), **34,** 101–108.
7. Karim, S. M. M., and Somers, K., *Renal and cardiovascular actions of prostaglandins* (1971). In: *Prostaglandins:* Medical and Technical Publishing Company (ed. S. M. M. Karim).
8. Bennett, A. *Effects of prostaglandins on the gastrointestinal tract* (1971). In: *Prostaglandins:* Medical and Technical Publications (Ed. S. M. M. Karim).
9. Bergström, S., Duner, H., Euler, U. S. von, Pernow, B., and Sjövall, J., Observations on the effects of infusion of prostaglandin E in man. *Acta Physiol. Scand.* (1959), **45,** 145–151.
10. Karim, S. M. M., and Filshie, G. M., Therapeutic abortion using prostaglandin $F_{2\alpha}$. *Lancet* (1970), **1,** 157–159.
11. Misiewicz, J. J., Waller, S. L., Kiley, N., and Horton, E. W., Effect of oral prostaglandin E_1 on intestinal transit in man. *Lancet* (1969), **1,** 648–651.
12. Karim, S. M. M., Effects of oral administration of prostaglandins E_2 and $F_{2\alpha}$ on the human uterus. *J. Obstet. Gynaec., Br. Commonw.* (1971), **78,** 289–293.
13. Bennett, A., and Flesher, B., Prostaglandins and the gastrointestinal tract. *Gastroenterology* (1970), **59,** 790–800.
14. Horton, E. W., Main, I. H. M., Thompson, C. J., and Wright, P. M., Effect of orally administered prostaglandin E_1 on gastric secretion and gastrointestinal motility in man. *Gut* (1968), **9,** 655–658.
15. Way, L., and Durbin, R. P., Inhibition of gastric acid secretion *in vitro* by prostaglandin E_1. *Nature, Lond.* (1969), **221,** 874–875.

16. Sweatman, W. J. F., and Collier, H. O. J., Effects of prostaglandins on human bronchial muscle. *Nature, Lond.* (1968), **217,** 69.
17. Large, B. J., Lesswell, P. F., and Maxwell, D. R., Bronchodilator activity of an aerosol of prostaglandin E_1 in experimental animals. *Nature, Lond.* (1969), **224,** 78–80.
18. Cuthbert, M. F., Bronchodilator activity of aerosols of Prostaglandins E_1 and E_2 in asthmatic subjects, *Proceedings of the Royal Society of Medicine* (1971), **64,** 15–16.
19. Haessler, H. A., and Crawford, J. D., Insulin-like inhibition of lipolysis and stimulation of lipogenesis by prostaglandin E_1 (PGE_1). *J. Clin. Invest.* (1967), **46,** 1065.
20. Vaughan, M., *An effect of prostaglandin E_1 on glucose metabolism in rat adipose tissue.* Nobel symposium 2 (1967), Prostaglandins, ed. S. Bergström and B. Samuelsson, pp. 139–142. Almqvist and Wiksell, Stockholm.
21. Mody, N. J., *Effects of prostaglandins on platelet function* (1971). In: *Prostaglandins:* Medical and Technical Publishing Company (ed. S. M. M. Karim).
22. Bygdeman, M., The effect of different prostaglandins on the human myometrium *in vitro. Acta Physiol. Scand.* (1964), **63,** Suppl. 242, 1–78.
23. Pickles, V. R., The prostaglandins. *Biol. Rev.* (1967), **42,** 614–652.
24. Karim, S. M. M., *Prostaglandins and human reproduction: Physiological roles and clinical uses of prostaglandins in relation to human reproduction* (1971a). In: *Prostaglandins:* Medical and Technical Publications (ed. S. M. M. Karim).
25. Milton, A. S., and Wendlandt, S., A possible role for prostaglandin E_1 as a modulator for temperature regulation in the central nervous system of the cat. *J. Physiol., Lond.* (1970), **207,** 76P–77P.
26. Ramwell, P. W., Shaw, J. E., and Jessup, R., Spontaneous and evoked release of prostaglandins from frog spinal cord. *Am. J. Physiol.* (1966), **211,** 998–1004.
27. Horton, E. W., and Main, I. H. M., Identification of prostaglandins in central nervous tissues of the cat and chicken. *Br. J. Pharmac. Chemother.* (1967), **30,** 582–602.
28. Sandler, M., Karim, S. M. M., and Williams, E. D., Prostaglandins in amine-peptide-secreting tumours. *Lancet* (1968), **2,** 1053–1055.
29. Kaley, G., and Weiner, R., Prostaglandin E_1: A potential mediator of the inflammatory response. *Ann. N.Y. Acad. Sci.* (1971), **180,** 338–350.
30. Greaves, M. W., Søndergaard, J., and McDonald-Gibson, W., Recovery of prostaglandins in human cutaneous inflammation. *Br. Med. J.* (1971), **2,** 258–260.
31. Ambache, N., Irin, a smooth-muscle contracting substance present in rabbit iris. *J. Physiol. Lond.* (1955), **129,** 65P–66P.
32. Ambache, N., and Brummer, H. C., A simple chemical procedure for distinguishing E and F prostaglandins, with application to tissue extracts. *Br. J. Pharmac. Chemother.* (1968), **33,** 162–170.

33. Waitzman, M. B., and King, C. D., Prostaglandin influences on intraocular pressure and pupil size. *Am. J. Physiol.* (1967), **212,** 329–334.
34. Beitch, B. R., and Eakins, K. E., The effects of prostaglandins on the intraocular pressure of the rabbit. *Br. J. Pharmac.* (1969), **37,** 158–167.
35. Embrey, M. P., and Hillier, K., Therapeutic abortion by intrauterine instillation of prostaglandins. *Br. Med. J.* (1971), **1,** 588–590.
36. Vane, J. R., Inhibition of prostaglandin synthesis as a mechanism of action for aspirin-like drugs. *Nature, New Biology* (1971), **231,** 232–235.

The techniques useful in the study of factors influencing infertility are discussed. A detailed description is given of the recent advances in the study of developing embryos *in vitro*. The factors influencing early human development and an analysis of the endocrinological and cellular factors in the menstrual cycle are presented.

Recent Advances in the Treatment of Infertility

by

P. C. Steptoe

Consultant Gynaecologist, Oldham Group of Hospitals.

The introduction of endoscopy into gynaecological practice has widened the scope of accurate and scientific diagnosis of the causes of infertility in the human female, and has improved the possibilities of treatment. In particular the laparoscope allows clarification of some of the causes of primary and secondary sterility conditional upon the state of (1) the ovaries, and (2) the oviducts.

At what point should the laparoscope be introduced into investigative procedures? The general plan of investigations is as follows:

A general medical history is taken together with a special gynaecological history including sexual activity. The husband's general and special history is assessed. These histories are taken with great care, because an important evaluation of the general psychology of the marital situation can often be made. Each of the couples are examined physically, and arrangements are made for a seminal analysis. The husband may be referred for a urological and endocrinological investigation.

The wife is subjected to a detailed pelvic examination including bacteriological and cytological tests of the cervix and vagina. The finding of pathogenic organisms will need treatment with specific antibiotics. At the first visit special investigations may be initiated, such as blood examinations, thyroid function tests, hormone assays, buccal smears as well as starting routine basal temperature records.

At the second visit, usually four to six weeks later, the results of the tests are analysed and a premenstrual endometrial biopsy is performed. The material is examined not only for evidence of secretory activity, but also for the presence of any pathological changes including tuberculous infection.

A twenty-four hour hospital admission is arranged for the third consultation. It is timed to take place at the anticipated day of ovulation, and the investigations carried out include evaluation of the cervical mucous and sperm penetration. Coitus is asked for some two hours before hospital admission in the early morning. A general anaesthetic is given with tracheal intubation and controlled automatic respiration.

After examination of the cervical mucous, laparoscopy is performed and may include carbon dioxide insufflation, pertubation with hydrocortisone/streptomycin solutions with or without dye, aspiration of the oviducts, perfusion of the oviducts with aspiration of the washings from the pouch of Douglas, tubal biopsy, ovarian biopsy, biopsy and/or diathermy of endometriomata, division of peritubal or periovarian adhesions.

These investigations and minor surgical procedures are quite safe in skilled trained hands. The full assessment can be completed in not more than three months, and often less. A programme of therapy can then be devised. Laparoscopy is an essential feature of these investigations and no plan of treatment can be considered adequate without it, and if it is left out there may be a waste of valuable time for the patients concerned. Laparoscopy has the disadvantage that it is usually performed under general anaesthesia, during which tubal peristalsis is inhibited.

Hysterosalpingography is reserved for those cases with suspected uterine deformation or pathology, and for the follow-up of certain treated cases. This investigation provides only limited information about diseased tubes, as the pelvis beyond the limits of tubal obstruction is not visualised and it is not informative about the periovarian and peritubal areas. It can be of value when there is equivocal evidence of cornual obstruction.

Insufflation with carbon dioxide without laparoscopy is reserved for treatment of tubal disorder rather than for diagnosis, since at best the investigator can only infer from it that at least one tube is patent, and it can give rise to false negative results and there are many ambiguous kymographic patterns. It is my experience that when infertility has been in existence for two years or more there is a high incidence of tubal or peritubal pathology, or of unsuspected early endometriosis. For example the combined incidence of these two factors in 1969 was 64 per cent. of 142 cases.

Behrman [1] estimated the range of tubal disorders from 15 to 25 per cent., Swolen [2] stated that the most common cause of infertility in women was disturbed function of the oviducts, and Frangenheim [3] found damage to the tubes in more than 50 per cent. of infertility patients, and pelvic adhesions in 30 per cent. of the others.

The extended postcoital test by laparoscopy was introduced by Sjovall [4], and this method has made possible the recovery of spermatozoa both from the pouch of Douglas and the oviduct. However, most of these investigations have been done on infertile women, and only a limited number of examinations have been done on fertile women. Ahlgren [5] from Lund has reported examinations in 177 women of infertile marriages examined after coitus or insemination for the presence of spermatozoa in the oviducts and abdominal cavity. Spermatozoa were recovered in 30 per cent. of cases only. A conclusive minimum time of 1 hour and 50 minutes for sperm migration to the human oviduct and the abdominal cavity was observed. With an increasing time interval between coitus and the examination of up to about 15 hours the recovery rate in women with patent tubes was reduced. Relatively few spermatozoa were found at the site of fertilisation, but blocked tubes greatly increased the numbers recovered. These patients with hydrosalpinges were investigated at laparotomy. Ahlgren [5] found that the prognosis of the infertile couple as regards subsequent pregnancy was *not* correlated to the demonstration of spermatozoa in the oviduct or in the abdominal cavity. He concluded that this extended postcoital test was of limited value, but might yield information on the basic physiology of spermatozoa in the oviduct.

I have confirmed that spermatozoa can be recovered from the oviduct, by examining aspirates from the tube, and also fluid from the pouch of Douglas. There is no doubt that spermatozoa do sometimes enter the abdominal cavity under normal conditions. Hypothetically, the occasional presence of spermatozoa in the abdominal cavity might induce sperm antibody formation. This hypothesis was not supported when screening part of the infertile group of women by the serum sperm agglutination test of Kibrick *et al.* [6] and the serum sperm immobilisation test of Isojima *et al.* [7]. This problem needs further investigation. Incidentally, on one occasion Trichomonas vaginalis were also recovered from the aspirate from the pouch after perhydrotubation, and Trichomonas were also recovered from the cervical canal. The patient came to no harm, but recalling the bacterial friends which the Trichomonas vaginalis has it may be asked how many enthusiastic insufflations or perhydrotubations have caused more harm than good. Obviously every precaution should always be taken against causing an ascending infection.

Laparoscopy and tubal morphology

Apart from establishing the facts about tubal patency and sperm penetration, laparoscopy has proved most valuable in establishing the causes of failure of ovum migration to the oviducts, and thence through them to the uterine cavity. Details of the diagnosis of developmental and pathological conditions have been described elsewhere (Steptoe, [8]). Biopsy can be performed of course, and peritubal adhesions can often be divided by laparoscopic technique. Special attention must be devoted to the condition and motility of the fimbrial end of the tube. A recent advance in technique is in the treatment of phimosis of the abdominal ostium. The ostium is dilated by means of an inserted forceps which is then opened to dilate the ostium gradually. Ahlgren [9] has also described salpingotomy at laparoscopy by using a slight modification of this technique with the employment of two organ forceps (Nordvall, [10]). In addition he introduces large doses of hydrocortisone acetate through the trocar-cannula, as advocated by Swolen [2]. In the course of five years he achieved three pregnancies in 12 women, which compares very favourably with the results of salpingostomy done at laparotomy. Clyman [11] performs a similar procedure after culdoscopy, which he follows with opening the pouch of Douglas through the posterior vaginal fornix.

Laparoscopy has a most important part to play in the assessment and selection of cases for tuboplastic surgery. In cornual obstruction it is absolutely essential, since only about 30 per cent. of cases are amenable to surgery (Palmer, [12]). This means that without preliminary laparoscopy there is a risk of performing a useless laparotomy in 70 out of every 100 cases of cornual obstruction.

In distal occlusion, while laparoscopy is not quite obligatory, nevertheless other investigations, including hysterosalpingography, give no indication of the nature of peri-tubo-ovarian adhesions, the state of the ovaries, the presence of small endometriomata or latent tuberculosis. The presence of heavy vascular adhesions makes operation more difficult and less likely to succeed.

Preliminary laparoscopy also allows diagnosis of subacute inflammation which requires prolonged preliminary treatment before attempting tuboplastic operations, and it is also valuable in the follow-up of the treated patients.

Endometriosis

Early endometriomata are being found in increasing numbers in young infertile women, when all other investigations are negative. Retrograde menstruation is undoubtedly a factor, which I believe is aggravated by the presence of uterine retroversion. The menstrual fluid lies for several days in the ovarian fossae, around the tubes and in the pouch of Douglas, and these are the sites of the early endometriomata. The ovaries themselves seem less commonly affected in these early cases. Correction of the retroversion by laparoscopic technique is indicated together with coagulation of small endometriomata and treatment with progestogens.

Small endometrial cysts of the ovaries should be incised and emptied at laparoscopy. The judicious combination of these techniques, ventro-suspension, coagulation dispersal of small lesions, and prolonged progestogen therapy should lead to successful pregnancy in about 40 per cent. of cases.

Disorders of ovulation

Certain disturbances of ovulation are revealed or clarified by laparoscopic assessment. It is emphasised that it is not enough to prove that ovulation occurs, as adjudged by the usual parameters. Disturbances of the mechanism of dehiscence of Graafian follicles may be present to a degree which interferes with the possibility of conception. For example, the presence of surface adhesions, of scars, of nearby endometriomata and of sclerosis of the ovaries, with or without ovarian enlargement, may distort or change the operculum to such a degree that the escaping oocyte with its surrounding corona will be damaged. With regard to sclerocystic disease, although laparoscopy allows a very accurate diagnosis, especially when combined with ovarian biopsy, there is disappointment with the results achieved by laparoscopic incision or resection. In 1969, 20 such cases were assessed and treated. One patient became pregnant after incision of the ovaries, three after treatment with clomiphene and Pregnyl (Organon), and six after treatment with Pergonal (Searle) and Pregnyl, 10 pregnancies in all. At the present time it would appear that inspection of the ovaries for the typical porcelain-like appearance, the small deep encysted follicles, the absence of recent or old corpora lutea is adequate to make a diagnosis in conjunction with the analysis of symptoms and signs and hormone assays, and the value of ovarian biopsy or incision by laparoscopy is still questionable.

Laparoscopy is valuable in the diagnosis of the causes of both primary and secondary amenorrhoea, and is useful in assessing those cases which are likely to respond to pituitary gonadotrophin therapy. The exhibition of these hormones to the patient can be monitored not only by measurement of total oestrogens or oestriol responses but also by direct observation of their effects upon the ovaries before exposure of the subjects to insemination by coitus. The ovarian response can be measured at laparoscopy by observation of the changes in volume of the ovaries and the number of follicles which develop. By this means, some partial control of hyperfolliculation can be achieved and so the risk of multiple pregnancies can be reduced.

Immunological factors and sterility

The immunological reaction is the principal system of defence against antigens. The introduction into an organism of a foreign molecule, known as antigen, whether it is part of a virus, a bacterium or a grafted tissue, induces the formation of antibodies which react specifically with it.

It has been shown that infertility may be related to antibodies found in husband or wife to antigenic material present in human sperm. Apparent normal results of examination of the husband and of the wife are associated in some cases with repeated absence of mobile spermatozoa in the cervical mucous a few hours after normal intercourse. In some cases agglutination of spermatozoa is seen, and this may be due to specific antibodies, or to non-specific factors causing auto-agglutination. Franklin and Dukes [13] described a technique for demonstrating the presence of anti-spermatozoal antibodies in women. They considered that vaginal contact with spermatozoa can lead to the production of circulating antibodies. If absence of contact could be obtained for six months agglutinations disappeared in 9/10th of their cases.

Is sterility encountered due to immunological mechanisms within the functioning of the ABO system? A great number of studies have sought to estimate the possible role of the difference in blood groups between partners in order to explain certain forms of sterility by agglutination of spermatozoa. ABO antibodies have been found in the cervical mucous of some women, more frequently in those of group O, but no definite conclusions can yet be drawn as to the part they play in causing sterility.

The errors of evaluation in this field have multiple causes: immunological tests vary too much from author to author, and some are satisfied with only one reaction. Auto-immunisation of male partners leads to a decrease in fertility but not necessarily to absolute sterility:

Immobilisation or agglutination of spermatozoa in the mucous of certain women are not necessarily of an immunological nature, and in the light of our present lack of knowledge it is more appropriate to speak of 'diminished fertility' of immunological origin rather than 'sterility'.

Absent or damaged oviducts

In 1967 a review of cases operated on in Oldham for tubal occlusion revealed a pregnancy success rate of only 21 per cent. A 'second look' laparoscopy in many cases revealed the presence of fimbrial phimosis, or adhesions, even though patency was observed by perhydrotubation, a recurrence of occlusion. What could be done for these cases, and what could be done for the unfortunate patients who had both tubes absent following surgical intervention, or who were found initially to have advanced peritubal pathology or healed tuberculosis? Many such women are attending our department in Oldham. All have at least one healthy ovary, most have two healthy ovaries and a healthy uterus. Should these women be treated by Estes' operation? Palmer (personal communication, [14]) reports 60 such operations without a single pregnancy, and this has been confirmed by my personal experience. Could these patients be given a tubo-uterine implant? The technical problems of rejection involved in this procedure appear formidable for the production of a healthy infant at present. Can tubal function be performed by a so-called artificial oviduct utilising the appendix for example, or a purely man-made substance? One has yet to learn of successful pregnancies by these methods.

Would it be possible to recover oocytes from the ovary with little disturbance to the patient, fertilise them with the husband's spermatozoa, initiate cleavage and replace the early embryo into the uterus?

Material and methods

The volunteer patients were women of infertile married couples, who were subjected to full investigation, including laparoscopic examination of the wife. The patients selected for oocyte recovery were those with advanced peritubal lesions, tubal occlusion, absence of the tubes and 'failed' tuboplastic surgery.

The objects of the proposed clinical research programme were discussed with the patients, including the possible results which might relieve their infertility, or might even benefit only the infertility of others. The risk of disappointments both in the progress of the research and in the ultimate outcome were described to the patients. The problems of recovering oocytes, of fertilising them with the husband's spermatozoa, of achieving normal development of early embryos *in vitro*, and of bringing about successful implantation were discussed, together with the opportunities and the dangers which might present.

The programme was started by Dr R. G. Edwards and myself in 1968.

In that year, oocytes which had been recovered from excised ovarian tissue were matured in culture media, and incubated with spermatozoa. Bavister [15], working in the Cambridge Physiological Laboratory, defined suitable conditions for *in vitro* fertilisation of hamster eggs, and succeeded in attaining very high rates of fertilisation. He also showed that tubal or follicular fluids play little or no part in the achievement of successful fertilisation in laboratory conditions, and that they may not capacitate spermatozoa directly, but simply create a suitable environment for spontaneous occurrence of this process. The successful use of Bavister's culture medium when applied to human oocytes matured *in vitro* was reported in detail by Edwards *et al.* [16].

However, the fertilisation rate of oocytes matured *in vitro* was low and it was considered vital to find a method of bringing oocytes to maturation *in vivo* in sufficient numbers to recover them by laparoscopic technique.

Recovery of pre-ovulatory human oocytes

Many rabbit oocytes matured outside their follicles and fertilised *in vivo* failed to form blastocysts, Chang [17]. Development to full-term was only obtained if the oocytes completed most of their maturation *in vivo* under the influence of exogenous gonadotrophins, Edwards (unpublished). Some of the human oocytes matured and fertilised *in vitro* displayed cytoplasmic fragmentation.

Several problems had therefore to be solved in order to obtain embryos capable of normal cleavage, including:

(1) The ovaries had to be primed so that controlled hyperfolliculation would occur, and mature pre-ovulatory oocytes would develop.

(2) These oocytes had to be recovered by laparoscopy, so disturbing the patient as little as possible, and offering the opportunity of repeating the process without harm to the patient.

(3) Media capable of supporting the cleavage of human ova had to be developed.

Human postmenopausal and chorionic gonadotrophins (HMG and HCG) were therefore given to women with cyclic bleeding in order to impose some control over the menstrual cycle and oocyte maturation, and laparoscopy was performed to aspirate follicles shortly before the expected time of ovulation. Fine control can be established over the maturation of oocytes in animals using similar methods of treatment, Edwards and Gates [18]. Based on the timings of the maturation of human oocytes *in vitro*, and on preliminary work by Jagiello *et al.* [19] on the treatment of patients with dysmenorrhoea, we estimated that human ovulation would occur about 36 hours after the ovulatory injection of HCG. Laparoscopy was therefore performed initially 28 hours after the injection in order to recover oocytes in diakinesis or metaphase-I of the first meiotic division. These characteristic and brief stages of meiosis offer an excellent guide to oocyte maturation, and their recognition in many oocytes confirmed that ovulation would occur some eight to 10 hours later. The recovery of oocytes was then re-timed for 32 to 33 hours after injection of HCG, in order to recover oocytes shortly before ovulation. Details of the dosages of HMG and HCG were published by Steptoe and Edwards [20] together with the technique adopted. During the work a special aspirator was designed by Purdy, Sekker, Edwards and Steptoe (unpublished results) and this facilitated the successful recovery of 133 oocytes from 49 patients. Of these, 42 were judged to be pre-ovulatory either in metaphase-I, metaphase-II or diakinesis. A dosage of 675 i.u. to 900 i.u. of HMG given in three divided doses on days 3, 5 and 8 of the cycle, followed by 5,000 i.u. of HCG resulted in a high recovery rate of pre-ovulatory oocytes. Increasing the doses above these levels has not yet given an increased number of pre-ovulatory oocytes. One mild case of hyperstimulation of the ovaries was encountered, and in this case the dosage of HMG given was 900 i.u. These observations showed that the necessary endocrinological and surgical methods for recovering pre-ovulatory oocytes had been achieved. Since fertilisation *in vitro* had been accomplished earlier, it was now necessary to produce media capable of supporting the cleavage of human embryos.

In certain animals the fertilisation of oocytes that completed most of their maturation *in vivo* has led to full-term foetal development after they were replaced in the oviduct as mentioned earlier. Recognition of the importance of pyruvate as an energy source for mouse embryos in early cleavage, Bavister [21] and perhaps embryos of other species, had led to the development of simple defined media based on a physiological saline solution, with added pyruvate and bovine serum albumin. Whittingham [22] obtained viable young mice using oocytes matured *in vivo* and fertilised *in vitro* with uterine spermatozoa in such a medium, and then transferring embryos at the two-cell stage to a recipient female. Mukkerjee and Cohen [23] fertilised mouse tubal oocytes *in vitro*, grew them in culture to blastocysts and obtained viable young when these embryos were transferred into uterine foster-mothers. Whitten [24] summarises the data on culture of mouse ova from their pronuclear stage and gives details of the development of various media to blastocysts. Fertilisation *in vitro* of rabbit tubal oocytes, followed by their early transfer into recipient females, has also yielded viable young, Chang [17].

We have grown human embryos in various culture media. Some were the simple defined media developed for mouse embryos, whereas others were more complex, namely Ham's F10 medium, Ham [25] Waymouth's MB752/1 medium, Waymouth [26], and medium 199, Parker (1950), which were supplemented with serum. These media are widely used in tissue culture. Pre-ovulatory oocytes obtained by laparoscopy were thus fertilised in Bavister's solution before transfer into culture media for cleavage. The complete series of steps is as follows, Edwards, Steptoe and Purdy [27].

Pre-ovulatory oocytes were incubated temporarily in droplets consisting of fluid from their own follicle when possible, and the medium being tested for fertilisation (now almost always Bavister's solution). They were then washed through two changes of the medium under test, and placed in suspensions of spermatozoa obtained from the husband. These suspensions were made to a concentration of between 8×10^5 and 2×10^6 per ml depending on the quality of the sample. The droplets used for fertilisation were of about 0·05 ml. Bavister's medium, adjusted to a pH of 7·6, was used extensively because of its success in sustaining fertilisation in previous work, Edwards *et al.* [16]; Bavister *et al.* [21]. Modifications made to various other media in tests for fertilisation included raising the pH to within the range 7·5 to 7·6, and adding bovine serum, albumin and pyruvate. The gas phase was either 5 per cent. carbon dioxide in air, or 5 per cent. carbon dioxide, 5 per cent. oxygen and 90 per cent. nitrogen. Cultures were incubated at 37°C. On November 21st, 1969, in Oldham, Lancashire, the first successful fertilisation of an oocyte recovered by laparoscopy was achieved. The criteria for fertilisation were:

(1) Observation by phase contrast microscopy of two pronuclei, polar bodies and a sperm tail in the cytoplasm.

(2) Identification of pronuclei using a stereoscopic low power microscope.

(3) Cleavage of the egg, after identification of pronuclei.

Fertilisation was found to occur in Bavister's medium, modified Waymouth's medium and modified Whittingham's medium. Low rates of fertilisation sometimes were a consequence of the poor quality of some samples of spermatozoa.

Twelve to 15 hours after insemination the oocytes were transferred to various media for cleavage. All media were adjusted to a pH of approximately 7·3, and a gas phase of 5 per cent. CO_2 in air, or 5 per cent. CO_2, 5 per cent. O_2 and 90 per cent. N_2. Initially the simple defined media known to support the cleavage of mouse embryos were utilised. The embryos were inspected regularly during culture, and left in culture until their development had obviously ceased. The first cleavage occurred before 38 hours post-insemination, the second between 38 and 46½ hours, the third between 51 and 62 hours and the fourth cleavage occurred before 85 hours. The embryos seldom cleaved beyond the 8-celled stage in these media, and some did not reach this far, Edwards *et al.* [27]. Lowering the osmotic pressure of the medium, as recommended for mouse embryos by Whitten [21] proved unsuitable for human embryos, for many of them displayed fragmentation of blastomeres or other forms of degeneration.

In view of these results, more complex media were tested, and Ham's F10 supplemented with foetal calf or human serum proved to be the most suitable. Embryos now developed to the 16-cell stage, and some were stained to examine their nuclear morphology. The blastomeres of many embryos that had cleaved normally possessed a single nucleus as judged by phase contrast microscopy. Whole mount or flattened preparations of two 12 to 16-celled, three 8-celled and two 4 to 5-celled embryos revealed the same number of nuclei as cells in each embryo. One of the 12 to 16-celled embryos was found to possess four mitoses. One embryo that reached at least the 16-celled stage possessed 21 nuclei; although some were smaller than others.

These results encouraged further work with Ham's F10 supplemented with serum, Steptoe, Edwards and Purdy [28]. Cleavage through the 32 to 64-celled stage has been observed, and several embryos developed into excellent blastocysts. The inner cell mass was distinctly protuberant in these embryos, the blastocoelic cavity was distinct and appeared to develop through the release of fluid from large secretory cells. The trophoblast formed a single layer of cells, and the zona pellucida became thinner. Some of the blastocysts have been found to contain at least 132 cells, and all of them possessed mitoses. Nuclear morphology appeared to be very good. Exact counts on the number of chromosomes have not proved possible since there are few mitoses for examination, yet it is clear that none of them were triploid. There is little doubt that the blastocysts were capable of further development. The availability of blastocysts grown in culture will permit the analysis of their metabolism. Does the early differentiating trophoblast secrete HCG or other hormones? This could indeed be the function of this tissue in order to maintain the conditions for continuing pregnancy. We have collected these secretions from around the embryos, and intend to analyse them for various hormones.

Identification of a Y chromosome in some embryos would furnish formal proof to confirm the morphological evidence of fertilisation. The quinacrine dyes might detect the Y chromosome in interphase nuclei and mitoses, as they do in somatic cells (Pearson, Bobrow and Vosa, [29]) although caution will be necessary since they fail to stain the Y in most spermatogonia (Pearson and Bobrow, [30]). Chromosomal analysis of the embryos should also reveal anomalies in early development, e.g. non-disjunction and especially triploidy arising through polyspermy or failure of polar body formation.

Follicular growth, and steroids in urine and follicular fluid

An aspect of human, and also animal reproduction that is too little understood concerns the selective growth of the ovulatory follicle, the steroids produced by this follicle, and the relationship between the number and size of Graafian follicles in the ovary and the urinary excretion of steroids. Careful counts have been made of the number of follicles in the ovaries of treated patients, their size has been measured approximately and fluids from these follicles collected whenever possible for analysis.

We were unable to do a detailed analysis of urinary steroids for each day of the treatment cycle. Twenty-four-hour samples were collected from some of the patients on certain days before, during and after laparoscopy, and these were analysed for total oestrogens and pregnanediol. Our preliminary observations indicate that there is a positive correlation between the number of large Graafian follicles and total urinary oestrogens, but not with the total number of Graafian follicles. It thus appears that the largest follicles contribute mostly to the oestrogen levels. In collaboration with Doctors G. Abraham and K. Fotherby [31] the levels of oestradiol 17β, progesterone, and of luteinising hormone have been measured in many of the follicular fluids obtained at laparoscopy, using radio-immunoassay or protein-binding assay. Levels of oestradiol in different follicles were between 12·5 and 1,700 ngms per ml, those of progesterone between 38 and 18,000 ngms per ml. A correlation existed between the size of a follicle and the levels of oestradiol and progesterone in the fluids. A regression line was calculated between the log concentration of oestradiol and of progesterone, and values for all follicles, whether ovulatory, atretic or unscorable were found to fall on this line. So were values from a few follicles collected from patients in their natural cycle. These data suggest that there is no major shift in the type of steroid synthesised by these different types of follicles, merely an increase in amount. If we can confirm this conclusion, our understanding of the biosynthesis of steroids by follicles approaching ovulation would be enlarged. Follicles punctured in response to treatment with HMG are synthesising steroids in a woman similar to those growing during the natural cycle, as shown by the similar correlation of oestrogens and progesterone in the two types. The correlation between urinary steroids and the number of large Graafian follicles that we have found should enable us to avoid laparoscopy on those patients likely to have no ovulatory oocytes.

Pregnanediol excretion in the second half of the cycle induced by treatment with HMG and HCG has indicated active luteinisation in almost all of our patients.

We have also found well developed secretory changes present in the endometrium seven days after the oocyte recovery, and with the dosage of HMG and HCG at present used, menstruation occurs 12 to 14 days after the injection of HCG in most patients. The existence of a secretory endometrium, a regular return to menstruation and the excretion of satisfactory levels of pregnanediol by most patients indicate that uterine conditions for implantation of an embryo appear to be suitable.

Discussion

Every gynaecologist is constantly faced with the problems of infertility. It is not a crippling disease, but nevertheless the sterile couple feel that they have a basic right, a powerful urge to have children, as an essential part of their marriage and human existence. The infertile should not be penalised for the sake of the over-fertile. A child born by these new methods will be conceived in a rational responsible manner. Gynaecologists who have been so much concerned with the control of over-population must still remain sympathetic to the plight of the infertile couple.

The advances that we have made already now offer an excellent opportunity to many childless couples to have their own children by means of embryo transfer. Couples where the wife has occluded oviducts should be able to benefit fairly soon, provided the husband has sufficient spermatozoa for fertilisation *in vitro*. Oligospermic men could well be the next to be helped. At present, we are obtaining cleaving embryos from approximately one half of our patients. The major difficulty lies in the response to hormones, for failure to obtain embryos appears due to the lack of oocytes distinctly recognisable as pre-ovulatory. This difficulty might be due to the well known variability in response to gonadotrophins that has been found in anovulatory patients (Crooke, [32]). It could be reduced by selecting patients excreting more than a certain amount of urinary oestrogens, and we are now establishing these levels. Alternatively, clomiphene could be used to replace the HMG, which would make the treatment both cheaper and more acceptable. Other causes leading to failure to develop pre-implantation embryos are failure to collect the oocytes by laparoscopy – although here the recovery rates from the larger follicles, i.e. those that are probably ovulatory, are higher than from small follicles (Steptoe and Edward, [20]). Failure of fertilisation is difficult to judge because it is impossible to classify an oocyte as definitely pre-ovulatory, i.e. ready for fertilisation, without destroying its capacity for further development. Nevertheless, it appears that the great majority of oocytes classified as pre-ovulatory from their appearance are actually fertilised if the sperm suspension is sufficiently active. Cleavage seems to be a minor cause of difficulty, for most embryos cleave well past the 16-cell stage, which is probably the stage when embryos normally enter the uterus. The rapid development of methods to monitor pregnancy such as amniocentesis, ultrasonic scans, etc., will permit the identification of many forms of anomalous development while the foetus is in utero.

In the field of human reproduction we must learn about basic factors involved in conception. The opportunities offered by the successful culture and fertilisation of human oocytes, and the subsequent growth

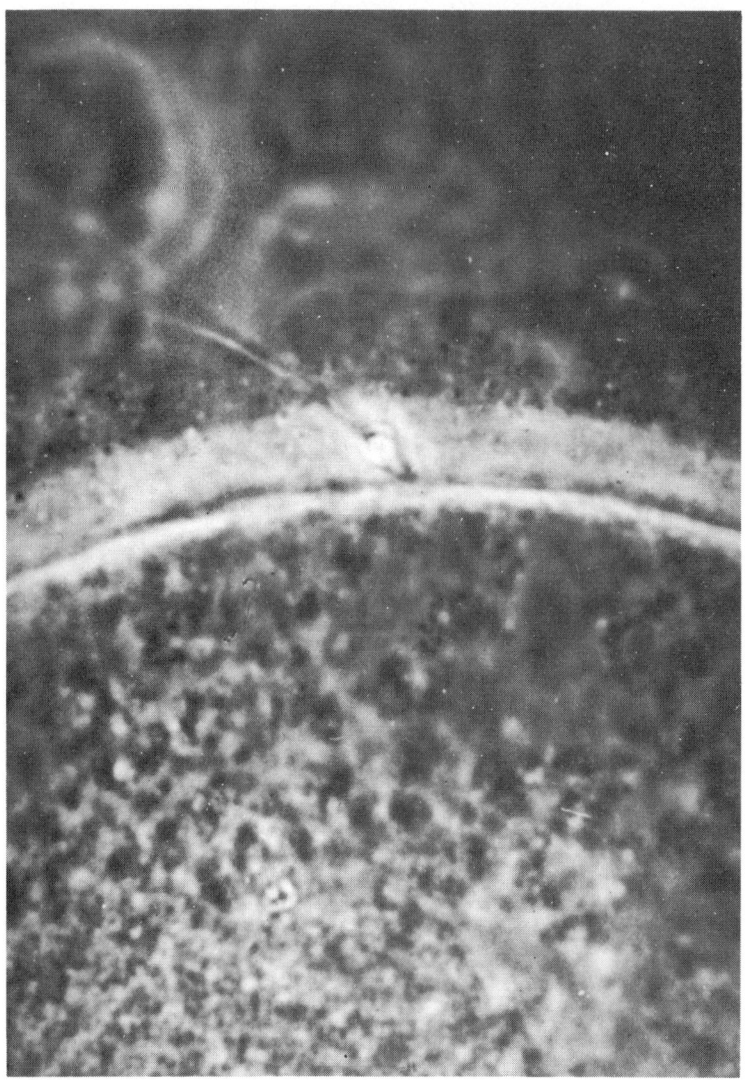

1. Spermatazoon having penetrated the vitellum is about to enter the oocyte.

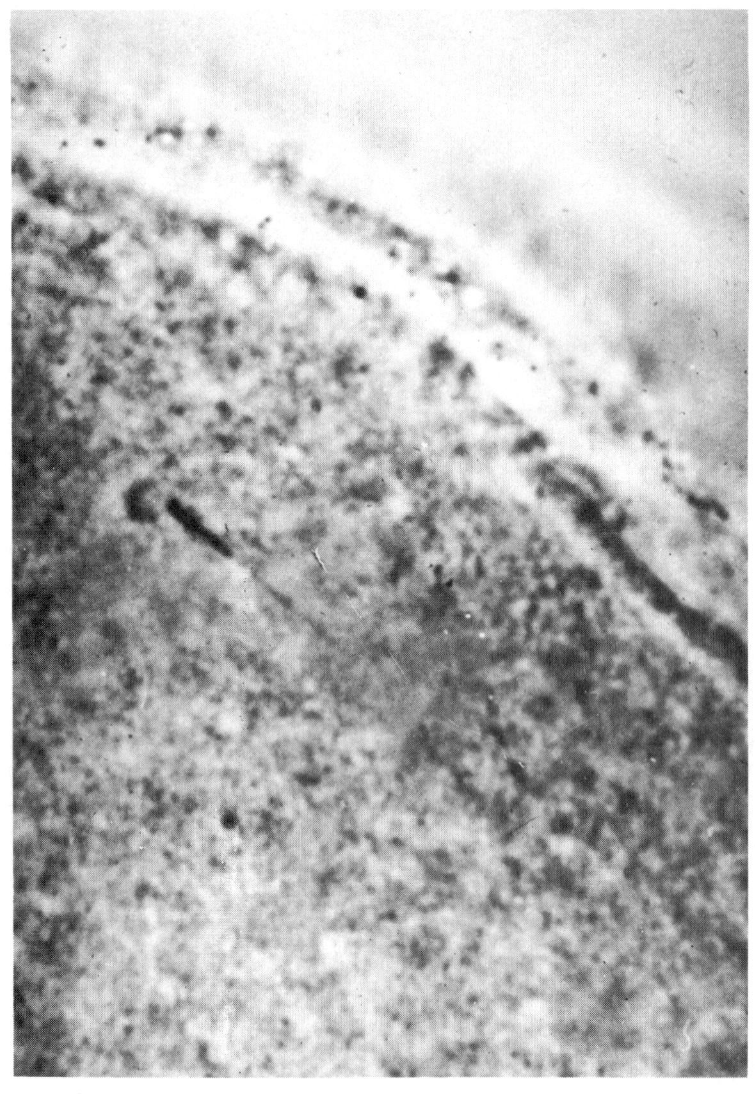

2. Spermatazoon in oocyte cytoplasm. Note the enlargement of the head and presence of the middle piece and tail.

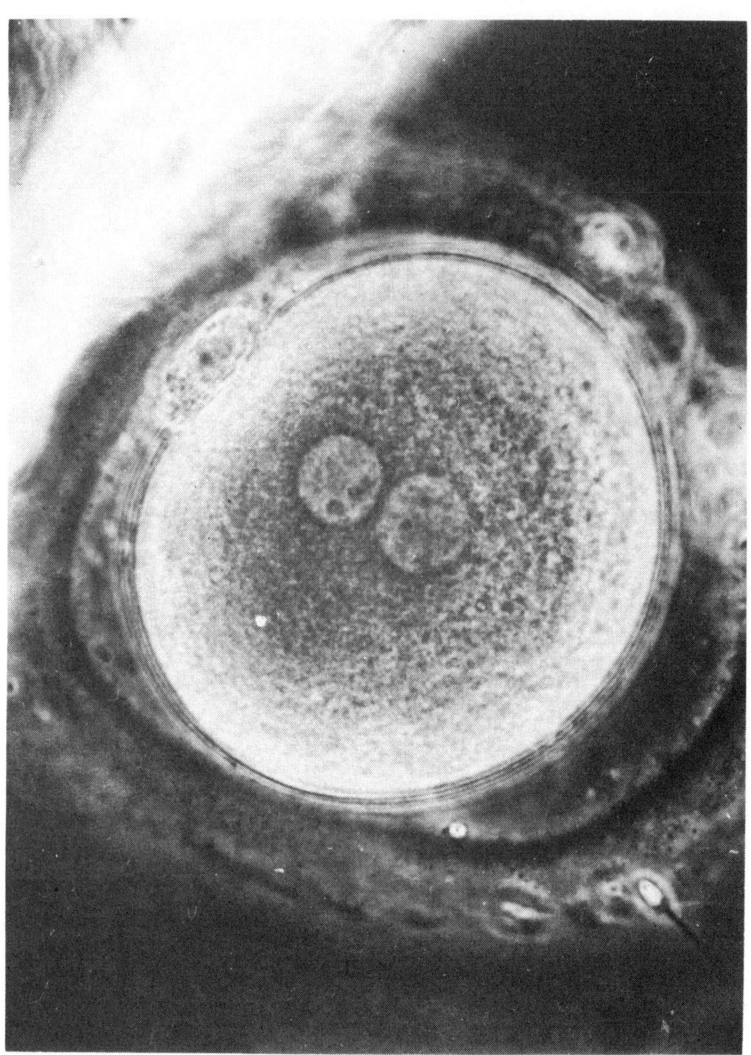

3. Male and female pronuclei, and extrusion of polar bodies.

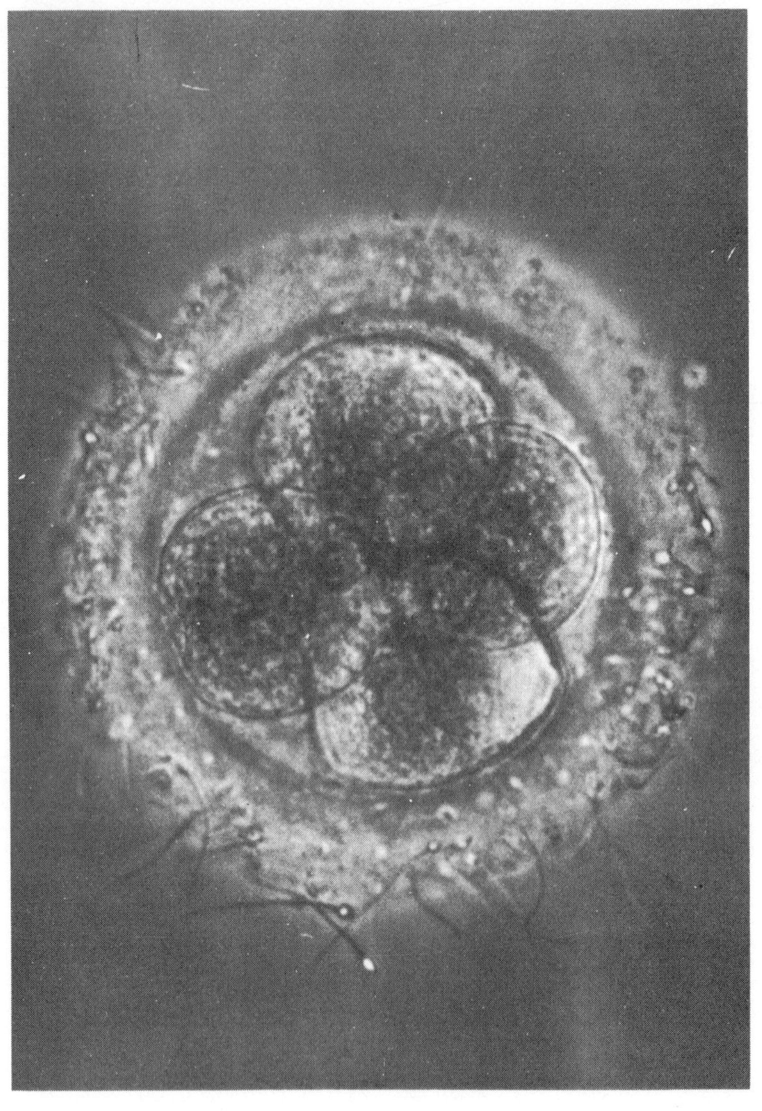

4. 4-cell human embryo.

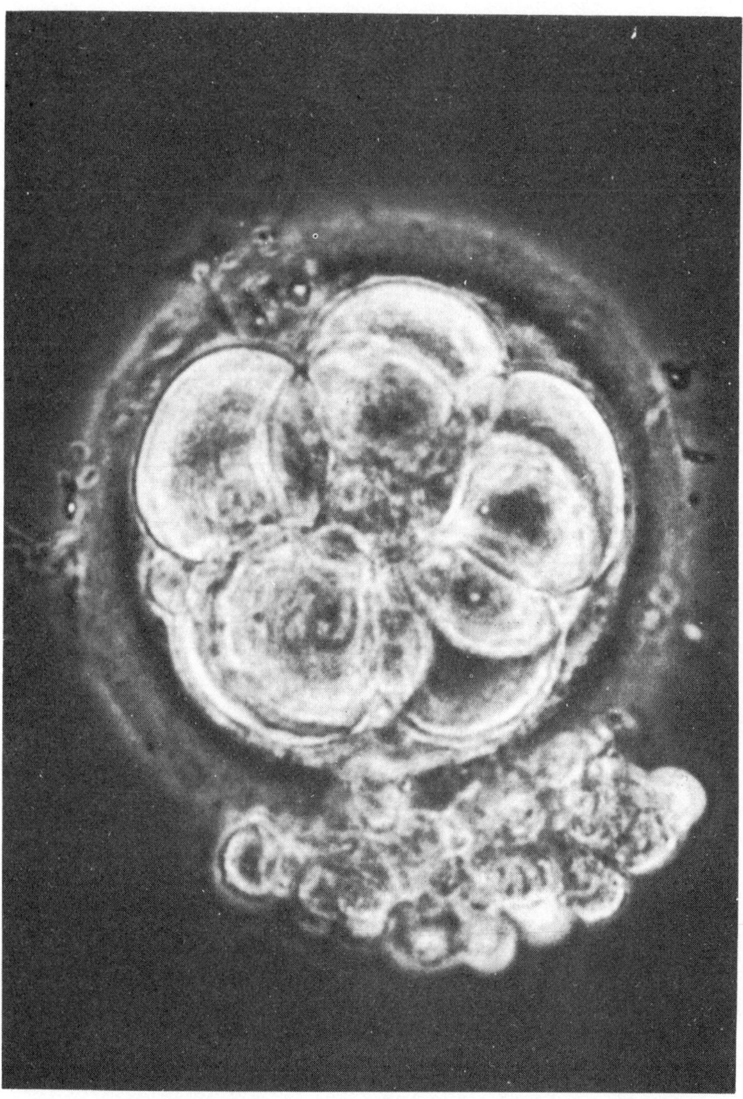

5. 8-cell human embryo. Note the excellent blastomeres and cumulus cells detaching themselves from the embryo.

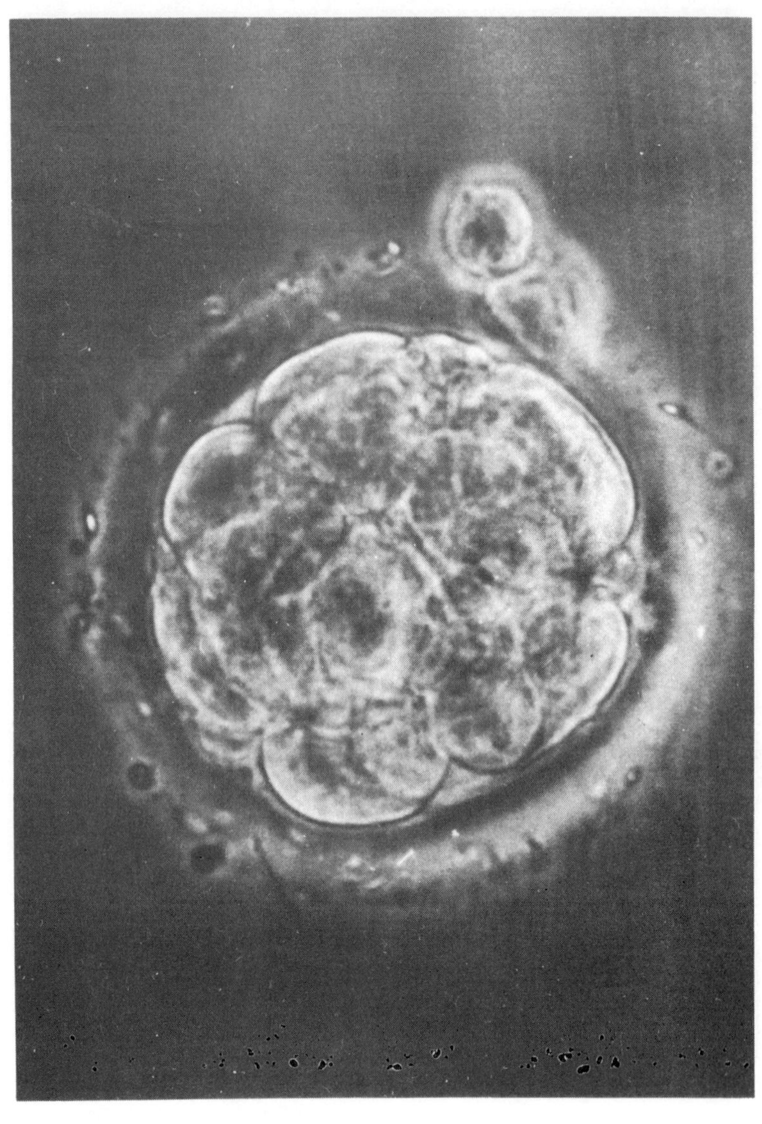

6. 16-cell plus human embryo – probably early mourula.

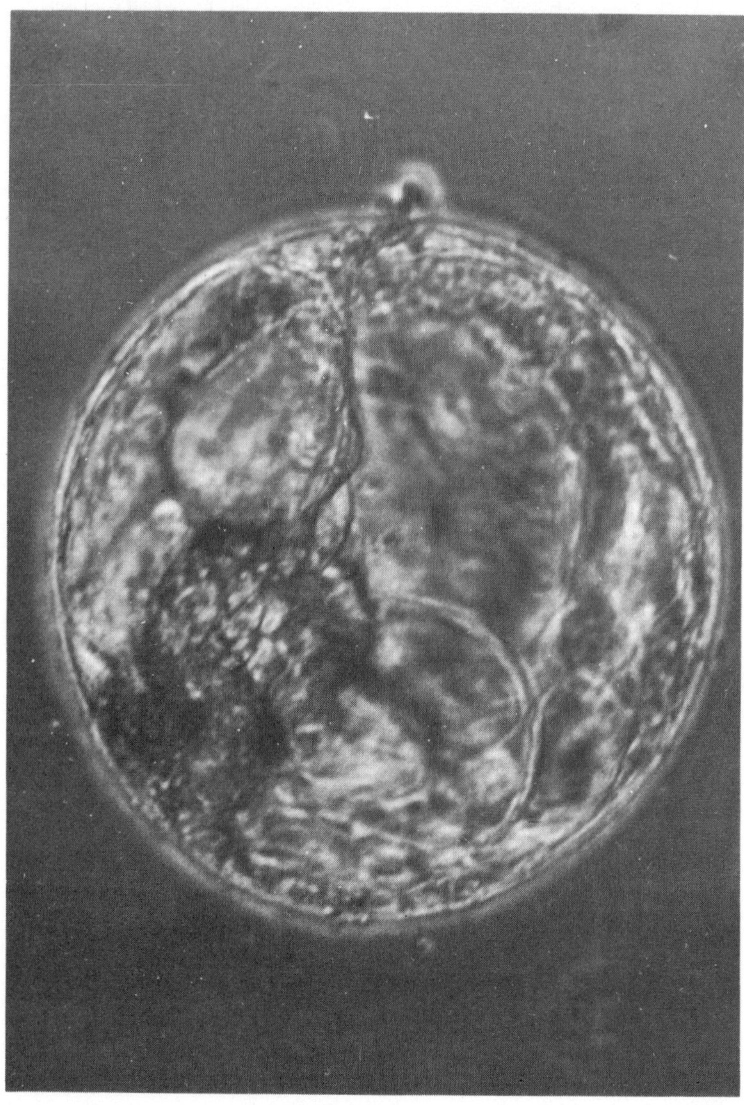

7. Early blastocyst showing differentiating trophoblast and inner cell mass. Some central cells have discharged their secretions to form central cyst.

of the embryos *in vitro* are abundant. Analysis of the factors influencing early human development are dependent on these methods. For example, capacitation of spermatozoa was believed to occur only while they were in the female genital tract. Attention has now shifted to the follicular fluid and the cells surrounding the oocytes as the source of the factors inducing capacitation. The metabolism of the granulosa cells and the secretions of the oviduct require further analysis to discover the components that become attached to spermatozoa, or remove substances from the surface of the gamete. Capacitation must occur in the immediate vicinity of the oocytes maintained *in vitro*, together with those detectable changes in the acrosome which probably lead to the release of hyaluronidase and other enzymes necessary for the penetration of the sperms between the cells and through the zona pellucida.

Another excellent opportunity afforded is to continue the analysis of underlying endocrinological and cellular factors involved in the menstrual cycle. Measurement of the steroidal and ovarian response of patients to exogenous gonadotrophins is possible by calculating the number and size of Graafian follicles, the patterns of steroid excretion by the patients and the contrasting steroid metabolism of ovulatory and non-ovulatory follicles. Our preliminary results show that large amounts of progesterone and oestradiol are present in follicular fluid, although so far there is no obvious correlation with the pre-ovulatory or atretic state of the follicle and the levels of these hormones.

Our initial task is to attempt to establish pregnancies in our patients. In addition, various studies of fundamental importance for genetics and immunology can now be carried out on the cleaving human embryos. Their karyotype can be determined and the effect of external agents or different media tested on the embryos. Various immunological phenomena such as the expression of transplantation antigens on the early trophoblast or the effect of antibiotics against spermatozoa on conception can be studied. Analysis of the chromosomes may reveal early chromosome disorders and permit study of the origins of human trisomy such as certain types of mongolism. We may learn how to correct or eliminate certain types of abnormal embryos, particularly those of sex-linked hereditary diseases, if the blastocysts can be sexed. The effect of various external agents on the embryos may lead to the discovery of new methods of contraception.

Studies are at present in progress of the possible methods of introducing early embryos into the uterus, and of the support which might be necessary to bring about successful re-implantation of these embryos.

These are but some of the opportunities offered, and they are the result of close collaboration between a scientist and a gynaecologist. Surely these methods of advancing medical knowledge and of applying such gains in clinical application are more than justified. May I close this chapter with these words which are written on the flyleaf of Cromwell's Bible in the British Museum:

'If we cease to get better, we cease to be good.'

References

1. Behrman, S. J., *Hosp. Pract.* (1966), **1**, 50.
2. Swolen, K., *Acta Obstet. Gynec. Scand.* (1967), **46**, suppl. 4.
3. Frangenheim, H., *Laparoscopy in Gynaecology* (1967), Livingstone, Edinburgh.
4. Sjovall, A., *Proc. First Int. Sympos. on Gynec. Celioscopy* (1964), Palermo, 14–15 Nov.
5. Ahlgren, M., *Studentlitteratur Lund.* (1969).
6. Kibrick, S., Belding, D. L., and Merrill, B., *Fertil. Steril.* (1952), **3**, 430–438.
7. Isojima, S., Li, T. S., and Ashitaka, Y., *Amer. J. Obstet. Gynec.* (1968), **101**, 677–683.
8. Steptoe, P. C., *Proc. First Int. Sympos. on Gynec. Celioscopy* (1964), Palermo, 14–15 Nov.
9. Ahlgren, M., *Acta Obst. Gynec. Scand.* (1971 *Vol. 50, supplement.* 9.56).
10. Nordvall, S., *Acta Obstet. Gynec. Scand.* (1970), **49**, 111.
11. Clyman, M. J., *Obstet. Gynec.* (1963), **21**, 343.
12. Palmer, R., *Bull. Fed. Soc. Gyn. et Obst.* (1968), **130**, 20.
13. Franklin, R. R., and Dukes, C. D., *Am. J. Obstet. Gynec.* (1964), **89**, 6.
14. Palmer, R., Personal communication (1970).
15. Bavister, B. D., *J. Reprod. Fert.* (1969), **18**, 544.
16. Edwards, R. G., Bavister, B. D., and Steptoe, P. C., *Nature, Lond.* (1969), **221**, 632.
17. Chang, M. C., *J. exp. Zool.* (1955), **128**, 379.
18. Edwards, R. G., and Gates, A. H., *J. Endocr.* (1959), **18**, 292–304.
19. Jagiello, G., Karnicki, J., and Ryan, R. J., *Lancet* (1968), **i**, 178.
20. Steptoe, P. C., and Edwards, R. G., *Lancet* (1970), **1**, 683.
21. Bavister, B. D., Edwards, R. G., and Steptoe, P. C., *J. Reprod. Fert.* (1969), **20**, 159.
22. Whittingham, D. G., *Nature, Lond.* (1968), **22**, 592.
23. Mukkerjee, A. B., and Cohen, M. M., *Nature, Lond.* (1970), **228**, 472.
24. Whitten, W. K., *Advances in the Biosciences* (1971), **6**, 129.
25. Ham, R. G., *Exp. Cell. Res.* (1963), **29**, 215.
26. Waymouth, C., *J. Nat. Cancer Inst.* (1959), **22**, 1003.
27. Edwards, R. G., Steptoe, P. C., and Purdy, J. M., *Nature, Lond.* (1970), **227**, 1307.

28. Steptoe, P. C., Edwards, R. G., and Purdy, J. M., *Nature, Lond.* (1971), **229,** 132–133.
29. Pearson, P. L., Bobrow, M., and Vosa, C. G., *Nature, Lond.* (1970), **226,** 78.
30. Pearson, P. L., and Bobrow, M., *J. Reprod. Fert.* (1970), **22,** 177.
31. Abraham, G. E., Odell, W. C., Edwards, R. G., and Purdy, J. M., *Acta Endocrin. Supp.* (1970), **147,** 332.
32. Crooke, A. C., *Br. Med. Bull.* (1970), **26,** 17.

Section B

A Concise Guide to Modern Treatment

Every doctor's problem is keeping up-to-date with his therapeutic armamentarium. With wider experience of drugs unwanted side-effects, hitherto unrecognised, may often reduce their usefulness whilst contraindications limit their exhibition. Professor Trounce and his team of specialists have produced the first really succinct and easily referrable section on Drugs in Current Use that has been published. In this Section will be found the pharmacological guide that any doctor, in any field of medical practice, needs.

Drugs in Current Use

by

J. R. Trounce
Professor of Clinical Pharmacology,
Guy's Hospital Medical School, London

Introduction

One of the major problems which face those who are engaged in treating patients is the large number of drugs available. These drugs are often powerful agents with potential to do harm as well as good.

This section is not a treatise on therapy and the particular drug or drugs which should be used in a given clinical situation will be found elsewhere. Once however the line of treatment has been decided it is the duty of the doctor to know as much as possible about the drugs which he intends to use. It has been our aim to provide a short account of most of the drugs in current use with particular emphasis on side effects and contraindications. There is also a short review of drug interaction at the end.

In some 50,000 words it has obviously not been possible to cover every aspect of every drug and a certain amount of selection of what is considered important has had to be made. However, it is hoped that nothing of real importance has been omitted. A few references have been included where they were considered useful. These will prove useful if the reader requires a more complete knowledge of a drug. In the case of drugs not covered by a reference, one of the many large textbooks of pharmacology should be adequate. The main difficulty is with very new drugs which are not yet in standard texts and further information about them can usually only be obtained from the literature.

It will be noted that only approved names of drugs have been used. It is arguable that trade names are widely known and easier to remember. However, many drugs have more than one trade name and if these were used or even given as an alternative in the text it would lead to considerable confusion and difficulty.

Category 1

Drugs Used in Neurological Disease

THE TREATMENT OF EPILEPSY

Many of the currently available anticonvulsant drugs belong to the ring or cyclic compounds, and share common characteristics. Absorption is usually complete in patients with normal alimentary function, but it may be slow, as in the cases of phenobarbitone and of phenytoin. Following absorption, distribution occurs throughout the body and there does not appear to be any selective concentration in the brain. The drugs are bound to a variable extent in the serum to protein molecules, and they are metabolised in the liver. The inactive metabolites and the active unchanged drug are excreted by the kidney, often quite slowly. This slow excretion accounts for the tendency of many anticonvulsants to be cumulative. Blood levels of the drug depend both on the dose administered and on variations in the activity of drug metabolising enzymes in the liver. Individual differences in the metabolism of the drug may result in its being metabolised so rapidly that it is impossible to achieve therapeutically effective blood levels; or metabolism may be so retarded that the active unmetabolised drug accumulates with the appearance of symptoms of overdosage. Variations in the metabolism of drugs may be genetic or acquired. Concurrent administration of another drug may interfere with the metabolism of anticonvulsants.

The mode of action of anticonvulsant drugs is uncertain. Some anticonvulsants appear to act by influencing abnormal neurones; others seem to protect normal neurones from abnormal discharges by influencing the transport of sodium from within the neurone across the cell membrane, thus decreasing intracellular sodium and increasing the threshold of seizure activity.

The side effects and toxic effects which may complicate anticonvulsant drug therapy are either due to embarrassment of the normal function of the brain (e.g. cerebellum) or of other systems (e.g. haemopoeietic system), or due to hypersensitivity reactions e.g. skin, gums.

Phenobarbitone

Pharmacological action. The drug is an effective anticonvulsant for generalised convulsive seizures and focal seizures. The neural synapse is probably its major site of action. It is thought that the drug slows or blocks cation transport of sodium and potassium across the cellular membrane and that this action damps down both excitatory and inhibitory post-synaptic potential generation. Barbiturates exert a markedly depressant effect upon repetitive activity in CNS pathways.

Therapeutic use [2]. The drug is used in the treatment of grand mal epilepsy and focal epilepsy. Temporal lobe epilepsy responds less satisfactorily. The usual starting daily intake for adults is about 100 mg per day, taken in three divided doses or in a single dose at bedtime. Daily doses are increased if seizures persist, but should rarely exceed 300 mg per day. Initial daily doses for children are smaller, usually 45 to 60 mg per day. If phenobarbitone must be discontinued after prolonged use, withdrawal should proceed slowly over a period of a week to avoid the possibility of withdrawal convulsions. However, this complication is uncommon with phenobarbitone because of its slow rate of metabolism and elimination.

Side effects and contraindications. 1. The sedative effect of the drug is a drawback. This can be circumvented by giving the total daily dose in the early evening and perhaps by medicating with central nervous system stimulants (amphetamines) during the waking hours.

2. Occasionally, for reasons as yet not clearly explained, phenobarbitone has a paradoxical exciting effect on children, the mentally retarded, and the elderly.

3. One or two per cent of patients receiving the drug develop dermatitis, which necessitates withdrawal of the drug. Rare instances of exfoliative dermatitis have been reported. The drug is contraindicated in hepatic failure, as it is normally metabolised by hepatic enzymes; in acute intermittent porphyria it may produce a precipitous and dangerous rise in the level of porphyrins which is associated with the development of symptoms of acute porphyria.

Primidone

Pharmacological action [2]. This drug is structurally closely related to phenobarbitone and its mechanism and site of action are probably the same. It is effective in the treatment of convulsive seizures refractory to other medications. However, its effectiveness against temporal lobe epilepsy and sometimes against petit mal suggests mechanisms of action additional to those of phenobarbitone.

Therapeutic use. The drug is of value in major epilepsy of either primary or secondary type. Preferably it should be used in combination with phenytoin, so that maximum anticonvulsant effect can be obtained in lower dosage and therefore with minimal sedation. The drug is approximately one-fifth to one-tenth as potent as phenobarbitone. The average daily dose for adults is 750 mg, and for children 150 to 250 mg.

Side effects. The effectiveness of the drug is limited by its sedative properties. This sedative property is particularly noticeable at the beginning of therapy, and for this reason it should be introduced at a very low dosage which is gradually increased over a few weeks.

A syndrome of vertigo and ataxia sometimes with diplopia may occur during the first few days of treatment. Skin rashes and leucopenia have been reported, but are rare.

Phenytoin sodium (Diphenylhydantoin, *USA*)

Pharmacological action. The mode of action of phenytoin is not fully understood. The drug appears to inhibit the spread of epileptic discharges, but it does not depress spontaneous discharge from the epileptic focus itself. It reduces neuronal irritability by decreasing intracellular sodium concentration and by stabilising membranes.

Therapeutic use. The drug is the most effective and widely used anticonvulsant in the treatment of generalised convulsive seizures and focal epilepsy. Therapy is usually started in the adult with 100 mg three times per day. Doses can be increased to the point of intoxication or of cessation of seizures. Lack of effect on seizures of prescribed daily doses above 500 to 600 mg suggests that the patient is not taking that amount of drug, or, in rare instances, that intestinal absorption is inadequate or that metabolism of the drug is over active. Doses above 500 mg per day are rarely necessary or tolerated.

Side effects. The drug is, in general, very safe, with low toxicity. The following side effects may, however, occur.

1. A small number of patients are hypersensitive to the drug, and become intoxicated with the usual doses. In some cases this hypersensitivity may be due to a defect of metabolism of the drug by the liver, or to interference with metabolism of the drug by other drugs. In such an event reduction of dosage is required.

2. A reversible syndrome of cerebellar dysfunction appears to be related to the serum concentration of phenytoin. The normal therapeutic blood levels of phenytoin are between 15 and 20 mg per litre. Above 20 mg/litre nystagmus, ataxia and dysarthria may occur. This is not uncommonly seen at the onset of therapy. Chronic intoxication and severe acute intoxication have resulted in Purkinje cell degeneration in the cerebellum.

3. Neuropsychiatric symptoms (e.g. depression, dementia, schizophrenic-like psychosis, peripheral neuropathy) may occur rarely due to prolonged administration over a number of years. These neurological states often respond well to combined therapy with folic acid and vitamin B_{12}.

4. Megaloblastic anaemia may occur rarely after prolonged administration of the drug for several years. This is due to interference with folic acid metabolism, and treatment of the anaemia should be with folic acid. Other blood dyscracias have been reported, but are rare.

5. Minor side effects include gastric upset due to the alkalinity of the drug; dermatitis, with the development of a morbilliform rash; gum hypertrophy – this occurs particularly in children and can be minimised by careful dental hygiene. The finding of a low serum protein-bound iodine in patients on the drug is due to the drug interfering with the binding of thyroxine to plasma proteins. The drug itself does not cause hypothyroidism.

Methoin (Mephenytoin, *USA*)

Pharmacological action. The drug is related chemically and pharmacologically to diphenylhydantoin. It simulates the activity of the anticonvulsant barbiturates, and it also acts as a hydantoin in preventing the tonic phase of major motor convulsions.

Therapeutic use. The drug should be used only if less toxic preparations fail to control grand mal seizures of primary or secondary type. It is of value in the treatment of generalised and major motor convulsions. It is also effective to some extent in preventing temporal lobe automatisms. It has little effect on petit mal seizures, and may make them worse. The dose is 100 mg daily, increased to 600 mg in accordance with the needs of the patient.

Side effects and contraindications. The drug possesses the disagreeable characteristics of the barbiturates (sedation and lethargy) often at less than optimum therapeutic levels. As a hydantoin it is considerably more toxic than diphenylhydantoin. The most dangerous toxic effects are leucopenia, pancytopenia, agranulocytosis, and aplastic anaemia. This hazard of bone marrow depression is considerably greater when methoin is given in combination with troxidone which itself affects the bone marrow adversely. Lymphadenopathy may occur.

Troxidone (Trimethadione, *USA*)

Pharmacological action. Troxidone is an anti-epileptic drug with specificity for the treatment of petit mal seizures. It is probable that troxidone blocks the propagation of an epileptic discharge from a cortical epileptic focus to the thalamus, while the local cortical spread of the epileptiform activity is only slightly reduced, if at all.

Therapeutic use. The drug is used for the treatment of petit mal epilepsy. For an adult the dose is 900 mg daily, in divided doses, increasing to 1·8 g. daily, according to the needs of the patient. For children the dose is 300 mg. daily, in divided doses, increasing to 900 mg.

Side effects and contraindications. A frequently observed side effect is hemeralopia or night blindness. This probably represents a drug action at the ganglion layer of the retina.

Skin rashes occur with troxidone; they indicate a sensitivity reaction and their occurrence is an indication for drug withdrawal.

Bone marrow depression may occur, usually during the first year of treatment.

Nephrosis, hepatitis and lupus erythematosus have been reported.

Ethosuximide

Pharmacological action. This is the drug of choice in the treatment of petit mal and myoclonic seizures. It is extremely effective.

Therapeutic use. The adult dose is 500 mg daily, in divided doses, increasing to 2 g., according to the needs of the patient.

Side effects and contraindications. The drug has a distinct tendency to evoke major seizures, and if there is any tendency to grand mal epilepsy (either clinical or electroencephalographic) the patient should also be given a drug effective in controlling grand mal in order to counteract this tendency. In other respects the drug is relatively non-toxic. Gastro-intestinal upset, headache, dizziness, skin rashes and blood changes may occur but are rare.

Sulthiame

Pharmacological action. This drug is a sulfonamide congener with weak carbonic anhydrase activity. It has reported success in the treatment of temporal lobe epilepsy, although its mode of action is not known and trials have not shown the drug to be convincingly superior to other available medications.

Therapeutic use. The main indication for sulthiame appears to be in the control of secondary cortical epilepsy. The adult dose is 100 – 200 mg twice or three times daily.

Side effects. As the drug is a carbonic anhydrase inhibitor it may produce features of metabolic acidosis such as over-breathing. It potentiates phenobarbitone and the hydantoins, and this may account for some of its therapeutic effect. Headache, nausea, vomiting, dizziness, drowsiness, visual blurring, gastric disturbances and rarely psychoses may complicate its use.

Diazepam

Pharmacological action. This drug is thought to exert an action upon the limbic system or its connections to reduce the intensity of emotional feeling. In addition, it has an anti-epileptic effect and in particular it appears to be extremely effective in arresting status epilepticus without producing overwhelming narcosis.

Therapeutic use [3]. The chief value of the drug in epilepsy is in the control of status epilepticus. The drug is given parenterally, either in a single dose of 10 mg by slow intravenous injection, or by intravenous infusion of 100 mg over a 12-hour period.

Side effects. Weakness, drowsiness and ataxia may be produced. Long-term usage may result in habituation and very rarely in dependence. The drug may 'normalise' an abnormal E.E.G. tracing and therefore should not be given in the 10 days preceding an E.E.G. examination.

THE TREATMENT OF MIGRAINE

This subject has recently been comprehensively reviewed [4,5,6]. The general principles in the management of the migrainous subject are discussed elsewhere in this book.

Treatment of the acute attack should be with analgesia in the first instance, before any other form of therapy is used; i.e., 300–600 mg of soluble aspirin, or 500 mg of paracetamol, taken at the beginning of the attack and repeated in two hours if necessary. Next in line is ergotamine tartrate. The autonomic effects of the acute attack on the gastro-intestinal tract which produce nausea, vomiting, diarrhoea and even abdominal pain are best treated with an antiemetic drug e.g. 50 mg cyclizine hydrochloride, or 10 mg thiethylperazine.

Preventive therapy with the serotonin antagonist methysergide is effective and relatively safe if carefully administered.

Ergotamine tartrate

Pharmacological action. The drug is thought to exert its beneficial action by causing vasoconstriction of the cerebral vessels.

Therapeutic use [5]. Ergotamine is extremely useful in the treatment of acute migraine. Ideally, it should be given in small doses, at the very onset of the attack. Larger doses often prove unsatisfactory due to the production of toxic effects. These side effects, notably nausea and vomiting, are very similar to those of an acute attack of migraine. The maximum dosage of ergotamine tartrate in any one week should not exceed 12 mg.

The following methods of administration are used:

1. By mouth. Ergotamine tartrate tablets B.P. 1 mg; the dosage should be 1–2 mg. There is some doubt whether tablets taken in the acute attack are properly absorbed. Cafergot Q tablets, which contain 1 mg of ergotamine tartrate and 100 mg of caffeine, may be chewed, and absorption is then thought to take place through the buccal mucous membrane. These tablets are, however, bitter, and therefore not acceptable to some patients.

2. By suppository. This is a satisfactory form of treatment for the patient who vomits in the attack. Absorption from the rectum is good. Difficulties arise in patients who have diarrhoea as a symptom of their attacks. Cafergot suppositories contain 2 mg ergotamine tartrate, 100 mg caffeine, 0·25 mg belladonna alkaloids, and 100 mg isobutalyl barbituric acid.

3. By inhalation. Medihaler-Ergotamine vials, which contain a suspension of ergotamine tartrate are used. The inhaler is calibrated so that each dose contains 0·36 mg ergotamine tartrate. This is rapidly absorbed, either through the buccal mucous membrane or through the epithelium of the respiratory tract. Usually one or two inhalations (0·36 or 0·72 mg) are enough.

4. By injection. Intramuscular injection of 0·25 or 0·5 mg ergotamine tartrate with an antiemetic such as 50 mg cyclizine lactate is probably the most effective means of treatment of a classical migraine attack. This is an effective dose and improvement should occur within two hours in over 90 per cent of patients.

Side effects and contraindications. The immediate toxic effects of argotamine tartrate are nausea and vomiting. Variability in tolerance to the drug is marked; some patients can tolerate large doses, and in others extreme sensitivity may be encountered.

Other side effects of the drug are numbness, tingling and chilling of the extremities, a rise in blood pressure and painful uterine contractions.

The contraindications to its use include peripheral vascular disease, hypertension, coronary, hepatic and renal insufficiency, pregnancy, and sepsis and infections which seem to sensitise to the drug. In migranous hemiparesis the drug may prolong arterial spasm and induce a true cerebral thrombosis.

Methysergide

Pharmacological action. The exact pharmacological action of methysergide in migraine is not known. This drug is the most powerful known antagonist to serotonin; it is structurally similar to serotonin and this antagonism is possibly due to competition for similar receptors. It is therefore possible that methysergide acts by competitively inhibiting the effect of serotonin on the carotid tree or by modifying its central vasomotor mechanism in the hypothalamus. However, it is quite probable that the pharmacological action of the drug may be completely independent of its ability to antagonise serotonin and bradykinin and that it is changed in the body in such a way as to acquire the long-acting, vasoconstrictor properties of ergot, or to increase the patient's sensitivity to endogenous and exogenous vasoconstrictor agents.

Therapeutic use [7]. The drug is used in the prophylaxis of migraine. 1–6 mg is used daily. A small dose of 1–2 mg is given at night for a week, during which time the patient is observed for untoward symptoms. If these do not occur the dose can be increased to a maximum of 6 mg daily. Continuous treatment for more than 6 months is undesirable without a drug-free interval for at least a month. The dosage should be decreased gradually for 2 or 3 weeks before withdrawing the drug to prevent the occurrence of a rebound phenomenon. The patient should be carefully examined at least every 3 months for the development of side effects. The prospect of serious side effects is greatly minimised when methysergide can be given intermittently for short periods only.

Side effects and contraindications. There is great individual variation in susceptibility to methysergide. Some 40 per cent of patients taking the drug experience side effects and these are so severe as to require stopping its administration in about 15 per cent.

The most common early side effects are a stimulant effect on the appetite; nausea, vomiting and diarrhoea, abdominal pain which may be due to vasoconstriction of the abdominal vasculature, peripheral oedema – probably due to constriction of veins and lymphatics; thrombophlebitis, and symptoms resulting from vasoconstriction of any artery in the body. These effects are quickly reversible when the administration of the drug is stopped.

The most important side effect of treatment with methysergide is the development of retroperitoneal fibrosis. This may develop after more than 4 months of treatment; most patients give the history of having taken the drug for many months or years. Presentation may be with low-grade fever, pain in the loins, oliguria, dysuria, and symptoms of uraemia, and confirmation is with pyelographic evidence of ureteric obstruction. About 1 per cent of patients taking the drug develop this complication; in these cases it should be withdrawn and not used again.

Methysergide is contraindicated in pregnancy, arterial and venous disease of all types, valvular heart disease, chronic pulmonary disease, impaired renal or hepatic function, peptic ulcer, and anything suggesting a diathesis of collagen disease, or a pathological tendency to fibrosis.

THE TREATMENT OF PARKINSON'S DISEASE

[8] There is good evidence now available that a disturbance of neurotransmitter systems occurs in the brains of Parkinsonian patients. Cholinergic drugs exacerbate parkinsonism, and clinical experience has shown that anticholinergic agents are beneficial. Pharmacological studies suggests that this beneficial action of anticholinergic drugs is at a central nervous level, and not peripheral in origin. Antihistamines are also useful in parkinsonism. However, these drugs also interfere with acetylcholine and it has not been established that their antihistamine properties are relevant.

The relief afforded by the conventional anti-parkinsonism drugs is limited, and at best a modest improvement in mobility, general motor performance and subjective well-being, and a slight decrease in tremor and mobility may be expected. A 30 per cent improvement in 80 per cent of patients is an optimistic estimate of the response that might be expected. The course of the disease is not altered, and there are prominent undesirable actions. In some cases sudden withdrawal of treatment may precipitate a marked deterioration in clinical status which is often out of proportion to the therapeutic benefit which had previously been noted.

The recent use of L-dopa in recent years has offered a significant advance in the treatment of patients with Parkinson's disease.

Artane hydrochloride (Trihexipleridyl hydrochloride, *USA*)

Pharmacological action. The actions of this drug on the central nervous system resemble those of the belladonna alkaloids. The evidence is that artane acts by blocking acetylcholine at certain central synaptic sites.

Therapeutic use [7]. The drug is used for the symptomatic control of all forms of Parkinsonism, including the postencephalitic, arteriosclerotic, and idiopathic types. The drug favourably influences rigidity and akinesia in the majority of patients. Tremor is generally improved as well, but in some instances of severe rigidity the tremor may be accentuated when the rigidity is diminished.

The drug is virtually devoid of serious systemic toxicity.

It is the drug of choice for initial therapy of the various types of Parkinson's disease. The initial doses should be small – 1 or 2 mg twice daily, with meals. The dose is gradually increased to 2 mg three or four times daily. In some cases, the total daily dose for optimal results is 15–30 mg. The factors which determine dosage are the patient's response to therapy and his tolerance for the drug.

Side effects and contraindications. The side effects of the drug resemble those of atropine. Five to ten per cent of patients cannot tolerate fully effective doses. Side effects such as dry mouth and blurred vision are common. Overdosage produces mental confusion, delirium, agitation and hallucination. When intolerable side effects occur the dose must be reduced and if necessary another drug used along with artane, or the drug must be withdrawn in favour of another drug.

Cycrimine hydrochloride

Pharmacological action. This drug closely resembles artane hydrochloride in its action and therapeutic use.

Therapeutic use. The drug serves as a substitute for artane in the event that that agent is not well tolerated. The dose is 1·25 or 2·5 mg four times daily, initially, and it is increased according to the patient's need. The total daily dose usually does not exceed 20 mg except in post encephalitic patients, who may require as much as 45 mg daily.

Side effects. These are similar to those of artane. Large doses cause excitatory effects.

Procyclidine

Pharmacological action. This drug closely resembles artane hydrochloride in its action and therapeutic use.

Therapeutic use. The usual dose of procyclidine is 2·5 mg three times daily. This may be increased according to the tolerance of the patient to as much as 45 to 60 mg per day. The indication for the drug is as for cycrimine hydrochloride.

Side effects. These resemble those of artane.

Biperiden

Pharmacological action. The drug closely resembles artane in its pharmacological action and therapeutic use.

Therapeutic use. The drug is given as biperiden hydrochloride. The initial dose is 2 mg three or four times daily.

Side effects. Resemble those of artane.

Benztropine mesylate

Pharmacological action. This drug contains both an atropine moiety (tropine base) and an antihistaminic element (benzohydryloxy moiety). The drug possesses atropine-like as well as antihistaminic properties.

Therapeutic use. The drug may be given orally, or by intramuscular or intravenous injection. Initially, single daily doses of 0·5 to 1 mg are employed. This may be increased by daily increments of 0·5 mg until the optimum response is obtained; the maximum dose rarely exceeds 8 mg per day.

It is useful in all types of parkinsonism, and it is an effective drug to replace artane and its congeners in patients who have become tolerant to these agents. A desirable feature of the drug is its long action. The drug produces mild sedation characteristic of the antihistamines, and it is therefore an appropriate drug for patients, particularly the aged, who are adversely affected by the agents which produce excitement. Benztropine mesylate is especially effective in relieving 'frozen states'. A significant effect of the drug is the amelioration of pain secondary to muscle spasm and cramping.

Side effects. These are usually mild, and mainly associated with the anticholinergic component of the drug. Occasionally, weakness in certain muscles necessitates reduction in dosage.

Orphenadrine hydrochloride

Pharmacological action. The drug exerts a central anticholinergic action on the nervous system.

Therapeutic use. This agent reduces the rigidity of parkinsonism but it has little effect on the tremor. With favourable response there is increased muscular power and endurance. The drug produces euphoria. The initial dose is 50 mg three times daily. Total dose may be increased to 300 mg per day if necessary.

Side effects. Drowsiness is a common side effect. The peripheral anticholinergic action of the drug is relatively weak.

Chlorphenoxamine hydrochloride

The pharmacological action, therapeutic use, dosage and side effects of this drug are similar to orphenadrine. The duration of action is however slightly greater.

Ethopropazine hydrochloride

Pharmacological action. The drug is a phenothiazine derivative which possesses anticholinergic actions on the central and the peripheral nervous systems. In addition, it exerts a slight antihistaminic effect.

Therapeutic use. The initial dose is 10 mg four times daily. The dose is increased as required, and total daily doses as high as 1 g. have been employed. The drug is effective against the tremor and rigidity of parkinsonism. Sialorrhoea is well controlled.

Side effects. The side effects characteristic of anticholinergic drugs are produced by ethopropazine. Dizziness and drowsiness are common.

L-dihydroxyphenyllanine (L-dopa)

Pharmacological action. The theoretical basis for the use of dopa in parkinsonism rests on the observation that dopamine, of which dopa is the precursor, is depleted in the corpus striatum of patients with this disease. It has been supposed that dopa administered to patients with Parkinson's disease may improve neurological function by increasing levels of dopamine in the striatum. Dopa must be used since dopamine will not pass the blood-brain barrier. It is possible that loading the central nervous system with dopa may have very much more complex and as yet obscure therapeutic effects in Parkinson's disease.

Therapeutic use [9]. Early studies indicate that most patients with idiopathic Parkinson's disease derive benefit from treatment with L-dopa.

The beneficial response appears to be chiefly noticeable in the akinesia. Rigidity is improved in most patients, but there is no consistent reduction in tremor. A mild euphoriant action may occur with treatment with L-dopa but this is not thought to account for its beneficial action in more than a small minority of patients. The optimum dose lies between 3 g. and 8 g. daily. Patients with post-encephalitic parkinsonism appear to respond best.

Side effects [10]. 1. Gastointestinal symptoms. In the early stages of treatment anorexia and nausea are encountered in the majority of patients. These effects are probably due to a central effect of the drug. The symptoms may be reduced by slowing the rate of increase in dosage, and by administering conventional anti-emetic drugs. Nausea can be reduced by taking L-dopa after food. It may take several weeks for the nausea to disappear.

2. Alterations in blood pressure. Falls in the erect systolic blood pressure induced by L-dopa average about 20 mms Hg. Symptoms such as giddiness are particularly likely to occur as patients build up their intake. It may be necessary to reduce the dose temporarily and patients may have to stay in bed for a few days. The symptoms usually clear, and intake may gradually be increased again. It is probably hazardous to give the drug to patients with coronary heart disease. The mechanism of the orthostatic hypotension produced by L-dopa is not known.

3. Dyskinesia. Involuntary movements complicating the use of L-dopa usually begin as dyskinesia of the tongue and jaw with grimacing of the face and choreoathetoid movements of the neck. The clinical picture closely resembles the dyskinesia which is occasionally induced by phenothiazines. Choreoathetoid movements may also appear in the limbs, and sometimes involuntary fexion-extension activity occurs, resembling myoclonus. The mechanism of these drug-induced involuntary movements is not understood. On high doses of L-dopa a fine postural tremor is sometimes seen, similar to that of thyrotoxicosis and anxiety states. These abnormal movements are often difficult to control and as a rule the drug has to be stopped for a few days, and then reintroduced at a lower dosage.

4. Psychiatric disturbances. Patients receiving L-dopa are sometimes aware of increased energy and this may be associated with elevation of mood and enhanced libido. Somnolence and unusually vivid dreams have also been recorded. Mental features such as restlessness, anxiety, agitation and insomnia are common. Some patients become confused or depressed. When such disturbances occur the drug should be with-

drawn. It is often difficult to reintroduce the drug in these patients. Caution should be exercised in treating a patient with L-dopa who has a background of psychiatric disturbances.

5. Other adverse effects induce various cardiac arrythmias, development of a positive Coomb's test (rare), headaches, and excessive sweating.

THE TREATMENT OF TRIGEMINAL NEURALGIA

Carbamazepine

Pharmacological action. This drug is an iminodibenzyl compound which is chemically related to imipramine. It has anticonvulsant activity.
Therapeutic use. Dose is 100 mg twice daily, gradually increasing to 200 mg three or four times daily as required. The majority of patients obtain relief within 48 hours of starting treatment.

Side effects are common. They include giddiness, nausea, anorexia, vomiting and skin rashes. Serious toxic effects have been reported; aplastic anaemia, lupus erythematosus, and the Stevens-Johnson syndrome. Adverse effects are most likely to occur when high doses of the drug are required.

References

1. Sutherland, J. M., and Tait, H., *The Epilepsies: modern Diagnosis and Treatment* (1969). Livingstone, London.
2. Schmidt, R. P., and Wilder, B. J., *Epilepsy* (1968), Blackwell, Oxford, 141.
3. Pryse-Phillips, W., *Epilepsy* (1969), 59. John Wright, Bristol.
4. Blau, J. N., *Br. med. J.* (1971), **2,** 751–754.
5. Wilkinson, M., *Br. med. J.* (1971), **2,** 754–755.
6. Carroll, J. D., *Br. med. J.* (1971), **2,** 756–757.
7. Goodman, L. S., and Gilman, A., *The Pharmacological basis of Therapeutics* (1965). Macmillan, New York, 241.
8. Calne, D. B., *Parkinsonism: physiology, pharmacology and treatment* (1970), Edward Arnold, London.
9. Godwin Austin, R. B., Tomlinson, E. B., Frears, C. C., Kok, H. W. L., *Lancet* (1969), **ii,** 165.

This chapter was written by Dr P. I. Folb (Dept of Clinical Pharmacology, Guy's Hospital Medical School) and edited by Professor J. R. Trounce.

Category 2

Hypnotics

The Barbiturates

Pharmacology. The group of barbiturate hypnotics have the general formula

```
HN———CO
|     |  R1
|     | /
O=C      C
|     | \
|     |  R2
HN———CO
```

Substitution can occur in the R_1 and R_2 position, producing a large number of compounds. For example:

	R_1	R_2
Quinalbarbitone	$CH_2CH{=}CH_2$	C_5H_{11}
Amylobarbitone	C_2H_5	C_5H_{11}
Phenobarbitone	C_2H_5	Phenyl

The introduction of a phenyl group confers anticonvulsant properties and also decreases conjugation in the liver, and thus prolongs action.

This group of drugs is well absorbed from the intestinal tract and penetrates widely through the tissues. They are largely conjugated in the liver and only phenobarbitone is excreted to any degree (30 per cent) unchanged in the urine. Renal excretion of phenobarbitone is enhanced in an alkaline urine, as this increases the ionised fraction in the urine and decreases back diffusion from the tubules to the blood [1]. With repeated dosage tolerance will develop, and it has been shown that barbiturates will induce enzymes in the liver which metabolise the drug. The enhanced production of glucuranyl transferase by barbiturates has been used in treating neonatal jaundice [2].

The effect of the very short-acting barbiturate is terminated by redistribution of the drug – a short while after administration a major portion passes from the brain to fat and muscle.

Barbiturates produce sleep by depressing both the cortex and reticular activating system. In larger doses they produce unconsciousness and the very quick acting ones can be used as anaesthetic agents.

In hypnotic doses the barbiturates have no effect on perception of pain, and in those suffering pain they must be combined with an analgesic.

Barbiturates lower the blood pressure by reducing cardiac output [3]. This is partially due to venous pooling and perhaps also to a direct effect on the myocardium.

The respiratory centre is depressed, especially with large doses, and this is an important feature of overdosage.

Therapeutic uses. Barbiturates can be classified in terms of their duration of action.

Long Acting Group: Phenobarbitone (Phenobarbital, *USA*) is the most important. Its action is generally considered too long for a hypnotic but unlike other barbiturates it is an anticonvulsant and is used in grand mal epilepsy. The usual anticonvulsant dose is 30–60 mg two or three times daily, but the top range of dose may well produce drowsiness. The sodium salt is also available for intramuscular injection in doses of 60–200 mg in status epilepticus. It is also used as a sedative in doses of 30 mg twice daily.

Medium Acting Group: This includes the commonly used hypnotics. Various members of the group vary a little in their speed of onset and duration of action, but generally they produce sleep in about half an hour, which lasts about six hours.

Most commonly used are:

UK	*USA*	*Dose*	
Pentobarbitone	Pentobarbital	100–200 mg	very rapidly metabolised
Quinalbarbitone	Secobarbital	50–200 mg	
Heptobarbitone	Heptobarbital	200–400 mg	
Amylobarbitone sodium	Amobarbital	100–200 mg	less rapidly metabolised
Butobarbitone	Butobarbital	100–200 mg	

The actual dose of barbiturate used will depend on the size of the patient and on any complicating factors which may modify the patient's sensitivity to the drug (see below).

Short Acting Group: This group includes thiopentone sodium (thiopental, *USA*) and hexobarbitone sodium (hexobarbital, *USA*).

They are used for short duration anaesthesia and also for induction of anaesthetics.

Contraindications and side effects. Barbiturates should not be given to those who have previously had a hypersensitivity reaction to them. Barbiturates will precipitate an acute attack of porphyria in those with this disease.

They should be used with great care if at all in those with decreased liver function or with chronic respiratory disease. In the elderly, barbiturates may produce confusion rather than sleep.

Skin rashes are the commonest side effect with barbiturates and may take a variety of forms from irritating erythemas to bullous eruptions.

The most important side effects are overdosage and dependence.

An overdose of barbiturates produces coma with respiratory depression. With very large doses there is also a falling blood pressure with circulatory, and ultimately, renal failure. The lethal dose is very variable, as is the fatal blood level. In general, a blood level of more than 3·0 mg per 100 ml with a short acting barbiturate or 10 mg per 100 ml with phenobarbitone, suggests a seriously ill patient. Blood levels are, however, a poor guide to prognosis. It must be remembered that the effects of barbiturates will be enhanced by other CNS depressant drugs, in particular alcohol.

Dependence on barbiturates is now recognised as a serious problem [4]. Continued taking of barbiturates in doses of 600 mg daily or more causes chronic intoxication [5] with psychological dependence, weakness, dizziness, slurred speech, nystagmus and sometimes orthostatic hypotension. Withdrawal symptoms can be severe and include anxiety, weakness, and in particular, convulsions.

NON-BARBITURATE HYPNOTICS

Glutethimide

Pharmacological action. Glutethimide is related to the barbiturates but is usually called a 'non-barbiturate' hypnotic. It is fairly well absorbed from the intestinal tract and is entirely metabolised in the body. It produces sleep lasting about 6–8 hours.

Therapeutic use. Glutethimide is a useful hypnotic in doses of 250–500 mg before retiring.

Contraindications and side effects. Contraindications are similar to those for the barbiturates. Side effects are skin rashes and nausea. Rarely it may produce convulsions. Glutethimide has some cholinergic blocking effect and may interfere with bowel or bladder function. Dependence can occur.

Overdosage differs from barbiturates in that although there is some respiratory depression failing circulation with low blood pressure is a prominent feature – the pupils are also widely dilated due to the drug's anticholinergic action.

Methyprylon

Pharmacological action. Methyprylon is a piperidinedione compound related to glutethimide. Its hypnotic action is very similar to that of the barbiturates and it is almost entirely metabolised by the liver. The usual hypnotic dose is 200–400 mg.

Contraindication and side effects. Death can occur from overdosage and as with the barbiturates, dependence and tolerance can develop.

Carbromal

Pharmacological action. Carbromal is a bromine-containing derivative of urea. It is a mild, short-acting hypnotic (about four hours) and is given in doses of 300–900 mg. It can however, cause rashes which may be purpuric, and bromism can occur after prolonged use.

Chloral hydrate

Pharmacological action. Chloral hydrate is well absorbed from the intestine. In the body it is rapidly converted to trichlorethanol which is the main active substance. Trichlorethanol is inactivated by conversion to the glucuronide, and to trichloracetic acid. These products are excreted in the urine. Chloral produces sleep lasting about eight hours.

Therapeutic use. Chloral is a gastric irritant and is therefore usually given well diluted in a solution such as chloral mixture BNF (10 mls contains 1·0 g.) or as syrup of chloral hydrate U.S.P. It has an unpleasant taste. The usual adult dose is 1–2 g. but some adults may require a larger dose. It is particularly useful and safe as a hypnotic or sedative in children when the dose is 15–30 mg/kg bodyweight. It is also said to be less liable than the barbiturates to cause confusion in the elderly.

Contraindications and side effects. Chloral should not be used in patients with peptic ulcer, in those with severe liver disease or in renal failure.

Chloral can occasionally cause rashes. Overdosage is rarely a serious problem.

There are a number of chloral compounds which are similar in action and uses to chloral. Unlike chloral however they are stable in tablet form and less liable to cause gastric irritation and are more palatable:

UK	*USA*	*Dose*
Dichlorphenazone		0·65–2·0 g.
Triclofos	Trichlorethylphosphate	1·0–2·0 g.
Chloral betaine		0·87–1·75 g.
Chloral hexadol		0·8–1·6 g.

The phenazone moeity of dichlorphenazone, which itself is a mild analgesic, can cause skin rashes and rarely agranulocytosis.

Ethchlorvynol

This mild hypnotic has a particularly rapid and short hypnotic effect. It has no special advantages but it is metabolised rather than excreted by the kidneys and might therefore be useful in renal failure. The dose is 250–750 mg orally.

Occasionally its use may be associated with some hangover and confusion.

Methylpentynol (Methylparafynol, *USA***)**

This drug is a mild, short-acting hypnotic with no particular advantages. It is a liquid and is given in capsule form and may produce a rather unpleasant tasting belch. The usual dose is 250–500 mg and large doses produce a state resembling alcoholic intoxication. Rashes may occur. Methylpentynol carbamate is similar but has a more prolonged action.

Paraldehyde

Pharmacological action. Paraldehyde is a fairly powerful and rapidly acting hypnotic. It is well absorbed from the intestinal tract and from the rectum and also after intramuscular injection. It produces sleep lasting about eight hours, and is also an anticonvulsant. It is largely metabolised in the liver but about 10 per cent is excreted unchanged by the lungs.

Therapeutic use. Paraldehyde can be used as a hypnotic in doses of 3–8 ml orally, or as a 10 per cent solution in normal saline rectally. It has however largely gone out of use for it tastes unpleasant, and the patient emits a particular smell for hours after administration, from the breath, urine and sweat.

It can also be given intramuscularly in doses of 4·0 ml and repeated as required to quieten noisy patients, or in status epilepticus. By this route however it is painful, and may lead to abscess formation, so again has been largely discarded.

Contraindications and side effects. Paraldehyde is nevertheless a safe drug and side effects are rare. However, dependence can occur. Paraldehyde also changes slowly to acetic acid when stored, and bottles more than six months old should be thrown away.

Nitrazepam

Pharmacological action. Nitrazepam is a fairly quick-acting hypnotic. It is believed to depress the reticular activating system rather than the cerebral cortex. It is relatively non-toxic and considerable overdosage can occur without serious effects [6].

Therapeutic use. Nitrazepam is a useful hypnotic, as effective as the short acting barbiturates. The hypnotic action of the drug usually lasts about six hours; rarely, patients complain of some drowsiness persisting into the next day. Nitrazepam is said to be less liable to cause confusion in the elderly. The oral dose is 5–10 mg at night. In old people 2·5 mg may be sufficient.

Methaqualone

Pharmacological action. Methaqualone is a hypnotic similar in effectiveness to the barbiturates. Its action may last for 6–12 hours. The usual dose is 150–300 mg and toxic side effects are rare, but sleep may sometimes be preceded by transient paraesthesia. It is contraindicated in liver disease.

A combination of methaqualone 250 mg and diphenhydramine 25 mg per tablet is an effective hypnotic. Dependence, however, is not uncommon. Larger doses produce a distinctive clinical picture with coma, combined with hypertonia, myoclonia and increased tendon reflexes [7].

Propiomazine

Pharmacological action. Propiomazine is related to the antihistamine promethazine but differs in that it has greater sedation and hypnotic properties. The usual dose is 200 mg.

Contraindication and side effects. Propriomazine is of low toxicity but dry mouth and rashes can occur.

Chlormethiazole

Pharmacological action and therapeutic use. Chlormethiazole is a sedative and hypnotic being related structurally to vitamin B1. It probably acts by producing cortical depression. It can be used as a hypnotic but has proved particularly valuable in treating withdrawal symptoms in alcoholics. It has been tried with success in pre-eclamptic toxaemia, when it produces minimal foetal depression.

As a hypnotic the dose is 2–4 tablets or capsules (500 mg of chlormethiazole). In the elderly it can be used as a sedative in doses of one capsule three times daily. In acute alcoholic withdrawal symptoms, three capsules four times daily and reduced as necessary, is usually satisfactory [8]. Chlormethiazole can also be given by intravenous infusion.

Contraindication and side effects. The most obvious side effect is an unpleasant tingling in the nose a few minutes after administration. Occasionally it can also cause nausea. Toxicity is generally low but the action is additional with other CNS depressants.

References

1. Bunn, H. F., and Lubush, G. D., *Ann. Intern. Med.* (1965), **62,** 246.
2. Ramboer, C., Thompson, R. P. H., and Williams, R., *Lancet* (1969), **i,** 966.
3. Tuckman, J., and Shillingford, J., *Brit. J. Pharm.* (1964), **26,** 206.
4. Bewlay, I. H., *Bull Narcotics XVIII* (1966), **4,** 1.
5. Isbell, H., Altschul, S., Kornetsky, C. H., Eisenmann, A. J., Flanary, H. G., and Fraser, H. F., *Archiv. Neurol. Psychiat.* (1950), **64,** 1.
6. Matthew, H., Proudfoot, A. I., Aitkin, R. C. B., Raeburn, J. A., and Wright, N., *Brit. med. J.* (1969), **2,** 23.
7. Lawson, A. A. H., and Brown, S. S., *Scot. med. J.* (1967), **12,** 63.
8. Glatt, M. M., George, H. R., Frish, B. P., *Brit. med. J.* (1965), **2,** 401.

This chapter was written by Professor J. R. Trounce.

Category 3

The Analgesics

These can be subdivided into (i) MAJOR or narcotic analgesics and (ii) MINOR or antipyretic analgesics. For certain kinds of pain other more specific measures may be indicated, e.g. carbamazepine for trigeminal neuralgia and ergot for migraine. Details will be found in the relevant section. Certain diseases may present initially with pain as the major or only symptom, e.g. hyperparathyroidism, myxoedema and depression, and prompt diagnosis and relevant treatment may give relief. The presence and nature of a pain is frequently of diagnostic help, and the administration of an analgesic should not, wherever possible, precede or overshadow history-taking, examination and diagnosis.

THE MAJOR OR NARCOTIC ANALGESICS

Opium was the earliest source of all narcotic analgesics. All the analgesic alkaloids (e.g. morphine, codeine and thebaine) were found to be phenanthrene derivatives, whereas other alkaloids (e.g. papaverine and narcotine) were inactive as analgesics (see table 1). Other semi-synthetic and synthetic substances have since been developed and used as analgesics, yet despite wide chemical differences the pharmacological actions of all the major analgesics are very similar. For this reason morphine will be taken as the central drug of this group and discussed in some detail; the actions of the other drugs being described in relation to it.

The narcotic antagonists will also be included in this section as they are closely related to the narcotic analgesics.

Morphine

Pharmacological action. A powerful analgesic and narcotic having various stimulating and depressant actions on the nervous system. Centrally it produces euphoria and depresses the cortex, thalamus, cerebellum, respiratory and cough centres. It stimulates the vagus, vomiting centre and spinal cord and also causes constriction of the pupil. Increased ADH secretion reduces the urine output and if hypercapnia develops intra-

Table 1 **The opiates**

Useful analgesics	Related drugs with other uses
Phenanthrene Derivatives	
Morphine	Apomorphine (emetic)
Diamorphine	Ethyl morphine (eye-drops)
Papaveretum	Nalorphine*
Hydromorphone	Thebaine (not used)
Oxymorphone	
Metopon	
Codeine	
Pholcodine	
Dihydrocodeine	
Hydrocodone	
Oxycodone	
Benzylisoquinoline Alkaloids	
	Papaverine (vasodilator)

*Narcotic Antagonist.

cranial pressure may be increased. Peripherally, morphine reduces secretions and increases tone in involuntary muscle. The latter effect is most marked in the muscle and sphincters of the gastro-intestinal and biliary tracts and similar effects have been described in the urinary tract. Skin vessels are dilated and there is increased sweating.

Tolerance develops within 2–3 weeks of continuous use, chiefly in relation to its depressant actions. Physical dependence may begin even earlier leading to a withdrawal syndrome on stopping the drug. If use of the drug is prolonged overt addiction may develop.

Morphine is metabolised in the liver and excreted chiefly into the urine but also into the gut via the bile. Its analgesic effect is maximal at about 1 hour and lasts for 3–4 hours.

Therapeutic uses. Morphine sulphate is the most frequently used preparation for oral or parenteral use but other salts are available:

Oral preparations:	Morphine sulphate
	Morphine hydrochloride
Parenteral preparations:	Morphine sulphate
	Morphine tartrate
	Morphine acetate

The dose for all these preparations is roughly the same and is usually 10–15 mg. Absorption from the gastrointestinal tract is often unreliable and subcutaneous or intramuscular injection is more effective. Morphine can also be given as a slow intravenous injection.

It is used to relieve pain which is not amenable to the milder analgesics and is of particular value when this is associated with anxiety and restlessness. Its use in patients suffering from haemorrhage, trauma or shock, who are not troubled by pain, is of doubtful merit in view of the well-documented tendency for morphine to lower the blood pressure. However, it is difficult to deny its good effect when given to patients with gastro-intestinal haemorrhage and other factors may play a part here. It relieves the dyspnoea of cardiac asthma and is also used to suppress unwanted coughing, to control diarrhoea and as a premedication (with hyoscine or atropine) before surgery.

The euphoriant effect is used in the management of terminal disease and where this is associated with severe pain chlorpromazine produces a useful synergistic effect as well as having a mild anti-emetic action. In cases where respiratory depression or undue somnolence becomes a problem an analeptic such as amiphenazole (q.v.) may be used with morphine to good effect.

Contraindications and side effects. Morphine should not be used in the presence of respiratory depression, cyanosis, obstructive airways disease, hepatic insufficiency, acute alcoholism, toxic confusional states, convulsive disorders or raised intracranial pressure. It is unwise to give it alone for cholecystitis, biliary disorders, pancreatitis or diverticulitis, but increased smooth muscle activity can be offset by combination with propantheline [1]. It is badly tolerated by patients with myxoedema and the elderly and debilitated. Its action is enhanced by mono-amine oxidase inhibitors, neostigmine, chlorpromazine, barbiturates and alcohol. Potentiation occurs with hypotensive agents.

Side effects include: nausea and vomiting (especially if not resting in bed), constipation, tremors, restlessness, insomnia and rarely convulsions. The nausea and vomiting can be readily prevented by the co-administration of an anti-emetic such as cyclizine tartrate (50 mg). Itching and urticaria occur as well as other rashes. Hypotension which may be postural is usually mild but is often pronounced when the drug is given to patients following myocardial infarction. Toxic doses produce respiratory depression, cyanosis, hypotension, pinpoint pupils and coma. These effects are best treated by an injection of one of the specific antagonists nalorphine or levallorphan (see below).

Diamorphine (Heroin, *USA*)

Pharmacological action. Slightly more potent than morphine. It has an earlier onset and shorter duration of action (about two hours). It more readily produces euphoria, is a powerful anti-tussive and respiratory depressant but is probably less likely to cause vomiting or constipation.

Therapeutic uses. It may be given as an elixir or linctus in a dose of 5–10 mg or by injection in a dose of 3–6 mg initially. It is not available in some countries because of the problem of addiction. It is favoured by some for the pain of acute myocardial infarction, but it has a similar effect on the blood pressure as morphine, and a recent study [2] suggests that pentazocine (see below) may be a better choice. It is most often used for terminal disease and occasionally for post-operative analgesia and sedation.

Contraindications and side effects. As morphine; it has often been thought to be more addictive than morphine but this point is still debated.

Papaveretum (total extract of opium)

Pharmacological action. Very similar to morphine which forms most of the active part of this preparation. However it is better tolerated and is said to cause less respiratory depression and vomiting.

Therapeutic use. As morphia. Dose: 10–20 mg orally or I.M.

Contraindications and side effects. As morphine.

Hydromorphone

Pharmacological action. Very similar to morphine, being slightly more potent and having a shorter duration of action.

Therapeutic use. As morphine. Dose: 2–5 mg orally; 2 mg by injection.

Contraindications and side effects. As morphine.

Oxymorphone

Pharmacological action. Slightly more potent than morphia and producing more euphoria, respiratory depression, nausea and vomiting.

Therapeutic use. Dose: 5–10 mg orally; 1·5–5 mg I.M. or S.C.

Metopon

Pharmacological action. A narcotic analgesic about twice as potent as morphine but in all other respects the same. Dose: 3–6 mg.

Codeine
Pharmacological action. Analgesic but much less potent than morphine. It is a mild hypnotic but does not depress the respiratory centre or constipate as much as morphine. It is an effective cough suppressant. Little of it is metabolised in the body, most appearing in the urine.

Therapeutic uses. It is used as the hydrochloride, phosphate or sulphate and the dose for all three salts is 10–60 mg. It is taken as a tablet, linctus or I.M. injection. It is most useful for the control of less severe pain, unwanted cough and diarrhoea. It does show a synergistic action with aspirin and is often prepared in combination with the antipyretic analgesics.

Contraindications and side effects. Less than morphine. Overdosage gives a different picture consisting of narcosis often preceded by exhilaration and excitement and followed by convulsions. Nausea and vomiting are prominent, the pupils constrict and there is a tachycardia.

Pholcodine
Pharmacological action. A derivative of morphine with almost no analgesic action. It does not suppress respiration but is an effective cough suppressant.

Dihydrocodeine
Pharmacological action. It has a shorter duration of action and is less potent than morphine. Is as good a cough suppressant as codeine.

Therapeutic use. Preparations:

Dihydrocodeine phosphate – dose 10–30 mg
Dihydrocodeine bitartrate – dose 10–60 mg

It can be given as a linctus, tablet, I.M. or S.C. injection. It has few side effects; contraindications as morphine.

Hydrocodone
Pharmacological action. Intermediate in action between morphine and codeine. It is chiefly used as a cough suppressant.

Therapeutic use. It is used as the phosphate, hydrochloride or acid tartrate. The dose for each is 5–15 mg orally but it can also be given as a S.C. injection.

Oxycodone

Pharmacological action. A moderately strong analgesic, slightly more potent and possibly more addicting than codeine.

Therapeutic use. Preparations:

Oxycodone Hydrochloride – dose 5–30 mg orally; 5 mg by injection
Oxycodone Pectinate – dose I.M. 10–20 mg

The latter acts for much longer (up to 10 hours).

Contraindications and side effects. As morphine.

Nalorphine

Pharmacological action. It is a specific narcotic analgesic antagonist reducing or abolishing most of the actions of morphine and all the major analgesics. It does not antagonise the depressant effect on the cough centre and hence there is little evidence of antagonism with pholcodine and other anti-tussives which have little analgesic effect. It acts within a few seconds of intravenous injection, increasing the rate and volume of respiration and can awaken a patient from a narcotic state. It reverses the rise in biliary pressure and miosis but has similar analgesic properties to morphine. It is not effective in reversing depression produced by barbiturates, cyclopropane or ether.

Therapeutic uses. Dose: 5–10 mg I.V. as either the hydrochloride or hydrobromide. It is used particularly to treat overdosage with narcotic analgesics and in severe cases much larger doses may be required [3]. It has also been used in a test for narcotic analgesic addiction in which the reversing effect on pupil size is noted. If given to an addict it will precipitate withdrawal symptoms.

It is also used to prevent respiratory depression in the newborn. It can be given I.V. 10 mg to the mother 10 minutes before delivery or injected directly into the umbilical vein immediately after birth (0·25–1 mg).

Table 2 **Phenylheptylamine derivatives**

Useful analgesics	Related drugs with other uses
Methadone	
Phenadoxone	
Propoxyphene (d-propoxyphene)	l-Propoxyphene (anti-tussive)
Dextromoramide	
Dipipanone	

Contraindications and side effects. If given on its own it may cause respiratory depression and disturbing psychotic effects. In addicts to morphine and its derivatives it will produce withdrawal symptoms. Side effects include drowsiness, irritability, miosis, nausea, pallor, sweating and hypotension.

Methadone

Pharmacological action. A potent analgesic similar to morphine but with less sedative effect and a longer duration of action. It is more reliably absorbed from the gastro-intestinal tract.

Therapeutic use. Dose: orally 5–10 mg; I.M. 5–10 mg; linctus 1–2 mg doses. It is not used intravenously. It is useful for severe pain and unproductive cough. It is not suitable as a premedication unless combined with a short-acting barbiturate or hyoscine. It has been used in the rehabilitation of morphine and heroin addicts as withdrawal from it is less unpleasant, probably because of its longer duration of action.

Contraindications and side effects. As with morphine nausea, vomiting, dizziness, respiratory depression and constriction of the pupils occur, although it less readily produces constipation. It may lower the blood pressure and children tolerate it poorly. It is not recommended for use in obstetrics as it significantly depresses foetal respiration.

Phenadoxone

Pharmacological action. An effective analgesic with a mild hypnotic effect. It reduces smooth muscle activity and does not cause constipation in normal doses. Orally it acts within 15–30 minutes and lasts for 1–3 hours. When used parenterally there may be considerable irritation at injection sites. It is not used intravenously.

Therapeutic use. Dose: orally 10–30 mg; I.M. or S.C. 5–15 mg.

Contraindications and side effects. As for methadone.

Propoxyphene

Pharmacological action. It is chemically similar to methadone but is only a mild analgesic having a similar onset, duration of action and potency to codeine. It is not anti-tussive.

Therapeutic use. Dose: 30–60 mg orally. It is used for mild to moderate pain associated with chronic and recurrent disease. It is often combined with aspirin or paracetamol for this purpose.

Contraindications and side effects. Nausea and vomiting occur less than with codeine although it does constipate as much. In large doses it causes drowsiness, dizziness, general excitement, mental confusion, twitching, respiratory depression, convulsions and coma. Local irritation occurs if given subcutaneously. It is only mildly addictive but can block the withdrawal effects of morphine and is antagonised by nalorphine.

Dextromoramide

Pharmacological action. A strong analgesic, slightly more powerful than morphine and with a similar duration of action. It is well absorbed by mouth.

Therapeutic use. Preparations: alone or as the acid tartrate (5 mg dextromoramide ≡ 6·9 mg D. acid tartrate). Dose: 5–20 mg orally or I.M. It may also be given by S.C. or I.V. injection or administered rectally.

Contraindications and side effects. As for morphine but respiratory depression is not evident with oral therapeutic doses.

Dipipanone

Pharmacological action. A potent analgesic of similar strength to morphine with a more rapid onset but a similar duration of action. There is less respiratory depression and it is effective orally.

Therapeutic use. Dose: 25–50 mg S.C. or I.M. Oral tablets of 10 mg are usually combined with cyclizine 30 mg.

Table 3 Phenylpiperidine derivatives

Useful analgesics	Related drugs with other uses
Pethidine or Meperidine	Diphenoxylate (costive)
Alphaprodine	
Anileridine	
Piminidone	
Fentanyl	
Phenoperidine	
Ethoheptazine	

Pethidine (Meperidine, *USA*)

Pharmacological action. An effective analgesic but less potent and with about half the duration of action of morphine. It is only a mild sedative, euphoria is less marked and dysphoric sensations are more likely to occur. It does not affect the size of the pupil in therapeutic doses and is a poor cough suppressant. It does not cause constipation but its effect on smooth muscle is similar to morphine. It reduces the severity of labour pains without diminishing the force of uterine contraction but like most other major analgesics it prolongs labour.

Therapeutic uses. Dose: orally 50–100 mg; S.C. or I.M. 25–100 mg and I.V. 25–50 mg. It is used as an alternative to morphine to relieve pain; for obstetric analgesia and in conjunction with barbiturates or hyoscine to produce obstetric amnesia. It is also used commonly for pre- and post-operative medication. Pethidine (50 mg) has been combined with levallorphan tartrate (0·625 mg) as an injection. This was primarily designed for use in obstetrics but is only of marginal benefit. In view of its effect on smooth muscle it should be given with propantheline for the treatment of visceral colic [1].

Contraindications and side effects. Nausea and vomiting are as frequent as with comparable doses of morphine but constipation is less. The blood pressure may fall after I.V. administration and this is especially noticeable in patients with acute myocardial infarction [4]. Pethidine can cause excitement and dysphoria especially with overdosage when inco-ordination, tremor, convulsions, respiratory depression and coma may supervene. Its action is potentiated by mono-amine oxidase inhibitors and phenothiazines. There is a danger of addiction.

Alphaprodine

Pharmacological action. It has a similar potency and action to pethidine but is more rapid in onset and of shorter duration. Given subcutaneously and with an adequate peripheral circulation it will have an analgesic effect within 5 minutes lasting for about 2 hours.

Therapeutic uses. Dose: S.C. 20–60 mg and I.V. 20–30 mg. It is used chiefly in obstetrics and for premedication and minor surgical procedures.

Contraindications and side effects. Dizziness, itching and sweating occur but nausea, vomiting and respiratory depression are less likely than with morphine. However, it will cause depression of foetal respiration if given within 2 hours of delivery.

Anileridine
Pharmacological action. Similar but less potent than morphine. It is rapidly absorbed by mouth and acts more quickly and for a shorter time than morphine.

Therapeutic uses. Preparations: orally anileridine hydrochloride dose 25 mg; S.C. or I.V. anileridine phosphate dose 25–50 mg. It is used as a shorter acting analgesic especially as a premedication and in obstetrics.

Contraindications and side effects. Similar to morphine but it tends to cause more restlessness and less nausea, vomiting and constipation.

Fentanyl
Pharmacological action. A very potent analgesic with a rapid onset and brief duration of action. It causes respiratory depression and has an emetic effect.

Therapeutic uses. Dose: 0·1–0·6 mg I.V. It has been primarily used in association with tranquillizers such as triperidol and droperidol to produce brief surgical anaesthesia especially in young, old and debilitated patients. They block the emetic effect and the general effects are antagonised by nalorphine.

Contraindications and side effects. As morphine.

Phenoperidine
Pharmacological action. A potent analgesic which in large doses produces sedation and respiratory suppression.

Therapeutic uses. I.M. or I.V. 0·5–1 mg for analgesia; 2–5 mg where respiratory depression is desired. It is used in similar situations to fentanyl in combination with a 'neuroleptic' agent, e.g. droperidol (q.v.) to produce surgical anaesthesia. It is of particular value for sedation during artificial ventilation.

Contraindications and side effects. As morphine.

Ethoheptazine
Pharmacological action. An analgesic of equivalent strength to codeine. It is not anti-tussive or a respiratory suppressant and does not sedate. It acts within 30 minutes and lasts for 4–5 hours.

Therapeutic uses. Dose: 75–150 mg orally. It is used chiefly in conjunction with aspirin or paracetamol.

Contraindications and side effects. Similar to morphine but appears not to be addictive.

Table 4 Morphinans and Benzmorphans

Useful analgesics	Related drugs with other uses
Morphinans	
Levorphanol (l-methorphan)	d-Methorphan (anti-tussive)
	Levallorphan*
Benzmorphans	
Phenazocine	
Pentazocine	

*Narcotic Antagonist.

Levorphanol

Pharmacological action. A potent analgesic similar to morphine but causing less drowsiness. It is as effective by mouth as it is by injection.

Therapeutic uses. Dose: orally 1·5–4·5 mg; I.M. or S.C. 2–4 mg and I.V. 1–1·5 mg. It is used as an alternative to morphine and can be used for premedication (2 mg S.C.) with atropine or hyoscine.

Contraindications and side effects. As morphine.

Levallorphan

Pharmacological action. A narcotic antagonist having similar effects to nalorphine but with a greater potency and longer duration of action. Small doses antagonise the respiratory depression of narcotic drugs – larger doses also antagonising the analgesic effect.

Therapeutic uses. Dose: 1–2 mg I.V. with further doses as necessary. It is often used to reverse respiratory depression in the newborn when it is given to the mother (1–2 mg) 10 minutes before delivery or directly into the umbilical vein (0·05–0·25 mg) of the infant.

Contraindications and side effects. As for nalorphine.

Phenazocine

Pharmacological action. An analgesic of similar potency and actions to morphine. It is less sedative but may cause more respiratory depression.

Therapeutic uses. Dose: orally 5 mg; I.M. or I.V. 1–4 mg. It may be superior for obstetric use but otherwise has been used as an alternative to morphine.

Contraindications and side effects. Similar to morphine but usually less marked. Facial pruritus may follow I.V. injection.

Pentazocine

Pharmacological action. This drug was developed as an antagonist to phenazocine and was found to be a powerful analgesic itself of a similar potency to morphine. It is also sedative and does depress respiration when given parenterally. However, it appears to be much less addictive and does not lower the blood pressure unlike most of the other strong analgesics.

Therapeutic use. Dose: orally 25–100 mg; S.C. or I.M. 30–60 mg and I.V. 20–30 mg. It can be used as an alternative to morphine and in a comparison with morphine, diamorphine methadone and pethidine [2] it was the only drug which did not tend to lower the blood pressure; other side effects being much the same for all these drugs. However, a significant rise in pulmonary artery as well as aortic pressure has been recorded after the administration of 30–60 mg I.V. [6] and a similar effect is seen with intramuscular doses. In view of this pentazocine would seem not to be the drug of choice for acute myocardial infarction despite its other advantages. There is no reason to suppose that these effects can cause harm in patients with a normal cardiovascular system.

Pentazocine has been shown to be equivalent to pethidine for the management of labour [5].

Table 5 Equivalent doses of the major analgesics* (in mg)

Morphine	10	Dextromoramide	5–7·5
Diamorphine	5	Dipipanone	20–25
Hydromorphone	2	Pethidine/Meperidine	75
Oxymorphone	1	Alphaprodine	40–60
Metopon	3·5	Anileridine	30–40
Codeine	120	Piminidone	7·5–10
Dihydrocodeine	60	Phenoperidine	1·5
Oxycodone	10–15	Levorphanol	3
Methadone	10	Phenazocine	2–3
Phenadoxone	10–20	Pentazocine	30

*These doses represent that dose which when given subcutaneously produces an analgesic effect approximately equivalent to 10 mg. subcutaneous morphine.

Contraindications and side effects. Similar to morphine apart from its low addiction potential. There have been several reports of transient but disturbing hallucinations. It is not antagonised by nalorphine and it is recommended that methyl phenidate (see below) be given as an antidote instead.

THE MINOR ANALGESICS AND ANTI-INFLAMMATORY AGENTS

Nearly all share analgesic, anti-pyretic and anti-rheumatic (anti-inflammatory) properties. These drugs are free of addiction potential, although patients can become habituated to their use. Their exact site of action is still not entirely clear. Vasodilatation, whether produced centrally or peripherally, causes much of the antipyretic activity. The analgesia may originate centrally or may be due to a direct effect on pain receptors. A direct antagonism of various chemical mediators of inflammation may explain most of the anti-inflammatory effect.

THE SALICYLATES

Acetylsalicylic acid (**aspirin**)
Pharmacological action. An effective minor analgesic with considerable antipyretic and anti-inflammatory properties. In large doses it is uricosuric. In smaller doses it causes uric acid retention. It also has a mild hypoglycaemic and hypoprothrombinaemic action. It is rapidly metabolised to salicyclic acid which is probably responsible for most of its effects. Both acids are excreted rapidly in the urine and the more so if this is kept alkaline. Its effect lasts for about 4 hours.
Therapeutic uses. Doses: 300–1,200 mg orally. It is the most effective and useful of the minor analgesics and is used for all kinds of less severe pain, e.g. headache, neuralgia, rheumatic and muscle pains. It is of particular use for acute and chronic rheumatism. In these conditions doses of up to 4–8 g. a day are used, although in the chronic situation much less will often suffice. It has been used for gout but is inferior to the other uricosuric agents.
Contraindications and side effects. Gastric irritation is the commonest problem and may be accompanied by occult blood loss. Occasionally frank haematemesis and melaena occur. With larger doses, dizziness, tinnitus, deafness, sweating, nausea and vomiting may develop. In

sensitive patients salicylates may precipitate attacks of asthma, angioneurotic oedema and other allergy. Therapeutic doses produce minor platelet abnormalities and long-term use has caused pancytopenia [7]. Toxic doses cause hyperthermia, hyperventilation, excitement, coma and convulsions. Complex and changing acid-base disturbances also accompany overdosage. Salicylates should not be given to patients having a history of dyspepsia or peptic ulceration, known sensitivity, asthma or severe renal disease.

Other preparations have been made to try and overcome the irritant effect on the stomach, e.g. aluminium acetylsalicylate and calcium acetylsalicylate. The latter is more soluble, better absorbed and less irritant than acetylsalicylic acid. It is the usual form of 'Soluble Aspirin', containing acetylsalicylic acid, calcium carbonate and citric acid, which on dissolving gives a solution of calcium acetylsalicylate. Aloxiprin is a polymeric condensation product of aluminium hydroxide and acetylsalicylic acid and is also better tolerated.

Various forms of buffered aspirin have been developed but they have little advantage over calcium aspirin. Enteric-coated preparations also cause less gastric irritation but absorption takes much longer and they are more suited to long term regular use.

Aspirin is often combined with other minor analgesics and Aspirin Compound or A.P.C. is one of the most used preparations. It contains approximately 230 mg aspirin with 150 mg phenacetin and 30 mg caffeine. Sometimes codeine is added or used as an alternative.

Sodium salicylate

Pharmacological action. Similar to aspirin but less analgesic and a more effective antipyretic. It is more irritant to the stomach.

Therapeutic uses. Dose: 600–2000 mg. It has been used for acute rheumatic fever in doses of 5–10 g. daily, but aspirin is more suitable for rheumatoid arthritis in view of its greater analgesic activity.

Contraindications and side effects. As aspirin.

PARA-AMINOPHENOL DERIVATIVES

Paracetamol (Acetaminophen, *USA*)

Pharmacological action. An effective analgesic and antipyretic of similar potency to aspirin. It has less anti-inflammatory activity, less side effects and does not cause gastric irritation. It is not uricosuric.

Therapeutic uses. Dose: 500–1000 mg as tablets or elixir. It is used widely for all kinds of mild pain and is the drug of choice when aspirin is contraindicated. It is contained in many combined analgesic preparations.

Contraindications and side effects. These are few and rarely troublesome It is still not certain whether paracetamol can cause the same kind of renal damage as phenacetin when taken in high dosage over long periods. Liver damage may occur with overdosage.

Phenacetin (acetophenetidin)

Pharmacological action. Similar to paracetamol. Most of its action is due to the formation of paracetamol in vivo.

Therapeutic use. Dose: 300–600 mg. It is a common constituent of analgesic combinations.

Contraindications and side effects. Its toxic effects are similar to acetanilide (see below) and are due to small amounts of aniline being formed. This may cause methaemoglobinaemia and a haemolytic anaemia. If large amounts of phenacetin are taken over a long period serious renal damage in the form of papillary necrosis and chronic interstitial nephritis may ensue. It seems that upwards of a kilogramme of phenacetin has to be ingested before this occurs but the changes may be reversible [8]. More recently the development of transitional-cell tumours of the renal pelvis has been implicated [9].

Acetanilide

Pharmacological action. As with the case of phenacetin its action is very largely due to the formation of paracetamol by the liver.

Therapeutic uses. Dose: 120–300 mg. It used to be included in most headache powders but has latterly been replaced because of its toxicity.

Contraindications and side effects. Toxicity is chiefly due to the liberation of aniline which causes methaemoglobinaemia. Large doses produce cyanosis, cardiovascular depression and collapse.

PYRAZOLONE DERIVATIVES

Phenazone (Antipyrine, ***USA*****)**

Pharmacological action. An effective minor analgesic having a more, rapid and transient action than phenacetin, although like the other drugs in this group it is more potent than the salicylates. It is anti-pyretic and anti-inflammatory and in large doses uricosuric. Like the other uricosuric agents it may cause uric acid retention in low dosage.

Therapeutic uses. Dose: 300–600 mg. It is used as an alternative to aspirin and forms part of many combined remedies.

Contraindications and side effects. Rashes are common and some types of erythematous eruption leave residual pigmentation. Methaemoglobinaemia and cyanosis is a rare complication. Toxic doses produce nausea, fainting and collapse. Prolonged administration has led to agranulocytosis. It is nevertheless one of the least toxic drugs of this group.

Aminopyrine (Amidopyrine, *USA*)

Pharmacological action and side effects. In action it resembles phenazone but this drug has been withdrawn from general use because of the high incidence of agranulocytosis.

Phenylbutazone

Pharmacological action. It is analgesic, antipyretic, anti-inflammatory and uricosuric. It is hydroxylated in vivo to form oxyphenbutazone.

Therapeutic uses. Dose: orally 200–400 mg daily in divided doses, taken with food or milk. It can also be given I.M. in a dose of 600 mg (prepared with xylocaine) and rectally as 250 mg suppositories. It is used particularly for arthritic pain in association with rheumatoid arthritis, osteo-arthritis, ankylosing spondylitis, psoriasis and gout.

Contraindications and side effects. Untoward reactions are common. They include nausea, stomatitis, epigastric pain, diarrhoea, vertigo and oedema. The latter is due to sodium retention and may be offset by a low salt diet or a diuretic. Reactivation of peptic ulcers with perforation, haematemesis and melaena may occur. Less often agranulocytosis, thrombocytopenia, aplastic anaemia and a macrocytic anaemia responding to folic acid have occurred and a possible link with leukaemia is still uncertain. Hepatitis, acute renal failure and skin rashes have also been described.

Severe hypoprothrombinaemia occurs in people who are also being treated with coumarin anticoagulants and this may give rise to serious complications [10]. This effect is due to competitive binding of these drugs to plasma albumin.

Phenylbutazone should not be given to patients with known cardiac, liver or renal disease, or to those with a history of peptic ulceration, blood dyscrasia or allergy. It should not be used with gold salts.

Oxyphenbutazone

Pharmacological action and uses. A derivative of phenylbutazone with similar effects and uses. It is less effective in relieving stiffness or pain in rheumatoid arthritis or ankylosing spondylitis, but it is better tolerated. Dose: 300–600 mg daily in divided doses, taken with meals.

Contraindications and side effects. Similar to phenylbutazone but less severe.

Sulphinpyrazone (see page 274)

Pharmacological action and uses. A marked uricosuric agent with little direct analgesic or anti-inflammatory effect. It has been used for chronic gout in an initial dose of 50 mg q.d.s. with meals. This is increased to 500 mg daily over a period of a week and reduced to about 200 mg daily when controlled.

Contraindications and side effects. Gastro-intestinal symptoms occur but are less severe than with phenylbutazone and blood dyscrasias are rare. It should not be used in the presence of impaired renal function or peptic ulceration. Salicylates reduce its effect.

Nifenazone

Pharmacological action and uses. A pyrazolone chemically resembling amidopyrine, having analgesic, antipyretic and anti-inflammatory effects. It is inferior to phenylbutazone or oxyphenbutazone. Dose: orally 250–500 mg 1, 2 or 3 times daily. 400 mg suppositories are available for rectal use.

Contraindications and side effects. Gastro-intestinal symptoms may occur and in view of its chemical relationships blood dyscrasias are a possibility.

Phenyramidol

Pharmacological action, uses and side effects. A moderate analgesic which like phenylbutazone can cause serious hypoprothrombinaemia in patients on anticoagulant therapy. Dose: 200–400 mg. It may also cause nausea, dyspepsia, drowsiness, pruritis and skin rashes. It is contraindicated in patients having salicylate sensitivity.

QUINOLINE DERIVATIVES

Cinchophen and Neocinchophen

Pharmacological action and uses. Both these extracts from quinine or cinchona bark are analgesic and antipyretic and of similar potency to the salicylates. Neocincophen is more uricosuric and they were both used for chronic gout although more effective agents are now available. Dose: 200–500 mg.

Contraindications and side effects. Similar to the salicylates. In addition even therapeutic doses can cause hepatitis.

COLCHICINE DERIVATIVES

Colchicine

Pharmacological action. An alkaloid from meadow saffron which is analgesic for acute gout. It is also anti-mitotic but has little effect in leukaemia, although demecolcine (see below) has been used for leukaemia.

Therapeutic uses. Doses for acute gout: 1 mg stat. followed by 0·5 mg 2-hourly until pain ceases or vomiting or diarrhoea develops.

Contraindications and side effects. Stomatitis, nausea, vomiting, abdominal pain, and diarrhoea. It should be avoided in the old and feeble and in those with gastrointestinal disorders.

AN INDOLE DERIVATIVE

Indomethacin

Pharmacological action. This indole derivative is an effective analgesic, antipyretic and anti-inflammatory agent of value in acute gout and various forms of arthritis [11]. It is not recommended as a general analgesic.

Therapeutic uses. Dose: orally starting with 25 mg daily and increasing to 25 mg three times daily. It can also be used as 100 mg suppositories. Its chief route of elimination is via the kidneys and the dose will therefore require modification in the presence of renal insufficiency. For acute gout 50 mg is recommended orally followed by 25 mg 6-hourly.

Side effects. These are frequent but usually less serious than those found with phenylbutazone. They include dizziness, headache, vertigo, drowsiness, confusion, psychiatric disturbances, anorexia, nausea, vomiting, dyspepsia, diarrhoea, gastro-intestinal bleeding and corneal and retinal changes which are usually reversible. Pruritus, rashes and oedema also occur and a reversible leucopenia has been described in patients with rheumatoid arthritis. Deaths have occurred in children treated with indomethacin and it is now only recommended for adult use.

THE FENAMATES

Mefenamic acid

Pharmacological action. A derivative of anthranilic acid which is analgesic, antipyretic and anti-inflammatory. Its analgesic effect is greater than aspirin or paracetamol and roughly equivalent to codeine. Its anti-inflammatory activity is less powerful than phenylbutazone. Its effect comes on 1 hour after an oral dose and lasts for up to 6 hours.

Therapeutic uses. Dose: 250–500 mg q.d.s. It is used as a general analgesic as well as supplementing other measures used for arthritic pain.

Contraindications and side effects. Diarrhoea is the most common side effect but is usually reversible. It occurs in 10–20 per cent of cases. Reversible leucopenia, haemolytic anaemia and maculopapular rashes have been described. Gastric irritation occurs but is much less frequent or troublesome than with aspirin. Elevation of the blood urea may occur and renal papillary necrosis has been described in animal studies.

Flufenamic acid

Pharmacological action. Similar to mefenamic acid but less analgesic and antipyretic and more anti-inflammatory. For further information see [12].

Therapeutic use. Dose: 100–200 mg t.d.s. It is most useful for arthritic pain.

Contraindications and side effects. It also tends to cause diarrhoea in some patients and occasionally produces dyspeptic symptoms.

PHENYLALKANOIC ACID DERIVATIVES

Ibuprofen

Pharmacological action. This is the propionic acid derivative of an earlier substance. Ibufenac (p-isobutylphenylacetic acid) which was withdrawn because of the development of jaundice as a side effect. These substances have analgesic, antipyretic and anti-inflammatory activity. Its potency is comparable to aspirin. Ibuprofen unlike ibufenac is not concentrated in the liver and does not cause jaundice.

Therapeutic uses. Dose: 200 mg t.d.s. A further tablet can be taken at night. It is recommended for arthritic pain and particularly for those intolerant to salicylates.

Contraindications and side effects. These seem to be few and although it may occasionally cause dyspepsia it does not seem to aggravate peptic ulcers.

GOLD

Sodium aurothiomalate, aurothioglucose and aurothioglycanide.

Pharmacological action and uses. These three preparations will be considered collectively. Their action is uncertain but they have a long-lasting effect on rheumatoid arthritis, especially in the early stages. Gold is ineffective in other kinds of arthritis.

Dose: after a test dose of 10 mg I.M., weekly injections increasing by an increment of 10 mg up to 50 mg are given, usually up to a total dose of 1 g. although injections may be continued indefinitely, preferably at a reduced dose. The dosage required with aurothioglycanide may be a little higher.

Contraindications and side effects. Toxic effects occur in at least 30 per cent of cases and include pruritus, urticaria, purpura, dermatitis which may exfoliate, stomatitis which may ulcerate and less commonly thrombocytopenia, aplastic anaemia, hepatic and renal damage, peripheral neuropathy and an encephalopathy may develop. The urine should be examined for protein before each injection and blood counts made every 2–3 weeks. Gold therapy should be stopped as soon as any toxic affect appears. Serious toxic effects should be treated with dimercaprol (q.v.). Corticosteroids may be useful, especially for a severe dermatitis.

Gold should not be used in the presence of known renal or hepatic damage, anaemia, blood dyscrasias, skin diseases or any serious illness.

ANTIMALARIALS

Chloroquine phosphate and Hydroxychloroquine sulphate

Pharmacological action. Their mode of action is unknown. They have a beneficial effect in up to 50 per cent of cases of rheumatoid arthritis.

Therapeutic use. Doses: chloroquine phosphate – orally 250–750 mg daily initially, and 150 mg daily for maintenance.

Hydroxychloroquine sulphate – orally 800–1,200 mg daily initially and 200 mg daily for maintenance.

Contraindications and side effects. Toxic effects include nausea, vomiting, dizziness, diarrhoea and blurring of vision. After continued use bleached hair, rashes, corneal opacities and retinal degeneration may develop. The latter may be irreversible.

During treatment a six-monthly ophthalmic examination is mandatory in order to detect presymptomatic corneal or retinal damage. Eighth nerve damage also occurs. These drugs should not be given during pregnancy.

CORTICOSTEROIDS

Some of these agents have a powerful anti-inflammatory effect which is discussed later.

References

1. Boulter, P. S., *Brit. J. Surg.* (1961), **49,** 17.
2. Scott, M. E., and Orr, R., *Lancet* (1969), **i,** 1065.
3. Wright, N., and Syme, C. W., *Brit. Med. J.* (1969), **3,** 596.
4. Rees, H. A., Muir, A. L., Macdonald, H. R., Lawrie, D. M., Burton, J. L., and Donald, K. W., *ibid.* (1967), **ii,** 863.
5. Mowat, J., and Garrey, *Brit. Med. J.* (1970), **2,** 757.
6. Jewitt, D. E., Maurer, B. J., and Hubner, P. J. B., *Brit. Med. J.* (1970), **1,** 795.
7. Wijnja, L., Snijder, J. A. M., and Nieweg, H. O., *Lancet* (1966), **ii,** 768.
8. Bell, D., Kerr, D. N.S., Swinney, J., and Yeates, W. K., *Brit. Med. J.* (1969), **3,** 378.
9. Editorial, *Lancet* (1969), **ii,** 1233.
10. Aggeler, P. M., O'Reilly, R. A., Leong, L., and Kowitz, P. E., *New Eng. J. Med.* (1967), **276,** 9.
11. Hart, F. D., and Boardman, P. L., *Brit. Med. J.* (1965), **ii,** 1281.
12. P. Hume-Kendall (Editor), *Fenamates in Medicine.* Suppl. to *Annals of Physical Medicine* (1967).

This chapter was written by Dr W. G. Reeves (Dept of Clinical Pharmacology, Guys Hospital Medical School) and edited by Professor J. R. Trounce.

Category 4

Psychotropic Drugs

ANTIDEPRESSANTS

These drugs fall into three groups, namely the tricyclic compounds, monoamine oxidase* inhibitors and amino acids. The former are discussed first.

Imipramine

Pharmacological action [1–2–3–4]. After absorption imipramine enters rapidly into the tissues from the blood stream. The highest concentration is in the brain and kidney, lowest in the liver except in overdosage. Its action is by inhibiting the uptake of noradrenaline and probably 5 hydroxy-tryptamine from synaptic clefts between cells of the CNS thus increasing the amount of monoamine available at the peripheral receptor. It has been recently suggested that tricyclic compounds exert a dual action on peripheral adrenergic receptors. There is potentiation of effects at lower levels of the drug, but disappearance or reversal at higher levels, due to blockade at the receptor, as is seen with phenothiazines. Small quantities of the drug are excreted unchanged by the kidneys, whilst the major portion is metabolised within the body by demethylation, hydroxylation and N-oxydation. Imipramine has anti-cholinergic and anti-histamine effects with weaker anti-emetic and hypothermic actions.

Therapeutic use [5–6]. Imipramine is used in endogenous and involutional depression with a consequent reduction in the number of electroconvulsive therapies required in severe forms. It is also used in the treatment of reactive depression and depression associated with schizophrenia and treatment of nocturnal enuresis. Oral starting dose for depression is 75 mg daily in divided doses, increasing gradually to 150–200 mg a day. There is minimal therapeutic effect for 14 days and it is not complete until six weeks; treatment is continued for four to six months when the drug should be gradually withdrawn. The dual action mentioned above, however, may account for failure to respond

* Henceforth abbreviations M.A.O. will be used.

to treatment or worsening of depressive symptoms. Consideration should be given in these circumstances to reduction of the dose rather than cessation of medication in an already established regime. It may be given intramuscularly – 100 mg daily.

Contraindications and side effects. Use with caution in elderly people.

Imipramine is contraindicated in glaucoma and urinary retention. Side effects include dryness of the mouth, tachycardia, postural hypotension, constipation, difficulties in micturition, insomnia, drowsiness and tremor. Some patients complain of increased sweating and there may be extrapyramidal symptoms with very large dosage and epilepsy in susceptible patients. Mild skin sensitivity to light, mild cholestatic jaundice and a few cases of agranulocytosis have been reported.

Disipramine [7]

Trimipramine [8]

Clomipramine [9]

These drugs resemble imipramine in most respects and should be given in dosage. Desipramine, a demethylated form, acts more rapidly with similar unwanted reactions but is less effective. Trimipramine is as effective as imipramine; it produces greater drowsiness but is less hypotensive. Clomipramine, with added chloride, has pharmacological action between imipramine and amitriptyline. Action is rapid and effective orally, with reduced side effects. It may be given in place of ECT by daily intravenous infusion, initially 25 mg in 250–500 ml isotonic dextrose over 3–4 hours, increasing the dose by 25 mg steps to an optimum level with a maximum of 125 mg. The optimum level should be maintained until there is improvement and then the dose reduced in steps. The average number of infusions is 10 but up to 20 may be required.

Oprimal

Dibenzapine

These two tricyclic drugs also have a range of pharmacological activity similar to imipramine. Opripramol, an iminostilbene derivative with a perperazine side chain, is more a sedative but less efficacious than imipramine. It should be given in doses of 150–300 mg daily. Dibenzapine acts more rapidly than imipramine and is less likely to produce giddiness but is probably less effective. The oral daily dose ranges from 240–480 mg.

Amitriptyline [10]

Pharmacological action. A dibenzocycloheptene derivative similar to imipramine but with greater antihistaminic, anticholinergic and sedative effects.

Therapeutic use. Amitriptyline is useful in all forms of depression either alone or as an adjunct to ECT and particularly in agitated, elderly patients. The oral daily starting dose is 75–125 mg, part e.g. 50 mg may be given at night to assist sleep and reduce autonomic side effects during the day. The onset of action is in seven to ten days – its sedative action much sooner. A sustained release-form given at night, a 50 mg capsule being equivalent to three 25-mg tablets, has the advantage of side effects occurring during sleep, whilst therapeutic effects continue throughout the 24 hours. Also intramuscularly 10–30 mg t.d.s.

Amitriptyline in tablets or syrup may be given to children in the treatment of nocturnal enuresis, usual starting dose being 25 mg at night.

Contraindications and side effects. As for imipramine but with greater autonomic manifestations. Drowsiness may be marked initially.

Dothiepin

A thio analogue of amitriptyline with similar antidepressant and sedative effects but reduced anticholinergic properties. Well tolerated by the elderly and producing better response in early depressive states than amitriptyline. Usual daily dose 75–200 mg.

Nortripytline

Similar to amitriptyline but is more potent. Daily dosage of 30–100 mg, greater part of dose may be given at night to take advantage of sedative effects.

Protriptyline

This drug has stimulant properties and should be given with caution, average daily dose 15–60 mg. It may be given as a single dose in the morning followed by amitriptyline for the remainder of the day and at night.

Iprindole [11]

Pharmacological action. Similar to imipramine but minimal autonomic effects and less sedative than amitriptyline; excretion in faeces and urine.

Therapeutic action. All forms of depression, action is rapid and side effects are few. Oral dose: 30–60 mg t.d.s.

Contraindications and side effects. Care with MAO inhibitors.

Doxepin

Pharmacological action: A tricyclic compound with oxygen included in the central ring structure producing activities analogous to those of amitriptyline with added spasmolytic and muscle relaxant properties.

Therapeutic use: As good an antidepressant as amitriptyline and as effective in the treatment of anxiety as the benzodiazepines. Mixed states of anxiety and depression, unless of minor degree, should however be treated with separate drugs as this allows a greater degree of flexibility. Daily dosage ranges from 30–300 mg, a higher proportion being given at night, as with amitriptyline, to assist sleep and reduce autonomic effects during the day.

Contraindications and side effects. As for amitriptyline but with slightly reduced unwanted effects. Its use in children has not yet been established.

Overdosage of tricyclic compounds. Caution is required in the use of these drugs in the elderly due to hypotensive side effects. Coma, respiratory depression, choreiform movements, convulsions, anomalies of cardiac conduction and hyperpyrexia may occur with toxic levels. Tricyclic compounds must be stored securely as overdosage is difficult to treat, especially in children. These drugs are slow to be excreted, resistant to dialysis and the cardiac irregularities produced by them are hard to control. Suicide is possible with as little as 2 g. of imipramine in an adult.

MONOAMINE OXIDASE INHIBITORS
HYDRAZINE DERIVATIVES

Iproniazid

Pharmacological action [12] Absorbed from the gastrointestinal tract into the bloodstream and distributed to the tissues before reaching a high level in the brain, where it inhibits the oxidation of monoamines. This action takes place in all areas of the brain with the probable exception of the corpus striatum. Within the cell action takes place at the level of the catecholamine storage vesicles.

Therapeutic use. Mainly in reactive depression and phobic anxiety states with a depressive element. A further use is in the treatment of ejaculatio praecox. Oral dosage of 50–150 mg a day, the greater part of the drug given in the morning and the rest at noon to prevent interference with sleep. Clinical response usually takes place within 5 days, but may take up to 3 weeks.

Contraindications and side effects (see below). The most serious side effect of this drug is hepatocellular jaundice, which has an appreciable mortality and is the reason for it being withdrawn in the USA.

Isocarboxazide

Pharmacological action. Similar to iproniazid, metabolism is chiefly by hydrolysis to benzylhydrazine and a carboxylic compound; large quantities of hippuric acid reaching the urine.

Therapeutic use [13, 14]. The indications are similar to iproniazid but this drug, although more potent, is less effective clinically. Oral dose: 10–30 mg a day given early as above. It has a latent clinical response similar to iproniazid.

Contraindications and side effects (see below). Much reduced hepatotoxic effect as compared with iproniazid.

Nialamide

Pharmacological action. Similar to isocarboxazidazide but at least half the drug is excreted unchanged in the urine within 24 hours.

Therapeutic use. Similar indications to isocarboxazide but less efficacious. Oral dose: 75–150 mg a day given early as above with similar latent clinical response.

Contraindications and side effects (see below). Side effects are generally reduced with this drug but it is more hepatotoxic than isocarboxazide and should be given with care to agitated patients.

Phenelzine

Pharmacological action. Similar to iproniazid but with more activity in the brain and less in the liver.

Therapeutic use. Its marked sedative effect makes it particularly useful in reactive depression and phobic states with prominent anxiety. Oral dose: 45–90 mg a day given early and with similar latent clinical response as above.

Contraindications and side effects (see below). Reduced in comparison with other MAO inhibitors.

Mebanazine

Pharmacological action. Similar to phenelzine.

Therapeutic use. Similar to phenelzine. Oral dose 5–20 mg a day given early and with latent clinical response as above.

Contraindications and side effects (see below). Unsuitable with past history of liver disease or with impairment of hepatic or renal function.

Contraindications and side effects of MAO inhibitors

MAO inhibitors potentiate the action of the following drugs: sympathomimetic agents such as adrenaline, ephedrine and amphetamine derivatives; morphine, pethedine and cocaine; guanethidine, reserpine and other hypotensive drugs; antiparkinsonian agents and barbiturates. Preferably these agents should not be given for at least a fortnight after cessation of medication with MAO drugs. Great care should be taken in prescribing in combination with tricyclic antidepressants.

The oxidative deamination of tyramine which takes place in the walls of the gastrointestinal tract is blocked by MAO inhibitors. The following foodstuffs and drinks are contraindicated due to their large content of tyramine; cheese, broad beans, bananas, pickled herrings, certain protein and yeast extracts such as Bovril and Marmite; alcohol, including beer and certain wines such as Chianti.

Autonomic side effects include orthostatic hypotension; blurring of vision, dry mouth, warmer extremities with reduced sweating; constipation, micturition difficulties and impotence. Headaches, exacerbations of migraine and ankle oedema are met with. In the CNS drowsiness tremors and muscle jerks occur, as do manic states, toxic psychosis and exacerbation of schizophrenic symptoms.

Hepatocellular jaundice is seen in this group but to a variable extent as mentioned above.

Retrobulbar neuritis which usually resolves when the drug is discontinued; allergic skin reactions and exacerbations of eczema and asthma have been reported.

NON-HYDRAZINE DERIVATIVES

Tranylcypromine

Pharmacological action. Absorption and distribution are similar to preceding MAO inhibitors. Action in the brain resembles iproniazid, with the addition of amphetamine-like effects, which are sympathomimetic and stimulant to the ascending reticular formation. Metabolism is in part to hippuric acid; with other moieties entering the urine, and a small quantity of the drug is passed unchanged.

Therapeutic use [15]. Tranylcypromine is most effective in reactive and mixed depression where tiredness and lack of energy are prominent; it is contraindicated with marked tension and agitation. Oral dose: 20 mg a day in two doses before noon. Clinical response is faster than with hydrazine derivatives, but special precautions are required due to side effects.

Contraindications and side effects. Tranylcypromine can cause a gross hypertensive reaction with resultant transient hemiparesis or a subarachnoid haemorrhage. Habituation and true addiction occur. It is otherwise similar in side effects to hydrazine derivatives (see above).

Pargyline

This drug has MAO inhibitor properties, weak antidepressant action and is used for its hypotensive properties.

Overdosage of MAO inhibitors. Chief signs are marked drowsiness, depressed respiration, hypotonicity, fluctuations in blood pressure; and in presence of pressor agents headache, excitement, hallucinations, hypertension subarachnoid haemorrhage and coma.

Suicide is possible with less than 2 g.

AMINOACIDS

Tryptophan

Pharmacological action: This naturally occurring aminoacid is given orally often with pyridoxine hydrochloride and ascorbic acid to aid its metabolism. It joins the metabolic pathway in the CNS and is hydroxylated to 5-hydroxy tryptamine – said to be depleted in depression.

Therapeutic use. Used in all forms of depression, but usually in those depressive illnesses which have failed to respond to tricyclic compounds or MAO inhibitors. Oral dose: 10 g t.d.s. and 30 g at night for a month, reducing over 3 months to 20 g a day. This dose may be then maintained as long-term therapy to prevent recurrence.

Contraindications and side effects. Tryptophan should not be used in conjunction with L-Dopa if it is combined with pyridoxine hydrochloride. Some preparations also contain dextrose and allowance should be made for this in diabetic patients. Drowsiness and nausea tend to occur initially.

Depression in Children [16].
Tricyclic compounds and less toxic MAO inhibitors may be used for treatment of anxiety and depression in older children and adolescents, in suitably adjusted doses.

LITHIUM

Lithium carbonate
Pharmacological action [17]. Lithium is widely distributed throughout the tissues following absorption from the gastrointestinal tract. Depressant action in the CNS probably depends upon the inhibition of enzymes and displacement of sodium. Balance within the body is usually obtained within one to two days but may take up to a week. Excretion is chiefly in the urine.

Therapeutic use [18]. Lithium is effective in mania, hypomania and for stabilisation of mood in recurrent depressive illness. In oral dosage the aim is to gain a serum level which lies between 0·7–1·3 mEq/1 in blood samples drawn 12 hours after last intake of lithium. Over 2·0 mEq/1 produces toxic signs. Weekly blood tests usually taken before the morning dose are required until stable serum levels are achieved. Thereafter serum levels should be checked every one to two months. When rapid response to treatment is necessary, as with mania, the starting dose of lithium carbonate is 1–2 g a day, maintainance usually 0·5–0·75 g a day varying with serum levels. Lithium carbonate may also be given once daily in sustained-release tablets. Chlorpromazine may increase the excretion of lithium.

Contraindications and side effects. Lithium is contraindicated in patients with heart failure, renal failure, Addison's disease or any tendency to electrolyte imbalance. Restriction of sodium decreases renal clearance of lithium. Although well stabilised in hospital, some patients may return to a poor diet, low in salt, thus increasing the risk of intoxication. Toxic signs include tremor, nausea, vomiting and diarrhoea, giddiness, ataxia, thirst, polyuria and drowsiness and coma. The drug should be withdrawn temporarily and serum level estimated at first signs of toxicity.

MAJOR TRANQUILIZERS

1. PHENOTHIAZINES

DIMETHYLAMINOPROPYL SIDE CHAIN COMPOUNDS

Chlorpromazine

Pharmacological action [19]. Chlorpromazine is rapidly absorbed from the duodenum into the portal vein and thus to the liver where it is excreted via the bile and passed back to the gut for reabsorption. This cyclic process may be repeated and accounts for early conjugation observed after oral administration. Peak serum levels are usually obtained in thirty minutes and within the CNS in an hour: with highest concentrations appearing in mid-brain, medulla and pons. Parenteral administration has earlier peak levels and largely by-passes the entero-hepatic route. Chlorpromazine depresses the brain stem reticular formation, its probable site of action being at the outer cell membrane of the receptor with inhibition of amine transport. The drug is metabolised in the liver by demethylation, N-oxidation, sulphoxidation and hydroxylation. The latter is the chief route in formation of phenolic derivatives which conjugate with glucuronic acid. Glucuronides may be found in the urine, which is the main route of excretion, for up to thirty weeks after medication. The remainder of the metabolites are excreted in the faeces, 1 per cent being excreted in the urine as unchanged drug.

Therapeutic use [20, 21]. Chlorpromazine is used in psychotic illness; schizophrenia, states of mania and hypomania, acute and chronic brain syndromes, puerperal psychosis, states of agitation, restlessness, excitement in psychoneuroses, and acute anxiety. Also in personality disorders with tension, and with aggressive and destructive outbursts; in delirium tremens and withdrawal syndromes. In the treatment of acute schizophrenia there is argument as to whether chlorpromazine is anti-psychotic or merely tranquillizing in action. In chronic schizophrenia it is valuable in controlling symptomatic exacerbations but is not thought to be useful on a long term basis with inactive and anergic patients. Oral dosage as sugar-coated tablets or syrup ranges from 65–600 mg a day although doses as high as 3,000 mg a day, in divided doses may be given for short periods. Dosage is highly individual and is not related to habitus or severity of symptoms but to metabolism. Oral administration is preferred but intramuscular injections in the range of 100 mg may be given to uncooperative patients, with due attention to physique, physical illness, prior medication and known sensitivity to this drug.

Chlorpromazine may also be used for treatment of psychotic states and acute anxiety in children. Oral dose: 1–3 mg/kg/24 hours; injections may be painful.

Contraindications and side effects [22]. Chlorpromazine should be avoided in patients with a past history of jaundice and in those with glaucoma or prostatic hypertrophy. Side effects include initial drowsiness, and extrapyramidal symptoms in the elderly and with large dosage; these are weakness, tremor, rigidity, ataxia, loss of facial expression, excess salivation, restlessness and shuffling. Extreme dystonic reaction with gross bodily and facial contortions, protrusion of the tongue and oculogyric crises may occur. Autonomic effects include dryness of the mouth, nasal congestion, blurring of vision, urinary retention, constipation, tachycardia, ECG abnormalities and postural hypotension, especially in the elderly. Some cases of inhibition of ejaculation and paralytic ileus have been reported. Many patients gain weight, there may be disorders of menstruation, breast enlargement and lactation. With prolonged therapy the skin may become photosensitive and appears greyish from melanin deposition. Maculo-papular rashes occur and contact dermatitis is common in nursing staff. High dosage of over 500 mg a day may result in a pigmented retinopathy and lens opacities. Some patients develop an acute intrahepatic cholestatic jaundice which usually clears up when the drug is stopped. It very rarely progresses to cirrhosis. Blood dyscrasias, leucopaenia, granulocytopenia and agranulocytosis are rare but acute complications with high mortality rates; usually heralded by sore throat, malaise and fever. Myathenia gravis may be precipitated or exacerbated.

Promazine

Pharmacological action. Similar to chlorpromazine; the chlorine atom of the phenothiazine nucleus is in this agent, replaced by hydrogen.

Therapeutic use [23]. As for chlorpromazine and in similar dose but less hepatotoxic and suitable for less acute cases.

Contraindications and side effects. As for chlorpromazine but greater tendency to agranulocytosis, and convulsions with large dosage and in patients with a past history of epilepsy.

Trifluopromazine

Pharmacological action. Similar to promazine but the carbon trifluoride radical reduces the tendency to fits.

Therapeutic use [23]. (Also suitable for less acute cases). Oral dose: 50–300 mg t.d.s.

Methotrimeprazine

Pharmacological action. Additional methyl group in side chain increases anti-anxiety and analgesic effects.

Therapeutic use. Indicated in alcoholic withdrawal, depressive agitation and confusional states. Oral dose: 5–50 mg t.d.s.

PIPERAZINE SIDE CHAIN COMPOUNDS

Trifluoperazine

Pharmacological action. Analogous to chlorpromazine, but substitution of piperazine side chain increases potency and carbon trifluoride radical reduces epileptogenic action.

Therapeutic use [23]. Chiefly in withdrawn, resistant cases of schizophrenia and especially with paranoid delusions; also in cases of chlorpromazine liver damage. Oral dose: 2–10 mg t.d.s.

Contraindications and side effects. Extrapyramidal effects may be marked and dystonic reactions are common.

Perphenazine

Pharmacological action. Similar to chlorpromazine, whose chlorine atom it retains but perphenazine is more potent.

Therapeutic action [23]. Acutely disturbed patients. Oral dose: 2–24 mg t.d.s.

Contraindications and side effects. As for chlorpromazine.

Pericyazine

Pharmacological action. Analogous to chlorpromazine but more potent with substituted cyanide radical.

Therapeutic use. Thought to be useful in adolescent behaviour disorders and psychotic states. Oral dose: 5–50 mg t.d.s. Well tolerated intramuscularly, 10–20 mg dose.

Fluphenazine [23]

Fluphenazine decanoate is useful in unreliable patients in form of a depot injection and has largely replaced fluphenazine enanthate in clinical practice as the latter tended to produce more marked extra pyramidal manifestations. A depot injection of 12·5–25 mg is given which lasts from 2–5 weeks. Oral dose 1–100 mg t.d.s. Severe depressive mood changes have been reported following depot injections and patients still require careful supervision.

Thiopropazate
The retained chlorine atom, provides little advantage over chlorpromazine except in treatment of Huntington's Chorea. Side effects often troublesome. Oral dose: 5–150 mg t.d.s.

PIPERIDINE SIDE CHAIN

Thioridazine [23]
Pharmacological action. Strongest acting member of this group and as effective as chlorpromazine but less extra-pyramidal manifestations and reduced photosensitivity.

Therapeutic use. Similar to chlorpromazine.

Useful in ejaculatio praecox; oral dose: 50–100 mg t.d.s.

Contraindications and side effects. Large dosage tends to produce pigmented retinopathy and lens opacities.

Overdose of Phenothiazine Group. Hypotension which may go on to circulatory collapse; hypothermia, dystonic reaction, oculogyric crises, convulsions and coma are also seen.

BUTYROPHENONES

Haloperidol
Pharmacological action. Related chemically to pethidine but with properties similar to phenothiazines.

Therapeutic use [24]. Haloperidol is indicated in psychotic states of mania, excitement and acute confusion. It is also used for habit spasm and tics, especially 'Giles de la Tourette' syndrome. The oral dosage is 3–10 mg a day in two to three divided doses; in uncooperative patients it can be given by intramuscular injection, 5–10 mg stat. and up to 15–45 mg total dose in a day.

Contraindications and side effects [25]. Extra-pyramidal symptoms can be troublesome and haloperidol should be given with care in the elderly and those affected by Parkinson's disease. It is usually combined with an anti-parkinsonian drug (see above). Its contraindications are glaucoma and urinary retention. Depression, loss of appetite and a symptomatic triad of sweating dehydration and hyperthermia have been described.

Triperidol

Pharmacological action. Similar to haloperidol.

Therapeutic action. This drug is more potent; oral dosage ranging from 1–3 mg a day.

Contraindications and side effects. Similar to those of haloperidol, but with greater extra-pyramidal effects.

DIPHENYLBUTYLPIPERIDENES

Pimozide [26]

Pharmacological action. After absorption this drug reaches a peak level in the plasma and the brain in 3–6 hours. This is followed by an initial fall to half peak level which is maintained for about 24 hours. 50 per cent of the drug is excreted unchanged within 24 hours in the urine and faeces. The remainder is excreted over 4 days as benzimidazolinone, butyric and acetic acids.

Therapeutic use. As this drug is long-acting it is chiefly used for maintenance therapy in schizophrenia. It is not suitable for treatment of symptoms in the acute phase of schizophrenia. A single oral daily dose of 2–10 mg is the most suitable regime.

Contraindications and side effects. The incidence of sedation and autonomic effects is extremely small and extra pyramidal manifestations are seldom encountered.

RAUWOLFIA ALKALOIDS

Reserpine

Canescine

Rescinnamine

Pharmacological action. A small quantity of the ingested alkaloids reach the central and peripheral nervous systems where they act by depleting the amine stores.

Therapeutic use. These drugs may be tried in the treatment of schizophrenia when other tranquillisers have failed. They tend to produce depression and their use is therefore limited. Oral dose: 0·5–1·0 mg t.d.s., increasing gradually until optimum effect is produced, to a maximum of 9–12 mg daily.

Contraindications and side effects. They should not be used in schizophrenia with a depressive colouring. Other unwanted reactions include sleepiness, nasal congestion, dizziness, diarrhoea, extrapyramidal symptoms and hypotension.

TRICYCLIC COMPOUNDS RESEMBLING PHENOTHIAZINES

Chlorprothixene

Pharmacological action. Tranquillizing properties similar to chlorpromazine with less central depressant activity but greater anti-cholinergic effect.

Therapeutic use. Similar to chlorpromazine and particularly indicated in psychomotor agitation. Daily oral dose: 30–150 mg.

Contraindications and side effects. Reduced as compared with chlorpromazine and extra pyramidal symptoms are infrequent.

Thiothixene

Pharmacological action. This thio derivative has tranquillizing properties similar to chlorpromazine but is less sedative and is capable of psychomotor excitation.

Therapeutic use. In psychotic illness where regression and withdrawal have led to inactivity and poor co-operation. Oral daily dose: 10 mg initially and then 20–40 mg in divided doses.

Contraindications and side effects. Used with care in patients with a history of epilepsy or blood dyscrasias.

Extra pyramidal symptoms. Restlessness and insomnia may prove troublesome.

Prothipendyl

An azothiazine derivative similar to chlorprothixene but less powerful and more suitable for use as a minor tranquillizer. Daily dose ranges from 40–960 mg, according to the severity of the illness, in divided doses. With improvement in symptoms dose may be reduced and maintenance therapy in form of 60-mg spansules.

Clopenthixol

Pharmacological action. Similar to chlorpromazine but with stronger extra-pyramidal effects than chlorprothizene.

Therapeutic use. Anxiety associated with obsessional states and depression. Oral dose: 10–30 mg a day.

Contraindications and side effects. Less but in general similar to phenothiazines.

Oxypertine

This drug is an indol derivative with a piperazine side chain.

Therapeutic use. In schizophrenia, especially in withdrawn or apathetic patients. Oral dose 80–120 mg a day.

Contraindications and side effects. This drug produces extra-pyramidal manifestations.

Treatment of drug induced extra-pyramidal effects. These can be controlled with orphenadrine and benztropine (see above).

MINOR TRANQUILLIZERS

These drugs have sedative, hypnotic and relaxant properties.

1. BENZODIAZEPINES

Chlordiazepoxide [27]

Pharmacological action. Following absorption from the gastrointestinal tract this drug is widely distributed via the blood stream to all tissues. It acts as a depressant in the brain probably on the limbic system and has anticonvulsant and muscle relaxant properties. Metabolism is by hydroxylation and splitting which is followed by excretion, primarily in the urine and secondarily in the faeces.

Therapeutic use. Chlordiazepoxide relieves tension and anxiety, and its anticonvulsant properties indicate its use in the treatment of anxiety in epileptics. It is also used to alleviate symptoms of alcohol and drug-withdrawal syndromes.

Anxiety is a frequent presenting symptom of depression and may mask the underlying illness. Chlordiazepoxide is not an antidepressant and should be used in conjunction with antidepressant drugs when a depressive element is present.

Chlordiazepoxide may be used in the treatment of anxiety in children, also in conjunction with antidepressants in depression; and to promote relaxation leading to sleep.

Oral dosage is usually 10 mg t.d.s. with a daily range of 15–45 mg. Older patients may require smaller doses to avoid sleepiness and dosage must be suitably adjusted in children. It may be given as a hypnotic at night.

Contraindications and side effects. Drug dependence is possible but rare with chlordiazepoxide and withdrawal may produce convulsions. Drowsiness, mild disorientation and periods of inattention may pose a problem over driving. Confusion and excitement, especially in the elderly, ataxia, pruritus, hypotension and loss of libido may occur. The appetite may be stimulated with consequent weight gain. There is potentiation of alcohol and barbiturates but suicide with this drug has not been reported.

Diazepam [27]

Pharmacological action. Similar to chlordiazepoxide but with stronger anticonvulsant and muscle relaxant properties.

Therapeutic use. Similar to chlordiazepoxide but more potent and particularly indicated in patients with marked tension producing muscle pains and headaches. Its [28] stronger anticonvulsant properties make it useful in the treatment of drug withdrawal and it may be given intravenously in status epilepticus. Usual oral dose: 2–10 mg t.d.s.

In children for treatment of anxiety and phobias, oral dose as tablets or syrup 1–5 mg/day; or for management of psychological disorders associated with brain injury and epilepsy, 2–40 mg/day.

Contraindications and side effects. Similar to chlordiazepoxide.

Oxazepam

Similar to chlordiazepoxide and most useful in the treatment of anxiety expressed as gastrointestinal, respiratory or cardiovascular symptoms. Sedative effects are said to be reduced. Oral dose: 15–30 mg t.d.s.

Nitrazepam

Pharmacological action. Similar to chlordiazepoxide but is said to have a selective depressant action on the limbic system and little effect upon the cerebral cortex and reticular formation.

Therapeutic use. Chiefly as a hypnotic but may be used as a sedative. Oral dosage: 5–10 mg at night or t.d.s.

Medazepam

Pharmacological action. This benzodiazepine hydrochloride, similar to chlordiazepoxide pharmacologically, is, however, claimed to have a more specific action on the amygalda – the seat of anxiety within the limbic system.

Therapeutic use. For the treatment of anxiety, especially anxiety associated with phobias and obsessions. It is also useful in the treatment of emotionally disturbed and mentally retarded children with behaviour disorders. Drowsiness is minimal and alertness tends to be maintained. Oral dose is from 5–6 mg a day.

Contraindications and side effects. As for chlordiazepoxide.

2. SUBSTITUTED DIOLS

Meprobamate

Pharmacological action [27]. Meprobamate is rapidly absorbed from the gastrointestinal tract with distribution via the blood stream, initially to the visceral organs, peak levels being reached in about two hours in the CNS. It acts as a depressant in the brain on the limbic system and thalamus. It is largely metabolised within 24 hours by hydroxylation and conjugation of the drug with glucuronic acid followed by urinary excretion.

Therapeutic use [29]. In the management of mild anxiety states and tension but is unsuitable for severe anxiety. Its efficacy is open to some doubt. The oral dose is 800–1,600 mg a day and usually 400 mg t.d.s.

Contraindications and side effects. Meprobamate should not be used where there is a risk of drug dependence. A withdrawal syndrome is seen after prolonged medication consisting of restlessness, tremors, and ataxia with the possibility of convulsions and delirium. A commoner side effect is drowsiness, but sensitivity reactions occur with rash, pyrexia and fever. More rarely gastro-intestinal upsets, excitement, blood dyscrasias and paralysis of the extra-ocular muscles are seen.

The following drugs resemble meprobamate and are said to have sedative and relaxant properties:

Drug	Dose
1. Tybamate	350 mg t.d.s.
2. Phenaglycodol	200 mg q.d.s.
3. Oxanamide	400 mg t.d.s.
4. Emylclamate	200 mg t.d.s.
5. Mephenesin	500 mg t.d.s.
6. Carisoprodol	350 mg t.d.s.
7. Styramate	200 gm t.d.s.

3. THIAZOLE DERIVATIVES

Chlormethiazole

Pharmacological action. Not well understood after absorption from the gastrointestinal tract.

Therapeutic use. Claimed to be effective in the treatment of delirium tremens and confusional states. Dosage is 2 g initially followed by 1 g hourly until sleep ensues. Up to 8 g may be given in 24 hours. Subsequent daily dosage should be gradually reduced, depending on the patient's state, and stopped in one or two weeks.

Contraindications and side effects. Sneezing and facial itching have been reported, hypotension and respiratory depression may occur.

4. DIPHENYLMETHANE DERIVATIVES

Azacyclonol

Pharmacological action. After absorption from the gastrointestinal tract azacyclonol is distributed primarily to brain, lungs and spleen. Site of action is uncertain; it is largely excreted in the urine within 24 hours.

Therapeutic use. Primarily for the treatment of hallucinations in schizophrenia but results have been disappointing. Average daily dose: 60–300 mg.

Contraindications and side effects. Rashes and hypotension may occur.

Benactyzine

Pharmacological action. Similar to azacyclonol.

Therapeutic use. Treatment of mild states of anxiety and depression. Oral dose: 3–6 mg daily.

Contraindications and side effects. Dryness of mouth, blurring of vision, poor concentration, feelings of mental retardation and increased anxiety have been reported.

Hydroxyzine

Pharmacological action. Similar to azacyclonol.

Therapeutic use. Mainly in states of anxiety and in psychogenic vomiting. Oral dose: 10–25 mg four times a day.

Contraindications and side effects. Headache, dry mouth and itching have been reported.

5. OCTADIENE RING STRUCTURE

Benzoctamine

Pharmacological action. This drug is said to exert a tranquilizing effect via the higher brain centres and to have a peripheral effect on the gamma-fibre system, thus inducing muscle relaxation. It is metabolised chiefly in the liver to phenolamines conjugated with glucuronic acid and is excreted in the urine.

Therapeutic use. Benzoctamine is claimed to be effective in anxiety states where there is a combination of emotional symptoms and somatic complaints. Oral dose 10 mg t.d.s.

Contraindications and side effects. This drug is not recommended for use alone in depressive illness as this may cause deterioration; it should be given with care in patients with hepatic or renal disease. Drowsiness and dry mouth may occur initially.

SEDATIVES

Barbiturates

These drugs are similar and will be described as a group.

Official Name

Phenobarbitone (Phenobarbital, *USA*)

Amylobarbitone (Amylobarbital, *USA*)

Pentobarbitone (Pentobarbital, *USA*)

Quinalbarbitone (Secobarbital, *USA*)

Pharmacological action. See above.

Therapeutic use. Barbiturates are used in minor states of anxiety, and the faster acting compounds in large dose in cases of acute disturbance. Individual response is wide and varied. They have been replaced in modern practice by the tranquillizers and particularly phenothiazines and butyrophenones in more acute states. However, intravenous barbiturates are still used as abreactive agents [30] often with methylamphetamine.

The following are the chief drugs in order of speed of sedative action:

Phenobarbitone, oral dose: 30 mg t.d.s.

Amylobarbitone, oral dose 15–45 mg t.d.s.

Amylobarbitone sodium, rapid action for acute anxiety, oral dose: 60–120 mg. In acutely disturbed patients by intramuscular or intravenous injection, 250–500 mg in 10 ml of water.

Pentobarbitone, oral dose: 100–200 mg.

Quinalbarbitone, oral dose: 100–200 mg.

Contraindications and side effects. Accumulation with subsequent depression may occur with phenobarbitone, and there are problems of tolerance and addiction for the group as a whole. Drowsiness, rash, and in the elderly, states of excitement and confusion may be troublesome.

PSYCHOTO-MIMETIC DRUGS [31]

Lysergide

Mescaline

Psylocybine

Piperidyl benzylate

Phencyclidine

Pharmacological action. These drugs are widely distributed following absorption, but there appears to be little correlation between brain concentrations and clinical effects. These may be divided into peripheral actions, including stimulation of muscle and vasoconstriction, and central actions such as stimulation of sympathetic centres with tachycardia, hypertension, hyperglycaemia, pilo-erection and eye ball protrusion. Metabolism varies, with dephosphorylation, deamination and hydroxylation; piperidyl benzylate being rapidly excreted unchanged in the urine.

Therapeutic use. Their value is in dispute but lysergide, mescaline and psilocybine have been used to produce abreaction and as an aid to psychotherapy. The group as a whole have been used in the production of model psychoses for research purposes.

Contraindications and side effects. Schizophrenia, depression and obsessional states may be exacerbated and manic states precipitated in aggressive psychopaths.

Warning

As drowsiness may occur whilst taking psychotropic drugs, patients should be informed of this and adequate warning given of the dangers of driving a car or operating machinery. They potentiate the action of alcohol, and should be used with care in the elderly.

References

1. Domenjoz, R., and Theobald, W., *Archs. int. Pharmacodyn, Ther* (1959), **120,** 450.
2. Holtz, P., and Westermann, E. (1965), *ibid.*, 1015.
3. Pare, C. M. B., *Lancet* (1965), **i,** 923.
4. Asberg, M., Crönholm, B., Sjögvist, F., Tuck, D., *Brit. med. J.* (1971), **3,** 331.
5. Kuhn, R., *Amer. J. Psychiat.* (1958), **115,** 459.
6. Medical Research Council, Report by Clinical Psychiatry Committee, *Brit. med. J.* (1965), **1,** 881.
7. Dimascio, Heninger, G., and Klerman, G. L., *Psychopharmacologia* (1964), **5,** 361.
8. Collins, G. H., *Brit. J. Psychiat.* (1970), **117,** 211.
9. Burns, B. H., *Brit. J. Psychiat.* (1965), **111,** 1155.
10. Angst, J., *Psychopharmacologia* (1963), **4,** 389.
11. Daneman, E. A., *Psychosomatics* (1967), **8,** 216.
12. Pscheidt, G. R., *Intern. Rev. Neurobiol.* (1964), **7,** 191.
13. Crisp, A. H., Hays, P., and Carter, A., *Lancet* (1961), **i,** 17.
14. Richmond, P. W., and Roberts, A. H., *Brit. J. Psychiat.* (1964), **110,** 469.
15. Bartholomew, A. A., *Med. J. Aust.* (1962), **149,** 655.
16. Frommer, *Recent Developments in Affective Disorders* (1968), Headley Bros., Ashford.
17. Gershon, S., and Yuwiler, A., *J. Neuropsychiat.* (1960), 229.
18. Baastrup, P. C., Poulsen, J. C., Schou, M., Thomsen, K., Amdisen, A., *Lancet* (1970), **ii,** 326.
19. Parkes, M. W., *in* Ellis, G. P., and West, G. B. (editors) *Progress in Medicinal Chemistry* (1961), **1,** Butterworths, London.
20. Freyhan, F. A., *Amer. J. Psychiat.* (1959), **115,** 577.

21. Malitz, S., *Ann. N.Y. Acad. Sci.* (1957), **66,** 717.
22. Hollister, L. E., *Clin. Pharmac. Ther.* (1964), **5,** 322.
23. Hanlon, T. E. *et al.*, *Psychopharmacologia* (1965), **7,** 89.
24. Trethowen, W. H., (editor), Proceedings of a Symposium on Haloperidol. *Clin. Trials J.* (1965), **2,** 133.
25. Gerle, B., *Acta Psychiat. scand.* (1964), **40,** 65.
26. Morris, P. A., Mackenzie, D. H., and Masheter, H. C., *Brit. J. Psychiat.* (1970), **117,** 683
27. Wittenborn, J. R., *The Clinical Psychopharmacology of Anxiety* (1966), Thomas Springfield, Illinois.
29. McNair, D. M. *et al.*, *Psychopharmacologia* (1965), **7,** 256.
28. Boyer, P. A., *Dis. Nerv. Syst.* (1966), **27,** 35.
30. Sargant, W., and Slater, E., *Physical Methods of Treatment in Psychiatry* (1963), Livingstone, Edinburgh.
31. Shepherd, M., Lader, M., and Rodnight, R., *Clinical Psychopharmacology* (1968), English Universities Press Limited, London.

This chapter was written by Dr J. R. Colville (Dept of Child and Adolescent Psychiatry, Guy's Hospital) and edited by Professor J. R. Trounce.

Category 5

Drugs Affecting the Autonomic Nervous System and Motor End-Plate

When considering the drugs which affect the autonomic nervous system and motor end-plate, it is useful to think in terms of four basic kinds of neuronal connection between the central nervous system and the end-organ. These are displayed diagrammatically below. The chemi-

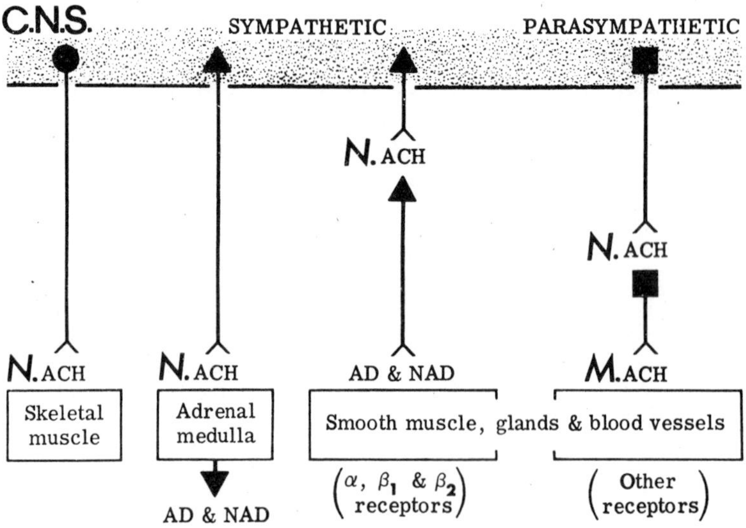

N=nicotinic; *M*=muscarinic; ACH=acetylcholine; AD=adrenaline; NAD=noradrenaline

cal transmitter at the first synapse in each case is acetylcholine. All these sites are 'nicotinic' as the effects of transmission can be mimicked by nicotine-like substances. The second synapse in the parasympathetic pathway is rather different and although dependent on acetylcholine as transmitter it is also stimulated by muscarine-like substances. In the sympathetic pathway adrenaline and noradrenaline are the second synapse transmitter and the various end-organ receptors have been classified into α and β chiefly according to whether their effect is an excitatory or inhibitory one. This classification has proved useful but has required a little modification [1]. For further discussion of this subject see references [2] and [3].

Table 1

α Effects	β Effects
VASOCOSITRICTION particularly in skin and gut producing a rise in systolic and diastolic blood pressure with reflex slowing of the heart.	β_1 increased rate and force of contraction of the HEART.
MYDRIASIS.	β_2 BRONCHODILATATION.
ADRENERGIC SWEATING.	VASODILATATION particularly of coronary vessels and vessels in skeletal muscle.

The drugs affecting the autonomic nervous system and motor end-plate will be discussed under the following headings:

1. Sympathomimetic Drugs.
2. Anti-adrenergic Drugs:
   (a) Post-ganglionic Neurone Blockers.
   (b) α and β Receptor Blockers.
3. Parasympathomimetic Drugs.
4. Anti-cholinergic Drugs:
   (a) Ganglion Blockers
   (b) Neuromuscular Blockers
   (c) Drugs blocking muscarinic sites, i.e. Atropine and related drugs.

SYMPATHOMIMETIC DRUGS

Adrenaline (Epinephrine, *USA*)

Pharmacological action. Both α and β receptors are stimulated, its action resembling the activity of the sympathetic nervous system itself. Its α effects are to constrict blood vessels in skin and viscera, dilate the pupil and release glucose from the liver. The β effects are to increase the rate and force of contraction of the heart, dilate blood vessels in muscle and heart and dilate the bronchi. Like noradrenaline, it is inactive by mouth but has a rapid onset and short duration of action after subcutaneous injection.

Therapeutic uses. It is generally used as the acid tartrate or the hydrochloride. Dose: S.C. or I.M. 0·4–1 mg. It is often used locally in dilute solutions of varying strengths from 1 in 200,000 to 1 in 1,000 depending on the situation. It is not given intravenously. It is used to stop or reduce capillary bleeding both during and after surgery; to reduce nasal congestion; in combination with local anaesthetics (e.g. procaine) to prolong their action; to produce bronchodilatation in asthma; to counteract anaphylactic shock and other less serious allergic manifestations, e.g. urticaria, hay fever and angioneurotic oedema and to reverse heart block with syncope or even cardiac arrest. In the latter case it is often given as an intra-cardiac injection. It is also used in eye drops for retinoscopy and for open-angle (chronic simple) glaucoma in which situation it lowers the intra-ocular pressure. In narrow angle glaucoma it may increase the pressure.

Contraindications and side effects. It may produce feelings of anxiety, restlessness, palpitations, tachycardia, tremors, weakness, dizziness, headache and cold extremities. In excess it can cause cardiac arrhythmias and gangrene of extremities. It should not be used in very nervous or anxious paitents or those with hypertension, ischaemic heart disease, hyperthyroidism, or in conjunction with trichlorethylene, halothane or cyclopropane. It is best avoided in patients who are receiving monoamine oxidase inhibitors.

Noradrenaline (Norepinephrine/Levarterenol, *USA*)

Pharmacological action. It has a predominant effect on α receptors causing vasoconstriction in muscle, skin and viscera, dilatation of the pupil, reduced muscular activity in the gastrointestinal and urinary tracts and glucose release from the liver. Both systolic and diastolic blood pressures rise and there is reflex slowing of the heart. It causes less cardiac stimulation than adrenaline.

Therapeutic uses. The acid tartrate is usually used, the dose being 2–20 μg/minute intravenously. Its chief use has been to treat hypotension in association with peripheral circulatory failure complicating myocardial infarction, the removal of phaeochromocytomas, the use of ganglion-blocking agents and many other conditions. The intense vasoconstriction usually restores the blood pressure but at the expense of adequate perfusion, especially of the kidneys. Latterly the trend has been to attach more significance to blood flow than pressure and to try and improve the former by using a combination of an α-adrenergic blocking agent and intravenous infusion of fluid [3]. Noradrenaline infusions should be stopped slowly as otherwise an abrupt fall in blood pressure may follow.

Contraindications and side effects. Gangrene of the extremities may follow prolonged infusions and severe phlebitis and necrosis around the site of injection has often been a sequel.

Isoprenaline (Isoproterenol, *USA*)

Pharmacological action. This is almost entirely on β receptors, producing a marked increase in the rate and force of contraction of the heart and relaxation of peripheral blood vessels, bronchi and most of the smooth muscle of the gut.

Therapeutic uses. It is usually given as the sulphate in a dose of 5–20 mg sublingually or by inhalation in an atomiser or as a pressurised aerosol. The hydrochloride is also used in a dose of 10 mg sublingually; or by inhalation or as a 0·02 per cent solution (1 in 5,000) subcutaneously. It can also be given I.M. or I.V. as an infusion. It is used widely in the control of bronchial asthma but has the disadvantage of stimulating the heart often to a considerable degree. It also produces ventilation/perfusion imbalance in the lungs and a fall in arterial oxygen tension [4]. The pharmacological separation of the β effects on heart and bronchial muscle [1] and the advent of drugs which have predominantly a β_2 effect, e.g. salbutamol, reduces this problem. It has been suggested that the combination of isoprenaline with phenylephrine will prevent the reduction in arterial oxygen levels [5]. However, such a manoeuvre does not get round the other untoward effects of isoprenaline. It is only given by injection in the management of complete heart block and for long-term control it is best given as an oral sustained-release preparation, e.g. saventrine.

Contraindications and side effects. These include tachycardia, praecordial pain, hypotension, dizziness, headache, tremor and weakness. It should not be given in the presence of acute coronary insufficiency, heart failure and only with caution in hyperthyroidism.

Orciprenaline

Pharmacological action. An analogue of isoprenaline having similar β_1 and β_2 effects and which is fully active when swallowed.

Therapeutic uses. It is used almost entirely as a bronchodilator. Dose: orally 10–20 mg; as a 5 per cent solution by inhalation or 0·5 mg S.C. or I.M.

Contraindications and side effects. As isoprenaline but usually less troublesome.

Salbutamol

Pharmacological action. A drug which stimulates β_2 receptors in bronchial muscle but which has little or no effect on β_1 receptors in the heart.

Therapeutic uses. This has considerable advantages over isoprenaline in the management of bronchial asthma as it is both longer acting and does not have the risk of precipitating untoward cardiac effects, e.g. arrhythmias [6]. It is given as a pressurised aerosol discharging puffs of 100 μg. Dose 100–400 μg. It can also be used as tablets in a dose of 2–5 mg b.d. or t.d.s.

Contraindications and side effects. So far remarkably few side effects have been seen although tremor is occasionally noticeable.

Terbutaline

Pharmacological action. Like salbutamol this new agent is chemically very similar to isoprenaline but also has the distinction of being a selective β_2 receptor stimulator [7].

Therapeutic uses and side effects. As salbutamol. Dose 2·5–5 mg t.d.s. It can also be given subcutaneously (0·25 mg) up to four times a day.

Isoetharine

Pharmacological action and uses. Another β_2 stimulator. Dose 10 mg t. or q.d.s.

Ephedrine

Pharmacological action. This is similar to adrenaline as it has both α and β effects, although its effect is slower and more sustained. It acts partly on the receptor directly but also by releasing noradrenaline from stores at adrenergic nerve endings. It may also work partly by inhibiting amine-oxidase. It has a greater stimulating effect on the central nervous system in adults although children may be sedated. It is effective orally.

Therapeutic uses. Dose: 15–60 mg orally or subcutaneously as the hydrochloride or sulphate. It is also used as a 1 per cent spray. Its chief use is as a bronchodilator. It is sometimes used to increase conduction in complete heart block, to alleviate narcolepsy and cataplexy and to augment the effect of neostigmine in myasthenia. It is also useful in the management of enuresis.

Contraindications and side effects. Large doses may cause headache, nausea, vomiting, palpitations, difficulty in micturition, muscular weakness, tremors, anxiety, restlessness and insomnia. It should not be given to elderly men and those in whom prostatism is suspected. It should not be used in the presence of ischaemic heart disease, hypertension and thyrotoxicosis.

Amphetamine

Pharmacological action. A sympathomimetic drug with a marked stimulating effect on the central nervous system. It lessens fatigue, gives a feeling of well-being and can easily produce a state of habituation or addiction, especially following indiscriminate use. It also suppresses appetite.

Therapeutic uses. Dose: orally 5–10 mg. It has been used in the management of narcolepsy and occasionally in epilepsy and parkinsonism. Other agents have now largely replaced it in all these situations in view of the very real danger of habituation. It should not be used as a tonic, to reduce appetite or to treat depression. It should not be given with MAO inhibitors.

Dexamphetamine

Pharmacological action and therapeutic uses. This has the same effects, uses and disadvantages as amphetamine.

Methylphenidate

Pharmacological action and uses. This has a similar action to amphetamine but is the recommended antidote for pentazocine (q.v.) overdosage as nalorphine is ineffective.

Hydroxyamphetamine

Pharmacological action and therapeutic uses. This has an effective vasopressor action without the central effects of amphetamine. It also has a direct stimulating action on the heart. It has been used to correct hypotension, bradycardia and as a nasal decongestant and mydriatic. Dose: orally 20–60 mg; I.M 10–20 mg and I.V. 5–10 mg.

Methylamphetamine (Methamphetamine, *USA*)

Pharmacological action and therapeutic uses. These are the same as for amphetamine with the exception that I.M. or I.V. it is an effective *α*-stimulator and produces a vasopressor effect in a dose of 10–30 mg. Its central stimulant effects are marked even in small doses and this has led to its vogue as a drug of addiction.

Methoxyphenamine

Pharmacological action and therapeutic uses. This drug has little vasopressor activity but does dilate bronchi and is used in the control of asthma. Dose: orally 50–100 mg every 3 or 4 hours.

There are many other sympathomimetic drugs which have been used as vasopressor agents. These include:

Cyclopentamine/Mephentermine/Metaraminol/

Methoxamine/Phenylephrine/Phenylpropranolamine

Most of them are *α* stimulators although metaraminol has both *α* and *β* effects and mephentermine has almost entirely a *β* stimulating effect.

ANTI-ADRENERGIC DRUGS

POST-GANGLIONIC NEURONE BLOCKERS

These are discussed in the section on HYPOTENSIVE DRUGS.

α BLOCKING AGENTS

Phentolamine

Pharmacological action. This is similar to tolazoline (q.v.) although it is rather more potent and has a shorter duration of action. It acts by competing with *α*-stimulating agents for the *α* receptors and its effects can be reversed by giving large amounts of these drugs. It is not reliably effective when given orally.

Therapeutic uses. Dose: orally 40–100 mg 4 to 6-hourly as the hydrochloride or I.V. 5–10 mg as the mesylate. The latter is used chiefly in the diagnosis of phaeochromocytoma. In this situation a fall in blood pressure of at least 32/25 mm Hg should occur within 2 minutes of giving 5 mg I.V. Orally, phentolamine has been given for the control of hypertension in phaeochromocytoma prior to surgery.

Parenterally it can also be used as an antidote to adrenaline or noradrenaline.

Contraindications and side effects. Orally it may cause nausea, vomiting, diarrhoea and gastrointestinal disturbances. Less often tachycardia, praecordial pain and postural hypotension are troublesome.

Phenoxybenzamine

Pharmacological action. A powerful α-blocker which acts for longer than phentolamine; its effect lasting for several days. It probably alters the receptor in some way rather than acting by competition and its effects cannot be reversed by noradrenaline. The maximum effect of an I.V. injection may take an hour to develop.

Therapeutic uses. Dose: orally 10–20 mg initially, subsequent doses to be determined according to the patient's response. It has been used for peripheral vascular disease but is not suitable for the control of hypertension, other than that due to phaeochromocytoma, because of side effects which usually develop with the dose levels required. Latterly it has been used in the management of peripheral circulatory failure in combination with the intravenous infusion of fluid and central venous pressure monitoring [8]. This is in preference to the previous vogue of giving α-stimulators, e.g. noradrenaline (norepinephrine) which produces marked vasoconstriction but at the cost of a severe reduction in flow and tissue perfusion. I.V. a total daily dose of 0·5–1 mg/kg bodyweight is given in 250–500 ml normal saline or dextrose injection over a period of at least 1 hour.

Contraindications and side effects. It should not be given where a fall in blood pressure would be dangerous. A single large dose can cause postural hypotension lasting for 2 days or more. Other side effects include nasal congestion, dry mouth, pupillary constriction, drowsiness, fatigue and weakness. Anorexia, nausea, vomiting and other gastrointestinal disturbances tend to occur more with oral therapy.

Thymoxamine

Pharmacological action. This is a potent and fairly specific α-blocking agent having a marked vasodilator effect. It produces its effect by a competitive and reversible blockade of the α-receptors.

Therapeutic uses. Dose: orally 5–10 mg 3 or 4 times daily; or 5–30 mg daily S C or I.M. or by slow I.V. injection. Its chief use is as a peripheral vasodilator.
Contraindications and side effects. These include nausea, diarrhoea, facial flushing, vertigo and headache, but are less severe than those seen with phentolamine.

Some phenothiazines, e.g. chlorpromazine hydrochloride, also have an α-blocking effect which is strong enough to cause hypotension. Some ergot alkaloids have α-blocking activity but this is usually masked by their powerful direct vasoconstrictor effect.

β-BLOCKING AGENTS

D.C.I. [Dichloroisoprenaline (*UK*), Dichloroisoproterenol (*USA*)] was the first drug of this class but in addition it had some of the sympathomimetic activity of isoprenaline and is not now used. Another drug pronethalol was withdrawn because it produced tumours in animals.

Propranolol

Pharmacological action. A powerful and fairly specific β-blocker which probably acts by competition with catecholamines for the β-receptors. This produces a reduction in the rate and force of contraction of the heart. It also has a quinidine-like and a local anaesthetic effect, reducing the rate of ectopic foci. Even in normal people it causes mild bronchial constriction which is much more marked in asthmatics.
Therapeutic uses. Its uses in the treatment of angina, cardiac arrhythmias and hypertension are discussed elsewhere. Propranolol has been shown to be of benefit in the control of anxiety in a dose of 20 mg q.d.s. This effect seems to correspond more with β-blockade [9] than the other activities of this drug. It is also used in the management of phaeochromocytoma in association with α-blocking agents which should usually precede its administration. For details see [10].

Several new β-blocking agents have recently been the subject of drug trials. These include practolol (I.C.I.50172), oxyprenolol (trasicor) and alprenolol.

Practolol

Pharmaceutical action. A recently developed drug which seems to block β_1 receptors in the myocardium without blocking β_2 receptors in bronchi or peripheral vessels [11, 12]. It also differs from propranolol in that it has no quinidine-like or local anaesthetic effect but does have weak sympathomimetic activity [13].

Therapeutic uses. It is effective in treating cardiac arrhythmias but is probably not so effective as propranolol or oxprenolol in angina of effort. It rarely induces broncho-constriction or cardiac failure and is especially useful in the management of arrhythmias following myocardial infarction [14]. Dose I.V. 5–25 mg, orally 50 mg b.d. A maximum dose of 600 mg daily for control of arrhythmias and 1 g. daily for angina has been used although the dose should always be tailored to the individual patient.

Contraindications and side effects. Any degree of atrio-ventricular block in association with a slow heart rate is taken as an absolute contraindication. Otherwise it seems to give rise to much fewer side-effects than propranolol.

Oxyprenolol

Pharmacological action and uses. Another β_1 blocker which also has some intrinsic sympathomimetic activity. Its uses and side effects are very similar to practolol although a fall in blood pressure is often seen after I.V. administration. Dose: I.V. 1–5 mg; orally 40–60 mg t.d.s. may be increased.

PARASYMPATHOMIMETIC DRUGS

CHOLINE ESTERS

Methacholine

Pharmacological action. Like acetylcholine it stimulates the parasympathetic nervous system but has predominantly a muscarinic effect. It chiefly affects the cardiovascular system causing bradycardia and dilatation of peripheral blood vessels. It increases salivation, sweating and bronchial secretion.

Therapeutic uses. Dose: orally 10–500 mg; S.C. 10–25 mg. It is not given intravenously. Methacholine bromide is sometimes used and has a similar action. Dose: orally 200–600 mg. Methacholine has been used to stop supraventricular tachycardias and to stimulate the bowel and bladder, although carbachol is probably better for the latter.

Contraindications and side effects. These include nausea, vomiting, flushing, increased salivation, involuntary defaecation, bradycardia, transient heart block, hypotension, dyspnoea and substernal discomfort. If given by injection it may give rise to a terrifying feeling of choking. It should not be given to patients with asthma, hypertension, ischaemic heart disease, Addison's disease or peptic ulceration. Serious reactions have resulted from the combined use of methacholine and neostigmine.

Carbachol

Pharmacological action. It has both muscarine and nicotinic effects but chiefly affects the gastrointestinal tract.

Therapeutic uses. Dose: S.C. 0·25 mg repeated up to 2 or 3 times at 30-minute intervals. It is also used in a 0·8 per cent aqueous solution as eye drops. Its most frequent use is for post-operative intestinal atony and retention of urine. It has also been used for supraventricular tachycardias and is occasionally used as a miotic. Unwanted side effects can be reversed with atropine 0·6 mg S.C.

Contraindications and side effects. It may cause sweating, nausea, faintness, colic and diarrhoea. It should not be used in the presence of mechanical obstruction in the gastrointestinal or urinary tracts or after gastrointestinal anatomosis. It is less safe in the elderly.

Bethanechol

Pharmacological action. This is similar to methacholine but it is not destroyed by choline-esterase. It is less toxic and less active than methacholine.

Therapeutic use. Dose: orally 5–30 mg up to 3 times a day; S.C. 2·5–5 mg at no less than 4-hourly intervals. It is the best tolerated of these three drugs for the treatment of postoperative intestinal stasis (e.g. after vagotomy) and distension, and is also useful for postoperative urinary retention.

Contraindications and side effects. As carbachol but less troublesome.

CHOLINE-ESTERASE INHIBITORS

Physostigmine

Pharmacological action. It potentiates the action of acetylcholine by inhibiting choline-esterase. It thus produces muscarinic and nicotinic effects as well as acting on the central nervous system. It is particularly useful as a miotic acting within 10 minutes of local application, the effect lasting for about 12 hours.

Therapeutic uses. It is now only used as eye-drops. It is useful for the relief of glaucoma and to counteract the dilation produced by atropine or cocaine. It is usually used as a 0·25 per cent solution, higher concentrations often causing irritation.

Neostigmine

Pharmacological action. This has a similar action to physostigmine although the nicotinic effects are more and the muscarinic effects less prominent. It is thus used chiefly for its effect on skeletal muscle.

Therapeutic uses. Preparations: N. bromide – orally, N. methyl sulphate–by injection. It is still the mainstay of treatment for myasthenia gravis and is used in a dose of 15–30 mg orally three or four times daily. It can be given by I.M. or I.V. injection 1–2·5 mg several times daily up to a total of 3 mg/day. It has also been used as a diagnostic aid for myasthenia in a dose of 1–1·5 mg I.M. or I.V. Increase in muscular power with improvement in symptoms should be noticeable within 15 minutes. Neostigmine is also used as an antidote to the muscle relaxants tubocurarine and gallamine. 2·5–5 mg is given I.V. after 0·5–1 mg atropine I.V.

Contraindications and side effects. Toxic effects include restlessness, weakness, nausea, vomiting, diarrhoea and abdominal pain. Increased sweating, salivation and lachrymation occur, and if excessive doses are given generalised muscular twitching convulsions and collapse may ensue. The muscarinic effects can be controlled with atropine. Neostigmine should not be used in patients with asthma, ischaemic heart disease, parkinsonism, epilepsy, bradycardia, hypotension, and intestinal or urinary tract obstruction. Its use during operation involving intestinal anastomosis is associated with an increased incidence of leaking from the intestinal suture line [15]. This effect seems to be considerably reduced if halothane is used as the general anaesthetic.

Pyridostigmine

Pharmacological action. Similar to neostigmine but with a quarter of the potency. It is slower in onset, acting within 30–45 minutes and lasting for 4–6 hours.

Therapeutic uses. It is used, often in association with neostigmine, for myasthenia gravis, in a dose of 60–240 mg orally and 1–5 mg S.C. or I.M.

Contraindications and side effects. As neostigmine.

Ambenonium

Pharmacological action and therapeutic uses. Similar to neostigmine but longer lasting. It is used for myasthenia gravis especially when neostigmine is poorly tolerated. Dose: 5–25 mg three or four times daily.

Contraindications and side effects. As neostigmine but less marked.

Benzypyrinium

Pharmacological action and therapeutic uses. Another very similar compound. Dose: 2 mg I.M.

Edrophonium

Pharmacological action. Similar to neostigmine but its effect on skeletal muscle is much more marked and most of its effect is probably due to a direct action on the muscle receptor rather than inhibition of choline-esterase. It has a rapid onset and short duration of action.

Therapeutic use. It is particularly useful in the diagnosis of myasthenia gravis. A test dose of 2 mg is given I.V. and if there has been no untoward effect after 30 seconds a further 8 mg is given. With myasthenia there is immediate improvement and increase in muscle power which disappears within 5 minutes. It is therefore not suitable for routine use. It is also suitable for deciding in a myasthenic patient between weakness due to too much or too little neostigmine.

Contraindications and side effects. As neostigmine but very short-lived.

Dyflos (DFP)

Pharmacological action. Causes prolonged inhibition of choline-esterase as do many of the organophosphates. Its effect may last for two weeks and thus it is not suitable for systemic use. Its action resembles neostigmine and physostigmine and its particular value is as a miotic.

Therapeutic use. Eye drops are made up as a 10 per cent solution in arachis oil. Dose: 1 drop t.d.s. It is used as a miotic for glaucoma.

Contraindications and side effects. Ocular pain often occurs initially and there may be a transient rise in intra-ocular pressure. After prolonged medication iris cysts may develop which usually regress after treatment has ceased. DFP can be absorbed through the skin, conjunctiva and respiratory and gastrointestinal tracts. Its vapour is very toxic and thus eye drops are made up in an oily substance. Systemic administration via one or more of these routes leads to ciliary and iris spasm, transient bronchial constriction, muscle fibrillation, salivation, diarrhoea, urinary retention, restlessness, headache, convulsions, and collapse.

Most of these effects of poisoning can be controlled by I.M. or I.V. injections of 1–2 mg atropine sulphate. This may be repeated every 10–30 minutes until signs of atropinisation appear. 20 mg or more may be required. A specific choline-esterase reactivor, e.g. Pralidoxime (UK and USA) should be given (dose: 1–2 g. daily, I.M. or I.V.) and repeated as necessary. Artificial ventilation may be required.

Contraindications are as for neostigmine, with the additional exclusion that it should not be used for acute congestive (narrow angle) glaucoma as here it may cause a further rise in pressure; neither should it be used in the presence of retinal damage.

Ecothiopate

Pharmacological action and therapeutic uses. Very similar to dyflos. It is used as a miotic. It is usually used as an 0·25 per cent aqueous solution. Dose: from 1 drop alternate days to twice a day.

Contraindications and side effects. As dyflos.

PILOCARPINE

Pilocarpine

Pharmacological action. An alkaloid having the muscarinic effects of acetycholine with little of its nicotinic effects. It is used chiefly as a miotic and has about half the activity of physostigmine and acts for a shorter length of time. It has also been used to counteract the side effects of ganglion-blocking agents.

Therapeutic uses. As a miotic it is used as a 1 per cent solution; orally it is given in a dose of 2·5–12 mg.

Contraindications and side effects. Increased salivation, sweating and production of tears predominate. With excessive doses nausea, vomiting, diarrhoea, dyspnoea, confusion, tremor and convulsions may occur.

ANTI-CHOLINERGIC DRUGS

GANGLION-BLOCKING AGENTS

Hexamethonium/Mecamylamine/Pempidine/Pentolinium/ Trimetaphan

These are now chiefly used for the rapid control of an elevated blood pressure and are discussed in the section on HYPOTENSIVE DRUGS.

NEUROMUSCULAR BLOCKING AGENTS

Depolarising Agents

Suxamethonium (Succinylcholine, *USA***)**
Pharmacological action. This drug acts by depolarising voluntary muscle in a similar way to acetylcholine but as suxamethonium (succinylcholine) is destroyed less quickly the depolarisation temporarily persists. The onset of relaxation is preceded by a short period of contraction which causes pain if the patient is conscious, and probably causes the muscle pain which occurs for up to 3 days after its use. The effect of this drug is not reversed by cholinergic drugs. It is destroyed by plasma pseudo-cholinesterase.
Therapeutic uses. Dose: 30–50 mg I.V. It is used as a short-acting muscle relaxant in conjunction with major and minor surgical and manipulative procedures.

Contraindications and side effects. Prolonged apnoea will occur in those with a low or atypical plasma pseudo-cholinesterase. The former may occur with liver disease, severe anaemia, malnutrition or after treatment with anticholinesterases, e.g. neostigmine. The latter is an hereditary defect. A prolonged effect may also follow if streptomycin or neomycin is given soon after the administration of suxamethonium. Repeated doses can cause bradycardia and arrhythmias. Generalised muscle pain is a common after-effect and can be prevented by giving a small dose of a competitive blocking agent before the suxamethonium.

Non-Depolarising Agents

Tubocurarine
Pharmacological action. This drug acts by competing with acetylcholine for the receptors on the motor end-plate. It does not cause depolarisation but prevents its occurrence due to acetylcholine. This causes a flaccid paralysis. It develops within a minute of I.V. injection and lasts for 20–45 minutes. Tubocurarine also has a ganglion-blocking effect and causes tissue histamine to be released. These effects explain the occasional occurrence of a fall in blood pressure and the development of bronchospasm.

The action of tubocurarine is reversed by anticholinesterase drugs, e.g. neostigmine methylsulphate 2·5–5 mg I.V. preceded by 0·5–1 mg atropine I.V. to prevent the parasympathetic effects of the neostigmine.

Therapeutic uses. Dose: initially 5 mg I.V. as a test dose followed in 5 minutes by 10–20 mg I.V. Additional dose of 2–4 mg can be given at 30 minute intervals up to a total dose of 45 mg.

Dimethyltubocurarine bromide, chloride or iodide can be used instead of tubocurarine chloride and these drugs are all roughly three times as potent requiring about a third of the above dose. This drug is used to produce muscular relaxation during surgery and is also used to control muscle spasm and convulsions in tetanus.

Contraindications and side effects. It is rarely toxic but may occasionally lower the blood pressure and cause bronchospasm. Administration of tubocurarine before or after the use of suxamethonium can cause a state of neostigmine-resistant curarisation. This will require continued ventilation but usually settles after a few hours. It tends to occur in patients who are dehydrated, hypokalaemic or otherwise metabolically disturbed. Tubocurarine should not be used in patients with myasthenia or those with respiratory, hepatic or renal disease. Patients with carcinomatous neuromyopathies often give abnormal and prolonged responses to muscle relaxants. Potentiation occurs with ether, chlorpromazine and some antibiotics (e.g. streptomycin, neomycin and polymyxin).

Gallamine

Pharmacological action. It is similar to tubocurarine but has little effect on autonomic ganglia. It does not produce histamine release and is less potent and shorter-acting. Relaxation starts within 2 minutes and lasts for about 20 minutes.

Therapeutic uses. Dose: 80–120 mg I.V. Up to half of the initial amount can be given as a second dose. It is used to obtain shorter periods of muscular relaxation during surgery and to minimise the convulsions of shock therapy. Premedication with atropine is necessary to prevent excessive salivation.

Contraindications and side effects. As tubocurarine. In addition it may produce allergic reactions in people sensitive to iodine and occasionally causes a tachycardia which persists for a while after the relaxant effect has disappeared.

ATROPINE AND RELATED DRUGS

Atropine (dl-Hyoscyamine)

Pharmacological action. Centrally it initially stimulates and later depresses the nervous system. It reduces tremor and muscular rigidity especially in people with parkinsonism and may help oculogyric crises although the mechanism is unknown. Peripherally it blocks the muscarinic effects of acetylcholine and thus antagonises all the effects of acetylcholine except for those at autonomic ganglia and the neuromuscular junction. It has an antispasmodic action on smooth muscle and decreases secretions. It depresses vagal activity causing slowing of the heart. It is also an antiemetic.

On the eye it has both a mydriatic and cycloplegic action and may cause a rise in intraocular pressure.

Therapeutic uses. Dose: 0·25–2 mg orally, S.C. or I.M. Its effect on the gut is utilised in the treatment of peptic ulceration and pylorospasm. In congenital hypertrophic pyloric stenosis it is usually given as atropine methonitrate (UK)/atropine methylnitrate (USA) in a dose of 2–6 ml of a 0·01 per cent aqueous solution half an hour before feeds. The methonitrate has less effect on the central nervous system and is less toxic to infants. It is also used to control bronchial asthma in a compound adrenaline and atropine spray or as the methonitrate alone in a pressurised aerosol. However atropine may make bronchial secretions extremely viscid and sympathomimetic agents are often preferred.

Atropine is often used for its effect on the heart, e.g. to prevent vagal syncope and to correct the bradycardia due to digitalis, opiates, choline esters, pilocarpine or anticholine esterases. It has also been used for partial heart block. It is used as a premedication in view of its ability to reduce secretions and protect the heart from vagal inhibition. It has been used in parkinsonism and will also reduce the sialorrhoea, but other atropine-like agents, e.g. benzhexol are probably more suitable.

Atropine has an antiemetic effect but other drugs, e.g. cyclizine, meclozine, etc. cause less side effects. As a mydriatic and cycloplegic it is used as 1 per cent eye drops. Dilatation occurs within 30 minutes and may last 2 weeks. For this reason homatropine is usually preferred.

Contraindications and side effects. These include dry mouth, thirst, dilatation of pupils with loss of accommodation and photophobia, flushing, difficulty with micturition and constipation. Toxic doses cause restlessness, excitement, confusion and hallucinations, tachycardia and hyperpyrexia. Later drowsiness, stupor and generalised central depression may occur. Side effects may even occur with eye drops. Atropine must not be used on patients with a narrow angle between the iris or cornea or those who have developed glaucoma. It should be used with care in those with prostatic enlargement, ischaemic heart disease or cardiac failure, and should not be used in paralytic ileus. The danger of hyperpyrexia should be considered in unduly hot weather or climates.

Hyoscine (**scopolamine**)
Pharmacological action. Similar to atropine although its effect on the central nervous system is between 3 and 10 times as potent. This is usually a depressant effect although excitement can occur especially in the elderly.

Mydriasis is quicker in onset and of shorter duration.

Therapeutic uses. Dose: as atropine. It has been used for acute mania, parkinsonism and as an hypnotic. It is also used as a premedication, usually in combination with an opiate, and as a mydriatic.

Contraindications and side effects. As atropine but it should be avoided in the elderly.

Hyoscine hydrobromide
Pharmacological action. Very similar actions and uses to hyoscine.
Therapeutic use. Dose: 0·3–0·6 mg S.C.

Hyoscine butylbromide
Pharmacological action. It is often ineffective orally but parenterally it is an effective smooth muscle relaxant and is used for this effect on the cardia, stomach, colon and biliary and renal tracts. It does not have much effect on gastric secretion and unlike hyoscine it also has a blocking action at ganglia. Dose: 20–40 mg S.C. or I.M.; 10–20 mg I.V.

Hyoscine methobromide (Methscopolamine bromide, *USA*)
Pharmacological action. A quarternary amine which thus lacks the central action of atropine and is a more selective inhibitor of gastric secretion. It is longer acting than hyoscine.

Therapeutic use. Dose: orally 2·5–5 mg 8-hourly; 0·25 to 1 mg S.C. or I.M. three or four times a day.

Homatropine hydrobromide
Pharmacological action. Similar to atropine but rather weaker. As a mydriatic its action is more rapid and less prolonged although it may

last for 24 hours. The dilatation is easily reversed with physostigmine. It is rarely used systematically although the methobromide has been used for its effect on the gastrointestinal tract.
Therapeutic use. Dose: 0·5–2 mg as a 1 or 2 per cent solution.

Cyclopentolate
Pharmacological action and use. A mydriatic and cycloplegic agent quicker and shorter-acting than homatropine. Mydriasis develops within 10–20 minutes and cycloplegia soon after; the effect lasting for 6–12 hours. Dose: 1–2 drops of a 0·5 or 1 per cent solution. Its effect is best reversed by pilocarpine.

Lachesine
Pharmacological action and uses. A mydriatic and cycloplegic agent having a slower onset of action which is less prolonged than atropine, achieving a maximum at 1 hour and disappearing within 6 hours. It does not cause conjunctival irritation and is a useful alternative for those patients who show a sensitivity to substances of the atropine group. Usual dose is 2 drops of a 1 per cent solution.

Propantheline
Pharmacological action. It is one of many synthetic anticholine drugs and has a marked peripheral atropine-like effect with little effect on the CNS. It is also a weak ganglion-blocker and at very high doses has a curare-like effect on the neuromuscular junction.
Therapeutic uses. Dose: 15–30 mg orally, I.M. or I.V. Its more frequent use is to reduce gastric intestinal secretion and motility. It is an effective antispasmodic and may be given with an opiate for visceral colic to reduce the stimulating effect of the former on smooth muscle.
Contraindications and side effects. As for atropine with the additional hazard that in toxic doses paralysis of voluntary muscle may occur.

There are many more anticholinergic agents which have been developed for systemic use, chiefly for their effects in reducing spasm, motility and secretion in the gastrointestinal tract. Four further drugs will be mentioned by name, although they differ little from propantheline in their actions, uses and side effects.

Poldine
Pharmacological action and uses. This is a potent inhibitor of gastric secretion with a prolonged action. Dose: 2–4 mg orally, 6-hourly, but this often requires adjustment as atropine-like side effects are common at the higher dose levels.

Dicyclomine

Pharmacological action and uses. It is an antispasmodic similar to but weaker than atropine. It has also a mild local anaesthetic action. Dose: 10–20 mg orally, three or four times daily.

Tricyclamol

Pharmacological action and uses. Similar to atropine; it also has ganglion blocking activity in large doses. Dose: 50–100 mg orally four- or six-hourly before meals.

Isopropamide

Pharmacological action and uses. Similar to tricyclamol except that it has a more prolonged action. Dose: orally 5 mg 8–12-hourly.

References

1. Lands, A. M., Arnold, A., McAuliff, J. P., Luduena, F. P., and Brown, T. G., *Nature* (1967), (London), **214,** 597.
2. Burn, J. H., and Dornhorst, A. C., *in Recent Advances in Pharmacology* (1968), J. & A. Churchill, London. Edited by Robson, J. M., and Stacey, R. S., 4th Edition.
3. Turner, P., *in Fifth Symposium on Advanced Medicine* (1969). Edited by Roger Williams, Pitman Medical.
4. Palmer, K. N. V., Legge, J. S., Hamilton, W. F. D., and Diament, M. L., *Brit. Med. J.* (1970), **2,** 23.
5. Harris, L. H., *Brit. Med. J.* (1970), **4,** 597.
6. Palmer, K. N. V., and Diament, M. L., *Brit. Med. J.* (1969), **1,** 31.
7. Legge, J. S., Gaddie, J., and Palmer, K. N. V., *Brit. Med. J.* (1971), **1,** 637.
8. Riordan, J. F., and Walters, G., *Brit. Med. J.* (1969), **1,** 155.
9. Bonn, J. A., and Turner, P., *Lancet* (1971), **i,** 1355.
10. Ross, E. J., Prichard, B. N. C., Kaufman, L., Robertson, A. I. G., and Harris, B. J., *ibid.* (1967), **1,** 191.
11. Turner, P., *Clinical Aspects of Autonomic Pharmacology*, (1969), Heinemann.
12. Palmer, K. N. V., Legge, J. S., Hamilton, W. F. D., and Diament, M. L., *Lancet* (1969), **ii,** 1092.
13. Wilson, A. G., Brooke, O. G., Lloyd, H. J., and Robinson, B. F., *Brit. Med. J.* (1969), **4,** 399.
14. Jewitt, D. E., Mercer, C. J., and Shillingford, J. P., *Lancet* (1969), **ii,** 277.
15. Wilkins, J. L., Hardcastle, J. D., Mann, C. V., and Kaufman, L., *Brit. Med. J.* (1970), **i,** 793.

This chapter was written by Dr W. G. Reeves (Department of Clinical Pharmacology, Guy's Hospital Medical School) and edited by Professor J. R. Trounce.

Category 6

Drugs Used in Cardiac Disease

Digoxin

Pharmacological action. Digoxin is a pure glycoside obtained from the leaves of Digitalis lanata.

The action of the digitalis glycosides at the cellular level is uncertain, but it is possible that they affect the movement of ions across the cell membrane in such a way as to reduce the sodium and potassium gradients, whilst conserving calcium within the cell. The result of the former is to lead to an increased ease of depolarisation of the cell membrane – this could explain the toxic effects on the heart – and of the latter is to improve the contractility of the muscle fibre. In addition to these direct cellular actions the cardiac glycosides are known to increase vagal control of the heart.

The effects of digitalis glycosides are most readily seen in patients with cardiac failure and tachycardia, in whom they lower the venous pressure and slow the heart rate. Part of this slowing can be blocked by atropine but part is due to a direct action on the SA node. A greater slowing effect can be produced in patients with atrial fibrillation due to diminished conduction from the atria to the ventricles; it has recently been shown that digitalis increases the normal delay in the activation of the AV node by the atrial action potential. A more indirect effect is the occurrence of diuresis which is due to the improvement in the circulation. There is no useful action on the healthy myocardium and digitalis is of no benefit, therefore, where the impediment to the circulation is a mechanical one (e.g. valve stenosis or regurgitation) unless this is complicated by secondary myocardial failure. Unfortunately, the margin between the dose required to achieve the desired therapeutic response and that which leads to toxic effects is small.

Therapeutic use. Digitalis glycosides have their greatest use in the patient with myocardial failure and atrial fibrillation. It is of value also in the management of either of these disorders alone. When used in patients with atrial fibrillation the response of the ventricular rate is usually a convenient index as to the adequacy of treatment. In patients with sinus rhythm it is necessary to give the drug until the desired therapeutic result is obtained or until evidence of toxicity necessitates reduction of dosage.

Digitalis is also of value in the management of other arrhythmias particularly as a prophylaxis against paroxysms of supraventricular tachycardia in young subjects. In atrial flutter it may convert the rhythm to atrial fibrillation and then control the ventricular rate; sometimes it may succeed in increasing the degree of atrioventricular block without change of rhythm, thereby controlling the tachycardia, but more often this is not achieved before serious toxic effects are apparent. Rather surprisingly digitalis may also abolish ventricular or supraventricular ectopic beats, even though in toxic doses it may stimulate them. Digitalis is often ineffective in slowing the heart rate when infection, hyperthyroidism or anxiety are responsible for the tachycardia.

In general, older patients require less digitalis than younger ones; impairment of renal function reduces excretion and therefore the required dose; potassium depletion, most commonly the result of diuretic therapy, potentiates the toxicity of digitalis and this must be watched for in patients on diuretics.

Digoxin has the same actions as digitoxin or prepared digitalis but it is absorbed more rapidly and has a quicker onset of action. It is also available for intramuscular or intravenous injection; the latter is to be preferred as the preparation is irritating and absorption from an intramuscular site is less reliable. By mouth it takes effect in about an hour and peak activity is reached in 6 to 7 hours; by injection onset of effect may be detected in 10 to 15 minutes and the full effect is obtained by 2 hours. After stopping the drug the effect lasts for several days.

Because of its more rapid onset of action digoxin has especial value in the urgent treatment of left heart failure with uncontrolled atrial fibrillation. It is also particularly useful in the management of infants in heart failure where its greater flexibility of use is an advantage.

For rapid effect the usual adult oral loading dose is 1·0 to 1·5 mg followed by 0·25 to 0·5 mg every 6 hours until the desired therapeutic response is achieved. Maintenance usually requires 0·25 mg once to thrice daily. Intravenously 0·5 to 1·0 mg may be given, provided no digitalis preparation has been given in the previous two weeks; if digitalis has been given, not more than 0·25 mg should be given at any one time and at least two hours should elapse between each injection for its effect to be assessed.

For children the loading dose can be calculated on the basis of 0·025 mg per kg bodyweight, either by mouth or injection every 6 hours, adjusted to an appropriate maintenance dose when the desired response is achieved. The administration of small fractional doses is facilitated by the availability of tablets of 0·0625 mg, i.e. one-quarter of the normal 0·25 mg tablet.

Contraindications and side effects. Although theoretically digitalis should not be given to patients with ectopic beats, ventricular arrhythmias or early after myocardial infarction, because of its known potentiating effect on depolarisation, in practice it should not be withheld on these grounds if its use is otherwise indicated.

Gastrointestinal disturbances, anorexia, nausea, vomiting, and sometimes diarrhoea, are usually the first manifestations of digitalis toxicity. Other, less common, non-cardiac manifestations include headache, facial pain, drowsiness, mental confusion, and blurring of vision and, rarely, disturbances of colour vision, so that objects seen by the patient take on a yellow or green hue.

The more serious toxic effects of the digitalis are related to its action on the heart. Ectopic beats, usually ventricular and characteristically coupled to the preceding normal beat are common. In some cases they occur so regularly that they produce pulsus bigeminus which can be readily recognised clinically. When this is not so it is important in patients with atrial fibrillation to ensure that the increased rate and irregularity of the heart beat is not misinterpreted as indicating a lack of control of the atrial fibrillation necessitating an increased dose. Patients previously in sinus rhythm may develop paroxysmal atrial tachycardia with varying atrioventricular block; and in patients with atrial fibrillation the occurrence of a regular ventricular rhythm due to AV junctional rhythm is usually an indication of toxicity; the continued or increased administration of digitalis in these situations is likely to be fatal. Ventricular tachycardia and later ventricular fibrillation are the usual fatal disturbances of rhythm. Other effects are sinus bradycardia and increased atrioventricular block, at first only detectable on the electrocardiogram but later leading to slowing of the ventricular rate. The use of recently developed techniques for estimating plasma digoxin indicates that toxicity is related to plasma levels; levels of less than 1·5 mg/ml are unlikely to be associated with toxic effects.

Prepared digitalis (Digitalis leaf)

Pharmacological action. As for digoxin.

Prepared digitalis is the dried leaf of the Foxglove, Digitalis pur-

purea, adjusted by dilution to a standard activity ascertained by biological assay. It contains a number of glycosides.

Therapeutic uses. The usual initial leading dose for an adult is between 1·0 and 1·5 g. given in divided doses over 24 hours; maintenance usually requires 100 to 200 mg daily. It is readily absorbed but its full effect takes some hours to develop; it is slowly excreted and once established the effect may take several days or even weeks to wear off. Now that pure glycoside preparations, which do not require biological assay, are readily available, prepared digitalis is little used.

Contraindications and side effects. As for digoxin.

Digitoxin

Pharmacological action. As for digoxin.

Digitoxin is a crystalline glycoside obtained from the leaves of several species of Digitalis.

Therapeutic use. Digitoxin has properties which are almost identical with those of prepared digitalis, including its slow onset of action and the persistence of its effect. Digitoxin is the most potent (weight for weight) of the cardiac glycosides and the most persistent in its effect; accumulation with prolonged administration may therefore be a problem. There is some clinical evidence that the gastrointestinal side effects are less pronounced than with some other glycosides. In general, however, its slow onset of effect and persistence outweigh this slight advantage and, although widely used in some countries, it would seem to be less convenient than digoxin.

Owing to its high potency the initial loading dose is about 1·0 mg in divided dose and the maintenance dose is between 0·05 and 0·2 mg daily. Preparations for intravenous administration are available but the onset of the effect when given by this route is no faster than when it is given by mouth.

Contraindications and side effects. As for digoxin.

Lanatoside C

Pharmacological action. As for digoxin.

Deslanoside is desacetyl-lanatoside C and is the active material used for intravenous preparations corresponding to the orally administered lanatoside C. Their properties are virtually identical. Lanatoside C is a glycoside obtained from the leaf of Digitalis lanata.

Therapeutic use. These preparations have virtually the same uses as digoxin but have a more rapid onset of action (10 minutes) and a more rapid clearance. They are also reputed to have a larger margin between the therapeutic and toxic dose. For these reasons the intravenous preparation particularly is sometimes of use in rapidly changing situations.

The initial loading dose of lanatoside C given by mouth is about 1·0 to 1·5 mg with a daily maintenance dose of 0·25–0·75 mg daily for adults and a loading dose of 0·025 to 0·05 mg per lb bodyweight for children. For deslanoside given intravenously, the corresponding doses are, for adults 0·8 to 1·2 mg followed by 0·4 mg doses every 2–4 hours as required and, for children 0·01 mg per lb bodyweight.

Contraindications and side effects. As for digoxin.

Aminophylline

Pharmacological action. Aminophylline is a mixture of theophylline and ethylenediamine; the latter helps to improve the solubility of the theophylline and also increases its pharmacological activity. The principal effect of aminophylline is to relax the tone of involuntary muscle, especially of the bronchial tree. It lowers the venous pressure in patients with congestive heart failure. It has a weak diuretic action and also appears to increase the sensitivity of the respiratory centre to increasing carbon dioxide tension.

Therapeutic use. When administered by intravenous injection it has a very rapid beneficial effect on bronchospasm. It is probably most often used for severe bronchial asthma but because of its combination of effects it is of great value in the management of cardiac asthma. The usual dose is 250 mg in 10 ml of solution injected *slowly*.

Aminophylline is not satisfactorily given by mouth because it is a gastric irritant. Several proprietary preparations of aminophylline or closely related substances have been developed to permit oral use; in general they do not have the same potency as the injected drug. It is well absorbed through the rectal mucosa so that, in the form of suppositories, patients can use it for the prevention or relief of attacks of paroxysmal nocturnal dyspnoea. In the UK the suppositories normally contain 360 mg but in the USA they are available with 125, 250 or 500 mg.

Contraindications and side effects. Side effects have been most commonly associated with too-rapid injection; this may lead to restlessness, palpitation, dizziness, nausea, or hypotension. Sudden death has been reported following intravenous injection in normal doses and again this has been associated with rapid injection.

Serious toxic effects appear to have been reported most frequently in children, which suggests that in them its use requires greater caution than in adults.

Quinidine

Pharmacological action. Quinidine is the dextro-rotatory stereo-isomer of quinine. Its principal therapeutic effect is prolongation of the refractory period of cardiac muscle, thereby reducing the rate at which successive contractions can occur. It does, however, have a powerful general depressive action on the myocardium, reducing excitability, contractility and conduction, and it also has some atropine-like action, reducing vagal tone. It has recently been shown that its effect on atrio-ventricular conduction is due to prolongation of the conduction of the impulse from the AV node to the ventricular myocardium (cp. action of digoxin on conduction).

Therapeutic use. Quinidine is a potent cardiac-depressant anti-arrhythmic drug, although considered by many to be too toxic for common use. The recent introduction of other less dangerous substances and the advent of the electric-shock correction of arrhythmias have now reduced its usefulness. It does, however, still have a place in the management of some patients with rhythm disturbance, especially if these are supraventricular. It is often effective in correcting or preventing atrial or ventricular tachy-arrhythmias and in abolishing atrial or ventricular ectopic beats. When used for the treatment of supraventricular tachycardias (e.g. atrial flutter) with some degree of atrioventricular block, digitalis should be given first to avoid a sudden, possibly dangerous, increase in ventricular rate which can result from one-to-one conduction developing as the rate of the supraventricular focus is slowed.

Although quinidine may be given intravenously with the protection of electrocardiographic control in urgent cases, e.g. to stop ventricular tachycardia when the patient's life is threatened, it is usually given by mouth. The desired therapeutic response is commonly obtained with a blood level of about 6–8 mg/l. Blood levels above 10 mg/l are associated with a high incidence of toxic effects. The effects of the drug are not, however, uniformly related to the blood level and electrocardiographic monitoring of the response is an alternative way of controlling the dose; the drug may be given until some prolongation of the PR interval and QT time are apparent and changes in the ST segment and T waves occur. An increase in these effects and a widening of the QRS complex are evidence of excessive dosage. Various dose schedules have been described using repeated doses at short intervals to build up higher blood levels each day on top of the residue left from the previous day; a common one uses 0·3 g. or 0·4 g. every 2 hours for 5 doses on successive days for about 3 or 4 days; if necessary the individual dose may be increased to 0·5 g. on the fourth or fifth day and to 0·6 g. on the sixth day. Before starting full therapeutic doses a test dose of 0·2 g. should be given to detect any hypersensitivity.

Contraindications and side effects. Quinidine is absolutely contraindicated by a history of serious reaction to the drug and is given with an increased risk to patients with heart block, or bundle branch block, severe congestive cardiac failure and renal failure, especially in the presence of hyperkalaemia. Individuals may show hypersensitivity to the drug by developing tinnitus, vertigo, blurring of vision or blindness, headache, confusion, rashes, bronchospasm, gastrointestinal disturbances, fever, collapse with hypotension or death from ventricular fibrillation. These reactions may also occur as dose-related side-effects; thrombocytopenic purpura has also been reported. Increase of the width of the QRS complex by more than 25 per cent of its control value, the development of bundle branch block, of second degree or complete heart block, of ventricular ectopic beats, or atrial standstill are all indications of cardiac toxicity and call for withdrawal of the drug before ventricular tachycardia, fibrillation or asystole occur.

Procainamide

Pharmacological action. Procainamide hydrochloride, has a depressant action on the myocardium, diminishing the excitability, conductivity and contractility of both atrium and ventricle, and prolonging the refractory period of the atrium. It has been shown that, like quinidine, its action on atrio-ventricular conductivity is distal to the AV node.

Therapeutic use. It is chiefly of use in suppressing ventricular ectopic beats or arrhythmias; it has some effect on atrial arrhythmias and may even convert atrial fibrillation to sinus rhythm, but it is less successful in the management of supraventricular arrhythmias. For the rapid correction of serious arrhythmias, such as ventricular tachycardia, it may be given intravenously but caution is required as it can precipitate depression of myocardial activity with severe hypotension and sometimes the initiation of ventricular fibrillation. It is more safely given by mouth and, when used for the correction of a rhythm disturbance, the dose is 1·0 g. followed by 0·25 to 1·0 g. every four to six hours. For the long-term prevention of ectopic beats the usual dose is 500 mg every four to six hours. Larger doses are sometimes required. When used intravenously the dose for the control of ventricular arrhythmias is 0·2 to 1·0 g. injected slowly in dilute solution.

Contraindications and side effects. Procainamide antagonises the action of sulphonamides. It should be avoided in patients subject to bronchial asthma and those known to be hypersensitive to it, in patients with renal failure and those with conduction defects of the heart.

Reported side effects include anorexia, nausea, vomiting and diarrhoea, with large oral doses, and severe hypotension when given intravenously. Prolonged or repeated administration may lead to a syndrome resembling systemic lupus erythematosus, leucopenia, granulocytopenia or, rarely, fatal agranulocytosis. Abdominal pain, hepatomegaly with evidence of liver damage, confusion, pruritis and hyper-sensitivity with fever and urticaria have also been described.

Lignocaine (Lidocaine, *USA***)**

Pharmacological action. Although primarily used for its local anaesthetic action, lignocaine decreases cardiac excitability. It differs, however, in having little or no depressant effect on myocardial contractility.

Therapeutic use. Lignocaine is not effective when given by mouth and is more useful in the treatment of ventricular rhythm disorders. Given intravenously it is used to suppress ventricular ectopic beats or to arrest and prevent ventricular tachycardia, especially after myocardial infarction or cardiac surgery. It may be given as a single dose of 1–2 mg per kg of bodyweight or by continuous intravenous infusion at a rate of 1–2 mg per minute.

Contraindications and side effects. Lignocaine should be used with caution in the presence of heart block as it can give rise to asystole. The development of serious tachycardia due to the development of 1:1 conduction as may happen with quinidine (see above) when used in the presence of atrial flutter has been reported. The earliest side effects are drowsiness, euphoria and muscular fasciculation; larger doses may produce hypotension, apprehension, confusion, nausea, vomiting, convulsions and ultimately respiratory and circulatory collapse.

Phenytoin sodium (Sodium diphenylhydantoin, *USA*)

Pharmacological action. In addition to its anticonvulsant action, phenytoin has been shown to have some anti-arrhythmic effect on the heart. The precise mode of action of phenytoin is uncertain, although it appears to have a depressant effect on pacemaker tissue and on myocardial function; unlike other anti-arrhythmic drugs it does not appear to delay activation of the AV node or slow conduction from the node to the ventricles.

Therapeutic use. It is said to be most effective in correcting supraventricular and ventricular arrhythmias resulting from digitalis intoxication and to be of use in preventing paroxysmal arrhythmias. It is not effective in the correction of atrial flutter or fibrillation. The true value of this drug as an anti-arrhythmic agent still remains to be determined.

It may be administered intravenously as a single dose of up to about 250 mg (or 5 mg per kg bodyweight), injected slowly, followed by maintenance doses of 200–400 mg orally, or by intramuscular injection.

Contraindications and side effects. As it may itself produce bradycardia or atrioventricular block it should not be used when either of these are already present; it probably has an additive effect with procainamide or lignocaine in depressing pacemaker tissue so should be used with caution in patients who have recently received these drugs. Sinus arrest has been reported after administration of 250 mg intravenously.

Intravenous injection can produce hypotension. Prolonged administration can, of course, produce the toxic effects which are better known in relation to its use as an anticonvulsant.

Propranolol

Pharmacological action. Propranolol hydrochloride is one of a series of compounds with structures related to that of the natural catecholamines, synthesised in a search for a substance which would block the effect of the stimulation of the β-sympathetic receptors. It slows the sinus rate and reduces myocardial contractility to some extent in the resting state but has a more obvious effect in reducing the tachycardia and increase in cardiac output which normally occurs in response to exercise. The subsequent demonstration that propranolol was a racemic mixture of stereoisomers, each of which has slightly different effects, and the preparation of other clinically related substances, each with its own differing spectrum of effects, suggests that the hypothetical concept of β-receptor blockade is an over-simplification; nonetheless, the observed effects mentioned above remain true. In addition, propranolol seems to have an action on the myocardial cell membrane resembling that of quinidine. Apart from its cardiac actions it also blocks the broncho-dilator sympathetic action.

Therapeutic use. Propranolol found its first application as an anti-arrhythmic agent; it is effective in abolishing ectopic beats occurring during anaesthesia and, with digitalis, will often reduce the ventricular rate in atrial fibrillation when digitalis alone fails to do so. It is very effective in controlling sinus tachycardia related to anxiety. It has also been found useful in controlling arrhythmias induced by digitalis intoxication and in hyperthyroidism, where the cardiovascular disturbance is mediated by sympathetic over-activity. It is an effective antidote to tachycardia or rhythm disturbance induced by sympathetic amines therapeutically administered or produced endogenously by a phaeochromocytoma.

Its effect of impairing myocardial contractility led to its trial in the management of patients with hypertrophic obstructive cardiomyopathy (muscular subaortic stenosis) and of patients with Fallot's tetralogy subject to cyanotic attacks, whose right ventricular outflow obstruction was presumably variable due to a muscular mechanism at infundibular level; in both groups it has proved of value in some cases.

For the above purposes it is usually given orally three or four times a day in doses from 10 to 40 mg each; initially the full desired effect is often obtained by a small dose but it is commonly necessary subsequently to increase this to maintain the response. In acute situations, and when used under anaesthesia, it may be given by intravenous injection; the initial dose then should be only 1–2 mg given slowly, followed by further doses, if required, as the effect of the drug can be assessed; it is recommended, particularly in patients with recent myocardial infarction, that intravenous administration should be preceded by 1–2 mg atropine injected intravenously or bradycardia may occur.

The reduction by propranolol of the normal increase in the cardiac output on exercise suggested that it might be of value in the treatment of angina pectoris by limiting the myocardial demand for oxygen. It has been found to be of considerable value in this respect but maintenance of the response is usually dependent upon considerable increases in the dose up to levels of over 80 mg four times a day. Initial reports that it is of value in the treatment of hypertension remain to be confirmed by subsequent studies (see page 183).

Contraindications and side effects. Because of its action on the sympathetic nervous control of the bronchiolar musculature it should not be used for patients subject to asthma or bronchospasm of any cause. Because of its myocardial depressant effect, it should not be used in patients with myocardial failure or heart block. Even in patients with no clinical evidence of myocardial failure beforehand, propranolol administration has been held responsible for its development subsequently, especially when given on a long-term basis in high doses, usually for the control of angina pectoris. Intravenous administration, especially if the initial dose is rather large (10 mg or more), has been followed by hypotension, extreme bradycardia and occasionally the precipitation of ventricular fibrillation.

Propranolol may also cause nausea, vomiting, diarrhoea, lassitude, depression or insomnia; these effects are reduced by initial low dosage. Less commonly it has produced rashes, non-thrombocytopenic purpura, hallucinations and paraesthesiae.

Practolol

Pharmacological action. Practolol is another of the compounds which can block β-sympathetic activity. It differs from propranolol (q.v.) in not having direct myocardial depressant activity, in having some intrinsic sympathetic stimulant activity and not having any blocking action on the sympathetic innervation of bronchial muscle.

Therapeutic use. Because it has no direct myocardial depressing effect and does not enhance bronchospasm, practolol is to be preferred to propranolol when treating patients with left heart failure or a tendency to bronchospasm. It is very effective in controlling supraventricular tachycardias and the ventricular rate in atrial fibrillation or flutter; for this it is used in an oral dose of 100 mg two or three times a day or it can be given intravenously in a dose of from 5–25 mg. In considerably larger doses (e.g. 1,200 mg a day) it is used for the management of angina pectoris. It has been recommended for the treatment of hypertension but does not seem to be very effective in this respect.

Contraindications and side effects. Compared with propranolol it has few side effects, though in large doses it may give rise to diarrhoea. It is contraindicated in patients who already have bradycardia or who have atrioventricular block.

Oxprenolol

Pharmacological action. Oxprenolol hydrochloride has actions similar to propranolol and practolol. It differs from propranolol, however, in possessing intrinsic sympathetic stimulating activity and it differs from practolol in being less cardio-selective so that it also has some blocking action on bronchiolar sympathetic endings.

Therapeutic uses. It is of value in the treatment of arrhythmias, particularly those of supraventricular origin or due to digitalis intoxication. The oral dose is 20–40 mg two or three times a day. It appears to be useful after myocardial infarction, having less myocardial depressant activity, and may suppress ventricular ectopic activity when lignocaine fails to do so; for this purpose it may be given by intravenous injections of 2 mg followed by infusion at a rate of 0·25 mg/minute. It has been reported to be particularly effective in the management of angina pectoris, but adequate comparative studies with other β-blocking agents are not yet available. The dose for angina pectoris starts with 40 mg twice daily, increasing after a few days to 120–200 mg a day (in divided doses); up to 800 mg daily has been used.

Contraindications and side effects. As with other β-blocking agents it is contraindicated in patients with atrioventricular block or bradycardia. Like propranolol, though not to so great a degree, it should be used with caution in patients with a tendency to bronchospasm. It may produce gastro-intestinal disturbances and a feeling of lassitude, but these can usually be avoided by starting with small doses and increasing the dose gradually. Hypertension and ventricular fibrillation have been recorded after intravenous administration in acute situations (e.g. ventricular tachycardia after myocardial infarction). Aggravation of angina or the development of status anginosus has been described following withdrawal of treatment with oxprenolol.

Bretylium Tosylate

Pharmacological action. Bretylium tosylate acts presynaptically and blocks all sympathetic nervous activity but does not block the effect of circulating catecholamines. It has a positive inotropic action on heart muscle but it is not clear how this is mediated. In animals it has been shown to raise the threshold for the electrical induction of ventricular fibrillation.

Therapeutic use. Originally introduced for the treatment of hypertension but since superseded by more satisfactory agents, bretylium tosylate has recently been advocated for the management of ventricular arrhythmias after myocardial infarction. It is reported to suppress ventricular ectopic beats and to prevent ventricular fibrillation whilst at the same time improving cardiac performance. Intravenous administration may cause nausea or vomiting so it is better administered by intramuscular injections or 300 mg, unless the situation is urgent; the dose can be repeated every 6–12 hours and supplementary doses of 100 mg may be given according to need at hourly intervals.

Contraindications and side effects. By all routes of administration it tends to produce loose stools. Its pharmacological action produces postural hypotension but this is not a problem in recumbent patients; supine hypotension occurs only occasionally. Nasal stuffiness is also reported but is not a serious problem.

Glyceryl trinitrate

Pharmacological action. Several organic nitrites and nitrates have a direct action on involuntary muscle, producing relaxation; this effect results in widespread vasodilatation. The distribution and degree of this varies with different compounds but in the case of glyceryl trinitrate is widespread and includes the coronary arterial vessels, but with relatively little effect on the skin vessels. Recent studies have demonstrated that it produces a reduction in the resistance of the coronary circulation but that this is offset by the fall in blood pressure which results from the more generalised vasodilatation so that the myocardial blood flow is diminished; the fall in systemic blood pressure, however, is such that the myocardial work is decreased by a proportion which is greater than that of the reduction of myocardial blood flow. The net result is an increase in myocardial blood flow relative to its work.

Therapeutic use. Glyceryl trinitrate, in the form of 0·5 mg tablets allowed to dissolve in the mouth so that it is absorbed through the oral mucosa, is used for the prevention and relief of angina pectoris. It acts within two or three minutes and the effect lasts for 15 to 30 minutes. Repeated use leads to the development of tolerance but a cessation of use for a few days re-establishes the normal effect.

Contraindications and side effects. Glyceryl trinitrate causes a rise in intraocular tension, so should be avoided in patients with glaucoma. It also causes widespread dilatation of the blood vessels of the head and neck and in some individuals this results in distressing headache or throbbing in the head; it should be used with caution in patients with cerebrovascular disease, intracranial lesions or recent head injury. In some patients the hypotensive effect produces a sensation of syncope which may be accompanied by nausea or vomiting.

Amyl nitrite

Pharmacological action. Similar to glyceryl trinitrate but with a greater effect on the skin vessels, especially of the face and neck.

Therapeutic use. Amyl nitrite is a highly volatile liquid administered by inhalation of the vapour released by crushing a glass capsule containing 0·2 ml of the liquid. It has an effect in about 10 seconds which lasts only 2–3 minutes. Its penetrating odour and the abruptness and intensity of the vasodilatation of the head and face make it objectionable to many patients.

Contraindications and side effects. As for glyceryl trinitrate.

Sorbide nitrate (Isosorbide dinitrate, *USA*)

Pharmacological action. As for glyceryl trinitrate.

Therapeutic use. When given as a 10 mg tablet dissolved in the mouth its effect is produced in about 10 to 15 minutes and lasts up to 4 hours. With this slower, but more prolonged action it is of little use for the immediate relief of angina pectoris but is recommended as a prophylactic; it is widely used for this purpose in the USA but the reported trials have mostly been uncontrolled and the results have been conflicting.

Pentaerythritol

Pharmacological action. As for glyceryl trinitrate.

Therapeutic use. When given by mouth pentaerythritol tetranitrate produces some fall in the blood pressure after about an hour, which lasts for about 5 hours. It is therefore of no value in the treatment of the acute attack of angina pectoris. It is commonly used as a prophylactic agent although many trials have failed to show any statistically significant benefit. The dose is from 20 to 30 mg.

Dipyridamole

Pharmacological action. Extensive studies in experimental animals and in man have established that dipyridamole has a remarkably selective, but powerful, vasodilator action on the coronary blood vessels, leading to a significant increase in coronary blood flow. It also appears to have an effect in inhibiting platelet clumping.

Therapeutic use. The pharmacological action of dipyridamole led to the expectation that it would be of value in the treatment of ischaemic heart disease; so far no study has shown that it is of any benefit in that condition. It can be given by mouth in a dose of 25 to 50 mg two or three times daily or by slow intravenous injection in a dose of 10 to 20 mg.

Contraindications and side effects. There do not appear to be any contraindications to its use; it may cause anorexia or nausea, headache, dizziness, or faintness and occasionally, after intravenous injection, facial flushing or some fall in the blood pressure.

Prenylamine

Pharmacological action. Like dipyridamole, prenylamine lactate has been shown to have a powerful coronary vascular dilating effect. It also has a slight hypotensive action which is probably mediated by an antagonistic effect against sympathetic activity.

Therapeutic use. The combination of coronary vasodilatation and sympathetic blockade suggests that this drug should be of value in the treatment of angina pectoris. Several trials have reported its successful use as a prophylactic agent in a dose of 60 mg two to four times a day.

Contraindications and side effects. Prenylamine is contraindicated in the presence of conduction defects, heart failure, or hepatic disease. Patients already receiving hypotensive agents may require some reduction in the dose whilst receiving prenylamine. Gastric intolerance has been reported occasionally when the drug is first administered; rashes rarely occur.

Cholestyramine

Pharmacological action. Cholestyramine is a basic anion-exchange resin which binds bile acids in the intestine and thereby prevents their resorption and interferes with the absorption of other lipids.

Therapeutic use. In total daily doses of between 12 and 15 g. cholestyramine has been shown to reduce the blood-cholesterol levels in patients with type II hyperlipidaemia and has been used to correct this biochemical deviation in the hope of reducing the risk of development of atheroma. It is also said to be effective in relieving itching in obstructive jaundice.

Contraindications and side effects. It may produce gastrointestinal discomfort.

Clofibrate

Pharmacological action. Clofibrate lowers elevated serum triglyceride and cholesterol levels by its effects upon low-density β-lipoproteins. These effects appear to result from the binding of clofibrate to specific sites on the plasma proteins which in turn leads to a redistribution between the plasma and liver of several factors which affect the blood-lipid pattern. It also seems to correct a number of factors which produce the hypercoagulability often associated with atherosclerotic disease.

Therapeutic uses. Prolonged administration is used in patients with atherosclerosis, especially if this is manifest by clinical evidence of coronary heart disease, cerebral or peripheral vascular disease and those with type IV hyperlipidaemia or diabetic arteriopathy in the hope of reducing progression of vascular disease. Recent reports state that in patients with angina it can reduce the risk of myocardial infraction and early death from coronary disease. The drug is introduced gradually and is then maintained at 20 to 30 mg per kg bodyweight daily in divided doses.

Contraindications and side effects. Clofibrate should not be given during pregnancy, or to patients with impaired renal or hepatic function. It potentiates the action of anticoagulant drugs and, in some patients, of insulin so that it should be introduced cautiously to patients receiving these. It may cause nausea, gastrointestinal discomfort, drowsiness or produce rashes; a gain in weight frequently follows its administration. A rise in serum transaminases and a fall in alkaline phosphatase levels may occur but are probably related to the action of the drug rather than to hepatotoxicity.

Isoprenaline (Isoproterenol, ***USA*****)**

Pharmacological action. Isoprenaline is a potent stimulator of the β-receptors of the sympathetic nervous system. It increases the heart rate, improves atrio-ventricular conduction, increases myocardial contractility and produces predominant vasodilation in the systemic circulation.

Therapeutic use. It is of considerable value in improving myocardial function in patients who have had recent myocardial infarction or undergone major cardiac surgery and thereby leads to improved tissue perfusion. For this purpose it is infused intravenously as 2 to 5 mg diluted in 500 ml of 5 per cent. dextrose at a rate of from 2 to 50 drops per minute, carefully controlled and adjusted according to the response of the patient whose electrocardiogram should be under continuous oscilloscope observation. In the form of tablets of 30 mg contained in a slow release base it can be given by mouth to increase the idioventricular rate or improve the conduction in patients with complete heart block.

Contraindications and side effects. Isoprenaline should not be given to patients with hyperthyroidism or who have any form of ventricular arrhythmia. It can provoke tachycardia, ectopic beats and ventricular fibrillation. Headache, palpitations, anginal pain, flushing, apprehension, tremor, nausea and weakness are common side effects of overdosage.

Atropine

Pharmacological action. In relation to the cardiovascular system atropine blocks the inhibiting effect of vagal activity on the sinus and atrioventricular nodes. If the heart is affected by increased vagal tone atropine increases the heart rate and reduces the atrioventricular conduction time.

Therapeutic use. It is the specific treatment for vagally mediated bradycardia with or without atrioventricular conduction defect such as may occur from digitalis intoxication or reflexly after myocardial infarction, DC shock correction of arrhythmias, or in response to procedures such as aortic catheterization or cardiac puncture. For this purpose it can be given by intravenous injection of between 0·25 and 1·5 mg.

Contraindications and side effects. See above.

Calcium chloride

Pharmacological action. In relation to the cardiovascular system it is a powerful stimulator of myocardial contractility.

Therapeutic use. The effect of calcium chloride is transient so that it is of no value for long-term treatment but a slow injection of 0·5 to 2 g. intravenously will often restore the contractility of an asystolic ventricle or improve that of a fibrillating ventricle so as to permit successful electrical defibrillation.

Contraindications and side effects. Calcium chloride should not be used if digitalis intoxication is a possible cause of the arrhythmia. Calcium chloride is irritating to the tissues so that care must be exercised during intravenous injection.

This chapter was written by Dr D. C. Deuchar (Physician to the Cardiac Dept, Guy's Hospital) and edited by Prof. J. R. Trounce.

Category 7

Drugs Used in the Treatment of Hypertensive Disease

RAUWOLFIA ALKALOIDS

This group of alkaloids are mild hypotensive agents. They may be used either as various crude fractions or as the pure alkaloids (reserpine, rescinnamine, deserpidine). Reserpine is the most widely used.

Reserpine

Pharmacological action. Reserpine lowers blood pressure by reducing the activity of the sympathetic nervous system and also by a tranquillizing and depressing action on the brain. Reserpine depletes catecholamines in both the peripheral sympathetic nervous system and in the brain and it seems probable its effects are due to this depletion.

Therapeutic uses. Reserpine in doses of up to 0·25 mg twice daily has a moderate blood pressure lowering action which is unrelated to posture, and which is due to fall in peripheral resistance. It is well absorbed from the intestine but it is usually four or five days before it begins to lower the blood pressure and it may be a week or two before it becomes fully effective. Likewise its activity will continue for several days after stopping the drug. At this dosage level side effects can be troublesome and a lower dose (0·25 mg daily) may be used, combined with a diuretic.

There are a number of other preparations available which contain reserpine or related alkaloids. They include:

Methoserpedine, 10 mg
Rescinnamine, 0·35 mg } equivalent to 0·25 mg of Reserpine
Deserpedine, 0·5 mg

There is no evidence that they have any advantage over reserpine.

The other actions of reserpine can be grouped:

(a) Sympatholytic effects: including bradycardia, nasal stuffiness and extrasystoles. There may also be increased gastrointestinal motor activity with a raised gastric acid secretion and occasionally peptic ulceration and diarrhoea.

(b) Central effects can be troublesome. Some drowsiness and general lack of 'go' with decreased libido is common, and occasionally a psychotic depression develops. With large doses a Parkinson-like state can be produced.

In addition, patients may show weight gain due to fluid retention.

Contraindications and side effects. Reserpine should not be used in depressed patients and should be used with care in those with intestinal disease, particularly peptic and ulcerative colitis. In a patient on reserpine, a general anaesthetic may provoke a considerable fall in blood pressure, though this is not universally accepted.

MISCELLANEOUS HYPOTENSIVE AGENTS

Hydrallazine

Pharmacological action. Hydrallazine [1] produces a widespread vasodilatation with a fall in blood pressure which is not usually affected by posture. The greatest fall is in the diastolic pressure. This is accompanied by a rise in pulse rate and cardiac output which to some extent neutralises the hypotensive action of the drug. How this rise in cardiac output is achieved is not known but it is possible that hydrallazine reflexly augments the actions of the adrenergic nervous system.

Hydrallazine is well absorbed and the drug is largely metabolised.

Therapeutic uses. Hydrallazine is a mild blood pressure lowering agent and its use is limited by the high incidence of side effects. The initial dose is 10 mg four times daily, and this is gradually increased to a total of 100–200 mg daily. In order to prevent the rise in pulse rate and cardiac output which accompanies its use hydrallazine may be combined with propranolol (see above). It increases renal blood flow and is therefore said to be particularly useful in hypertension complicating renal disease.

Contraindication and side effects. Headaches are particularly common at the start of treatment, but usually disappear after a week or so of continued treatment. They may be accompanied by nausea and diarrhoea. In the higher dose range (over 400 mg daily) and after prolonged treatment about 10 per cent of patients show a rheumatoid-like syndrome, sometimes accompanied by a positive L.E. phenomena. This may take a considerable time to subside after stopping the drug.

Hydrallazine may also produce skin rashes and rarely a peripheral neuropathy.

The rise in pulse rate and output caused by hydrallazine may precipitate anginal pain in those with coronary disease. Under these circumstances it should be combined with propranolol.

Clonidine (Catapres)

Pharmacological action. In acute experiments clonidine causes a fall in blood pressure associated with a drop in cardiac output. With long term administration, however, the fall in blood pressure is probably due to a depressing action on the vasomotor centre and is not related to posture.

Resistance to the hypotensive action of clonidine can develop. It appears to be due to associated sodium retention and can be reversed by a diuretic.

Therapeutic use. Clonidine will lower blood pressure effectively in hypertensives. The lack of postural fall is an advantage and impotence is not a feature of its action. However, side effects are rather common. Its place in treating hypertension is probably as a substitute for methyldopa when that drug for some reason is unsatisfactory. The initial dose is 200 micrograms daily and increased as required.

It has also been found useful in preventing attacks of migraine. The initial dose should be small and it may take several weeks to become effective.

Contraindication and side effects. The most frequent are sedation and a dry mouth. Peripheral vasoconstriction with 'cold hands' has been reported. It should be avoided in those with manic or depressive tendencies as it may cause psychological disturbances.

THE GANGLION BLOCKERS

Pharmacological action. The ganglion blockers were the first effective blood pressure lowering agents. They interfere with transmission at the relay ganglia of both the adrenergic and cholinergic nervous system. At these sites they compete with acetylcholine and thus prevent depolarisation of the membrane of the postsynaptic nerve cells.

The actions of these drugs can be grouped according to the system involved:

1. *Cardiovascular system.* Loss of adrenergic tone leads to arterial and venous vasodilatation. This causes pooling of blood with a decreased

venous return to the heart and a fall in cardiac output. The drop in cardiac output and the arteriolar dilatation are responsible for the fall in blood pressure which is largely postural (i.e. only seen on standing and abolished by lying flat).

2. *Gastrointestinal.* Loss of cholinergic activity causes a dry mouth, slows intestine transit, and leads to constipation and occasionally ileus.

3. *Genitourinary.* Retention may occur especially if there is some bladder neck obstruction and impotence is an occasional complication.

4. *Eyes.* Pupils may dilate with paralysis of accommodation.

These drugs are largely excreted by the kidney and with impaired renal function, accumulation will occur.

Therapeutic uses. Although they are potent hypotensive agents, the widespread pharmacological effect of these drugs, and the fact that the fall in blood pressure is postural, has led to their being replaced by other agents and they are now rarely used.

The chief individual ganglion blockers available are:

Hexamethonium bromide was the prototype drug. It is irregularly and poorly absorbed from the intestine and was not therefore very satisfactory for the long-term treatment of hypertension.

Pentolinium tartrate is slightly better absorbed orally, but is now largely used in hypertensive crises when it is given by subcutaneous injection. The initial dose is 2·5 mg (1·25 mg in the elderly) and then a further 1·0 mg is given every fifteen minutes until a satisfactory fall in blood pressure is produced. (Note the blood pressure must be taken sitting or standing.)

Mecamylamine is well absorbed from the intestine and the initial oral dose is 2·5 mg twice daily. This is increased every four days until a satisfactory fall in blood pressure is produced. Mecamylamine is only slowly excreted in an alkaline urine and because of this should not be combined with acetazolamide. In addition to the side effects of ganglion blockade, mecamylamine may produce tremor and weakness due to an action on voluntary muscle.

Pempidine is also absorbed and the initial dose is 2·5 mg three times a day and increased as required.

Trimetaphan is a very rapidly acting ganglion blocker. It is given by intravenous infusion in a 1 in 1000 solution. Its effects pass off rapidly after stopping infusion. It is largely used to produce controlled postural hypotension.

Contraindications. Ganglion blockers should be used with care or not at all in patients where a sudden fall in blood pressure could be dangerous. This will include those with severe myocardial or cerebral ischaemia.

In patients with renal failure a blood urea of over 100 mg%, usually contraindicates as a large fall in blood pressure may cause a further disastrous deterioration in renal function and there is also the problem of impaired excretion.

Patients on these drugs are unduly sensitive to sympathomemetic amines.

THE ADRENERGIC BLOCKING AGENTS

(a) THOSE BLOCKING THE POST GANGLIONIC NERVES [2]

This group of drugs is the most widely used to lower blood pressure. They all produce this effect by interfering in some way with the release of noradrenaline at the adrenergic nerve ending. In general, they also cause a fall in blood pressure, which is largely postural. This is largely due to loss of vasomotor tone causing peripheral pooling of blood with decreased venous return and a lowered cardiac output. Prolonged treatment may result in some increase in blood volume and thus some decrease in efficiency of the hypotensive agent [3].

They all have side effects which are referable to adrenergic blockade. There are however minor differences in both the duration of action and in the incidence of side effects.

The main drugs of this type in use at present are:

Guanethidine

Pharmacological action. Guanethidine decreases a release of noradrenaline at adrenergic nerve endings. If injected intravenously it causes a transient rise in blood pressure, because it inhibits re-uptake of noradrenaline by nerve endings. Guanethidine also causes some depletion of peripheral noradrenaline stores. It is only moderately well absorbed from the intestines and is only slowly excreted by the kidneys, and it is several days before a single dose is cleared from the body. This means that one dose daily is adequate.

Therapeutic uses. Guanethidine is given initially in a dose of 10 mg in the morning. The dose is increased at weekly intervals until a satisfactory control of blood pressure is produced, usually with around 20–60 mg daily. The rather prolonged action of guanethidine makes it difficult to control the blood pressure if it varies widely throughout the day. Tolerance does not usually develop to any marked extent with guanethidine, but can be due to sodium and water retention and is controlled by using a diuretic.

Contraindications and side effects. Diarrhoea is the most troublesome side effect but can be controlled with codeine phosphate or with the addition of a ganglion blocking agent. Bradycardia is usual but is not important. Other results of adrenergic blockade are failure of ejaculation and parotid pain.

As with the ganglion blockers guanethidine must be used with great care in those with marked cerebral or myocardial ischaemia or in renal failure.

Guanoxan

Pharmacological action. Guanoxan is a combination of the guanethidine ring with benzodioxane. It blocks release of noradrenaline and also depletes peripheral stores. In addition, presumably due to its benzodioxane moiety it has some direct blocking action on circulating adrenaline and noradrenaline. The fall in blood pressure is postural but less markedly so than guanethidine.

Therapeutic uses. Guanoxan is administered in an initial dose of 20 mg daily and increased every four days as required [4].

Contraindications and side effects. Guanoxan causes diarrhoea and failure of ejaculation. In addition it may cause drowsiness, particularly early in treatment. Changes in liver function tests are not uncommon and occasionally they may be followed by jaundice.

It would seem that the risk of liver damage should limit the use of the drug.

Guanochlor

Pharmacological action. Guanochlor interferes with noradrenaline release and storage and may also interfere with the conversion of dopamine to noradrenaline. It produces a postural fall in blood pressure.

Therapeutic use. Guanochlor is given in an initial dose of 10 mg b.d. [5] and this is increased every third day until a satisfactory fall in blood pressure is produced.

Contraindications and side effects. In a few patients guanochlor causes some urea retention but there does not appear to be any interference with overall renal function. It may also cause salt and water retention and may have to be combined with a diuretic. Guanochlor causes pain in skeletal muscle in a small number of patients; the reason for this is unknown [6]. Other side effects are similar to those of the adrenergic blocking group as a whole.

Bethanidine

Pharmacological action. Bethanidine lowers blood pressure by blocking noradrenaline release from the adrenergic nerve endings. It has no peripheral depleting action and no blocking action on circulating noradrenaline. It is rapidly and well absorbed producing a peak effect within four to five hours. It is excreted via the kidneys and entirely eliminated within about twelve hours.

Therapeutic use. The relatively short action of bethanidine enables the blood pressure to be controlled more flexibly as the dose can be modified to meet fluctuation during the day [7].

The initial dose is 10 mg twice daily and this is increased by adding 5 or 10 mg to each dose until adequate control is obtained. If the blood pressure is very variable during the day bethanidine can be given three or four times daily. Some tolerance may develop.

In severe hypertension it appears to have some synergistic action with methyldopa [8].

Contraindications and side effects. The fall in blood pressure is markedly postural. However, diarrhoea is unusual.

Other side effects are similar to guanethidine, but it occasionally causes depression. It should not be used when a phaeochromocytoma is suspected and should not be combined with the amphetamine group of drugs.

Debrisoquine

Pharmacological action. Debrisoquine prevents release of noradrenaline at adrenergic nerve endings without depleting peripheral stores and produces a postural fall in blood pressure. It is relatively rapid in action and is very similar to bethanidine.

Therapeutic uses. The initial dose is 10 mg twice daily and this is increased every three or four days until a satisfactory fall in blood pressure results.

Contraindications and side effects. Debrisoquine is fairly free of side effects [9]. When they occur they include diarrhoea, failure of ejaculation, muscle weakness and tiredness. Contraindications are the same for any agent which can cause a considerable fall in blood pressure.

(b) THOSE INTERFERING WITH NORADRENALINE SYNTHESIS

Methyldopa

Pharmacological action. Methyldopa differs from all the other drugs which inhibit the adrenergic nervous system. It is believed to be converted to methylnoradrenaline at the adrenergic nerve endings and this substance which is only a weak vasoconstrictor acts as a 'false mediator'. It seems that the peripheral action of methyldopa cannot entirely explain its blood pressure lowering properties and it is probably that there is a central component to its action. The important result of these is that with methyldopa the fall in blood pressure is almost as great lying as standing.

Methyldopa is well absorbed but its hypotensive effect is delayed for 4–6 hours. It is excreted via the kidneys and about half the dose is cleared from the body in twelve hours, and excretion is complete in 48 hours.

Therapeutic use. Methyldopa is very widely used in the treatment of hypertension. The initial dose is 250 mg twice daily and this is increased every fourth day until a satisfactory response is obtained. The usual dose being 250 mg four times daily. It is not worth giving more than 2·0 g. daily as further increases in dose will not usually increase the hypotensive effect. Methyldopa has a tendency to provoke sodium and water retention and its action can be augmented by combining it with a diuretic.

Contraindications and side effects. Methyldopa produces drowsiness in 20–30 per cent of patients, although this may diminish with continued treatment. Other side effects include dry mouth, nasal congestion and lactation. Marked water retention is rare but can cause oedema. It responds to a diuretic.

Methyldopa can also provoke hypersensitivity phenomena. About 20 per cent of those on long term treatment at high dosage levels develop a positive direct Coombs test [10] and occasionally a frank haemolytic anaemia. Other hypersensitivity phenomena have been described, including drug fever, skin rashes and rarely, liver damage. In patients with renal failure, retention of the drug can give rise to a parkinson-like state.

Methyldopa should therefore not be used in liver disease, and with care in those with impaired renal function.

(c) BETA-ADRENERGIC BLOCKING AGENTS

Propranolol

Pharmacological action. (See page 166.)

Therapeutic use. Propranolol has been used with success in hypertension [11]. The fall in blood pressure is not postural. It is tentatively suggested that as a result of β blockade of the heart, transient rises in cardiac output and blood pressure are prevented. The aortic arch baroreceptors become readjusted and the blood pressure is 'set' at a lower level.

The initial dose is 10 mg four times daily and this is increased at fortnightly intervals by 25 per cent of the dose until blood pressure is controlled. It may take two months before the full effect is seen.

Contraindications and side effects. (See page 167.)

(d) ALPHA-ADRENERGIC BLOCKING AGENTS (see above)

Phentolamine **Phenoxybenzamine**

(e) MONOAMINE-OXIDASE INHIBITORS

Pargyline

Pharmacological action. The drug is a monoamine-oxidase inhibitor and also lowers blood pressure, probably by blocking the post-ganglionic part of the adrenergic nervous system. The fall in blood pressure is partially postural.

It is only slowly excreted and one dose daily is adequate.

Therapeutic uses. Pargyline [12] is given in an initial dose of 25 mg orally. It takes about two weeks to produce its full effect and the dose is thereafter increased by 10 mg at two-weekly intervals.

Contraindications and side effects. Pargyline has all the side effects and dangers of other MAO inhibitors (see above). The inherent dangers limit its use as a hypertensive agent. It is also contraindicated in liver or kidney failure, in thyrotoxicosis and in pregnancy.

DIURETICS

Pharmacology. A wide variety of diuretics will lower blood pressure. In the early stages of treatment this appears related to the decrease in circulating blood volume which follows naturesis. However, after some weeks treatment both blood volume and cardiac output return to normal but the hypotensive action continues.

Therapeutic use. The fall in blood pressure produced by diuretics is relatively small but they are particularly useful when combined with other hypotensive agents when they increase and smooth out the hypotensive action of these drugs. They may also prevent the development of resistance to some hypotensive drugs, in particular the adrenergic blocking agents.

In theory, the longer-acting diuretics, such as chlorthalidone should be most suitable in hypertension, but in practice any of the benzothiadizines, or even the relatively short-acting frusemide are satisfactory. The choice of diuretics and side effects are considered later.

Diazoxide

Diazoxide is related to the benzothiadiazine diuretics. It is a powerful blood pressure lowering agent when given intravenously, probably by a direct action on the arterial wall. The dose by this route is 5 mg/kg I.V., given undiluted, and it is not so effective if given diluted in an intravenous drip. The fall in blood pressure lasts 6–24 hours.

Unfortunately the drug is not effective orally and further repeated use leads to rise in blood sugar levels. This latter action has been used in the treatment of hypoglycaemia [13].

PERIPHERAL VASODILATORS

Tolazoline

Pharmacological action. Tolazoline produces peripheral vasodilatation, mainly of skin vessels. This is largely due to a direct action on the vessel wall but it is also a weak α receptor blocker. Tolazoline also increases both heart rate and output, and so may actually increase blood pressure. It also stimulates gastric secretion. It is well absorbed and rapidly excreted via the kidneys.

Therapeutic uses. Tolazoline is used in doses of 25–50 mg three times a day in the treatment of peripheral vascular disease. There is no good evidence that it has any benefit in atherosclerotic disease but may help in Raynaud's phenomena.

Contraindications and side effects. Tolazoline may cause tachycardia and cardiac arrhythmias, flushing and diarrhoea. It may also exacerbate peptic ulceration.

It should not be used in heart failure, angina of effort, or in those with peptic ulceration.

Cyclendelate

Pharmacology and therapeutic use. The drug produces vasodilatation by acting directly on the arterial wall. It has been used for peripheral vascular disease and is also claimed to increase cerebral blood flow. There is little evidence that it is of benefit in vascular disease of the limbs or the brain.

The usual dose is 400 mg three times daily. Side effects include flushing, dizziness and headaches.

Inositol nicotinate

A mild vasodilatator. The initial dose is 200 mg four times daily and it can be increased. It appears free of ill effects.

Isoxsuprine

This drug causes a combination of peripheral vasodilatation with an increase in cardiac output. The dose is 10 mg four times daily. Its efficiency in peripheral vascular disease is doubtful.

References

1. Schirger, A., and Spittell, J. A., *Amer. J. Cardiol.* (1962), **9,** 854.
2. Pritchard, B. N. C., Johnston, A. W., Hill, I. D., and Rosenheim, M. L., *Brit. med. J.* (1968), **1,** 135.
3. Romnov-Jersen, V., *A. ta med. Scand.* (1963), **174,** 300.
4. Peart, W. S., and MacMahon, M. I., *Brit. med. J.* (1964), **1,** 398.
5. Peart, W. S., and MacMahon, M. I., *ibid.*, 402.
6. Hodge, J. V., *ibid.* (1966), **2,** 981.
7. Montuschi, E., and Pickens, P. T., *Lancet* (1962), **ii,** 897.
8. Breckenridge, A., and Dollery, C. T., *ibid.* (1966), **i,** 1074.
9. Athanassiadis, D., Cranston, W. I., Juel-Jensen, B. F., and Olives, D. O., *Brit. med. J.* (1966), **2,** 732.
10. Carstairs, K. C., Breckenridge, A., Dollery, C. T., and Wolledge, S. M., *Lancet* (1966), **ii,** 133.

11. Pritchard, B. N. C., and Gillam, P. M. S., *Brit. med. J.* (1969), **1,** 7.
12. Moser, M., Brodoff, B., Miller, A., and Goldman, A. G., *Amer. med. Arch.* (1964), **187,** 192.
13. Graber, A. L., Porte, D., and Williams, R. H., *Diabetes* (1966), **15,** 143.

This chapter was written by Professor J. R. Trounce.

Category 8

Diuretics and Cation Exchange Resins

DIURETICS

Diuretics are indicated in any patient who has adequate renal function and who has oedema arising from a central rather than a local cause [1, 2]. They play a major part in the management of cardiac failure and of oedema attributable to a low plasma protein level whether this arises on a nutritional, hepatic, or renal basis. In addition they have a valuable supplementary role in the treatment of hypertension [1, 3] and are sometimes useful in the treatment of acute-on-chronic respiratory failure and of some cases of poisoning.

The power of modern diuretics has diminished the therapeutic value of dietary sodium restriction. This still has a place, however, and its effect may be increased by the oral administration of a cation exchange resin in the potassium, ammonium or calcium phase.

Benzothiadiazines and related drugs

Pharmacological actions and therapeutic use [1, 2]. There are at least twelve drugs of this type in use [1] (Table 1). They differ in their intestinal absorption and diuretic potency and in their solubility in fat which determines their rate of excretion, and duration of action.

In addition there are a number of closely related drugs (Table 2) which have a different heterocyclic moiety but common side chains, similar actions and identical side effects.

All these drugs increase the urinary excretion of sodium and have secondary effects on the excretion of water, chloride and potassium. They are weak inhibitors of carbonic anhydrase and may impair the ability to excrete an acid urine.

Some doubt exists concerning their sites of action on the kidney. Stop-flow studies indicate an effect on the proximal convoluted tubule but recent micropuncture work suggests that the most important action is on the proximal part of the distal convoluted tubule [5]. They are all given orally and, in addition, there is a preparation of chlorothiazide that is suitable for intravenous injection (dose: 500 mg). The shorter

Table 1 The Benzothiadiazines

Approved name		Duration of action (hours)	Dose (mg)
Chlorothiazide		12	500 –2000
Cyclopenthiazide		12	0·25–2·0
Cyclothiazide		24	1·0 –8·0
Bendrofluazide	Bendroflumethiazide (USA)	18	2·5 –10·0
Benzthiazide		12	25 –200
Flumethiazide		12	250 –2000
Hydrochlorothiazide		14	25 –200
Hydroflumethiazide		14	25 –200
Methyclothiazide		24	2·5 –10·0
Polythiazide		48	1·0 –8·0
Teclothiazide		10	110 –220
Trichlormethiazide		24	1·0 –8·0

Table 2 Diuretics which resemble the Benzothiadiazines

Approved name	Duration of action (hours)	Dose (mg)
Chlorthalidone	72	50–200
Clorexolone	48	25–100
Quinethazone	24	50–200
Clopamide	36	20–80
Mefruside [4]	24	25–100

acting drugs are given daily, usually in the mornings, but the longer acting ones need be given only on alternate days.

In addition to their conventional uses, the benzothiadiazines have been shown to lower the urinary excretion of calcium and may prove to be of value in the prevention of renal calculi.

Contraindications and side effects. The benzothiadiazines and related drugs are all fairly safe but have a number of well recognised side effects.

Early in treatment, potassium excretion rises due to the increased amount of sodium available for exchange in the distal tubule. Later, relatively less sodium and more potassium ions appear in the urine and, eventually, potassium may become the major urinary cation with the development of potassium depletion and an extracellular alkalosis. Ultimately oedema may be completely resistant to treatment and the serum sodium concentration falls. Intracellular potassium depletion contributes to this state [6] and it is advisable to stop the diuretic and replace potassium while restricting the intake of sodium and water. Although the serum potassium level is a poor index of potassium depletion, it is worth measuring it regularly in those on prolonged treatment especially with large doses of diuretic. In such patients supplements of potassium chloride are indicated (see below).

Secretion of uric acid by the distal tubule is inhibited with retention of uric acid and the production of hyperuricaemia [1]. Occasionally this is associated with episodes of acute gout which subside when the drug is withdrawn or when uricosuric drugs (e.g. probenecid) are used. Most patients develop some impairment of carbohydrate tolerance and a few become frankly diabetic; improvement occurs on stopping the drug but a few patients continue to require treatment for diabetes. Finally, occasional patients develop thrombocytopaenic purpura, leucopenia, photosensitivity, macular-papular rashes or jaundice.

Frusemide (Furosemide, *USA***)**

Pharmacological actions and therapeutic use. Frusemide has some chemical similarity to the benzothiadiazines but produces a substantially greater diuretic effect [1, 2,]. This is not increased by the addition of a benzothiadiazine suggesting that frusemide acts at the same sites in the tubule plus another site which is thought to be the ascending limb of Henle's loop [5]. Absorption from the gut is rapid and complete, and excretion is by the kidney.

A diuresis begins within two minutes of intravenous administration (dose: 20–60 mg) and lasts only two hours. This makes it ideal for the treatment of acute pulmonary oedema.

After oral administration (dose: 40–120 mg) the diuretic effect lasts about four hours. This transient action makes it relatively unsuitable for maintenance therapy unless weaker drugs have proved ineffective. Its great power makes it useful in the treatment of patients with impaired renal function when very large doses (500 mg) may be given.

Contraindications and side effects. The main problems derive from its potency, and it is easy to produce acute hypovolaemia and chronic electrolyte depletion. It is logical to start treatment with a small dose and to take particular care when the oedema is associated with hypoproteinaemia and hypovolaemia. In these circumstances it may be necessary to maintain the blood volume by the intravenous administration of salt poor albumin or an osmotic diuretic (see below). Apart from this, the drug is fairly safe; potassium depletion and hyperuricaemia occur frequently but carbohydrate intolerance is seen less often than with the benzothiadiazines. Leucopenia, thrombocytopenia and diarrhoea have been reported. On rare occasions, patients given large intravenous doses have developed transient cardiac arrhythmias and it is therefore wise to monitor the E.C.G. in these circumstances.

Ethacrynic acid

Pharmacological actions and therapeutic use. Chemically this drug differs substantially from frusemide and the benzothiadiazines. It has a powerful diuretic action which is not increased by frusemide and which lasts about eight hours [1, 2, 8]. It is well absorbed from the gut (dose: 50–400 mg) and may also be given intravenously (dose: 50 mg). Excretion is via the kidneys and liver.

Contraindications and side effects. Electrolyte depletion and hypovolaemia are real hazards and it is essential to start treatment with small doses. Potassium supplements are necessary during maintenance therapy. Hyperuricaemia, thrombocytopenia and skin rashes may also occur and there is a rather high incidence of gastro-intestinal symptoms. Patients have been reported who developed deafness when treated with large doses of ethacrynic acid in the presence of renal failure.

Organic mercurials

Pharmacological actions and therapeutic use. These drugs were the first effective diuretics and remain among the most powerful [1]. Unfortunately they are poorly absorbed from the gut and are usually given by intramuscular injection; in view of this inconvenience they have been largely replaced by oral diuretics. Excretion is via the kidneys. They inhibit sodium and chloride reabsorption in the proximal convoluted tubule but also act on the distal part of the nephron [5]. Chlormerodrin and mercurophylline may be given orally but are not as powerful as mersalyl and mercaptomerin which are given by injection. Mersalyl Inj. B.P. (dose: 2 ml I.M.) contains a small amount of theophylline which is itself a weak diuretic (see below) but which is included because it improves absorption from the injection site. The action lasts twenty-four hours and it is usual to repeat the dose every 2–4 days. Diuresis is enhanced by the administration of ammonium chloride (dose: 2–6 g daily). This may be attributable to the chloride ion but it is possible that the acidifying effect releases active mercuric ion within the tubular cell.

Contraindications and side effects. Intravenous injection is rarely followed by circulatory collapse and this route of administration should never be used. However even after intramuscular injection some patients develop hypersensitivity reactions with bronchospasm and urticaria. Stomatitis and anorexia may also occur with prolonged courses. Other side effects are rare but include proteinuria, the nephrotic syndrome and acute renal failure. Mercurials are not given to patients with established renal disease and it is advisable to test the urine regularly during treatment. If a patient becomes resistant to mersalyl there is a risk of mercury poisoning and therapy should be reviewed; if there is a severe alkalosis responsiveness can be restored with ammonium chloride but if this fails treatment should be stopped. Significant potassium depletion is rare and it is unnecessary to give supplements routinely although it is wise to measure the plasma potassium level occasionally.

Triamterene

Pharmacological actions and therapeutic use. This drug has a relatively weak action and is not given alone. It inhibits sodium/potassium exchange in the distal convoluted tubule and supplements the effect of diuretics which act higher up the nephron. It is given orally, the usual dose being 100–300 mg daily. Excretion is via the kidneys.

Contraindications and side effects. Potassium retention and hyperkalaemia occur frequently, and reversible impairment of renal function may also be seen. Plasma levels of urea and potassium should be measured regularly and the drug should not be given to patients with renal failure. Other side effects include anorexia, abdominal discomfort and skin rashes.

Amiloride

This drug is not yet available for general use in the USA.

Pharmacological actions and therapeutic use. Chemically it has a minor resemblance to triamterene, and like it acts on the distal convoluted tubule to produce a sodium and water diuresis with conservation of potassium [9]. It is a more powerful diuretic but is most useful for its effect on potentiating the actions of ethacrynic acid, frusemide and the benzothiadiazines and in removing the need for potassium supplements. The oral dose is 10–40 mg daily and the action is complete within twenty-four hours.

Contraindications and side effects. Occasional patients develop gastro-intestinal disturbances. However the only important problem is the development of severe hyperkalaemia in some patients with renal functional impairment.

Spironolactone

Pharmacological actions and therapeutic use. The majority of oedematous patients, particularly those with hypoproteinaemia, have evidence of hyperaldosteronism. Spironolactone is a competitive inhibitor of the action of aldosterone and has a weak diuretic effect with conservation of potassium. It is used in combination with drugs acting higher up the nephron and has a definite place in the treatment of resistant oedema when its effect on potassium excretion is particularly valuable. The original preparation was poorly absorbed from the gut and has been replaced by a microcrystalline form which is absorbed better. The dose is 25 mg q.d.s. and it is common to observe a delay of two or three days before the diuretic effect appears. In the treatment of primary hyperaldosteronism very large (100 mg q.d.s.) doses must be used.

Contraindications and side effects. These are rare but include gynaecomastia, hirsutism, headache, mental confusion and drowsiness. Hyperkalaemia may develop and spironolactone should not be given to patients with renal failure.

Carbonic anhydrase inhibitors

Pharmacological actions and therapeutic use. As diuretics, these drugs [1, 2,], which include acetazolomide, ethoxzolomide, methazolomide, and dichlorphenamide, are now only of historic interest. They prevent bicarbonate reabsorption and the excretion of hydrogen ions, leading to an increased excretion of sodium and potassium ions. However, the effect is transient as the development of a metabolic acidosis leads to a fall in the filtered bicarbonate.

Contraindications and side effects. These include potassium depletion, renal calculi, drowsiness, paraesthesiae, thrombocytopenia and skin rashes.

Xanthines

Pharmacological actions and therapeutic use. The xanthines are weak diuretics and are not used alone. Caffeine, theophylline and amiso metradine act when given orally but aminophylline, the most effective, is inactivated by gastric acidity and is given either as suppositories (360 mg) or intravenously (250–500 mg). Aminophylline increases the cardiac output and may be given at the peak of a diuresis produced by other diuretics when it produces a further increase in urine flow.

Contraindications and side effects. Cardiac arrest has been observed following rapid intravenous injection of aminophylline and this drug must therefore be given slowly over several minutes. Despite this precaution, vomiting and hypotension may occur.

OSMOTIC DIURETICS

Mannitol

Pharmacological actions and therapeutic use. Osmotic diuretics are believed to act by increasing the solute load per nephron, which in turn decreases the tubular transit time and the time available for reabsorption of water and electrolytes. In addition sodium and water reabsorption in the proximal convoluted tubule is limited by the relative hypertonicity of the tubular contents.

Mannitol may be used in the treatment of resistant oedema associated with hypoproteinaemia and hypovolaemia. It is given at the same time as a conventional diuretic and leads to a further increase in urine flow while the patient is protected from the expected fall in blood volume. It also has a place in the treatment of poisoning with drugs such as phenobarbitone and the salicylates, which are filtered at the glomerulus and partially reabsorbed by the tubules. The usual dose is 25–50 g. followed by continuous intravenous administration of 10–20 g/hour, the rate being adjusted according to the response observed.

There is good evidence that under certain circumstances, the pre-operative prophylactic administration of mannitol protects patients from the development of acute renal failure. However, the value of mannitol therapy in the treatment of patients with incipient acute renal failure is not yet proved. Providing there are no signs of circulatory overload a formal trial of mannitol is justified; occasionally there is a dramatic response but if there is none, the treatment must be stopped.

Contraindications and side effects. Two principal dangers arise from treatment of this type. Circulatory overload may be avoided by regular observation, careful fluid balance, and the cessation of treatment in the absence of a diuresis. The second danger is of fluid and electrolyte depletion; the composition of the urine passed must be measured and any losses which are not required must be replaced intravenously.

POTASSIUM SUPPLEMENTS

The majority of diuretics produce significant potassium loss and, unless spironolactone, triamterene or amiloride are being used, the administration of potassium supplements should be considered. A high potassium intake in the form of fresh fruit is advisable. However, many potassium rich foods such as milk and meat extracts are also rich in sodium and may be contraindicated. Potassium depletion is usually associated with chloride depletion [10] and it is therefore essential to replace potassium as the chloride salt. Solutions of potassium chloride are unpalatable and the salt is usually given as a capsule or tablet. The administration of simple tablets of potassium chloride, particularly in combination with a benzothiadiazine, has been associated with the development of jejunal ulceration. Recently there have become available in the U.K. three commercial preparations from which the salt is released slowly; these are Slow K (Ciba) and Kloref (Cox-Continental) which contain 600 mg (8 mEq. of potassium) and 500 mg (6·5 mEq. of potassium) of potassium chloride respectively. Tablets of Sando K (Sandoz) may be dissolved in water immediately before use and yield a solution containing 12 mEq. of potassium and 8 mEq. of chloride. Usually the patient requires 25–50 mEq. of potassium daily.

CATION EXCHANGE RESINS

These are synthetic polymers which act as weak, insoluble acids and bind cations relatively loosely according to their relative concentrations and the pH of the medium. Generally speaking, they have an affinity in decreasing order for calcium, potassium, sodium and ammonium ions. They are given in a particular phase with the object of removing other cations present in excess.

Ammonium polystyrene sulphonate

Pharmacological actions and therapeutic use. This resin is used in the treatment of resistant oedema. It is usually given orally in a dose of 15 g three times a day but may be given as an enema in doses of 50–100 g in 10 per cent. dextrose. It is unpalatable and may be partially disguised

if given in a flavoured drink or mixed with honey. Sodium ions exchange for ammonium ions and the patient may be spared rigorous dietary sodium restriction.
Contraindications and side effects. The resin may aggravate a severe acidosis and is therefore contraindicated in the presence of renal failure. Potassium ions will be removed along with sodium ions and potassium depletion should be anticipated. This may be overcome with the help of potassium supplements or by giving some of the resin in the potassium phase. Katonium contains 75 per cent ammonium polystyrene sulphonate and 25 per cent potassium polystyrene sulphonate. Minor gastrointestinal disturbances are common.

Sodium polystyrene sulphonate

This resin is used in the treatment of hyperkalaemia in renal failure and is given in the same way as ammonium polystyrene sulphonate. Potassium ions exchange for sodium ions and there is a risk of sodium overload. This has led to the introduction of resin in the calcium phase (calcium polystyrene sulphonate) but hypercalcaemia has been reported after prolonged use and it has been suggested that resin in the aluminium phase is used if prolonged administration becomes necessary.

References

1. Lant, A. F., and Wilson, G. M., *Diuretics in 'Renal Disease'* (1967). Editor Black, D. A. K. Publ. Blackwell Scientific Publications Ltd.
2. Mudge, G. H., *in The Pharmacological Basis of Therapeutics* (1970). Chapter 8. Eds. Goodman, L. S., and Gilman, A. Publ. Macmillan, New York.
3. Cranston, W. I., Juel-Jansen, B. E., Semmence, A. M., Handfield-Jones, R. P. C., Forbes, J. A., and Mutch, L. M. M., *Lancet* (1963), **ii,** 966.
4. Wilson, C. B., and Kirkendall, W. M., *J. Pharmacol. exp. Therap.* (1970) **171,** 288.
5 Dirks, J. H., and Seely, J. F., *Ann. Rev. Pharmacol.* (1969), **9,** 73.
6. Fuisz, R. E., *Medicine* (Balt.) (1963), **42,** 149.
7. Hutcheon, D. E., Mehta, D., and Romano, A., *Arch. Intern. Med.* (1965), **115,** 542.
8. Cannon, P. J., Heinemann, H. O., Stason, W. B., and Laragh, J. H., *Circulaion* (1965), **31,** 5.
9. Lant, A. F., Smith, A. J., and Wilson, G. M., *Clin. Pharmacol. Ther.* (1969), **10,** 50.
10. Schwartz, W. B., de Strihou C. van Y., and Kassirer, J. P., *New Eng. J. Med.* (1968), **279,** 630.

This chapter was written by Dr C. S. Ogg (Renal Physician, Guy's Hospital) and edited by Prof. J. R. Trounce.

Category 9

Drugs Used in Haematology

Iron

Iron is commonly administered orally and less often parenterally. Therapeutically, the important consideration is the elemental iron content of the preparation and not simply the total weight of the iron complex in the dose. To achieve a complete response in most cases 1,000–2,000 mg elemental iron must enter the body.

ORAL IRON THERAPY

On average about 20 per cent of the oral dose of an iron preparation is absorbed. Thus to ensure the absorption of 2 g. iron a course of therapy must supply 10 g. iron – the amount of the iron salt used to provide this dose will depend on its iron content. These iron preparations are taken daily and a course should last at least six months.

Ferrous sulphate

Pharmacological action. Haemoglobin biosynthesis.

Therapeutic use. The preferred iron preparation for the treatment of iron-deficiency anaemia. Each tablet contains 200 mg ferrous sulphate of which 60 mg is elemental iron. The usual dose is 1–2 tablets taken three times a day by mouth after meals. For children and those who have difficulty in swallowing tablets liquid preparation in the form of syrups or elixirs are used: 5 ml contains 45 mg elemental iron and the dose is 5–10 ml three times a day after meals. Used prophylactically in pregnancy in a dose of 200 mg daily.

Contraindications and side effects. Like other oral iron preparations, it may irritate the bowel and so exacerbate symptoms in patients with ulcerative colitis or with regional ileitis or in those with a colostomy and is therefore generally contraindicated in these conditions. In some patients oral iron produces nausea and dyspeptic symptoms which can often be avoided or lessened by taking the tablets after meals with a drink of water and by halving the dose. Constipation is not uncommon but if the dose is excessive there may be diarrhoea. Exceptionally an itchy skin rash may develop. All iron preparations blacken the faeces. Patients who are intolerant of ferrous sulphate may do better on either ferrous gluconate or ferrous fumarate or a slow release preparation (see below).

Other iron preparations are only used in those intolerant to ferrous sulphate. Contraindications and side effects are the same as for ferrous sulphate.

Preparation	Elemental iron per tablet	Dose
Ferrous fumarate	65 mg	1–2 tabs t.d.s. after meals
Ferrous gluconate	36 mg	1–2 tabs t.d.s. after meals
Slow Release Preparations		
Ferrogradumet	105 mg	1 tab daily before breakfast
Feospan	45 mg	2–3 caps before meals
Slow Fe	50 mg	1–2 tabs daily

PARENTERAL IRON THERAPY

This form of therapy is reserved for those few patients who fail to respond to adequate doses of oral iron because of intestinal malabsorption or who are intolerant of oral preparations, or for those who are unwilling or cannot be relied on to take tablets regularly for a period of several months. Oral iron should be discontinued at least 48 hours before an injection of iron is given to minimise the danger of generalised reactions.

Iron dextran

Pharmacological action. Haemoglobin biosynthesis.

Therapeutic use. Used intramuscularly usually but can also be given intravenously. 1 ml contains 50 mg elemental iron. Intramuscular injections should be deep and should be confined to the upper outer quadrant of the buttock. A test dose of 0·5 ml should be injected first to detect hypersensitivity. Not more than 100 mg (2 ml) should be injected at any one time and to avoid local pain the injection should be made slowly and smoothly. Injections are given at intervals of 1–2 days, alternating the buttocks, until a total dose of 1–2 g (20–40 ml) has been given. The total dose required can be calculated from the haemoglobin deficit – for every gram of haemoglobin/100 ml in deficit 300 mg iron is given.

Alternatively the total dose of iron dextran can be given as a single intravenous infusion over about 8 hours. The calculated dose of iron-dextran is added to 500 ml normal saline: the infusion rate should not exceed 5–10 drops/minute for the first 30 minutes since reactions will usually be evident in this time and if there is no reaction the infusion rate is increased to 20–30 drops/minute.

Contraindications and side effects. Iron dextran should not be used in patients with a history of allergy or asthma. The skin around the injection site may be stained, sometimes permanently. Intramuscular injections may produce severe local pain if given rapidly. If administered intravenously there may be thrombophlebitis at the infusion site; leakage outside the vein causes intense local pain and an inflammatory reaction follows. Occasional side effects are fever, allergic reactions, enlargement of lymph nodes and arthralgia. Although local sarcomata have been produced in rabbits by the long-term intramuscular injection of large doses of iron dextran there is no evidence that its use in the recommended clinical dosage carries any such risk for man.

Iron-sorbitol

Pharmacological action. Haemoglobin biosynthesis.

Therapeutic use. Used intramuscularly only and the method of administration is similar to that described for iron dextran. About 36 per cent of the injected dose is excreted in the urine and the calculated total dose should be increased by that amount.

Contraindications and side effects. Iron-sorbitol injections may be followed by fever, vomiting, disorientation, a metallic taste and local urticarial reactions. It should not be used if there is a history of allergy or asthma.

Vitamin B_{12}

Pharmacological action. Vitamin B_{12} is an essential co-factor in DNA and protein synthesis and is required for cell division and growth, particularly in rapidly proliferating tissues such as bone marrow and gastrointestinal epithelium. The synthesis and preservation of myelin in nerve tissue is also dependent on an adequate supply of vitamin B_{12}.

Therapeutic use. Used in megaloblastic anaemias due to vitamin B_{12} deficiency: pernicious anaemia, postgastrectomy states, diseases involving the terminal ileum, small intestinal blind loops, infestation with the fish tape worm and in strict vegetarians (vegans). Vitamin B_{12} in the form of hydroxocobalamin is preferred to cyanocobalamin because of better retention and is given by intramuscular injection. For initiating therapy 1,000 μg is given on alternate days for the first week. Thereafter maintenance therapy is essential (except when the cause can be eliminated), and consists of 1,000 μg hydroxocobalamin every two months.

Contraindications and side effects. Vitamin B_{12} should not be used in megaloblastic anaemias due to folic acid deficiency and it is of no value in anaemias not due to vitamin B_{12} deficiency. Very occasionally hypersensitivity reactions may occur.

Folic acid

Pharmacological action. Folic acid is converted in the body into its biologically active form tetrahydrofolic acid by the enzyme folic acid reductase. Its prime roll is to accept and transfer 1-carbon fragments, such as methyl groups, for biosynthesis of purines and thymine and thus of DNA, RNA and proteins. The methyl group is transferred to homocysteine to form methionine and this step requires vitamin B_{12}.

Therapeutic use. It is used in megaloblastic anaemia due to folic acid deficiency. Folic acid is usually administered orally in tablet form. For the treatment of established anaemia a daily dose of 5 mg is given until the blood picture is normal or until the dietary deficiency or malabsorption has been corrected. In pregnancy it is used prophylactically in a daily dose of 400 μg in combination with an iron salt. Folic acid is given by intramuscular injection in a dose of 15 mg if there is vomiting. The reduced form of folic acid, folinic acid, is used to treat toxicity due to folic acid antagonists and a dose of 15 mg is given by intravenous injection.

Contraindications and side effects. Folic acid should not be used in pernicious anaemia. Nor should it be used in other anaemias associated with B_{12} deficiency unless there is also a superadded folic acid deficiency: side effects are almost unknown.

Pyridoxine

Pharmacological action. Pyridoxine is one of the forms of vitamin B_6. It is required for the biosynthesis of haemoglobin. Synthesis of haem is reduced in its absence and consequently utilisation of iron and thus haemoglobin synthesis is impaired.

Therapeutic use. Some cases of congenital and of idiopathic acquired sideroblastic anaemia respond to pyridoxine. It is given by mouth in doses of 500 mg daily and treatment is continued indefinitely. Folic acid deficiency may also be present in such cases if there are associated megaloblastic changes when folic acid and pyridoxine are given together.

ANABOLIC STEROIDS

Methendienone

Pharmacological action. Anabolic steroids increase the sensitivity of erythropoietic stem cells to the action of erythropoietin.

Therapeutic use. Testosterone or a non-virilising anabolic steroid such as methendienone may sometimes stimulate erythropoiesis in hypoplastic anaemia and in myelofibrosis and are worth a trial. The dose is 5 mg t.d.s. daily.

ANTICOAGULANT DRUGS

Heparin

Pharmacological action. In conjunction with a plasma co-factor heparin exerts a direct and immediate anticoagulant effect, both *in vitro* and *in vivo*, by suppressing the activation of prothrombin and inhibiting the action of thrombin. Heparin also has a lipaemia-clearing action via activation of lipoprotein lipase but this effect occurs only *in vivo*.

Therapeutic use. Heparin is used in the prevention and treatment of intravascular thrombosis and embolism, either alone or combined with oral anticoagulant drugs. It cannot be given by mouth since it is destroyed in the gastrointestinal tract and is administered parenterally, usually intravenously. For preventing intravascular coagulation as in cardiac-bypass surgery heparin is used alone in a dose of 300 U/kg and supplemental doses of 150 U/kg are given every 45 minutes during the period of bypass. For treating established thrombosis an initial intravenous dose of 15,000 U is given followed by 10,000 U every 6 hours through an indwelling catheter or needle with a diaphragm. Heparin is also given by continuous infusion: 40,000 U are added to 500 ml saline and infused over 24 hours. Continuous infusion gives a uniform but relatively low level of heparin in the blood and it is important to ascertain that a satisfactory anticoagulant effect is obtained by doing whole blood clotting times on several occasions during the day – the clotting time should be about twice normal. In established thrombosis heparin is usually used in combination with oral anticoagulant drugs which are started at the same time: the heparin is given for 5 days by which time the oral anticoagulant will have reached a therapeutic level. Heparin has been given by deep subcutaneous injection using a concentrated solution of heparin (25,000 U/ml): a priming intravenous dose of 12,500 units is given followed by 25,000 U subcutaneously every 12 hours. Intramuscular administration is not recommended because of the danger of formation of large painful haematomata. The use of heparin in small doses commencing pre-operatively appears safe and effective in preventing post-operative deep-vein thrombosis.

Contraindications and side effects. Heparin should not be used in the immediate postoperative period because it may cause serious bleeding from the operation site. Otherwise there is little or no danger of serious haemorrhage when the period of heparin administration does not exceed 48 hours. Treatment for longer periods carries a definite risk of haemorrhage which increases with the duration of treatment. Side effects due to hypersensitivity are rare: local wheal formation, erythema, urticaria, macular skin rashes, facial flushing, fever and bronchospasm have been reported. Severe itching and burning of the feet coming on about a week after starting treatment with heparin has also been described. Long-term heparin therapy extending over weeks, although not generally used now has produced alopecia and osteoporosis.

Neutralisation of heparin. This can be rapidly accomplished by giving protamine sulphate intravenously: 1·5 mg, protamine sulphate will neutralise 100 units of heparin. Protamine sulphate is supplied as a solution containing 10 mg/ml and the appropriate volume diluted in isotonic saline is injected slowly over a period of 10 minutes. Rapid injection or excessive doses may cause hypotension. If possible the amount of heparin to be neutralised and the effectiveness of neutralisation should be checked by appropriate tests.

ORAL ANTICOAGULANTS

Apart from different dose requirements their pharmacological actions and therapeutic uses are similar and much of what is written about phenindione is applicable to the other preparations as well.

Phenindione

Pharmacological action. Phenindione decreases the coagulability of the blood by depressing the synthesis in the liver of the four vitamin-K dependent plasma clotting factors (prothrombin and factors VII, IX and X). It acts as a competitive inhibitor of vitamin K. With suitable doses of phenindione the plasma concentration of these clotting factors is reduced to the therapeutic level of 5–15 per cent. in 36–48 hours. Unlike heparin, phenindione is inactive *in vitro*. It is rapidly and completely absorbed from the bowel within three hours of ingesting the dose. It also has a uricosuric effect.

Therapeutic use. Phenindione is used for the prevention and treatment of thrombosis and embolism. The drug is taken by mouth and dosage is regulated by appropriate tests, usually the prothrombin time test of Quick or the Thrombotest, both tests being carried out on citrated plasma. For safe and effective therapy the prothrombin complex of factors should be maintained between 5 and 15 per cent of the normal level: levels below 5 per cent increase the risk of haemorrhage while levels above 15 per cent are less effective. Very ill patients, those in the early postoperative period or in congestive cardiac failure, those with liver or renal failure and old patients in general, tend to be more sensitive to the anticoagulant action of these drugs than do patients in good general condition. Large and overweight patients usually require higher doses than small and thin patients. The prothrombin time is done before starting treatment. To initiate therapy in patients whose general condition is reasonably good a single dose of 200 mg is given on the first day followed by 100 mg (50 mg b.d.) on the second day. No further doses are given until the results of the 'prothrombin' test, which is done on the third day, is known. The size of subsequent doses for maintenance therapy is dependent on this result: most patients will require a maintenance dose of 50–100 mg daily, given in divided doses in the morning and evening, but some may require doses as high as 175 mg. For patients who may be unduly sensitive the induction doses are halved and daily maintenance doses may be as low as 10 mg: as their general condition improves these patients will require higher doses to keep them in the therapeutic range. If heparin has also been used it is important to ensure that the blood sample for the prothrombin test is taken not less than 8 hours after the cessation of heparin therapy – the presence of heparin will itself prolong the prothrombin time. Some patients can be maintained on a constant daily dose while others are more easily controlled by varying the daily dose, e.g. alternating doses of 50 mg and 75 mg, or a constant dose for 5 days during the week with a lower or higher dose on the remaining days. Tests are done frequently until a stable anticoagulant level has been achieved: thereafter for patients in hospital tests are done once or twice a week, and, for outpatients on long term therapy, once or twice a week for the first two weeks after discharge and then monthly. Patients on long-term treatment should be advised not to vary their diets too much since the amount of vitamin K in the diet will vary with its composition.

Barbiturates and tranquillizing drugs tend to reduce sensitivity to oral anticoagulant drugs. Atromid, phenylbutazone, aspirin and anabolic steroids tend to increase the sensitivity. In general patients on anticoagulant drugs should not take aspirin or drugs like phenylbutazone.

For elective surgery in patients on long term anticoagulant therapy, the drug is stopped 48 hours before the operation and restarted on the third postoperative day. Postpartum prophylaxis can also be started on the third day.

Contraindications and side effects. Because of the danger of bleeding anticoagulant therapy is potentially dangerous in patients with peptic ulceration or other gastrointestinal lesions which may bleed. Most patients tolerate phenindione very well but a few (1–2 per cent) develop a skin rash which in occasional cases takes the form of a severe exfoliative dermatitis. Haematuria is not uncommon and can usually be brought under control by reducing the dose temporarily. Patients who are otherwise well controlled may develop melaena and this should prompt a search for a local lesion in the gastrointestinal tract. Haemorrhage into the wall of the bowel may give signs of intestinal obstruction and retroperitoneal haemorrhage may lead to ileus. A very occasional side effect of phenindione is agranulocytosis and there are isolated reports of hepatic and of renal damage. Occasional patients develop diarrhoea during phenindione therapy. Drug fever has been reported.

The urine may be coloured pink during phenindione therapy and this should not be mistaken for haematuria.

Intramuscular injections should be avoided in patients on anticoagulant therapy since they may cause painful haematomata.

Warfarin

Pharmacological action. See phenindione. The drug has a longer action than phenindione.

Therapeutic use. See phenindione. For starting treatment a single dose of 40–50 mg is given by mouth. No further doses are given until the third day when the prothrombin time is done. Maintenance doses are usually from 5–10 mg taken as a single dose at about the same time each day. Very ill patients tend to be difficult to stabilise on warfarin but can be controlled more easily with phenindione. For long term therapy, however, warfarin is preferable to phenindione. Warfarin is also used in those patients who have developed hypersensitivity or other reactions to phenindione. Warfarin can be administered intravenously if a patient is vomiting: the intravenous dose is the same as the oral dose.

Contraindications and side effects. See phenindione. Warfarin appears to cause fewer side effects than phenindione. A few patients may develop nausea, vomiting, or diarrhoea. Occasional patients are completely resistant to the anticoagulant effect of warfarin but they will respond if changed to another drug such as phenindione or nicoumalone.

Nicoumalone (Acenocumarol, *USA*)

Pharmacological action. See phenindione.

Therapeutic use. See phenindione. The drug is administered orally and the induction dose is about 12 mg given in a single dose. Therapeutic levels are reached in 36–96 hours. The results of the prothrombin test on the third day will determine the maintenance dose, which is usually about 4 mg.

Contraindications and side effects. See phenindione. Skin rashes have been reported.

Vitamin K_1

Pharmacological action. An essential co-factor in the biosynthesis of four plasma clotting factors: prothrombin, and factors VII, IX and X.

Therapeutic use. An antidote to the action of oral anticoagulant drugs. Used to treat bleeding due to excessive hypoprothrombinaemia. An intravenous dose of 10–20 mg will usually be effective in stopping the bleeding and reducing the prothrombin time in 12–24 hours. Excessive doses should be avoided in patients in whom anticoagulants are to be resumed since they may then be temporarily refractory to treatment. Vitamin K_1 is also used in treating the hypoprothrombinaemia associated with obstructive jaundice or severe intestinal-malabsorption; — in these cases intravenous doses of 5–10 mg are given.

ε-aminocaproic acid (EACA)

Pharmacological action. EACA is a competitive inhibitor of plasminogen activation.

Therapeutic use. EACA has been used in the treatment of bleeding associated with severe fibrinolysis. Major surgical operations, particularly on the heart and lungs, may be complicated by serious bleeding associated with marked fibrinolysis which leads to digestion of fibrinogen and other clotting factors. In such cases intravenous injection of 5 g. EACA may improve haemostasis but fibrinogen may also have to be administered at the same time if the plasma fibrinogen concentration is below 50 mg/100 ml. Spontaneous bleeding due to fibrinolysis and fibrinogenopaenia occurring in disseminated malignant disease, particularly prostatic carcinoma, may also respond to EACA given either orally or intravenously in a dose of 5 g. which can be repeated for 2–3 doses at intervals of 6 hours. Menorrhagia, in the absence of a local lesion in the uterus, has been reported to respond to oral EACA therapy. EACA has been of value in severe haematuria following prostatic surgery, the dose being 5 g. given orally or intravenously and repeated for not more than 1–2 doses at 6-hourly intervals if necessary. EACA is also used prophylactically in conjunction with AHG concentrates in haemophiliac patients undergoing dental surgery.

Contraindications and some side effects. EACA should not be used in chest surgery after closure of the chest since blood clots formed in the pleural or pericardial cavity may be unlysable and then become organised. It should also not be used in bleeding from the upper renal tract because the unlysed clots may lead to permanent obstructive nephropathy. The use of EACA in surgical patients carries the risk of subsequent thrombosis in the postoperative period. EACA is contraindicated in fibrinolysis secondary to disseminated intravascular coagulation. Oral EACA therapy may produce diarrhoea in some patients.

FIBRINOLYTIC AGENTS

Streptokinase

Pharmacological action and therapeutic use. Streptokinase is a streptococcal exotoxin. It reacts with the plasminogen in the blood, liberating plasmin which is a proteolytic enzyme. If it is injected after a thrombosis it breaks down fibres within the thrombus, forming soluble degredation products.

Streptokinase is the drug of choice in the treatment of deep vein thrombosis and pulmonary embelism. Its place in the management of coronary occulsion is not clear. There are several schemes of dosage. A loading dose of 250,000 units intravenously can be given over half an hour, which will neutralise any anti-streptokinase due to previous streptococcal infection and willconvert all the plasminogen to plasmin. The maintenance dose is around100,000 units hourly. Plasmin is destroyed by anti-plasmins and the effect of streptokinase passes off about three days after stopping the drug.

Contraindication and side effects. Streptokinase can cause bleeding from granulating surfaces and should not be used for four days after an operation. It can also increase menstrual loss. Excess dosage can also cause bleeding. Use for longer than seven days may cause rashes as, being a protein, it can provoke allergy.

References

Haematinics

Barkhan, P., *Chapter on Diseases of the Blood in Medical Treatment* (1969), edited by J. MacLean and G. Scott, **II,** p. 281, J. & A. Churchill Ltd., London.

Anticoagulants

Ingram, G. I. C., and Richardson, J., *Anticoagulant Prophylaxis and Treatment* (1965), Charles C. Thomas, Springfield, U.S.A.

Vigran, I. M., *Clinical Anticoagulant Therapy* (1965), Lea and Febiger, Philadelphia, U.S.A.

Douglas, A. S., *Management of Thrombotic Disorders, Seminars in Haematology* (1971), pp. 95–139. Henry M. Stratton, Inc. U.S.A.

This chapter was written by Dr P. Barkhan (Consultant Haematologist, Guy's Hospital) and edited by Prof. J. R. Trounce.

Category 10

Antimicrobials

Benzylpenicillin

Pharmacological action. Like all penicillins benzylpenicillin acts upon dividing bacteria by interfering with cell wall synthesis; it is bactericidal. Inactivated by gastric acid its absorption from the intestine is incomplete. Injected parenterally it is distributed throughout all tissues except bone, nervous tissue and serous spaces. Optimal blood levels are obtained 30–60 minutes after injection, very little being detectable after 6 hours. Sixty per cent is excreted by the kidneys – mainly via the tubules. This route of excretion can be inhibited by probenecid, increasing the blood level for a given dose.

Therapeutic use. Benzylpenicillin is highly effective against infections caused by susceptible organisms principally the Gram-positive cocci (pneumococcus, streptococcus pyogenes, and non-penicillinase producing staphylococcus), Gram-negative cocci (meningococcus and gonococcus), Gram-positive bacilli (clostridia and actinomyces) and Treponema pallidum. Resistance to benzylpenicillin has become a serious problem with penicillinase – producing Staphylococcus aureus.

Ideally it should be given 6-hourly to maintain optimal blood levels. For most infections the dose is 150 mg to 600 mg (250,000–1,000,000 units) intramuscularly every 6 hours until the infection is controlled. In subacute bacterial endocarditis where the organism is less sensitive and relatively inaccessible high doses 6–18 g. daily may be required and this is best given via continuous intravenous infusion. It may be injected into the pleura, pericardium or joints for infections at these sites. Intrathecal injections (not more than 12 mg) have been used in meningitis but inflamed meninges probably allow enough to pass from the blood into the cerebrospinal fluid.

Contraindications and side effects. Benzylpenicillin is virtually free from toxic effects when given intramuscularly in the usual doses although pain at the site of injection is common. Convulsions can follow intrathecal injection and very large intravenous doses in the presence of renal failure may cause encephalopathy. Since benzylpenicillin is supplied either as the sodium or potassium salt, retention of these cations will be important in, for example, bacterial endocarditis or severe renal disease.

The combination of benzylpenicillin with a bacteristatic antibiotic may greatly reduce its efficacy by preventing the former from acting upon dividing bacteria.

Hypersensitivity reactions occur most often in patients with a history of allergy such as eczema and asthma, and when repeated courses of treatment are given. Patients should not, except in extreme illnesses (and then only with suitable precautions), be given penicillin if they have a history of hypersensitivity to it. The common manifestations of this are urticaria, other rashes (including erythema multiforme) and drug fever. Less frequent but more serious effects are wheezing, laryngeal oedema and shock. Others include exfoliative dermatitis, haemolytic anaemia and thrombocytopenia. The Jarisch-Herxheimer reaction should be anticipated in the treatment of tertiary syphilis. Penicillin should not be used topically because of the risk of sensitising the patient and producing resistant organisms.

Procaine penicillin

Pharmacological action. Procaine penicillin differs from benzylpenicillin only by the addition of procaine, thereby slowing absorption and maintaining blood levels for 12–24 hours.

Therapeutic use. It is useful where fewer injections are desired or required on grounds of expediency as in domiciliary practice or in children. The dose is usually 900 mg (1,500,000 Units) once a day or 600 mg (1,000,000 Units) 12-hourly. In order to achieve an optimal blood level quickly it is wise to give with the first injection a dose of benzylpenicillin.

Contraindications and side effects. As for benzylpenicillin. The duration of its effect makes procaine penicillin potentially more dangerous in hypersensitivity reactions. Rare psychotic reactions have been reported after administration of procaine penicillin possibly due to inadvertent intravenous injection.

Phenoxymethylpenicillin

Pharmacological action. Phenoxymethylpenicillin being resistant to gastric acid absorption from the intestine is more reliable and complete than with benzylpenicillin. After absorption the action of the two penicillins is virtually identical although renal excretion is slower.

Therapeutic use. The oral route possesses obvious advantages, particularly in children. For most susceptible infections phenoxymethylpenicillin can be given instead of benzylpenicillin although some clinicians prefer to begin a course of treatment with 'priming' injections of the latter. Tablets are of 125 mg or 250 mg which should be given 6-hourly on an empty stomach. A flavoured oral suspension is available containing 125 mg in 5 ml. Oral penicillin is appropriate in pneumococcal and streptococcal infections of the upper respiratory tract and middle ear. It is also useful in prophylaxis against recurrence of rheumatic fever and glomerulonephritis – the dose being 125 mg or 250 mg daily.

Contraindications and side effects. These are similar to those mentioned for benzylpenicillin although allergy is less frequent. Looseness of the bowels is often encountered and, owing to alteration of the bacterial status quo in the alimentary tract, oral and perineal monilia infection may arise.

Phenethicillin

Phenethicillin is another orally active derivative of 6-amino-penicillinic acid which has no therapeutic advantage over phenoxymethylpenicillin. It is more expensive.

Cloxacillin

Pharmacological action. Cloxacillin is a synthetic penicillin unaffected by penicillinase which is resistant to gastric acid and can therefore be taken by mouth.

Therapeutic use. It is much less active than benzylpenicillin against most organisms except penicillinase producing staphylococci. It should be reserved exclusively for serious systemic infections caused by these organisms which are usually acquired in hospital. It is expensive.

The dose is usually 500 mg every 4 to 6 hours until the infection is under control. It can be given by intramuscular injection when 250 mg 4–6-hourly is usually adequate.

Contraindications and side effects. It is free from direct toxicity. Allergic reactions occur as with other penicillins. Looseness of the bowels and oral or perineal monilia overgrowth are common.

Flucloxacillin

Pharmacological action. Flucloxacillin is a new penicillin related to cloxacillin. It is well absorbed from the gut and higher free serum levels are achieved than with cloxacillin.

Therapeutic use. It has the same range of antibacterial activity as cloxacillin. Its place is therefore in the treatment of infections caused by penicillin-resistant organisms. The oral dose is 250 mg six hourly. For serious infections the parenteral route is preferable when 250–500 mg 4–6-hourly should be given.

Contraindications and side effects. These are similar to those mentioned for cloxacillin.

Ampicillin

Pharmacology. Ampicillin is a derivative of 6-amino-penicillanic acid which is resistant to gastric acid and therefore effective by mouth although absorption from the intestine is variable. Sustained blood levels are usually obtained and it is concentrated in the bile and urine. It is rapidly destroyed by penicillinase.

Therapeutic use. Ampicillin differs from other penicillins by being bactericidal to some Gram-negative bacilli including E. coli, some Proteus strains, Salmonellae and Haemophilus influenzae. Urinary tract infections due to susceptible organisms are treated with 500 mg 6-hourly for 10–14 days. In acute exacerbations of chronic bronchitis (frequently associated with Haemophilus influenzae) 500 mg 6-hourly is usually effective, but a very high dose 1 g. 6-hourly for a week reduces the likelihood of subsequent relapse. Typhoid and paratyphoid organisms are very susceptible *in vitro* but infections need to be treated with 1 g. 6-hourly for 14–28 days. Certain coliform organisms produce penicillinase making them resistant to ampicillin.

Contraindications and side effects. Sensitivity rashes are more frequent than with other penicillins and may appear 4–5 days after withdrawal of the drug. Nausea and heartburn are often experienced. Looseness of the bowels may occur and oral and perineal monilia is encountered.

Carbenicillin

Pharmacology. Carbenicillin is a semi-synthetic penicillin active against Ps. aeruginosa and certain Gram-negative organisms including strains of proteus. It is inactivated by penicillinase. Parenteral administration is necessary, high blood and urinary levels are obtained.

Therapeutic use. Carbenicillin may be used in the treatment of severe systemic infections (septicaemia, endocarditis), meningitis and urinary tract infections caused by susceptible organisms which are usually Gram-negative. It may also be used in the treatment (or prophylaxis) of infection in burns. The intramuscular dose is 1–2 g 6-hourly but it may be given by slow intravenous injection (3–4 g) 4-hourly. The dose for children and when renal function is impaired is smaller. Higher blood levels are obtained by the concurrent use of probenecid.

Contraindications and side effects. Pain is common at the site of intramuscular injection and may be relieved by adding a local analgesic. It should not be given to patients known to be hypersensitive to penicillin.

Cephaloridine

Pharmacology. Cephaloridine is a semi-synthetic preparation related to penicillin. Injection is necessary since it is not absorbed from the intestine. After intramuscular injection adequate blood levels are obtained for 8 hours and it is excreted unchanged in the urine.

Therapeutic use. It is highly active against certain streptococci (pneumoniae, pyogenes and viridans) and Staphylococcus aureus even when penicillin resistant. It is also active against E. coli, Proteus mirabilis and some shigella species. The dose is 250 mg or 500 mg 6-hourly for 5–14 days. The intravenous dose is 250 mg. It may be given intrathecally diluting 25 mg in 10 ml of fluid.

Contraindications and side effects. It is not toxic in usual dosage although intrathecally it may cause drowsiness. Skin rashes may occur and caution is required in patients known to be hypersensitive to penicillin since cross sensitivity occurs between these related substances. Renal damage may occur with doses exceeding 6–8 g daily.

Cephalothin is similar to cephaloridine in its action and range of antibacterial effect. Nephrotoxicity is not a problem in man so that cephalothin is preferable to cephaloridine in the presence of impaired renal function. The usual dose for susceptible infection is 0·5 to 1·0 g six hourly by intravenous or intramuscular injection. For serious and more resistant infections 4–12 g daily may be required intravenously.

Cephalexin is a Cephalosporin which is well absorbed from the gut. The oral dose is 0·5–1·0 g four times daily.

It has a wide anti bacterial activity similar to cephaloridine.

Sodium fusidate

Pharmacology. Sodium fusidate is well absorbed from the intestine and becomes widely distributed in most tissues though not the cerebrospinal fluid. It is active (bactericidal) against penicillinase producing staphylococci.

Therapeutic use. Its use is virtually confined to the treatment of infections due to penicillin resistant staphylococci. Combined with benzylpenicillin it may be more effective but the result is unpredictable. The dose for appropriate infections is 500 mg 3 times daily with or before meals. For children a suspension is available and the dose 23–33 mg/kg daily. Resistance to its action may occur during therapy.

Contraindications and side effects. No serious toxic effects have been reported. Nausea, heartburn and diarrhoea may occur. At present it is extremely expensive.

Tetracyclines

tetracycline	oxytetracycline
chlortetracycline	demethylchlortetracycline
lymecycline	methacycline
chlormethylencycline	tetracycline-phosphate complex.

Pharmacology. The antibacterial activity of the various tetracyclines is virtually identical. They are bacteristatic against a wide range of organisms including most of the pathogenic Gram-negative and Gram-positive bacteria (except some strains of proteus and Ps. aeruginosa), certain rickettsiae, large viruses and Entamoeba hystolytica. Absolute cross resistance exists between members of the tetracycline group.

Tetracyclines are usually given by mouth, absorption from the intestine is good and diffusion takes place through most tissues though not well into the cerebrospinal fluid. The liver partly inactivates them by producing protein binding and some metabolic breakdown. Concentration and excretion is high in the bile; the kidneys excrete appreciable amounts.

Good blood levels are obtained for up to 6 hours with tetracycline, oxytetracycline and chlortetracycline. Because of slower excretion demethylchlortetracycline gives adequate blood levels for up to 12 hours.

Therapeutic use. In hospitals there is a growing population of tetracycline resistant organisms, particularly some Gram-negative species and Staphylococcus aureus. Outside hospital the widest use for tetracyclines is in acute exacerbations of chronic bronchitis where the organism is usually either Haemophilus influenzae or Streptococcus pneumoniae. They are the first choice in rickettsial and certain viral infections and the most effective form of therapy for brucellosis. Although effective against E. coli they are not the most appropriate choice for urinary tract infections as they are bacteristatic and resistance often develops.

Tetracycline, oxytetracycline and chlortetracycline are given orally in tablet or capsule form, the dose being 250 mg 6-hourly for most susceptible infections but for more serious ones 500 mg 6-hourly will be necessary. For children a flavoured suspension is available the dose being 30 mg/kg bodyweight daily in divided doses.

The dosage of demethylchlortetracycline is usually 300 mg 12-hourly, methacycline 150 mg 6-hourly and lymecycline 300 mg 6-hourly (100 mg four to six hourly I.M.).

Topical preparations are available for the treatment of skin infections.

Although there are many varieties of tetracyclines the minor differences in absorption and excretion do not offer significant therapeutic advantage.

Contraindications and side effects. Epigastric burning, anorexia, nausea and vomiting are sometimes experienced. Allergy and marrow dyscrasias have been very rarely encountered. Tetracyclines cross the placenta and are deposited in developing bones and teeth of the foetus giving yellow discoloration. They should therefore be avoided in pregnancy and preferably not given to children less than eight years old. Large parenteral doses given in pregnancy have also caused fatal hepatic damage. Infants developing hydrocephalus due to tetracyclines have been reported, and exacerbations of myasthenia gravis may occur when these are given. Renal lesions have followed their use. Phototoxicity is frequent with demethylchlortetracycline and occasionally seen with others.

The most frequent side effects are due to the overgrowth of potentially pathogenic organisms in the alimentary, respiratory and genito-urinary tracts. Many patients develop candidiasis of the mouth and gut. In hospital severe staphylococcal infection of the bowel or lung may ensue. Loose stools are commonplace. Pain at the site of injection is relieved by concurrently giving Procaine.

Chloramphenicol

Pharmacology. Chloramphenicol is prepared synthetically. It is well absorbed when given by mouth, readily diffusable into tissues and body fluids including the cerebrospinal fluid. Good blood levels are obtained for up to six hours. It is bacteristatic.

Therapeutic use. The use of chloramphenicol is governed by the fact that it can cause fatal damage to the bone marrow although this is rare.

Its range of activity is similar to the tetracyclines but it is particularly effective against salmonellae and other Gram-negative organisms. It is the antibiotic of first choice in typhoid fever when it should be given for 14 days, the dose usually being 500 mg 6-hourly. It is also used in Haemophilus influenzae meningitis in children when it can be given as the succinate parenterally if necessary. It is doubtful if its use can be justified in other infections except Klebsiella pneumoniae.
Contraindications and side effects. Blood dyscrasias include granulocytopenia, thrombocytopenia and aplastic anaemia. Many fatalities have occurred and are apparently related to the total dose or repeated courses. Circulatory collapse (the 'grey syndrome') causing death may occur in neonates and infants given large doses. Other toxic effects that have been noted are Jarisch-Herxheimer reactions, jaundice, optic neuritis and skin rashes.

Erythromycin
Pharmacology. Several preparations of erythromycin exist which include the base, stearate, ethylcarbonate, estolate which are given orally and the lactobionate which is used parenterally. The range of activity is very similar to that of benzylpenicillin but the erythromycins are usually bacteristatic. The differences between the preparations are mainly in the rate of absorption and the serum levels obtained. The estolate gives somewhat higher and more predictable blood levels and may be bactericidal.
Therapeutic use. With the discovery of newer antibiotics the role of erythromycin has diminished considerably. It is used in common Gram-positive infections in patients known to be allergic to penicillin Some strains of staphylococci acquired outside hospitals are susceptible but resistance develops rapidly. The dose is 250 or 500 mg 6-hourly depending upon the severity of the infection. Infants and children require 4 to 11 mg per kg 6-hourly. The lactobionate is given by intramuscular injection 2–5 mg per kg three times daily.
Contraindications and side effects. Toxicity is low except with erythromycin estolate which may cause hepatitis and cholestatic jaundice. Heartburn, nausea and looseness of the bowels are common. Acute abdominal pain has been reported. Allergic reactions are uncommon.

Lincomycin
Pharmacology. Lincomycin resembles erythromycin in its properties although chemically it is unrelated. There is evidence that *in vivo* it readily penetrates bone and into the eye.

Therapeutic use. Its ability to penetrate bone makes it useful in the treatment of acute or chronic suppurative osteomyelitis or joint disease caused by penicillin resistant Staphylococcus aureus. It has the advantage that it can be given orally. For acute infections the dose is 500 mg 6-hourly by mouth, the duration of therapy depending on the response. In chronic infections the same dose may be given for 4–6 weeks and then reduced to 8-hourly for as long as a year if necessary.

Contraindications and side effects. Minor gastrointestinal disturbances such as looseness of the bowels are common. Other side effects are few but include skin rashes, granulocytopenia and headache.

Streptomycin

Pharmacology. Streptomycin is bactericidal to certain Gram-negative bacteria and particularly Mycobacterium tuberculosis. It is not absorbed from the intestinal tract and is given therefore by intramuscular injection. Maximum blood level is reached in 1–2 hours and this falls to low levels in about 6 hours. It is distributed in extra cellular fluid (except the CSF) and excreted in the bile and the urine.

Therapeutic use. The principal role of streptomycin is in the treatment of tuberculosis where, to avoid the development of resistant organisms, it is always given in combination with other antituberculous drugs. The usual dose is 1 g. daily I.M., but it may be given 2 or 3 times per week. It may be used in the treatment of urinary tract infections but many organisms are now resistant. It is more effective in alkaline urine. Combined with penicillin in the treatment of Streptococcus viridans endocarcitis synergistic enhancement takes place with improved results. It is useful in the treatment of certain bowel infections namely the dysentery organisms and E. coli. A 5-day course of 1–2 g. daily usually suffices.

Contraindications and side effects. Damage to the inner ear is the most common and serious toxic effect of streptomycin. Both vestibular function and hearing may be involved though the latter is less common. Some individuals are particularly susceptible and the risk is greater in the elderly or patients with impaired renal function. Dihydrostreptomycin is more likely to produce hearing loss. Neuromuscular block leading to respiratory paralysis has been reported following injection of streptomycin into the pleural space.

Skin hypersensitivity reactions are common in persons handling the drug. Allergic reactions by patients are usually of the delayed type (although anaphylactic shock has been reported) manifested as fever, skin rash, arthritis and lymphadenopathy.

Kanamycin

Pharmacology. Kanamycin is similar to streptomycin and neomycin in its antibacterial activity and its pharmacology. Its use is usually confined to parenteral therapy. Peak serum levels are achieved one hour after I.M. injection and it is not detected after six hours. Appreciable quantities are excreted in the urine, very little in the bile.

Therapeutic use. Its main use is in Gram-negative infections. Almost all strains of E. coli and proteus are inhibited by 8 mcg/ml or less *in vitro* and these levels are readily achieved *in vivo*. Many other micro-organisms are susceptible but resistance develops rapidly in Staphylococci.

In adults the standard dose is 250 mg I.M. 6-hourly. For children it is 12·5 to 15 mg per kg bodyweight depending on the severity of the infection. Fulminating infections with septicaemia usually require intravenous therapy when the dose is the same as with I.M. injections. It can be given into the peritoneum (250 mg in 500 ml of saline twice daily for 2–3 days) for severe peritoneal infections.

Kanamycin should be reserved for serious infections such as septicaemia resulting from urinary tract infection in pregnancy or the puerperium, proteus septicaemia, E. coli meningitis in the newborn or Gram-negative infections of the peritoneum.

Contraindications and side effects. Ototoxicity occurs particularly in the presence of renal insufficiency when the dose must be reduced. Estimation of the blood concentrations of the drug are useful in these circumstances. Nephrotoxicity in man is relatively low but albuminuria and urinary casts have been reported; tubular damage may occur if therapy is prolonged. Kanamycin shares with streptomycin and neomycin the ability to interfere with neuromuscular transmission particularly after intraperitoneal administration. Allergic reactions are rare.

Neomycin

Pharmacology. Neomycin is closely related to streptomycin and has similar antibacterial activity. Highly toxic parenterally it is used in topical preparations for the eye, ear or skin and may be given by mouth since absorption from the intact intestine is generally low.

Therapeutic use. In tablet form or for children as an elixir it is used for so-called bowel sterilisation before colonic surgery, for the treatment of bacillary dysentery and for certain types of E. coli enteritis. For adults the dose is 500 mg 6-hourly for 5 days for infection and for 3 days pre-operatively. The dose for infants and young children is 50 mg/kg bodyweight daily divided into four doses.

Numerous topical preparations are available for use in infections of the conjunctivae, external ear and skin. It is combined with bacitracin and polymixin in aerosols or fine powders for wounds or operation sites.

Contraindications and side effects. The high degree of ototoxicity precludes its use parenterally. Neomycin may damage the intestinal mucosa causing malabsorption. While usually hardly any of the drug is absorbed, in certain circumstances this may be important. Kidney damage has been reported after oral use. It shares with streptomycin a curare-like action enhanced by the use of muscle relaxants and certain types of general anaesthesia. Topical use of neomycin has led to an increasing incidence of skin hypersensitivity.

Gentamycin

Pharmacology. Gentamycin is related to streptomycin chemically and in its range of action against Gram-negative organisms. It is also effective against Ps. aeruginosa. It is given by intramuscular injection and excreted by the kidneys.

Therapeutic use. Its use has been largely confined to urinary tract infections by susceptible organisms. Serious systemic infections have been successfully treated. The dose is 0·8–1·2 mg/kg daily given in 3 equal doses 8-hourly.

Contraindications and side effects. The main toxic effects are upon the inner ear and labyrinthine damage is more frequent when renal function is impaired. Hypersensitivity has so far been uncommon.

Polymixin B

Pharmacology. Polymixin B is poorly absorbed from the alimentary tract and is therefore given parenterally when it is excreted in the urine. It is also used topically for ophthalmic and skin infections.

Therapeutic use. Polymixin B is active against Ps. aeruginosa and other Gram-negative organisms but is used when resistance to safer antibiotics has been demonstrated. Infections of the urinary tract or meningitis due to Ps. aeruginosa are the situations where it is most useful. The dosage is 50 mg (500,000 Units) 8-hourly by intramuscular injection combined with procaine to relieve local pain. It is effective topically in the treatment of infected burns and otitis externa where it is often combined with bacitracin.

Contraindications and side effects. Topical therapy is safe and hypersensitivity uncommon. Parenterally it is toxic to the kidneys and neurological disturbances (paraesthesiae, neuromuscular block, convulsions) have been reported.

Colistin

Pharmacology. Colistin which is identical to polymixin E is very similar in its pharmacological properties to polymixin B.

Therapeutic use. The indications for the use of colistin are the same as those for polymixin B, namely infections (particularly of the urinary tract) due to Ps. aeruginosa. The preparation for injection is called Colistin Sulphomethate and in the USA this is combined with a local analgesic. The dosage is usually 1,000,000 Units 8-hourly.

Contraindications and side effects. These are similar to those with polymixin B.

Sulphonamides

Pharmacology. Although there are numerous sulphonamide preparations with different properties certain generalisations can be made. Some are insoluble and when taken orally remain within the intestine but most are readily absorbed from the gastro-intestinal tract. After absorption there is variable protein binding, acetylation and excretion by the kidney. The rate of excretion and the degree of penetration into the cerebrospinal fluid are related to the amount of protein binding. Their action is to inhibit folic acid synthesis of bacteria by competing with its precursor para-aminobenzoic acid to which they are chemically related. This action is bacteriostatic.

Therapeutic use. Sulphonamides are active against Gram-positive and Gram-negative cocci and certain Gram-negative bacilli. They are inhibited by the presence of pus. Clinically they are most useful in treatment of infections of the urinary tract and meningococcal meningitis (although resistant meningococci have been reported in the USA). Formerly used in bacillary dysentery they are now less useful as resistant strains are common. Occasionally a particular sulphonamide may be useful in bacterial conjunctivitis, trachoma, toxoplasmosis, nocardiosis and dermatitis herpetiformis.

For systemic infections sulphadiazine or sulphadimide are used most often with a loading dose of 3–6 g. followed by 1–2 g. 4- or 6-hourly. For children a quarter or half this dosage applies. These preparations can be used for urinary tract infections, half the above adult dose is then adequate.

Other sulphonamides are used in urinary tract infections such as sulphamethizole (0·2 g. then 0·1 g. 4-hourly) or sulphafurazole. The choice is wide but the effects of the various preparations is similar. The long acting sulphonamides include sulphamethoxypyridazine and sulphadimethoxine the dosage of these being 1 g. daily.

Sulphonamides are sometimes used parenterally in the treatment of bacterial meningitis particularly in the UK when sulphadiazine is usually chosen. Other soluble sulphonamides are equally effective. These are best given via an intravenous saline infusion since it is important to ensure adequate hydration. The dose is usually 6 g. per 24 hours.

Contraindications and side effects. Numerous adverse effects have been described and the reported incidence varies between 1 and 15 per cent. Hypersensitivity reactions are fairly common and include fever and a variety of mild or serious skin eruptions. Almost all types of haematological disorders can occur. Gastrointestinal disturbances are usually minor but are very common; jaundice may be encountered. Crystalluria may occur if the urine is acid and concentrated. Other effects include arteritis and certain neurological disturbances.

Trimethoprim

Pharmacology. Trimethoprim has a similar range of action to the sulphonamides. It inhibits the enzyme which reduces dihydrofolic acid to tetrahydrofolic acid – a stage in purine synthesis which follows that arrested by sulphonamides. The combination of trimethroprim with a sulphonamide produces a synergistic action which is much more effective than either substance alone. Trimethoprim is well absorbed after oral administration. It is slowly excreted by the kidney and adequate blood levels are obtained by 12-hourly doses. It penetrates to the cerebrospinal fluid.

It is available in combination with sulphamethoxazole, each tablet containing 80 mg Trimethoprim and 400 mg of the sulphonamide.

Therapeutic use. The combination of trimethoprim and sulphamethoxazole is active against most of the pyogenic cocci (but have no advantage over the penicillins in this respect) and many Gram-negative organisms. The principal use is in infections of the urinary tract and for acute exacerbations of chronic bronchitis. The dose is usually two tablets twice daily. Gonorrhoea has also been effectively treated. The scope of this combination has not yet been fully discovered.

Contraindications and toxic effects. Toxic effects have so far been rare but leucopenia has been reported. Trimethoprim should not be given early in pregnancy as teratogenic effects have been observed in experimental animals.

Isoniazid

Pharmacology. Isoniazid (Isonicotinic acid hydrazide, INAH) is a synthetic substance very active against Mycobacterium tuberculosis. It is well absorbed after an oral dose and is distributed throughout body fluids including cerebrospinal fluid. The ability to acetylate (inactivate) the drug is genetically determined and varies considerably between racial groups.

Therapeutic use. Isoniazid is only used in the treatment of all forms of tuberculosis but since resistance develops if it is used alone it should always be used in combination with at least one other antituberculous drug – usually PAS. The usual dosage is 300 mg daily in two or three doses. It is presented in many forms either alone or in combination with PAS. It can be given intramuscularly and intrathecally but these routes are rarely required.

Contraindications and toxic effects. The incidence of side effects is low but allergic reactions have occasionally been reported. The most important toxic effect is peripheral neuropathy which is commonest among slow inactivators. Rare adverse reactions include jaundice, psychosis, endocrine disturbances and a lupus erythematosus-like syndrome.

Para-aminosalicylic acid (PAS)

Pharmacology. PAS is usually administered as the sodium or calcium salt. It is active against Mycobacterium tuberculosis although less so than streptomycin or INAH. It is well absorbed from the alimentary tract and distributed throughout body fluids but with poor penetration into the cerebrospinal fluid. Excretion via the kidneys is rapid.

Therapeutic use. Its use is confined to the treatment of tuberculosis always in combination with at least one other drug since resistance develops if it is used alone. Many preparations are available in tablet, powder or granular form usually in combination with INAH. The daily dose should ideally be 20 g but in practice 12 g. is usually the maximum that is tolerated. It should be given with food. The main purpose of combining PAS with INAH is to ensure that patients take both (or neither) to mitigate the risk of resistance developing to one drug alone.

Contraindications and side effects. Nausea, anorexia, and abdominal discomfort are common. Diarrhoea may occur. Hypersensitivity in the form of fever, skin rashes and lymphadenopathy are encountered. Desensitisation is often possible. Other reactions include pulmonary infiltration with eosinophilia, goitre with hypothyroidism, jaundice and haematological abnormalities.

Rifampicin

Pharmacology. Rifampicin is a new antibiotic active against Gram-positive bacteria and some Gram-negative bacteria as well as Mycobacterium tuberculosis where its activity is similar to that of isoniazid. It is well absorbed by the oral route and readily diffusable into the tissues. It is mainly excreted in the bile.

Therapeutic use. The role of rifampicin has not yet been defined but it is useful in the treatment of tuberculosis. At present it should be used only when organisms are resistant to first line drugs. The dose is 450–600 mg daily as a single dose. It should be given in combination with at least one other drug to prevent emergence of resistant strains.

Contraindications and side effects. Toxicity in man has not yet been fully studied but hepatic function may be impaired. Eosinophilia and leucopenia have been reported. Nausea occurs occasionally. It causes red discoloration of the sputum and urine. Patients with hepatic disease should not be treated with rifampicin and until further information is available it should be avoided in pregnancy.

Pyrazinamide

Pharmacology. Pyrazanamide is very active against mycobacterium tuberculosis. It is well absorbed when taken orally, and diffuses into the body fluids. It is excreted by the kidneys.

Therapeutic use. Pyrazinamide is a second line drug for the treatment of tuberculosis. The dosage is 30 mg per kg bodyweight daily in four doses, but this should not exceed 3 g per day.

Contraindications and side effects. Liver damage is common and may be fatal. Estimations of the serum transaminases should accompany its use. It may precipitate gout and cause skin rashes.

Ethionamide

Pharmacology. Ethionamide is chemically related to INAH but not as effective. Absorption by mouth is good and distribution takes place throughout body fluids including the cerebrospinal fluid.

Therapeutic use. Ethionamide is used in the treatment of tuberculosis when organisms are resistant to the safer and more effective drugs. The dose is 0·5 g twice daily.

Contraindications and side effects. Side effects are common and include vomiting, diarrhoea, peripheral neuropathy, convulsions and hepatic damage.

Cycloserine

Pharmacology. Cycloserine is well absorbed from the intestine and freely diffusable throughout tissue fluids including the cerebrospinal fluid. It is excreted by the kidneys.

Therapeutic use. It is used as a second line drug in the treatment of tuberculosis. The dosage is 1 g daily in two doses but therapy should begin with 250 mg twice daily, increasing slowly by increments of 250 mg each week.

Contraindications and side effects. Serious toxic effects are relatively common and include psychoses, depression and convulsions.

Ethambutol

Pharmacology. Ethambutol is well absorbed by the oral route and excretion is predominantly via the kidney.

Therapeutic use. This is a relatively new second line antituberculous drug. The dose is usually 25 mg per kg bodyweight daily.

Contraindications and side effects. The most important toxic effect of ethambutol is optic neuritis producing diminished visual acuity and central scotoma. Patients should have complete ophthalmological examination before therapy and visual acuity should be checked regularly during treatment. Other effects include rare instances of gastrointestinal disturbance and allergy.

Nalidixic acid

Pharmacology. Nalidixic acid, a synthetic preparation, is well absorbed after oral administration and largely excreted (80 per cent.) in the urine where it appears in high concentrations.

Therapeutic use. The role of nalidixic acid is confined to the treatment of urinary tract infections where it is effective against many Gram-negative organisms. It must be used in high dosage (at least 4 g per day) but resistance frequently occurs during therapy. Successful treatment is less likely in the presence of abnormalities of the urinary tract and deep seated infections of the kidney respond poorly.

Contraindications and side effects. Adverse effects are few and mild but include allergic reactions (rashes, fever) haemolytic anaemia, skin photosensitivity, respiratory depression, a variety of disturbances in the nervous system and occasional nausea or vomiting. It causes positive reactions in the urine to 'Clinitest'.

Nitrofurantoin

Pharmacology. Nitrofurantoin is a synthetic preparation which is absorbed from the gut and excreted in high concentration in the urine. Excretion is enhanced if the urine is acid. Blood levels are low at the usual dosage. It is effective against a large number of Gram-negative and Gram-positive organisms.

Therapeutic use. Its use is confined to the treatment of infections of the urinary tract by susceptible organisms. It is often useful against E. coli and some proteus infections. The dose for adults is 100 mg 6-hourly after food or, for prophylaxis, 50 mg 12-hourly. In renal failure its efficacy is reduced since less is excreted.

Contraindications and side effects. Nausea and vomiting occur frequently. Pulmonary infiltration and asthma have been reported. Nitrofurantoin has caused megaloblastic anaemia, and haemolytic anaemia – particularly in glucose-6-phosphate dehydrogenase deficiency. Peripheral neuropathy has been encountered, chiefly where there is impaired renal function.

Amphotericin B

Pharmacology. Amphotericin B is poorly absorbed from the alimentary tract. It is given by intravenous infusion. Urinary excretion is slow and adequate blood levels persist for long periods.

Therapeutic use. It is the drug of choice in systemic fungal disease and is indicated in serious infections due to candidiasis, histoplasmosis, coccidioidomycosis, cryptococcosis and blastomycosis. The dose is 1·0 mg/kg daily given by infusion over a period of 6 hours. The duration of therapy depends on severity of the infection and the response but it may be necessary to continue for several weeks.

Amphotericin B is available in tablet (10 mg) form for the treatment of oral candida infection.

For fungal meningitis 0·5 mg mixed with 20 mg of hydrocortisone can be given intrathecally.

Contraindications and side effects. Kidney damage occurs in nearly all patients given amphotericin B intravenously. The renal lesion, which may be permanent, consists of tubular swelling with calcification. Fever, nausea, vomiting, anorexia and severe malaise are common. They are to some extent mitigated by giving 50 mg hydrocortisone at the start of each infusion. Nearly all patients develop a normocytic normochromic anaemia. Intrathecal injection often produces severe headache.

Nystatin

Pharmacology. Nystatin is an antifungal antibiotic which is poorly absorbed from the alimentary tract.

Therapeutic use. It is used principally in the treatment of infections by Candida albicans. Lesions in the mouth respond to 500,000 units in the suspension given 8-hourly. Monilial vaginitis is treated with pessaries (100,000 units) inserted once or twice daily. Candidiasis of the intestine is treated by tablets or the suspension. It may be given as an aerosol or inhaled in powder form for pulmonary candidiasis and aspergillosis.

Contraindications and side effects. Toxicity is low and side effects are few. It has an unpleasant taste and nausea, vomiting and diarrhoea occasionally occur.

Griseofulvin

Pharmacology. Griseofulvin is partly but adequately absorbed from the alimentary tract and is then selectively taken up by precursors of keratin. It is particularly effective against superficial fungal infections of the hair, nails and skin.

Therapeutic use. It is the treatment of choice in ringworm of the nails and hair. Treatment is usually necessary for weeks or months since new keratin, free from the fungus, may be reinfected by the old keratin before this has been shed.

Dosage for adults is 0·5 g. daily either as one or two doses. Children require 125 to 250 mg daily. The course of therapy should be continued until after the fungus has disappeared from scrapings of previously infected tissue.

Contraindications and side effects. Nausea and abdominal discomfort are occasionally experienced. Depression of the white count has been reported and griseofulvin antagonises the action warfarin. Skin rashes and, rarely, photosensitivity may occur. Other infrequent adverse effects include allergic reactions, transient proteinuria, mood change, gynaecomastia in children and disturbances in porphyrin metabolism. The drug should be avoided in porphyria.

This chapter was written by Dr R. K. Knight (Physician, Guy's Hospital) and edited by Prof. J. R. Trounce.

Category 11

Drugs Used in Tropical Medicine

THE TREATMENT OF AMOEBIASIS

Dehydroemetine hydrochloride

Pharmacological action. This drug is lethal to the parasites in the tissue phase of amoebic infection. It does not affect the organisms in the intestine.

Therapeutic use [1]. The daily dose is 60 mg given intramuscularly; for children the daily dosage is calculated as 1 mg/kg of bodyweight. Treatment is given daily for up to 10 days. Because of the cardiotoxic effect of the drug the patient is kept in bed during the treatment, and he should avoid strenuous activity for a further three or four weeks. At least two weeks must elapse between courses if administration is repeated.

Side effects and contraindications. 1. Local pain and sterile abscess formation may result from tissue necrosis. A fresh site should be chosen for each injection.

2. The drug has a direct toxic action on the myocardium. Tachycardia, a fall of blood pressure and the development of a gallop rhythm may occur. Electrocardiographic changes consisting of T-wave change, prolongation of the PR interval, widening of the QRS complexes, and alterations in rhythm may be noted. The drug should be stopped if there is evidence of heart block.

3. Nausea and vomiting may be produced.

4. Toxic effect on skeletal muscle. Pain, tenderness and stiffness may occur in the muscles of the legs, arms and neck.

Contraindications. Heart disease, particularly if there is danger of heart failure or arrhythmia; pregnancy, due to toxic effect on the foetus; polyneuritis of recent development.

Emetine bismuth iodide

Pharmacological action. This is a derivative of emetine which is administered orally and, being only partially absorbed, it acts in the intestinal lumen as well as in the intestinal wall. It has a direct lethal effect on the organisms.

Therapeutic use [1]. The dose is 60 mg three times a day; it often produces considerable nausea, so that it should be given at night. Phenobarbitone or some other antiemetic preparation may be required.

The effect in the tissues is slow and rather weak so that ideally a 10-day course by mouth should be preceded by treatment with emetine by injection for 3 or 4 days.

The patient's activity should be strictly restricted but confinement to bed is not necessary. The pulse rate and blood pressure should be recorded daily. Unusual changes call for electrocardiography.

Side effects and contraindications. The drug is liable to cause nausea and vomiting; it is therefore prescribed in gelatin capsules or as enteric-coated tablets to lessen these side effects; an antiemetic may also be used.

Chloroquine

Pharmacological action. This drug is effective against the extra-intestinal phase of the infection, and is indicated when it is considered that the parasite has extended beyond the intestinal lumen. Its particular value is in the treatment of hepatic amoebiasis.

Therapeutic use. 150 mg of chloroquine base twice daily for 20 days.

Side effects. See section on malaria.

Diiodohydroxyquinolone (diiodoquin)

Pharmacological action. This is an intraluminal amoebicide and is essential if re-invasion of the tissues is to be avoided and if the patient's stools are to be rendered non-infectious. This drug is one of many intraluminal amoebicides; it is not the only effective one, but it is the best established.

Therapeutic use. 600 mg three times daily for 20 days, given orally.

Side effects and contraindications. The drug is usually free from unpleasant side effects; rarely it may produce mild iodism. The drug should not be given if there is a history of idiosyncrasy to iodine.

Metronidazole

Pharmacological action. This is an imidazole compound which has amoebicidal properties. It is active against amoebae in the liver as well as in the bowel. This is its advantage over most of the other amoebicidal drugs.

Therapeutic use. 800 mg three times a day orally for 10 days.

Side effects and contraindications. The drug is relatively non-toxic. Nausea occurs in some cases.

THE TREATMENT OF VISCERAL LEISHMANIASIS (syn. Kala-azar)

Pentavalent compounds of antimony

Pharmacological action. The mode of action of these compounds is not certain; they probably inhibit essential enzymes in the parasite by reacting with free thiol groups. Pentavalent antimony is rapidly excreted, principally via the kidneys.

Therapeutic use [2]. (a) **Sodium stibogluconate (Solustibosan)** is the most widely used preparation and is also the least toxic. It is issued in ampoules of sterile isotonic neutral solution in water so that 1 ml contains 20 mg of antimony. It can be given intramuscularly or intravenously. The initial dose is 6 ml for sensitivity test. Thereafter it is given in the dose of 15 mg/kg of bodyweight intravenously or intramuscularly for from 10 to 30 days. On account of the danger of allergic reactions it is advised that a break of ten days should be made between the fifth and sixth injections, if any untoward symptoms have been observed. To effect a cure this course of treatment may have to be repeated after an interval of a month.

(b) **Urea-stibamine.** This preparation is undoubtedly efficient and often succeeds where other pentavalent salts fail. In resistant cases it may be given in combination with neostibosan. The total amount to effect a cure is about 3 g. intramuscularly or intravenously in doses of 100 to 200 mg on alternate days for about one month; if, for some reason or other, intermission in treatment takes place, the parasites tend to become antimony-fast.

(c) **Ethylstibamine (neostibosan)**

Side effects and contraindications. Sodium stibogluconate is virtually free from side effects. However, all antimonials can produce a metallic taste in the mouth and throat, and mild gastrointestinal symptoms such as vomiting, diarrhoea and abdominal discomfort. These symptoms are uncommon.

Urea-stibamine may rarely give rise to such symptoms as an urticarial rash, a sense of suffocation following each injection, and collapse due to an anaphylactic reaction.

THE TREATMENT OF TRYPANOSOMIASIS

Suramin

Pharmacological action. This drug is effective against both Trypanosoma gambiense and Trypanosoma rhodesiense present in the blood and in the lymph nodes. The drug does not cross the blood-brain barrier. Suramin-resistant strains do not occur, so that this drug is given as first choice.

Therapeutic use. The drug is used for the early stage of trypanosomiasis, before these are signs of central nervous system involvement and with a normal cerebrospinal fluid. The adult dose is 1 g. intravenously each week for five weeks. Each injection is freshly prepared prior to administration. A test dose of 0·2 g. is given intravenously at the onset of treatment; if there is no untoward effect the patient is given 0·8 g. on the following day. For patients weighing less than 50 kg the weekly dose can be calculated as 20 mg/kg of bodyweight.

Side effects and contraindications. These include idiosyncrasy, with collapse after injection, renal damage with proteinuria, skin rash, conjunctivitis, stomatitis, hypotension, peripheral neuropathy and bone marrow depression. The drug is contraindicated in renal disease or in adrenal insufficiency.

Pentamidine

Pharmacological action. The pharmacological action and indications for use of this drug are much the same as for suramin. However, the development of pentamidine-resistant strains of Trypanosomes has been noted in East Africa. Like suramin, pentamidine does not cross the blood-brain barrier.

Therapeutic use. A course of treatment consists of 10 daily injections intramuscularly of 4 mg/kg of bodyweight. The solution must be freshly made. Local tissue reaction may occur at the site of injection; for this reason care must be taken to select a fresh site for each injection. (Some clinicians prefer the intravenous route.)

Side effects and contraindications. These are unusual and may occur irrespective of the route by which the injections are given, viz. faintness, hypotension, bradycardia, vertigo, sweating, salivation, nausea, vomiting, diarrhoea, epigastric discomfort, pruritus and urticaria.

Intravenous injections may cause syncope associated with a sudden fall in blood pressure, and there may be dyspnoea and constricting pain in the chest.

Tryparsamide

Pharmacological action. This drug is a pentavalent arsenical which is able to cross the blood-brain barrier and has consequently been used for many years for cases of trypanosomiasis with signs of involvement of the central nervous system and/or with an abnormal cerebrospinal fluid.

Side effects and contraindications. There are several disadvantages to its use:

(a) it has numerous serious toxic effects; notably optic neuritis and dermatitis;
(b) it is ineffective against T. rhodesiense infections;
(c) T. gambiense is becoming increasingly resistant to the drug;
(d) to be effective it needs to be given in combination with suramin.

On this account its place has largely been taken by melarsoprol.

Melarsoprol (Mel. B)

Pharmacological action. This drug is a combination of a trivalent arsenical with dimercaprol (BAL). It has the capacity of penetrating the blood-brain barrier and is given for cerebral forms of the disease. Both T. rhodesiense and T. gambiense respond. A 90 per cent cure rate and 5 per cent relapse rate has been reported with this drug.

Therapeutic use [3]. Some physicians have found the drug uncomfortably toxic and special care is advocated in its administration.

(a) For mild invasion of the nervous system three injections of 3·6 mg per kg of bodyweight to a maximum of 200 mg are given intravenously on alternate days.

(b) If the nervous system is seriously affected, two courses (as above) are given at an interval of three weeks.

(c) Relapses should be treated with a repeat course.

Side effects and contraindications. (a) Minor side effects include headache, abdominal discomfort, colic, vomiting, diarrhoea, urticarial rash, pyrexial reactions of the Herxheimer type.

(b) Exfoliative dermatitis.
(c) Toxic hepatitis.
(d) Arsenical encephalopathy.

Treatment of serious side effects should be by withdrawing the drug and giving a course of dimercaprol (BAL) as soon as possible.

THE TREATMENT OF LEPROSY

Damino-diphenysulphone (dapsone, DDS)

Pharmacological action. This is the parent drug of the sulphone group. It is effective, but cure even in favourable cases is slow. It is recognised as being the drug of choice, though some patients show intolerance. However, there are indications that resistance to dapsone may appear in leprosy bacilli (the number of cases in which this has been demonstrated is still small), and there is a possibility of relapse in lepromatous leprosy.

Therapeutic use. Dapsone is given in gradually increasing doses; for adults, 25 mg twice a week or 10 mg daily for 6 days each week (200 mg twice a week may be enough, especially in field work). For children the doses must be correspondingly lowered. Treatment should be taken regularly for 2–4 years.

Side effects. Most toxic reactions occur during the initial weeks of treatment.

1. Generalised dermatitis – patients can be desensitised by giving very small and gradually increasing doses.
2. Erythema nodosum leprosum, an allergic reaction sometimes seen in lepromatous or dimorphous leprosy, may be precipitated. Treatment of this form of leprous reaction requires experience. Corticosteroids may be necessary.

THE TREATMENT OF BILHARZIASIS (syn. Schistosomiasis, bilharzia)

Niridazole (Ambilhar)

Pharmacological action. This drug is effective against S. haematobium, S. Mansoni and S. japonicum.

Therapeutic use. It is administered orally. Dosage is 25 mg/kg of body-weight daily in two or three divided doses for 7–10 days. Tablets of 500 mg are available for adults, and of 100 mg for children. Maximum adult daily dosage is 2 g./day.

The drug is equally effective in urinary and intestinal bilharziasis. In urinary bilharziasis and mild intestinal infections the patient need not be confined to bed during the course of treatment, and may continue at work or at school. However, in the presence of hepato-splenic bilharziasis patients should be confined to bed because of the risk of neuropsychiatric disturbance.

Side effects and contraindications. Side effects are usually mild. They are more likely to occur in adults than in children. The minor toxic effects are gastrointestinal irritation and tachycardia. Neuropsychiatric disturbances have been recorded in patients with heavy intestinal infections; these include episodic excitement, euphoria, hallucinations, disorientation, generalised convulsions, localised muscle tremors and spasms. The urine takes on a cola-colour during treatment. ECG and EEG changes have been described.

Niridazole is incompatible with isoniazid (INH).

Sodium antimony tartrate

Pharmacological action. The pharmacological actions of antimony are in general similar to those of arsenic. This drug affects schistosomes by interfering with a glycolytic enzyme in the parasite. It affects all forms of schistosomiasis.

Therapeutic use [4]. A course consists of twelve intravenous injections on alternate days. Each injection is given in 10 ml of saline and the solution must be freshly prepared. The initial dose is 30 mg, the second 60 mg, the third 90 mg; subsequently 120 mg may be given. The full dose for children is 2 mg per kg of bodyweight. The injection should be given slowly.

Side effects and contraindications. 1. The drug is a tissue irritant and must be given intravenously; great care should be taken to ensure it is not injected outside a vein.

2. Gastrointestinal irritation may be produced.

3. Cough is thought to be due to minute emboli to the lungs; rarely pulmonary oedema and pneumonia have complicated its use.

4. The drug is a cardiac depressant; bradycardia and even severe hypotension may follow its use, so that the patient should lie down during the injection and for one hour subsequently.

5. Occasionally exfoliative dermatitis may occur. This is an indication for Dimercaprol therapy. Herpes zoster occurs quite commonly with the intensive use of antimony.

The drug is contraindicated in febrile patients and in cases of cardiac, respiratory, renal or hepatic disease.

Lucanthone (Miracil D)

Pharmacological action. This drug has a limited field of use in the treatment of bilharziasis (S. haematobium infection), for it is not as successful in curing S. mansoni infection. A cure rate of about 60 per cent may be anticipated.

Therapeutic use [5]. A daily adult dose of 1–2 g. in two divided doses is given for three consecutive days (children 25 mg per kg bodyweight daily).

Side effects. Nausea and mental depression may be produced. The skin and tongue may become yellow and the palms and soles reddish brown in colour.

Caution should be used in patients with impaired renal function.

ANTHELMINTICS

Hydroxychlorobenzamide (Niclosamide, *USA*)

Pharmacological action. The drug is a derivative of salicylamide.

Therapeutic use. The drug has eclipsed all older methods in the treatment of taeniasis. It is effective against the beef tapeworm (Taenia saginata), the pork tapeworm (Taenia solium) and the fish tapeworm (Diphyllobothrium latum).

On waking in the morning two tablets of 0·5 g. are chewed thoroughly and swallowed with a little water. One hour later this is repeated. There is no need for fasting or purgation. Two hours after the last dose a light breakfast can be taken, and the patient can eat normally thereafter. Children under 4 years require half a tablet at each dose, and those between 4 and 8 years require 1 tablet.

In the unlikely event of failure, the drug can be given the following time for two days instead of one, i.e. a total of 8 tablets.

Piperazine

Pharmacological action. The drug is highly effective against both Ascaris lumbricoides and Enterobius vermicularis. The effects of piperazine on ascaris have been investigated extensively. The gross effect of the drug on the ascaris is a paralysis of muscle that results in expulsion of the worm by peristalsis. The drug has been shown to block the response to acetylcholine of ascaris muscle. Orally administered piperazine is well absorbed but it is almost devoid of pharmacological activity in the host.

Therapeutic use. The official preparation is piperazine citrate. In ascariasis a single daily dose of 3·5 g is given for two consecutive days; this is the maximum dose. Children should be treated with 75 mg/kg. This dosage will cure almost 100 per cent of patients. In oxyuriasis, single daily doses of 65 mg/kg with a maximum of 2·5 g given for 8 days will result in 95–100 per cent cure.

It is unnecessary to supplement treatment with cathartics or enemas. Prior fasting is not necessary.

Side effects. Very occasionally gastrointestinal upset, transient neurological effects, and urticarial reactions have attended its use.

Piperazine has been used without ill effect during pregnancy. There are no contraindications to its use.

Thiobendazole

Pharmacological action. This drug is effective in hookworm, roundworm (ascaris), threadworm and whipworm infestations. The drug has specific anthelminthic activity.

Therapeutic use. Given as an emulsion or as chewable tablets of 500 mg; the dosage is 25 mg/kg of bodyweight twice daily for 2 days. The emulsion is put up in bottles of 15 ml and for an adult weighing over 60 kg, the dose is 7·5 ml twice daily for 2 days. The drug should be taken immediately after food to reduce gastric irritation. No purgation is required.

Side effects and contraindications. These are mild but common, and occur in about one-third of patients; they include dizziness, anorexia, nausea, vomiting, diarrhoea, headache, visual disturbance. There are no contraindications to its use.

Bephenium

Pharmacological action. The drug is very effective against Ascaris lumbricoides and hookworms, and moderately effective against whipworms. Very little of the drug is absorbed. It is of particular value in mixed ascaris and hookworm infestation.

Therapeutic use. The drug should be taken on an empty stomach, and food may be taken one hour later. The dose is 5 g. for adults or children; half of this dose for infants.

Side effects. Nausea, vomiting, diarrhoea, dizziness and headache may occur.

Diethyl carbamazine

Pharmacological action. The drug is used in the treatment of filariasis. It removes the microfilariae of Wucheraria bancrofti rapidly, but its action on the adult worms is less certain. In onchocerca infection caused by the filarial worm – Onchocerca volvulus – the microfilariae are killed but the adult worms survive. In sandworm disease (larva migrans) it is effective. Good results have been obtained in cases of tropical eosinophilia.

Therapeutic use. In Wucheraria bancrofti infestation 150–500 mg is given daily; for Onchocerca volvulus the dose is 2 mg per kg once on the first day, twice on the second day, then thrice daily for 30 days. In tropical eosinophilia the drug is given three times a day for five days.

Side effects. Headache, anorexia, nausea and vomiting occur in some patients. The release of proteins from the death of the worms in the tissues can produce allergic reactions.

THE TREATMENT OF MALARIA

Chloroquine

Pharmacological action. The drug has the ability to enter the red blood cells in high concentration, and it is effective against the asexual erythrocytic forms of plasmodium vivax and plasmodium folciparum, and against the gametocytes of plasmodium vivax. It is not effective against the exoerythrocytic tissue stages of plasmodia. The mechanism of the plasmodicidal action of chloroquine is not certain. The selective accumulation of the drug within parasitised erythrocytes may be abetted by the metabolic activity of the parasite itself.

Therapeutic use [6]. 1. In the acute malarial attack chloroquine rapidly controls parasitaemia and clinical symptoms; most patients become completely afebrile within 24–48 hours after administration of therapeutic doses, and thick smears of peripheral blood are generally negative by 48 to 72 hours.

Chloroquine phosphate or chloroquine sulphate are recommended; an initial loading dose of 600 mg (base) is given followed by an additional 300 mg (base) after 6 hours and a further single dose of 300 mg (base) on each of two consecutive days, so that a total of 1·5 g. is given in 3 days.

2. If parenteral therapy is required for the treatment of coma due to falciparum malaria, chloroquine hydrochloride is given by injection intravenously or intramuscularly. The equivalent of 200 mg of chloroquine base should be given immediately, and this may be repeated at intervals of 6 hours, but the total dose for the first 24 hours should never exceed the equivalent of 900 mg of base.

3. In the chemoprophylaxis of malaria, or for long-term suppression following an acute attack, 0·5 g. of chloroquine phosphate is given weekly, either alone or in combination with primaquine.

Side effects and contraindications [6]. 1. The amounts employed for therapy of the acute malarial attack may cause mild and transient headache, visual disturbances, gastrointestinal upset and pruritis.

2. Prolonged chronic medication for suppressive purposes causes few significant untoward effects, and only rarely must the drug be discontinued because of intolerance. None of the symptoms is serious and all readily disappear when the drug is withheld. In a small percentage of patients prolonged treatment with chloroquine may cause a mild, reversible lichenoid skin reaction which subsides promptly when the drug is stopped.

3. Prolonged high-dosage therapy of diseases other than malaria (e.g. 250 to 750 mg daily for many months or even years) may cause retinopathy characterised by loss of central visual activity, granular pigmentation of the macula, and retinal artery constriction. The visual loss is irreversible. This complication of chloroquine therapy is extremely rare when it is given for malaria.

4. The drug is contraindicated in pregnancy as it crosses the placenta and it has caused neurological damage in the foetus.

Resistance to chloroquine has become a great problem in parts of South America and Southeast Asia. Many of these strains are cross-resistant to other drugs such as pyrimethamine. Not infrequently, even quinine cannot be relied upon to effect a radical cure in such cases. Schedules of treatment must, therefore, depend on the strains involved and local experience. A combination of trimethoprim and a long-acting sulphonamide seems to be effective in the management of the resistance strain.

Quinine

Pharmacological action. Quinine is still obtained entirely from natural sources. Its primary action in malaria is schizonticidal, and no lethal effect is exerted on sporozoites or pre-erythrocytic tissue forms. In addition, quinine is gametocytocidal for P. vivax and P. malarial but not for P. falciparum.

The drug is both a suppressive and a therapeutic agent, but it is much less well tolerated and less effective than chloroquine. It passes into the red cell from the plasma with some difficulty, so that high doses are required for it to be effective. It is rapidly metabolised by the body and excreted, so that six- to eight-hourly dosage is necessary to maintain effective drug levels in the plasma.

Therapeutic use [7]. Quinine is particularly valuable in the following conditions:

(a) the treatment of severe illness due to certain multi-resistant strains of P. falciparum.

(b) cerebral malaria due to P. falciparum.

(c) it is useful in combination with primaquine for the radical cure of relapsing vivax malaria.

The oral route should be employed for quinine administration wherever possible. Intravenous injection of quinine is reserved for emergencies such as cerebral malaria. Quinine sulphate is most commonly used for oral administration, and the dihydrochloride is employed for the intravenous injection. The injection should be made very slowly, preferably by infusion through an intravenous drip.

The usual dose of quinine is 0·3 to 0·6 g., and the total daily dose is ordinarily not more than 2·0 g. Tolerance does not develop.

The total oral dose of quinine for adults is approximately 8 g.

Side effects and contraindications. When quinine is repeatedly given a typical group of symptoms occurs to which the term cinchonism is applied. In its mildest form this consists of ringing in the ears, headache, nausea, and slightly disturbed vision; however, larger doses may produce severe disturbance of hearing and vision, gastrointestinal symptoms such as nausea, vomiting, abdominal pain and diarrhoea due to the local irritant action of the drug, and neurological symptoms such as excitement, confusion, delirium and syncope. Renal damage may complicate quinine therapy, and anuria and uraemia may ensue.

When small doses of quinine cause toxic manifestations the individual is usually hypersensitive to the drug. For example, cinchonism may appear after a single dose of quinine.

The drug is contraindicated in patients who have manifested hypersensitivity to it. It should not be employed in patients with tinnitus.

Primaquine

Pharmacological action. Primaquine is highly active against the primary exo-erythrocytic forms of P. vivax and P. falciparum, especially the latter. It is less effective against erythrocytic parasites. Its great clinical value lies in the radical curative treatment of vivax malaria. In effecting radical cure of P. vivax infection primaquine is most frequently administered concurrently with a fast-acting schizonticide such as quinine or chloroquine. The mechanism of the antimalarial action of the drug is not clear.

Therapeutic use. For the propylaxis of malaria 45 mg of primaquine base is given weekly together with 300 mg of chloroquine. This regimen has been particularly successful against vivax malaria, but it is less successful in preventing overt falciparum malaria. For the radical cure of relapsing vivax malaria the equivalent of 15 mg of primaquine base is given daily for 14 days.

Side effects and contraindications. When given to Caucasians in the normal therapeutic doses primaquine has proven quite innocuous. Abdominal cramps have developed in subjects when given larger doses and occasionally mild anaemia, methaemoglobinoemia and tachoytosis have been observed.

The toxicity of primaquine in Negroes is essentially the same, except for the fact that the incidence and the degree of anaemia and intravascular haemolysis are greater at daily dose levels of 20 mg (base) and higher. The incidence of acute haemolytic anaemia is related to the genetic red cell deficiency of the enzyme glucose–6–phosphate dehydrogenase (G–6–PD). The exact mechanism of the haemolysis is not known.

The drug should not be given together with quinacrine or sulphadiazine which enhance its toxic effects.

Proguanil

Pharmacological action. The action of this drug is slow as it acts in the body only after being changed to an active metabolite. It is effective against both erythrocytic and extra-erythrocytic parasites; its fundamental action is to inhibit the nuclear division in the developing schizont.

Therapeutic use. For suppressive purposes the dose for adults is 100–300 mg daily.

Side effects and contraindications. Proguanil is practically non-toxic. Large doses may cause vomiting. Prolonged use may cause loss of appetite, weight and energy.

Pyrimethamine

Pharmacological action. This drug has schizonticidal activity. It is an antimetabolic of folic acid; it may in this way inhibit the nuclear division of the developing schizont.

Therapeutic use. As a suppressant of malaria with prolonged action; the recommended dose is 25–50 mg weekly. The action is too slow for treatment of an acute attack of malaria.

Side effects and contraindications. Pyrimethamine may produce leucopenia and thrombocytopenia. Megoloblastic anaemia has been described. The rapid development of drug resistance has been reported.

References

1. Wilmot, A. J., *Clinical Amoebiasis* (1962), Oxford, Blackwell.
2. Manson-Bahr, P., *Manson's Tropical Diseases* (1966), 125, Baillière, Tindall and Cassell, London.
3. WHO Expert Committee on Trypanosomiasis, 1962.
4. Maclean, K., and Scott, G., *Medical Treatment* (1969), 458, Churchill, London.
5. Sapeika, N., *Actions and uses of Drugs* (1966), 171, Balkema, Cape Town.
6. Goodman, L. S., and Gilman, A., *The Pharmacological basis of Therapeutics* (1970), Macmillan, New York.
7. Berberian, D. A., *Amer. J. Med.* (1969), **46,** 96.

This chapter was written by Dr P. I. Folb (Dept of Clinical Pharmacology, Guy's Hospital) and edited by Prof. J. R. Trounce.

Category 12

Cytotoxic Drugs

Although there is as yet no drug capable of entirely eradicating cancer (with the exception of choriocarcinoma), interesting developments are taking place in the strategy of managing neoplastic disease, in particular the lymphomas and acute leukaemias.

There are now quite a number of drugs which are partially effective against these neoplasms and at present research is in progress as to how these drugs are best deployed. In the treatment of advanced Hodgkin's disease evidence is accumulating that repeated courses of combinations of these drugs is more effective than using them singly. In the acute leukaemias, drugs may again be used in combination and further some drugs appear more useful for induction of a remission and others for maintenance therapy. This means that in the text only approximate doses of individual drugs can be given as much will depend on whether the drug is used alone or as part of a combination regime.

THE ALKYLATING AGENTS

These compounds have the general formula:

$$R—CH_2CH_2^+$$

They are capable of combining with a number of chemical groupings found in the cell. These include thiols, carboxyl, phosphate, amino and nucleic acid groups. Their effect on tumours is probably due to their linking with guanine in the DNA chain. It seems that cross linkage between the DNA strands by alkylating agents is of particular importance. Alkylating agents thus interfere with mitosis and they may also produce abnormalities of the chromosomes.

The various alkylating agents, although having the same general action differ considerably in their solubility, absorption, penetration and speed of action. It also seems that certain alkylating agents are particularly effective in certain types of tumour; the reason for this is not known.

All this group of drugs damage normal cells, particularly those of the bone marrow and intestinal tract, and this is one of the main limitations of their use.

NITROGEN MUSTARDS

Mustine (Mechlorethamine, *USA*)

Pharmacological action. Mustine is a highly reactive alkylating agent. It is rapidly transformed in solution into an ethyleneimmonium ion which is the active alkylating agent *in vivo*. Mustine is a highly irritant substance and can therefore only be given intravenously. After injection it rapidly combines with various groups and is cleared from the blood within a few minutes.

Therapeutic use. Mustine must be freshly made up before administration: it rapidly combines with water in solution. It is important to avoid extravasation of the drug around the vein and it is safest to set up an intravenous infusion of 5 per cent dextrose and to inject the dose of mustine through the tubing with the drip running rapidly.

Mustine often causes nausea and vomiting for some hours after administration. The patient will suffer less upset if it is given in the evening combined with chlorpromazine 25–50 mg I.M. and a hypnotic.

The usual total dose of mustine is 0·4 mg/kg. It can be given as a single injection, or the course can be spread over several injections – usually 0·1 mg/kg on alternate days for four injections. Larger doses have been used but this causes a considerable increase in side effects [1]. Mustine produces a rapid response in those with susceptible tumours.

Mustine can also be given intrapleurally or intraperitoneally in patients with recurrent malignant effusions. The usual dose is 20 mg as a single injection and the volume of the effusion should be reduced if possible to around 500 ml to produce optimal results. Little systemic absorption occurs and bone marrow depression is rare. Mustine may cause a temporary increase in the effusion but it should be effective within three weeks; if not it can be repeated.

Neoplasms which usually respond well to mustine are:

- Hodgkin's disease
- Lymphosarcoma
- Reticulum celled sarcoma

Neoplasms which sometimes show response to mustine are:

- Carcinoma of the bronchus
- Carcinoma of the ovary
- Carcinoma of the breast
- Seminomas.

Side effects and contraindications. Depression of the bone marrow is the most important toxic action of the drug. It affects the granulocytes and sometimes the platelets, and rarely it also causes erythrocyte depression. These effects are maximal about 10–14 days after giving the drug and they may clear up in 3–4 weeks.

Mustine usually produces severe nausea and vomiting (see above) and may also cause diarrhoea and even ulceration of the gut. Rarely it causes rashes.

Great care must be taken if mustine is given to those with existing bone marrow depression. If it is essential to give the drug, a considerably smaller dose should be used and the bone marrow examined regularly. Facilities should also be available to nurse patients with severe leucopoenia.

Mustine should also be avoided (as should all cytotoxic agents) in the first three months of pregnancy. Although evidence from human sources is scanty, there is good experimental evidence that it can cause foetal abnormalities.

Degranol

Degranol is a mannitol-mustine compound. It is given intravenously and does not appear to have advantages over mustine.

Chlorambucil

Pharmacological action. Chlorambucil is a mustine-phenylbutyric acid compound. It is relatively non-irritant and is satisfactorily absorbed after oral administration.

Therapeutic use. The usual dose is 0·1–·02 mg/kg daily as a single dose in the morning. It is usually two or three weeks before a response is seen and the course of treatment lasts three to five weeks. This may be followed by maintenance treatment at a dose of 2·0 mg daily.

Neoplasms which respond well to chlorambucil are:

Chronic lymphatic leukaemia

Hodgkin's disease and reticulum-celled sarcoma

Neoplasms which occasionally respond to chlorambucil are:

Carcinomas of the ovary and testicles.

Because of its predominant action on the lymphocyte series of cells chlorambucil has also been used as an immunosuppressive agent, and in the treatment of macroglobulinaemia.

Side effects and contraindications. Bone marrow depression can occur especially if the bone marrow is depressed or infiltrated. Weekly white counts are therefore required. Nausea occurs in about 10 per cent of patients and it can rarely cause rashes.

Cyclophosphamide

Pharmacological action. Cyclophosphamide is inactive *in vitro*; in the body it is split by the enzyme phosphoramidase, liberating an alkylating agent. It was originally hoped that this would occur predominantly in tumours, but it is now realised that activation occurs throughout the body. It is well absorbed from the intestine and partially excreted in the urine where it may set up a chemical cystitis.

Therapeutic uses [4]. The dose of cyclophosphamide is between 3–6 mg/kg daily and it can be given orally or intravenously. The high dose level should not be continued for more than five days and this may be followed by an oral maintenance dose of 2·0 mg/kg per day.

Neoplasms which often respond well to cyclophosphamide are:

Hodgkin's disease and other lymphomas
Multiple myeloma
Burkitt's tumour*
Maintenance therapy in acute lymphoblastic leukaemia.

Neoplasms which may show some response are:

Carcinoma of the breast and ovary
Neuroblastomas.

Cyclophosphamide in doses of around 100 mg per day can also be used as an immunosuppressive.

Side effects and contraindications. Cyclophosphamide will produce leukopoenia and regular white counts are required. However, it rarely causes platelet depression. About a third of the patients develop some degree of alopecia which is reversible. A few patients develop a chemical cystitis with haematuria and a high fluid intake is advisable. Other side effects include rashes and nausea.

Melphalan

Pharmacological action. Melphalan is a compound of phenylalanine and mustine. It was hoped that the combination of mustine with a naturally occurring substance would increase its activity. It is well absorbed from the intestinal tract. It differs from mustine in that after absorption it remains active for several hours.

Therapeutic uses. Melphalan is largely used in treating multiple myelomatosis [5]. It has also been used with some success in seminomas and ovarian carcinomas and in treating melanomas by local perfusion, about

*Africans appear to tolerate cyclophosphamide very well and large doses are given (30 mg/kg for 5 days).

half the patients showing some response. The usual dose is 5–8 mg daily for 10 days. When the bone marrow has recovered this may be followed by a maintenance dose of 1–2 mg daily.

Side effects and contraindications. Melphalan is a powerful depressive of the bone marrow, producing leukopoenia, and in particular, platelet depression. It may also cause nausea and with large courses some degree of alopecia.

THE ALKYL SULPHONATES

Busulphan

Pharmacological action. Busulphan is well absorbed from the intestine. It appears to react particularly with thiol groups and the major portion is excreted as sulphur-containing metabolites.

It depresses the myeloid series of cells and has much less effect on the lymphocytes.

Therapeutic uses. Busulphan is used in chronic myeloid leukaemia where it nearly always produces remission. It is also occasionally used in polycythaemia rubra vera. It is the drug of choice for treating thrombocythaemia.

The initial dose is between 3·0–6·0 mg daily. This is continued until the total white count reaches 20,000/cu.m.m. The drug is then stopped and the white cell count usually continues to fall for 2–3 weeks.

If the white cell count then rises rapidly a continuous maintenance dose of busulphan is required; usually 2·0 mg daily, with the object of keeping the white count at about 10,000 per cu.m.m. If the white count only rises slowly further treatment is delayed until the white count rises to about 50,000 cu.m.m. or troublesome symptoms develop. Intermittent courses are used in such cases. Blood counts are done at 2–4 week intervals.

Side effects and contraindications. Depression of the myeloid of cells has already been discussed, and it is important to remember that it is occasionally irreversible and may also affect the platelets. Pigmentation of the skin is quite common with prolonged treatment and is thought to be due to a disturbance of tyrosine metabolism.

A few patients complain of weakness, nausea and hypotension, reminiscent of adrenal failure – but adrenal function is normal.

Diffuse interstitial pulmonary fibrosis has been reported; its cause is unknown.

Mannitol myleran

Mannitol myleran is given orally but nausea is common. Its uses are similar to those of mustine and it has no particular advantages.

THE ETHYLENAMINES

Triethylene melamine

Triethylene melamine has been used in lymphomas. However its absorption is variable, and therefore the therapeutic dose varies between patients, and sometimes severe toxic effects may be produced. It is rarely used at the present time.

ThioTEPA

ThioTEPA is given by intramuscular or intravenous injection as it is rapidly hydrolysed in the stomach when given orally.

It appears most effective in carcinomas of the ovary and breast, and it has been suggested that this is due to depression of endocrine function rather than a direct action on the tumour.

ThioTEPA can be given:

1st week:	10 mg daily for 5 days
2nd week:	10 mg daily for 4 days
3rd week	10 mg daily for 3 days
Thereafter	2 mg weekly.

ThioTEPA produces bone marrow depression in a very arbitory manner and as it has little advantage over other alkylating agents, it is now rarely used.

ANTIMETABOLITES

These drugs resemble substances used by cells for their metabolism and growth.

They compete with the normal substrates of cell metabolism and thus may prevent cell growth and ultimately cause cell death.

The action of antimetabolites is not confined to malignant cells but they are useful in certain types of malignant disease, probably because they have their greatest effect on rapidly dividing cells. Ultimately their usefulness is limited by their toxicity to normal cells, particularly those of the bone marrow, or to the development of resistance.

FOLIC ACID ANTAGONISTS

Methotrexate

Pharmacological action. Methotrexate competes with folic acid for the enzyme dihydrofolic reductase. It has a very much greater affinity for the enzyme than folic acid and thus effectively blocks the synthesis of tetrahydrofolic acid, an important substance in the synthesis of purines.

This block can be circumvented by giving folinic acid, which is 5 formyl-tetrahydrofolic acid, a stage further on in purine synthesis.

About half a normal dose is absorbed and largely excreted unchanged in the urine within forty-eight hours. Only a small quantity penetrates the blood-brain barrier (see below).

Therapeutic uses. Methotrexate will produce a remission in about 50 per cent of children with acute leukaemia. It is also used for maintenance treatment when a remission has been induced by other drugs. It is best used for maintenance rather than induction of a remission in acute lymphoblastic leukaemia.

To induce a remission the dose is 2·5–5·0 mg daily in children, and 2·5–10·0 mg daily in adults. Although methotrexate can be given by injection it is usually given orally as a single dose on an empty stomach. This is important, as multiple doses during the day may not produce the same effect. This regime is continued for 3–4 weeks, until a remission is induced or toxic effects appear.

There are a variety of schemes for maintenance treatment. One method is to give 20 mg/m^2 of body surface twice weekly.

Methotrexate can also be used in meningeal leukaemia. It is given intrathecally in doses of 0·2 mg/kg on alternate days for a total of four doses, and this should be combined with folinic acid 5·0 mg I.M. to reduce systemic effects.

Methotrexate is also used with considerable success in the treatment of chorionepithelioma [6]. Higher doses are used and treatment requires special facilities.

Side effects and contraindications. In addition to bone marrow depression methotrexate causes oral ulceration which is preceded by patches of hyperaemia. It may also cause nausea, diarrhoea and alopecia.

Methotrexate should be used with care in patients with impaired renal function, as a high proportion of the drug is excreted via the kidneys.

PYRAMIDINE ANTAGONISTS

5-Fluorouracil

Pharmacological action. This drug interferes with the synthesis of nucleic acid. It is poorly absorbed after oral administration, and is usually given intravenously. Most of the drug is metabolised, and about 20 per cent is excreted in the urine.

Therapeutic uses. 5-Fluorouracil is of some benefit in about 30 per cent of patients with carcinoma of the ovary, stomach, intestinal tract and breast [7].

The usual dose is 15 mg/kg*/day for 5 days – the daily dose should not exceed 1·0 g. If there is no sign of toxicity a further four doses of 7·5 mg/kg can be given on alternate days.

Side effects and contraindications. Early signs of toxicity are nausea, anorexia and diarrhoea. If mouth ulceration develops the drug should be stopped.

Bone marrow depression is common and usually starts within a few days of starting treatment. Reduced dosage should be used in those with bone marrow depression or jaundice.

5-Fluorouracil is contraindicated in patients who have had an adrenalectomy as they are particularly sensitive to the diarrhoea and vomiting produced by this drug.

Cytarabin (Ara-C)

Pharmacological action. Cytarabin is a pyrimidine nucleoside which is incorporated in D.N.A. and inhibits D.N.A. synthesis. It is effective in acute leukaemias and also suppresses D.N.A. viruses.

Therapeutic uses. Cytarabin is most effective in producing remission in acute leukaemia. It is usually combined with one or several other cytotoxic agents, most commonly 6 M.P., cyclophosphamide, daunarubicin or thioquanine. In combination it produces a remission in about 25–50 per cent of patients with acute myeloblastic leukaemia, but the remission is usually brief. Dosage is variable, depending on other cytotoxic drugs being given but is in the range of 3·0 mg/kilo body weight.

Contraindication and side effects. Gastrointestinal upsets with nausea, vomiting and diarrhoea are common. Bone marrow depression is usual.

★ This is ideal body weight.

PURINE ANALOGUES

6-Mercaptopurine

Pharmacological action. 6-Mercaptopurine interferes with the synthesis of DNA.

The essential stage is probably the conversion of 6-mercaptopurine to its ribose phosphate derivative which either prevents DNA synthesis or leads to the formation of abnormal DNA.

6-Mercaptopurine is well absorbed and widely distributed in the body. However, penetration into the CSF is poor. It is rapidly metabolised and the metabolites are excreted in the urine.

Therapeutic uses. 6-mercaptopurine is used in treating acute leukaemia, producing a remission in about 30 per cent of children and a smaller proportion of adults. The dose is 2·5 mg/kg daily by mouth and is given as a single dose. The initial course should not exceed six weeks and is continued until a remission is produced or toxic effects appear. It is usually used in combination with other drugs in producing a remission. 6-mercaptopurine can be used for maintenance therapy, the usual dose being 1·0 mg/kg daily.

6-mercaptopurine in combination with other cytotoxic agents is used in treating chorionic carcinoma.

Side effects and contraindications. In addition to bone marrow depression 6-mercaptopurine occasionally causes nausea, vomiting and diarrhoea. Jaundice, which can be either cholestatic or due to cellular damage, has been reported.

The concurrent use of allopurinol with 6-mercaptopurine increases the toxicity of 6-mercaptopurine and the dose should then be halved.

Azathioprine

Pharmacology and therapeutic uses. Azathioprine is a 6-mercaptopurine derivative. It has been widely used to suppress rejection of transplanted organs and in the treatment of diseases (nephrotic syndrome, systemic lupus, and some types of haemolytic anaemia) which are believed to have an autoimmune basis. It is given orally in doses of 2–4 mg/kg bodyweight. Azathioprine can cause bone marrow depression with leucopenia and more rarely thrombocytopoenia. It is therefore desirable in patients on this drug to have white cell and platelet counts at regular intervals.

PLANT PRODUCTS

Vinca alkaloids

A number of alkaloids have been isolated from the periwinkle and two of them, *vinblastine* and *vincristine*, have been shown to have useful cytotoxic action.

Pharmacological action. Both of these alkaloids inhibit cell division at the metaphase but this does not appear to be their chief mode of antitumour action.

They are poorly absorbed from the intestine and are usually given intravenously.

They are rapidly excreted by the liver and therefore any biliary obstruction will increase the effect of the drug.

Therapeutic uses. **Vinblastine** is used in treating Hodgkin's disease, and chorionepithelioma.

The initial dose is 0·1 mg/kg intravenously; this is increased by 0·05 mg/kg each dose being given at weekly intervals until a remission is produced or toxicity occurs. Weekly dosage should not exceed 0·3 mg/kg. Maintenance treatment can be given weekly at a dose level which is found by trial not to produce leucopenia. A blood count should be performed before each dose.

Side effects and contraindications. Vinblastine can cause depression of the bone marrow. It usually occurs within a week of the dose, and is short lived.

Vincristine is used as the initial drug in treating acute leukaemia. It can also be used in Hodgkin's disease and related conditions; it is particularly useful when there is bone marrow infiltration as it has little depressing effect on leucocyte or platelet formation. The initial dose is 0·01 mg/kg intravenously; this is increased by 0·01 mg/kg given at weekly intervals until a remission is produced or toxicity appears.

Side effects and contraindications. The toxic effects of vincristine are mainly on the nervous system. Muscle weakness effects, particularly the dorsiflexors of the feet, the hands and larynx. This is followed by loss of reflexes and paraesthesiae. The autonomic nervous system is also affected, causing constipation and signs suggesting intestinal obstruction. Nerve damage usually recovers if the drug is stopped, but may persist indefinitely.

Vincristine also produces some alopecia. Depression of the bone marrow can occur but is usually preceded by neurotoxicity.

ANTIBIOTICS

Several antibiotics have been found to have antitumour activity.

Actinomycins probably produce their effect by interference with DNA and protein synthesis.

Actinomycin D (Dactinomycin, *USA*) is used in the treatment of Wilms' tumour in association with surgery and radiotherapy. It is given intravenously in doses of 15 micrograms/kg body weight daily for 5 days.

Toxic effects include dryness of skin, nausea, vomiting and bone marrow depression.

Actinomycin C can be used in Hodgkin's disease in doses of 200 μg daily until a total of 1·5 mg has been given.

Daunarubicin (Daunomycin, *USA*)

Pharmacological action and therapeutic use. Daunarubicin is believed to exert its cytotoxic effect by inhibiting DNA synthesis, forming a complex with preformed DNA. It is used in acute lymphoblastic and myeloblastic leukaemias. The dose is 30–60 mg/sq. metre body surface/per day for up to 5 days and it is usually used in combination with other cytotoxic agents.

Toxic effects include rapidly developing marrow depression (daily white counts are required), nausea, vomiting and ulceration of the mouth. Heart failure is produced by large doses.

MISCELLANEOUS COMPOUNDS

Procarbazine (Methylhydrazine, *USA*)

Pharmacology and therapeutic uses. Procarbazine is most useful in Hodgkin's disease when it induces a remission in about 60 per cent of patients. It may also produce some benefit in other lymphomas. Its mode of action is unknown. The initial dose is 50 mg daily orally, and this can be increased to 200 mg daily. A course usually lasts three weeks unless the white count or platelets become depressed.

Procarbazine can be used for maintenance treatment in doses of 100 mg daily.

It can also be given intravenously but this is rarely necessary.

Side effects and contraindications. Procarbazine depresses the bone marrow.

In addition it may produce nausea and vomiting. It is an amine oxidase inhibitor and potentiates phenothiazine which should therefore be used in half the normal dose if given concurrently.

Crasniton (L Asparaginase)

Pharmacological action. Crasniton splits the amino acid asparagine. Normal cells can manufacture this essential amino acid for themselves but certain types of leukaemic cells are unable to do so. They then become deficient in aparagine and die. Crasniton is usually obtained from E coli but can also be obtained from Erivinia carotorora. It is worth noting that there may not be cross hypersensitivity between Crasniton from these two sources. (See below.)

Therapeutic use. Crasniton is given intravenously in doses of 17,000 units/sq. metre body area in 10·ml of saline twice daily. Preliminary testing with a small dose for hypersensitivity is advisable. The course may be continued for up to four weeks but will depend on the response of the patient. Crasniton is most effective in acute lymphatic leukaemia and is frequently combined with other cytotoxic agents.

Side effects. Crasniton is often antigenic and hypersensitivity reactions of various types are common. Bronchosparm is an absolute indication to stop the drug

Hormones. Oestrogens and steroids are used in various neoplastic conditions.

References

1. Weisberger, A. S., *Ann. N.Y. Acad. Sci.* (1958), **68,** 1097.
2. Ezdwill, E. Z., and Schutzman, L., *J. Amer. med. Ass.* (1965), **191,** 444.
3. Galton, D. G., Wiltshaw, E., Szur, L., and Dacie, J. V., *Brit. J. Haemat.* (1961), **7,** 73.
4. Hamilton Fairley, G., and Simester, J. M., Editor *Cyclophosphamide* (*Endoxance*) (1964), J. Wright, Bristol.
5. Galton, D. G., and Peto, R., *Brit. J. Haemat.* (1968), **15,** 331.
6. Bagshawe, K. D., *Brit. med. J.* (1963), **2,** 1303.
7. Ansfield, F. J., Schroeder, J. M., and Currer, A. L., *J. Amer. med. Ass.* (1962), **181,** 295.
8. Bosen, E. G., Davis, W., *Cytotoxic Drugs in the Treatment of Cancer* (1969), Edward Arnold Ltd., London.

This chapter was written by Prof. J. R. Trounce.

Category 13

Drugs Used in the Treatment of Hormonal Disorders

PITUITARY HORMONES

Growth hormone

This is only available in small amounts for the treatment of children with hypopituitary dwarfism.

Gonadotrophins

Preparations	*Source*
Chorionic gonadotrophin injection.	Extract of pregnancy urine.
Human follicle stimulating hormone.	Extract of post-menopausal urine.

Therapeutic uses. Female infertility [1]. An accurate diagnosis is essential before treatment is begun, because primary ovarian failure and mechanical causes are not amenable to treatment with gonadotrophins. The essence of treatment is the intitial treatment with FSH injection to induce maturation of the follicle, followed by the administration of HCG to induce ovulation. There are many different treatment regimes, but the treatment must always be monitored carefully with one or more of the following serial measurements: urinary oestrogens, vaginal smears, basal body temperatures and pregnanediol.

Male infertility. This is less well established than female infertility, but successful results have been reported in patients with hypopituitarism and some types of testicular abnormalities.

Undescended testes and delayed puberty. HCG in doses of 1,000–2,000 units, two to three times weekly in six weekly courses are commonly used, but the exact indications and optimum ages are controversial.

Side effects. Allergic reactions may occur.

Hyperstimulation syndrome during the treatment of female infertility with ovarian enlargement abdominal pain and even ascites and pleural effusion.

Clomiphene

Preparation. Clomiphene citrate tablets, 50 g.

Pharmacology. Clomiphene is a non-steroid compound related to the oestrogen chlorotrianisene. It has weak oestrogenic properties but its principle property is the ability to cause increased secretion of gonadotrophins to the pituitary. Clomiphene may exert this effect by blocking the inhibitory effect of other oestrogens on the hypothalamus.

Therapeutic uses [2]. Clomiphene citrate is used for the treatment of infertility due to disorders of ovulation. It is ineffective, however, in cases of complete pituitary or ovarian failure. The usual dose is 50 mg daily for five days; if this induces ovulation then the course is repeated until a pregnancy occurs. If not, then the dose is increased to 100 mg daily for five to ten days.

Side effects. Hot flushes due to the increased level of gonadotrophin are frequent; ovarian enlargement occurs, but with careful supervision the incidence can be reduced. Headache, diplopia, dizziness, transient scotomata, constipation, allergic skin reactions, and reversible hair loss have been reported and there is a higher incidence of multiple pregnancy.

Thyroid stimulating hormone

Preparation. Thyrotrophin injection.

Therapeutic uses. TSH, in conjunction with radioiodine uptake measurements is used diagnostically to differentiate between primary and secondary hypothyroidism, to diagnose myxoedema in patients already receiving thyroid medication, and also to confirm hypothyroidism when the results of radioiodine investigations are borderline. It is sometimes used to increase the uptake of a therapeutic dose of radioiodine in the treatment of functioning thyroid carcinomas.

The dose is 2·5 to 10 units I.M. daily.

Side effects. Local allergic reactions. In adrenal insufficiency TSH should not be given before appropriate steroid replacement therapy.

Vasopressin

Pharmacology. Apart from its effect on smooth muscle causing a rise in arterial blood pressure and other manifestations of smooth muscle contraction, vasopressin is also the antidiuretic hormone increasing the permeability of the collecting ducts of the kidneys to water and thereby producing a hypertonic urine.

Side effects and contraindications. Vasoconstriction leads to skin pallor and a rise in arterial blood pressure.

Smooth muscle contraction may cause nausea, intestinal cramp and uterine contractions.

Constriction of the coronary vessels may occur and therefore should not be given if there is evidence of coronary artery disease.

Posterior pituitary snuff may cause local allergic reactions with nasal congestion, and allergic pulmonary infiltration has been described.

Preparation	Main use	Dose
Vasopressin injection	Diagnosis of diabetes insipidus Treatment of bleeding oesophageal varices	0·1 unit I.V. 20 units in I.V. infusion in 10 mins.
Vasopressin tannate injection	Diagnosis and treatment of diabetes insipidus	2·5–5 units I.M.
Lypressin injection★	Diagnosis of pituitary-adrenal insufficiency	10 units I.M.
Lypressin nasal spray★	Treatment of diabetes insipidus	10 units 3–6 times daily
Pituitary (posterior lobe) insufflation	Treatment of diabetes insipidus	5–20 mg t.d.s.

★ Synthetic preparations

More recently chlorpropamide (250–500 mg daily) and also thiazide diuretics (e.g. chlorothiazide 500–1500 mg daily) have been used in the treatment of diabetes insipidus. These drugs are dealt with in more detail elsewhere.

THYROID HORMONES

Preparations	*Equivalent doses*
Thyroid extract tablets	30 mg
U.K. Thyroxine sodium BP (Sodium levothyroxine, USA)	0·05 mg
Sodium liothyronine	10 μg.

Pharmacology. The main action of the thyroid hormones is to uncouple oxidative phosphorylation in mitochondria, but they undoubtedly also stimulate a large number of other enzyme activities.

The principal difference between thyroxine and liothyronine is in the duration of action; thyroxine has a peak action occurring at nine days and lasting for about eighteen days, whereas liothyronine has a peak action at two to three days and lasts for only eight days.

Therapeutic uses. Thyroxine is used in the treatment of primary or secondary hypothyroidism. The starting dose should be low (0·025–0·05 mg daily) and gradually increased at fortnightly intervals to a full replacement dose of 0·2–0·4 mg daily. Thyroxine is also used in the treatment of simple goitres, acute and chronic thyroiditis, and has been used in suppressive doses in the treatment of functioning thyroid carcinomas.

Liothyronine is used in the treatment of myxoedema coma; the dose is 25μg every six hours.

Side effects. Excessive dosage is characterised by many of the features of thyrotoxicosis, in particular tachycardia, nervousness, tremor and sweating. During the initial stages of the treatment of myxoedema, there may be precipitation of coronary insufficiency, cerebrovascular disease or failure of the pituitary adrenal axis.

ANTITHYROID DRUGS [3]

Thiocarbamides

UK and USA	Initial dose	Maintenance dose
Methimazole	10 mg (5–20) 8-hourly	5–10 mg daily
Carbimazole	15 mg (5–20) 8-hourly	5–20 mg daily
Methylthiouracil	150 mg (100–200) b.d.	50–150 mg daily
Propylthiouracil	200 mg (100–300) b.d.	50–200 mg daily

Pharmacology. The thiocarbamides act by inhibiting the oxidation of iodide to iodine, and interfere with the coupling of iodotyrosines in the production of triiodothyronine and thyroxine. They are rapidly absorbed by the gastrointestinal tract and excreted in the urine. They also cross the placenta and are excreted in breast milk.

Therapeutic uses. They are used to treat thyrotoxicosis, either as the primary treatment or in preparation for thyroidectomy. The initial dose is high until the patient is euthyroid (three to six weeks). Thereafter a smaller maintenance dose is required.

Side effects and contraindications. Skin rashes which may be associated with arthralgia and lymphadenopathy. Mild gastrointestinal upsets, leucopenia, agranulocytosis (which is usually reversible) have been reported.

The incidence of side effects is lowest with methimazole and propylthiouracil.

These drugs should be used with caution if there is tracheal compression, and thyrotoxicosis associated with pregnancy.

Other antithyroid drugs

Potassium perchlorate acts by competitive inhibition of the thyroidal iodine concentrating mechanism, and also releases any unbound intrathyroid iodine.

Therapeutic uses. In view of the unacceptable toxicity in therapeutic doses, it is only used for diagnostic purposes: 600 mg of perchlorate will discharge radioiodine from the thyroid affected by some forms of dyshormonogenesis.

Side effects include nephrotic syndrome, aplastic anaemia, neutropenia skin rashes, pancytopenia, gastrointestinal upsets.

Iodine

Preparations. Aqueous iodine solution (Lugols) 5 per cent iodine, 10 per cent potassium iodide.

Iodobrassid tablets (USA) containing 293 mg iodine.

Pharmacology. Iodine in thyrotoxicosis arrests the cellular hyperplasia, increases the storage of colloid and decreases the release of thyroxine. The vascularity of the gland is diminished. The maximum effect of iodine occurs at about ten days, but is only maintained for two to three weeks, in spite of continued administration.

Therapeutic use. After preparation for surgery with one of the thiocarbamide group of drugs, iodine may be used for ten to fourteen days preoperatively to diminish the vascularity of the gland. The dose is 0·3–1 ml of aqueous iodine solution daily in milk. Larger doses are used in the treatment of thyrotoxic crises (2–3 ml daily).

Side effects. Gastric irritation and rarely there is hypersensitivity to iodine with fever and skin rashes.

DRUGS AFFECTING CALCIUM METABOLISM

Parathyroid hormone

Preparation. Parathyroid injection (containing 100 units/ml).

Pharmacology. Parathyroid hormone increases calcium absorption from the gut, increases calcium resorption from bone, and decreases renal excretion of calcium. It also increases the renal excretion of phosphate. The peak effect of one injection occurs at about eighteen hours and lasts for up to thirty-six hours.

Therapeutic use. The only use is in the acute treatment of hypoparathyroid tetany. The initial dose is 100–300 units I.M. or S.C., followed by 20–100 units hourly, depending on the serum calcium level. Prolonged treatment is associated with the development of tolerance.

Side effects. Hypercalcaemia, and allergic reactions.

Vitamin D

Preparations	
Calciferol injection	300,000 units/ml
Calciferol solution	3,000 units/ml
Calciferol tablets	50,000 units/1·25 mg tablet
Cholecalciferol	40,000 units/1 mg tablet
Dihydrotachysterol	0·25 mg/ml.

Pharmacology. Vitamin D is absorbed orally or by intramuscular injections, it is fat soluble and requires bile acids for absorption from the gut. The principle action is to increase the absorption of calcium from the gut and the resorption of calcium from bone, effects which are mediated through changes in protein metabolism and closely linked to the action of parathyroid hormone.

Therapeutic uses and dosages of Calciferol

Prevention of rickets	400 units per day
Treatment of rickets	3,000–4,000 units per day
Treatment of osteomalacia	5,000–50,000 units per day
Treatment of vitamin resistant rickets	up to 500,000 units per day
Hypoparathyroidism	50,000–500,000 units per day.

Dihydrotachysterol has only 25 per cent of the antirackitic activity of calciferol, but the same serum calcium raising ability, and is therefore the treatment of choice in hypoparathyroidism. The dose is 3 ml daily until the serum calcium is normal, thereafter reducing to a maintenance dose of about 1 ml daily.

Side effects. Overdosage with vitamin D will produce metastatic calcification and renal failure, early symptoms are lassitude, thirst, nausea and vomiting. Convulsions and coma are also complications of acute hypercalcaemia.

Calcium

Preparations

Oral:	Parenteral:
Calcium gluconate tablets	Calcium gluconate injection I.M. or I.V.
Effervescent calcium gluconate	Calcium chloride I.V. only
Calcium lactate tablets	Calcium lactate S.C., I.M. or I.V.

Therapeutic uses. Tetany (associated with hypoparathyroidism, rickets, chronic renal disease and coeliac disease). Hypoparathyroidism, Acute colic associated with lead poisoning, Hypocalcaemic convulsions, Asystolic cardiac arrest, Osteporosis.
The dose is 5–20 ml of a 10 per cent solution parenterally for emergency use, or 3–15 grams orally.

Contraindications. Intravenous calcium should be given with caution to a patient on digitalis.

Side effects. Symptoms of hypercalcaemia, metastatic calcification which may progress to renal failure.

HYPOGLYCAEMIC DRUGS

Insulin preparations

Pharmacology. Insulin causes a fall in blood glucose concentration by increasing the entry of glucose into cells, and by reducing the output of glucose by the liver. In addition, insulin stimulates fat and glycogen synthesis, and decreases protein synthesis. It is not absorbed orally, being broken down by the gastric secretions.

Therapeutic uses. Insulin sensitive diabetes mellitus.

Diabetic hyperglycaemic coma.

In the insulin tolerance test to assess the integrity of the pituitary gland.

In the emergency treatment of hyperkalaemia.

Insulin has been used in the treatment of myocardial infarction, but its place is not established.

The dose in diabetes mellitis will vary from person to person, depending on the amount of endogenous insulin production, the diet and

Preparation	Animal Source	Onset (Hours, approx.)*	Peak	Duration
Short acting				
Insulin injection (soluble) (UK) / Regular insulin (USA)	Beef/pork or mixture	½	3–6 hrs	6–8 hrs
Neutral insulin injection (Actrapid)	Pork			
Insulin zinc suspension (Amorphous) (semi lente)	Beef	½	1–3	12–16
Medium acting				
Globin zinc insulin injection	Beef	1–2	6–12	18–24
Isophane insulin injection (BP) / Isophane insulin suspension (USA) } NPH	Beef/pork or mixture	1–2	10–20	up to 28
Insulin zinc suspension (lente)	Beef/pork or mixture	2	4–4	24–28
Long acting				
Protamine zinc insulin injection (BP) / Protamine zinc insulin suspension (USA) } PZI	Beef/pork or mixture	4–6	8–20	24–36
Insulin zinc suspension, crystalline (Ultra lente)	Beef	several hours	7–10	30+
Biphasic				
Biphasic insulin injection (Rapitard)	Mixture	½–1	4–6 8–24	12–24

*N.B.—An increasing dose increases the duration of action, but the figures given are representative. Individual patient variation may be over a wide range.

the amount of exercise taken. The requirements will increase in pregnancy, fever, thyrotoxicosis, infections and diabetic acidosis.

Side effects. Hypoglycaemia.

Local allergic reactions, including skin rashes, urticaria and angioneurotic oedema.

Local lipoatrophy or lipohypertrophy.

Sulphonylureas

Preparations	Relative potency	Average daily dose
Tolbutamide tablets	1 g.	0·5–3 g in divided doses.
Chlorpropamide	100 mg	100–500 mg daily
Tolazamide	100 mg	250–750 mg daily
Acetohexamide	200 mg	250–1,500 mg daily
Glibenclamide	5 mg	2·5–20 mg daily

Pharmacology. These preparations are absorbed by the gut, partially bound to protein and excreted via the kidney. Their main action is to release insulin from the pancreatic islet cells although in addition they may potentiate the peripheral action of insulin.

Therapeutic uses [4]. The sulphonylureas are used in the treatment of mild uncomplicated diabetes mellitus without ketonuria. They are particularly suitable for the adult type maturity onset diabetics, but should not be used to replace adequate dietary therapy. Tolbutamide given intravenously is also used as a diagnostic acid in the differential diagnosis of hypoglycaemia.

Contraindications. They are unsuitable in diabetes following total pancreatectomy, diabetes with ketosis or ketonuria, and are best avoided in children with diabetes and patients with coexistent hepatic or renal disease.

Side effects. Hypoglycaemia, particularly in the elderly and patients with hepatic or renal disease.

Leucopenia and agranulocytosis.

Skin rashes, including exfoliative dermatitis.

Cholestatic jaundice.

Gastrointestinal upsets.

Transient ataxia and muscle weakness.

Vasomotor disturbances with flushing, giddiness, tachycardia and breathlessness which may be precipitated by alcohol.

Eosinophilic pulmonary infiltrations.

Microgranulosis of the heart, liver and kidney have been described.

There may be biochemical evidence of hypothyroidism, but clinical myxoedema is rare.

Biguanides

Preparations	*Average daily dose*
Phenformin hydrochloride tablets	25–150 mg in divided doses
Phenformin hydrochloride SA tablets	50–150 mg
Metformin hydrochloride	1–3 g. in divided doses
Buformin hydrochloride tablets	50–300 mg in divided doses
Buformin hydrochloride SA tablets	100–300 mg

Pharmacology [5]. The exact mode of action is not established but probably the increased peripheral utilisation of both insulin and glucose is the major one.

The action of phenformin lasts 6–8 hours and that of metformin 8–12 hours, they are both excreted largely unchanged in the urine.

Therapeutic uses. As for sulphonyl ureas. In addition, the biguanides have been used as an adjuvent to insulin therapy, where smooth control has proved particularly difficult, and in the treatment of obesity in diabetics. The starting dose should always be low and gradually increased to control the blood sugar.

Contraindications. As for sulphonylureas.

Side effects

Gastrointestinal upsets, a metallic taste in the mouth, general malaise and weight loss, ketonuria without hyperglycaemia, skin rashes, lactic acidosis with phenformin.

CORTICOSTEROIDS

Pharmacology. The steroids produced by the adrenal cortex and the synthetic products can be classified into three groups on the basis of their predominant physiological effects. These are the glucocorticoids (i.e. principally affecting carbohydrate metabolism), mineralocorticoids (i.e. mainly affecting sodium and potassium metabolism), and the sex hormones which will be dealt with in a later section.

Preparations name	Equivalent oral dose	Route	Salt retaining activity
Hydrocortisone (UK) / Cortisol (USA)	20 mg	Oral/I.M./I.V.	++
Cortisone	25 mg	Oral/I.M./I.V.	++
Prednisolone	5 mg	Oral/I.M./I.V.	+
Prednisone	5 mg	Oral	+
Methyl prednisolone	4 mg	Oral/I.V./I.M.	
Paramethasone	2 mg	Oral	
Dexamethasone	0·75 mg	Oral/I.V./I.M.	
Betamethasone	0·75 mg	Oral/I.V./I.M.	
Fludrocortisone		Oral	++++
Aldosterone		I.M./I.V.	++++

The glucocorticoids increase gluconeogenesis, inhibit peripheral utilisation of glucose and increase glycogen deposit in the liver. In addition to these effects on carbohydrate metabolism, they help to maintain normal renal function and raise the arterial blood pressure. In normal pharmacological doses they reduce the inflammatory responses, decrease antibody production, and stimulate production of gastric and peptic secretion.

Corticosteroids with predominant mineralocorticoid activity increase the transport of sodium into cells in exchange for potassium. The principle effect of this is an increased urinary loss of potassium, with sodium retention within the body.

Therapeutic uses [6]. The corticosteroids are used therapeutically in three main categories.

1. *As substitution therapy.* In adrenocortical failure, in hypopituitarism and in congenital adrenal hyperplasia. The doses required are those which maintain normal health, electrolyte balance and arterial blood pressure. In primary adrenocortical failure, a powerful mineralocorticoid such as fludrocortisone (0·05–0·2 mg daily) is normally required in addition to cortisone (25–75 mg daily), whereas in hypopituitarism and congenital adrenal hyperplasia, cortisone alone is sufficient.

2. *In the treatment of some haematological disorders*, such as autoimmune haemolytic anaemia, idiopathic thrombocytopenic purpura, and some forms of leukaemia, especially in children.

3. *To suppress unwanted inflammatory responses* in a wide variety of disease processes. These include systemic lupus erythematosus, asthma, dermatomyositis, polymyalgia rheumatica, cranial arteritis, polyarteritis nodosa, selected cases of rheumatoid arthritis and the nephrotic syndrome, and occasionally in tuberculosis.

The preparation chosen in the latter two categories is one having the minimal mineralocorticoid activity. The dose may be very high for a short period (e.g. Prednisone 60–100 mg daily) in the early phase of the disease or during a relapse. But the correct dose at all times is the smallest dose necessary to produce a therapeutic response.

Side effects

Endocrine. Production of iatrogenic Cushing's syndrome.
Hyperglycaemia with accentuation or precipitation of diabetes.
Retardation of growth rate in children.
Salt and water retention with hypertension.
Potassium loss.
Mobilisation of calcium with osteoporosis.
Aseptic necrosis of the femoral head.
Suppression of the pituitary adrenal axis.

Infections. Reactivation or aggravation of tuberculosis.
Increased susceptibility to viral, bacterial, fungal and parasitic infections.

Eyes. Exacerbation of infections which may lead to corneal perforation.
Precipitation of glaucoma.
Cateract formation.

Skin. Atrophy with the production of striae.
Purpura.
Hypertrichosis and acne.

Gastrointestinal. There is an increased incidence of peptic ulceration and perforation.
Acute pancreatitis.
Increased incidence of toxic megacolon and perforation of ulcerative colitis.

Nervous system. Euphoria and psychosis.
Precipitation of latent epilepsy.
Raised intracranial pressure and papilloedema in children.
Pelvic girdle myopathy, especially with steroids having a F^+ ion at the 9α position.

Contraindications. The contraindications are all relative, depending on the severity of the disease for which they are to be used. However, they should rarely be used when the following conditions are present:

Peptic ulcer	Diabetes
Osteoporosis	Active or possibly active tuberculosis
Psychosis	
Congestive cardiac failure	Acute systemic viral or bacterial infections

Corticotrophin

Preparations

Short acting:
Corticotrophin injection (UK) – I.V. or I.M. preparation.
Corticotropin injection (USA) – I.M. preparation.

Long acting
Corticotrophin gelatin injection (UK).
Repository Corticotropin injection (USA).
Corticotrophin zinc hydroxide injection (UK).
Sterile Corticotropin zinc hydroxide suspension (USA).
Corticotrophin-carboxymethyl cellulose complex (ACTH/CMC).

Synthetic
Tetracosactrin (B^{1-24} corticotrophin).
Tetracosactrin depot.

Pharmacology. Corticotrophin stimulates the production and release of adrenal steroids. It also has some melanocyte stimulating action by virtue of the structural similarity to MSH, and suppresses corticotrophin releasing factor both by the production of high levels of corticosteroids and by direct action on the hypothalamus.

Therapeutic use. Stimulation of the adrenals following long-term corticosteroid therapy.

Asthma in children during the growing period
Bell's palsy
Multiple sclerosis.

Corticotrophin is always given parenterally. A maximal response is obtained with 40 I.U. twice daily, but the dose should always be the minimal needed to control the disease. It is better to give a larger dose less frequently (e.g. twice weekly) than a small dose daily.

Diagnostic uses [7]. Corticotrophin is used to assess the function of the adrenal cortex by measuring either the plasma cortisol or the urinary

17-hydroxycorticoids response following stimulation with corticotrophin. More recently the synthetic preparations have been used with more consistent results.

Contraindications and side effects. As for corticosteroids with the addition of pigmentation, which may occur during treatment with both natural and synthetic corticotrophin, and the occasional allergic response.

ANABOLIC STEROIDS

Preparations	Dose (mg/kg)	Route
Nandrolone phenylpropionate	0·75–1·0/week	I.M.
Nandrolone decanoate	1·0 –1·5/4 weeks	I.M.
Methenolone oenanthate	1·0 –2·0/10 days	I.M.
Norethandrolone	0·5 –1·0/day	Oral
Methandienone	0·2 –0·3/day	Oral
Methendone acetate	0·4 –0·6/day	Oral
Oxymetholone	0·25–0·5/day	Oral
Stanozolol	0·1 –0·15/day	Oral
Ethyloestrenol	0·05–0·1/day	Oral

Pharmacology. These compounds result from attempts to alter the chemical structure of the androgens, so as to reduce the androgenic effect and retain their protein anabolic function. At the present time all these drugs retain some virilising properties. Apart from causing nitrogen retention they also increase the retention of calcium sodium, potassium, chloride and phosphate ions and increase bone growth and maturation.

Therapeutic uses. There is no universal agreement regarding the indications for the anabolic steroids. Generally they are less effective in men than in women, they are rarely useful in acute catabolic diseases, and there is no indication for their use as a 'tonic'. They may contribute to nitrogen retention and protein anabolism in chronic debilitating diseases post-menopausal and senile osteoporosis and chronic renal failure [8]. They should be used with care in growth retardation, as epiphyseal closure may exceed increase in bone growth. Their place in the treatment of corticosteroid osteoporosis, burns and acute renal failure is not established.

Side effects

Virilising. This may occur in females with any preparation, and some patients appear to be excessively sensitive to this effect.

Hepatic. As with the androgens, those which have 17*a* alkyl substitution (the orally active preparations) cause liver impairment and may produce a reversible cholestatic jaundice.

Others. The oral preparations may also cause a rise in serum cholesterol and lipids, especially in conjunction with corticosteroids or in non-insulin requiring diabetics. Contraindications are the same as for androgens.

PROGESTOGENS

Preparations	Dose to produce a secretory endometrium
Progesterone injection (UK) Progesterone suspension (USA)	50–100 mg I.M. daily for five days
Progesterone derivatives	
Dydrogesterone tablets (UK) Didrogesterone tablets (USA)	10 mg daily orally for 10–15 days
Hydroprogesterone Caproate	250 mg I.M.
Chlormanidone acetate	2 mg orally for 2 days
Medroxyprogesterone acetate	10 mg daily for 10 days orally. 50 mg I.M. once
19 *Nortestosterone derivatives*	
Norethisterone (UK) Norethindrome (USA)	10–30 mg daily orally for 10 days
Norethynodrel tablets	10–30 mg daily orally for 10 days
Dimethesterone tablets	15–40 mg daily orally for 10 days
Ethynodial diacetate	1–2 mg daily orally for 10 days

Pharmacology. The progestogens produce the secretory changes in the endometrium, maturation of breast prior to lactation, and progesterone is responsible for the rise in basal temperature following ovulation, and the maintenance of normal pregnancy.

Therapeutic uses. The treatment of functional uterine bleeding.

Premenstrual tension.

Contraception.

Endometriosis.

In the diagnosis of amenorrhoea.

Progestogens have also been used in the treatment of habitual and threatened abortion, but their value is doubtful.

Side effects. All progestogens may cause nausea, vomiting and weight gain. The nortestosterone derivatives are variably androgenic, and consequently can cause hirsutism, acne and deepening of the voice. If given during pregnancy, virilisation of the foetus can occur. The progestogens with an alkyl group in the 17α position (Norethisterone, Norethynodrel) may cause cholestatic jaundice, and should be avoided in patients with liver disease.

OESTROGENS

Pharmacology. Oestrogens stimulate the development and maintain the secondary sexual characteristics including stromal and duct growth in the breast. They are responsible for the proliferation of the endometrium, and for the cyclic changes of the cervix and vagina. The pubertal growth spurt and epiphyseal closure is also an oestrogenic effect. There are a number of other general metabolic effects involving protein, fat, glucose and phosphate metabolism, and salt and water retention. Oestrogens increase the proteins which bind corticosteroids and thyroxine, which may give rise to difficulty in interpreting plasma levels of cortisol and protein bound iodine. There are also effects on the blood clotting factors.

Therapeutic uses. Replacement therapy in primary or secondary ovarian failure.

Suppression of lactation.

Suppression of ovulation in dysmenorrhoea.

With progestogens as a contraceptive.

With progestogens in the treatment of endometriosis.

Metropathic uterine bleeding.

Delayed puberty.

To encourage epiphyseal closure when there is excessive growth in girls.

Preparations	Usual dose	Route
Ethinyl oestradiol (UK) Ethinyl Estradiol (USA)	0·05–0·2 mg daily	Oral
Oestradiol (UK) Estradiol (USA)	0·25–10 mg daily 50–300 mg 4–6 monthly	Oral By im-plantation
Oestradiol benzoate (UK) Estradiol benzoate (USA)	1–5 mg 1–3 times weekly	I.M.
Oestradiol cypionate (UK) Estradiol cypionate (USA)	1–5 mg every 3–4 weeks	I.M.
Oestradiol Dipropionate (UK) Estradiol Dipropionate (USA)	1–5 mg weekly	I.M.
Oestradiol Valerate (UK) Estradiol Valerate (USA)	5–20 mg every 2–4 weeks	I.M.
Piperazine Oestrone Sulphate (UK) Piperazine Estrone Sulphate (USA)	0·75–4·5 mg daily	Oral
Oestrogenic substances, conjugated	0·125–2·5 mg daily 20 mg	Oral I.V.
Non-steroidal Oestrogens		
Stilboestrol (UK) Diethyl stilboestrol (USA)	0·5–10 mg daily	Oral or I.M.
Stilboestrol Diphosphate (UK) Diethyl stilboestrol Diphosphate (USA)	250 mg–1 g. (Treatment of prostate carcinoma)	I.V.
Dienoestrol (UK) Dienestrol (USA)	0·1–5 mg daily	Oral
Chlorotrianisene	12–48 mg daily	Oral
Methallenoestril (UK) Methallenestril (USA)	3–9 mg daily	Oral

Control of menopausal symptoms.

Treatment of carcinoma of the breast and prostate.

The dose will depend on the condition and will also vary with the patient. Examples of ethinyl oestradiol are 0·01 –0·05mg daily for menopausal symptoms; 0·05–0·25 mg daily in replacement therapy and the treatment of primary amenorrhoea; to control metropathic bleeding 0·5–2 mg daily should be given until the bleeding stops, or

20 mg of conjugated oestrogens may be given intravenously in an emergency; 0·1 mg three times daily is given to terminate lactation. The highest doses are given in the treatment of carcinoma of the prostate, when doses up to 10 mg or more are given daily.

Side effects. Nausea, headache, breast tenderness and weight gain due to sodium and water retention are frequent, usually transient, effects. More serious is the occurrence of thromboembolic phenomena. Oestrogens should be avoided in patients particularly liable to thromboembolism, in renal disease congestive cardiac failure and neoplasms of the female genital tract.

Androgens

Preparations	Dose/Route and frequency
Testosterone implants (UK) Testosterone pellets (USA)	200–1000 mg by subcutaneous implantation every 4–8 months
Testosterone propionate	5–25 mg intramuscularly one to two times each week
Testosterone phenylpropionate	10–100 mg weekly intramuscularly
Testosterone oenanthate (UK) Testosterone enanthate (USA)	100–200 mg intramuscularly every 2–4 weeks
Testosterone cypionate	10–100 mg intramuscularly every 1–2 weeks
Methyl testosterone tablets	25–50 mg sublingually daily
Fluoxymesterone	5–20 mg sublingually daily

Pharmacology. Testosterone and other androgenic steroids are responsible for the normal development of secondary sexual characteristics in the male. They also produce marked nitrogen retention and protein anabolism, which results in the growth spurt at puberty. They also cause maturation of bones, with fusion of the epiphyses.

Therapeutic uses. The only clear cut indication of the use of androgens is in the treatment of primary or secondary male hypogonadism. Either a long acting preparation such as testosterone oenanthate or testosterone implants are the most suitable preparations. While it is possible to get good sexual development there is rarely any improvement in spermatogenesis.

Androgens have also been used in the treatment of carcinoma of the breast in females, aplastic anaemia, osteoporosis and growth disorders, but the value and indications are not well established.

Side effects and contraindications. A reversible cholestatic type of jaundice may occur with the androgens which are substituted in the 17α position (methyl testosterone and Fluoxymesterone). This is a dose related not a sensitivity effect.

Other side effects include the suppression of spermatogenesis, sodium and water retention, hypercalcaemia and virilisation if administered to females.

Androgens are absolutely contraindicated in pregnancy and carcinoma of the prostate. They should be used with special care in children, and when there is hepatic or renal disease.

References

1. Gemzell, C. A., Roos, P., and Loeffler, E. E., *J. Reprod. Fertil* (1966), **12,** 49–64. The clinical use of pituitary gonadotrophins in women.
2. Roy, S., Greenblatt, R. B., Mahesh, V. B., and Jungck, E. C., *Fertil and Steril* (1963), **14,** 575. Clomiphene citrate: Further observations on its mode of action.
3. Astwood, E. P., *Thyrotoxicosis.* Proceedings of symposium Edinburgh (1969), Editor Irvine, W. J., Livingstone.
4. Madsen, J., *Acta med. Scand.* (1967), Suppl. 476, 108. The intrahepatic and extrapancreatic actions of sulphonylureas: A review.
5. Butterfield, W. J. H., *Ann. N.Y. Acad. Sci.* (1968), **148,** 724.
6. Picton, T., *Guide to Steroid Therapy* (1968), London, Lloyd-Luke.
7. Mattingly, D., *Proceedings of the Fourth Symposium on advanced medicine,* (1968), (ed. O. Wrong), London, Pitman.
8. Wynn, V., *Anabolic steroids and protein metabolism* (1967). In modern trends in endocrinology, (ed. Gardner-Hill), London, Butterworths.

This chapter was written by Dr. M. N. Maisey (Dept of Endocrinology, Guy's Hospital) and edited by Prof. J. R. Trounce.

Category 14

Miscellaneous Drugs

THE CHELATING AGENTS

Desferrioxamine

Pharmacological action. This drug is an iron-free compound obtained from ferrioxamine, a metabolite of *Streptomyces pilosus.* It is an iron-complexing agent capable of eliminating iron from the body. It does not remove iron from haemoglobin or iron-containing enzymes. The iron complex formed with such substances as ferritin, haemosiderin and transferrin is rapidly excreted by the kidneys. The serum iron concentration quickly decreases. The drug has almost exclusive affinity for iron.

Therapeutic use [1]. The drug is of value in secondary haemochromatosis, e.g. in aplastic anaemia, transfusion haemosiderosis, sickle cell anaemia and severe chronic acquired haemolytic anaemia. The dose is 1 g. daily in one or two intramuscular injections; for maintenance purposes 500 mg is given daily.

Desferrioxamine is of great value in the treatment of children who have taken an overdose of iron tablets. After gastric lavage with bicarbonate solution desferrioxamine should be instilled into the stomach, suggested doses being 3–7 g. in 50–200 ml of water or saline. This will prevent absorption of any iron still present in the gastrointestinal tract. At the same time an intravenous drip should be set up and desferrioxamine infused in a maximum dose of 15 mg/kg of bodyweight/hour to a total of 80 mg/kg bodyweight. Desferrioxamine is rapidly absorbed from muscle and it may be wise to give 2 g. I.M. before starting the time-consuming gastric lavage and intravenous infusion.

Side effects. Pain occurs at the site of intramuscular injection. The volume of urine may be temporarily decreased. The serum calcium is sometimes decreased.

Dimercaprol (British Anti-Lewisite)

Pharmacological action. The drug rapidly enters the circulation within five minutes after intramuscular injection; it is rapidly distributed and eliminated within a few hours. The greater part of the drug is quickly metabolised and excreted in the urine. The dithiol forms relatively stable chelated complexes with arsenic, mercury, gold, and certain other metals. It is also highly effective locally.

Therapeutic use. The drug has been shown to be of value in arsenical intoxication, mercuric chloride poisoning and in toxic reactions due to gold.

In hepatolenticular degeneration it increases the already high copper output in the urine, causing some improvement in the disease.

The drug is given as a 5 per cent solution of dimercaprol in arachis oil with benzylbenzoate as solubiliser. Administration is by intramuscular injection 8–16 ml in divided doses on the first day; 4–8 ml in divided doses on the second and third days; and 2–4 ml in divided doses on subsequent days.

Side effects. Reactions are of minor importance, reversible, and of short duration; they usually occur with doses exceeding 3 mg per kg of bodyweight. They may be prevented by giving an antihistaminic drug or ephedrine beforehand. Paraesthesiae, pains or burning of the mouth, eyes, feet, sweating, lacrimation, salivation, vomiting, weakness, rise in systolic and diastolic blood pressure; these features last thirty to sixty minutes.

Care is required in patients with impaired liver function. Renal damage may be produced due to excretion of the drug with chelated metal. The intramuscular injection may cause severe local necrosis. Intravenous injection may cause cardiac collapse.

Sodium calcium edetate

Pharmacological action. The drug forms strong un-ionised complexes with cations. The calcium compound is used to avoid producing low-calcium tetany.

Therapeutic use [2, 3]. The drug is effective in acute and chronic lead poisoning; it produces a marked increase in the urinary excretion of lead. In hepatolenticular degeneration it has been given with dimercaprol to increase the copper output in the urine. In digitalis intoxication and certain other arrhythmias sodium edetate has been used to bind calcium ions.

It is given by intravenous infusion, a maximum of 40 mg per kg bodyweight being given daily usually in two doses given over a period of one hour. A course of treatment usually lasts three days.

Pencillamine

Pharmacological action. This chelating agent consists of a portion of the penicillin molecule, which is an analogue of the aminoacid cysteine. In copper, lead and iron poisoning it appears to increase the excretion of these metals.

Therapeutic use. The drug is effective in hepatolenticular degeneration in promoting cupruresis. It has been used in copper, lead and iron poisoning.

Penicillamine hydrochloride is given in capsule form, 0·9–1·5 g daily, in divided doses, before meals.

Side effects. It may produce morbilliform skin rashes, and renal damage has been reported. Agranulocytosis may occur.

DRUG USED TO LOWER BLOOD URIC ACID

Allopurinol

Pharmacological action. Allopurinol inhibits the enzyme xanthine oxidease, which converts hypoxanthine and xanthine to uric acid. This results in a lowering of plasma uric acid levels and uric acid excretion. Hypoxanthine and xanthine, which accumulate, are rapidly cleared from the blood by the kidney and being more soluble do not form stones except occasionally in the rare Lesch-Nyhan syndrome.

Allopurinol is rapidly absorbed from the gut and is converted into alloxanthine and excreted via the kidney.

Therapeutic use. Allopurinol is used in the treatment of chronic gout and also in hyperuricaemia complicating polycythaemia and leukaemias. The usual dose is 100 mg two or three times daily.

Contraindications and side effects. The most important side effects are hypersensitivity reaction causing rashes and drug fever. Leucopaenia has been reported and patients may complain of headaches and nausea. An acute attack of gout may occur soon after starting treatment due to the initial moblisation of uric acid.

URICOSURIC AGENTS

These drugs lower the plasma uric acid level by increasing excretion by the kidney. Uric acid is filtered by the glomerulus and a large proportion is then reabsorbed in the proximal tubule. At the same time a certain amount of secretion of uric acid into the urine also occurs at this level. Uricosuric drugs produce their effect of blocking reabsorption at the proximal tubule.

The main drugs are:

Probenecid

Pharmacological action and therapeutic use. Probenecid inhibits the transport of organic acids both into and out of the tubular fluid. It prevents the reabsorption of uric acid from the tubule and thus increases loss in the urine. Penicillin is partially secreted by the tubular cells into the urine, by blocking this process probenecid reduces penicillin loss in the urine and thus raises penicillin blood levels.

In treating gout it is usual to start with 250 mg in a single dose daily and increase weekly to 250–500 mg four times daily. To prevent penicillin excretion the dose is 500 mg four times daily.

Contraindications and side effects. Hypersensitivity reaction may occur and occasionally gastrointestinal upsets.

Sulphinpyrazone (Sulfinpyrazone, *USA*)

Pharmacological action and therapeutic use. Sulphinpyrazone blocks tubular reabsorption of uric acid. Its uricosuric action lasts about ten hours. The initial dose being 100 mg daily and increased slowly to 100–200 mg twice daily.

Contraindications and side effects. Sulphinpyrazone should not be combined with salicylates as this will reduce its uricosuric action. Gastrointestinal upsets can be troublesome and the drug should be taken with a meal. Finally, hypersensitivity reactions occur.

The sudden rise in urine uric acid levels following the use of the foregoing drugs in treating gout may cause stone formation or the precipitation of gravel in the urinary tract. In the early weeks of treatment their use should be combined with a large fluid intake and alkalinisation of the urine will make the uric acid more soluble.

ANALEPTICS

This group of drugs are central stimulants with a marked effect on the medulla. They were formerly used to reverse the effect of medullary depressive drugs, in particular with barbiturates, but it is now realised that their use is of doubtful value in treating barbiturate overdosage.

They are also occasionally used in increasing ventilation in those with respiratory failure.

The main members of the group are:

	Dose	Uses
Picrotoxin	In barbiturate poisoning 6·0 mg at a rate of 1 mg/minute I.V.	Powerful central stimulant can produce convulsions, very short-acting.
Leptazol	In barbiturate poisoning up to 1·0 ml of a 10 per cent solution I.V.	Powerful central stimulant can produce convulsions, very short-acting.
Nikethamide	2–8 ml of 25 per cent solution I.V.	Less powerful central effect. Also sensitises carotid body. Very short-acting.
Amiphenazole	100–200 mg t.d.s., oral or 100 mg I.M.	Milder and longer-acting.
Bemegride	In barbiturate poisoning 50 mg I.V. repeated if necessary at intervals of 10 minutes to a total of 1·0 g.	Longer-acting.

APPETITE SUPPRESSORS

Phenmetrazine

Diethylpropion

Pharmacological action and therapeutic uses. These drugs are powerful suppressors of appetite with minimal adrenergic effect. They are used in the treatment of obesity. The dose is

Phenmetrazine	12·5–25 mg b.d.
Diethylpropion	25 mg t.d.s.

Contraindications and side effects. Dependence can occur with both these drugs. They should not be used in the early part of pregnancy, for there is some circumstantial evidence [4] that one of them (phenmetrazine) may affect the foetus.

Fenfuramine

Pharmacology and therapeutic use. Fenfluramine depresses appetite without apparently any stimulating effect on the central nervous system. In fact it sometimes has a mild sedative action. It is fairly long-acting and the recommended dose in obesity is 1 tablet (20 mg) two hours before the evening meal and 1 tablet mid-morning, but up to six tablets can be given daily. The main side effect is diarrhoea, with occasional nausea. Overdosage however, can produce agitation, confusion, convulsions and death.

THE ANTIHISTAMINES

The antihistamines are a large group of drugs, which in general are very similar in their actions, although they differ as to which particular action predominates.

Pharmacological action. The antihistamines are well absorbed from the gut and largely metabolised in the liver.

Their main pharmacological actions are:

1. They are competitive blockers of all the actions of histamine except they do not prevent histamine induced gastric secretion.
2. They are usually CNS depressors, producing some drowsiness and also are antiemetics.
3. They have some mild peripheral anticholinergic action.
4. They have a weak effect on the heart, similar to that of quinidine.

Therapeutic uses. Antihistamines are used in various allergic conditions, including urticaria and hay fever. They are rarely effective in bronchial asthma. Their effect on the CNS is used to prevent vomiting and they also may reduce the symptoms of Parkinson's disease.

(a) Useful as antihistamines:

Individual preparations

Promethazine: long-acting 25–50 mg at night often sufficient. Sedation marked.

Diphenhydramine: 25–50 mg four times daily. Sedation marked.

Mepyramine: 100–200 mg three times daily.

Chlorpheniramine: 4 mg three times daily or 10 mg I.M. Good antihistamine effect, some sedation.

Phenindamine: 25–50 mg three times daily. Little if any sedation.

(b) Useful as antiemetics:

Dimenhydrinate: 50 mg four times daily. Sedation marked.

Cyclizine: 50 mg three times daily. Mild sedation.

Meclozine: 50 mg daily. Mild sedation.

Promethazine chlorotheophyllinate: 25 mg three times daily.

Quite marked sedation.

Vomiting in pregnancy. All drugs should be avoided in early pregnancy, if possible. However, it is fair to say that the antiemetics listed above have not been shown to produce foetal abnormalities.

Contraindications and side effects. Troublesome sedation is the commonest side effect. The anticholinergic action of these drugs may produce dry mouth and gastrointestinal upsets. Rarely they produce bone marrow depression. It is interesting that both systemic and local use can produce sensitisation rashes.

Disodium cromoglycate

Pharmacology. Disodium cromoglycate is thought to relieve bronchospasm in asthma by inhibiting the release of bronchoconstrictor substances which follows an antigen-antibody union. It is not an antispasmodic. It is poorly absorbed from the gut and is given by inhalation.

Therapeutic use. Disodium cromoglycate is used to prevent attacks of asthma. It is given by inhalation and there are two formulations: either 20 mg disodium cromoglycate per Spincap capsule or 20 mg of disodium cromoglycate and 0·1 mg of isoprenaline per Spincap capsule. Initial treatment is one capsule night and morning and at 4–6-hourly intervals – this can be reduced when a satisfactory response is obtained. Disodium cromoglycate can be given concurrently with steroid or antispasmodics and may enable the dose of steroids to be reduced. If disodium cromoglycate is suddenly withdrawn in those whose steroid dose has been reduced the dose of steroids must be returned to their previous level or a severe relapse of asthma can occur.

Metoclopramide

Pharmacological action. Metoclopramide is an antiemetic but not an antihistamine. Its mode of action is not clear, but it decreases gastric emptying time, probably by stimulation of autonomic ganglia, and relaxes the duodenum.

Therapeutic use. Metoclopramide has been used in many types of vomiting and success has been claimed, although most of these studies are not very satisfactory. The oral dose is 10 mg and can be given three times daily. It can also be given intramuscularly in doses of 10 mg.

Contraindications and side effects. Metoclopramide can produce drowsiness with large doses. Dystonia has been reported and it should not be combined therefore with the phenothiazines. It should not be given in the first three months of pregnancy.

ANTACIDS

Antacids are used to relieve the pain of peptic ulcers. There is no evidence that they alter the rate of healing of an ulcer. They act by raising the pH of the gastric contents and thereby reducing the irritant effect of the gastric acid on the ulcer and decreasing the activity of pepsin. This is achieved if the pH of the gastric content is raised to around 4·0. The most widely used antacids are:

Sodium bicarbonate

Sodium bicarbonate is a rapidly acting antacid, but passes quickly through the stomach so its action is transient. It is absorbed and can thus produce alkalosis, although this does not occur with usual doses if renal function is normal. It is usually given in a dose of 1·0 g. mixed with a little water.

Magnesium oxide

This salt is rather longer acting than sodium bicarbonate. There is no danger of alkalosis but all magnesium salts cause diarrhoea due to the poor absorption of the magnesium ion. The dose of magnesium oxide is 0·3–0·6 g.

Magnesium trisilicate

A white powder given orally in a dose of 1·0 g. mixed with milk or water. Much slower in action and longer activity than the previous magnesium salts. In order to spread the action of magnesium salts they are often combined in a single tablet.

Calcium carbonate

This is an efficient antacid in doses of 1–2 g. It is important to remember that calcium carbonate combined with excessive milk intake can cause hypercalcaemia in some individuals leading to thirst, polyurea and renal damage.

Aluminium hydroxide

Aluminium hydroxide is a useful antacid and can be given either as a gel or in tablet form. It is said to have some inhibiting effect on pepsin.

Carbenoxolone

Pharmacology and therapeutic use. Carbenoxolone is a turpene. There is good evidence that it increases the rate of healing of gastric ulcers in ambulant patients. Its usefulness in duodenal ulcers is not as yet proven. Its mode of action is not known but it provides increased secretion of mucous by the stomach and this may protect the ulcer. The usual dose is 50–100 mg t.d.s. It can cause sodium and water retention and should not be used in those in or near cardiac failure, and care should be taken in the elderly. It can also rarely cause potassium depletion and muscle weakness. Carbenoxolone should not be used for more than two months.

PURGATIVES

Liquid paraffin. Acts by its lubricating action. It is useful particularly in the elderly and in painful conditions of the lower bowel. The dose is 15 ml twice daily or 5·0 ml, hourly for a few hours. Prolonged administration can cause vitamin A and D deficiency and inhalation by the very young or very ill can cause a paraffinoma in the lung.
Bulk purges. These act by increasing the bowel contents. There are a number of preparations available containing agar (dose: 4–8 g.) or methylcellulose (dose: 1–1·5 g.).
Saline purges. Magnesium sulphate is widely used in a dose of 8·0 g. in 150 ml of water before breakfast.

IRRITANT PURGES

Phenolphthalein

Pharmacology. Phenolphthalein is absorbed from the intestine and stimulates the colon. It is re-excreted via the bile and so a certain amount of recirculation occurs.

Therapeutic uses and side effects. Phenolphthalein in a dose of 120 mg at bedtime produces a purge the next morning. It is relatively free of side effects but can produce rashes.

Anthracene purges

Pharmacology. This group of purges contains a number of substances including emodin, which stimulates the colon.

Therapeutic uses
Senna – best given as the Senokot containing the purified active principles. The adult dose is 2–4 tablets or 1–2 teaspoonfuls of granules.
Cascara – Tablets of cascara (BP) 125–250 mg.

OTHER PURGATIVES

Bisacodyl

This purgative stimulates the colon when it comes into contact with the bowel wall. The dose is 5–10 mg.

Dioctyl-sodium sulphosuccinate

This substance is a wetting agent and softens the bowel contents. It is useful in faecal impaction in doses of 40–60 mg three times daily.

MUCOLYTIC AGENTS

The removal of sputum from the bronchial tree is an important aspect in treating a variety of chest disorders. For many years expectorants which usually contain *ammonium chloride*, *potassium iodide* or *sodium bicarbonate* were used. Although in emetic doses these substance would be expected to increase bronchial secretion and thus loosen sticky sputum, in the usual therapeutic dose it seems unlikely that they have much pharmacological effect. Among the older remedies the inhalation of steam is probably the most effective.

More recently however agents have been introduced which are claimed to liquify sputum.
Chymotrypsin may be given by inhalation but its use has not obtained wide acceptance.
Acetylcysteine and *methylcysteine* can be given by inhalation or orally. They are effective in liquifying sputum *in vivo*, but are less useful in a clinical context.
Bromhexine is believed to liquify sputum by breaking down mucopolysaccharide fibres, probably within the mucous secreting cell.
Clinical use. In doses of 8·0 mg three times daily bromhexine has been shown to produce some changes in sputum in asthmatic and bronchitics, although the effect on the clinical state of the patient is variable. Side effects are low but occasionally it can cause epigastric discomfort and nausea.

References

1. Williams, R., *Recent advances in medicine* (1968), Churchill, London.
2. Sapeika, N., *Actions and uses of drugs* (1966), Balkema, Capetown.
3. Browning, E., *Toxicity of industrial metals* (1969), 2nd ed., Butterworth, London.
4. Powell, P. D., and Johnstone, J. M., *Brit. med. J.* (1962), **ii**, 1327.

This chapter was written by Prof. J. R. Trounce.

Category 15

Vitamins

Vitamin A (Retinol, *USA*)

Pharmacological action. Vitamin A is required for the formation of visual purple which is essential for the eye to see in dim light. Vitamin A also directly affects the metabolism of all epithelial tissues; it appears to be necessary for the normal formation of mucopolysaccharides.

Therapeutic use [1]. Vitamin A is used for the treatment of zerophthalmia and of night blindness when this is due to dietary failure. It should also be given to malnourished people who show evidence of follicular keratosis.

Cod liver and shark liver oils are good natural concentrated sources of the vitamin. The prophylactic dose for children is 3,000 I.U. and for adults 5,000 I.U. daily. A therapeutic dose totalling 250,000 I.U. of retinol given in capsules over a period of one week usually achieves maximum therapeutic benefit.

Side effects. High doses taken by early Arctic explorers caused drowsiness, headache with increased cerebrospinal fluid pressure, vomiting and extensive peeling of the skin. Sporadic cases in children in recent years have generally been due to over-enthusiastic administration of fish liver oils. Rapid recovery follows withdrawal of the vitamin.

Vitamin D (Cholecalciferol, *USA*)

Pharmacological action. The vitamin probably has a direct action on bone; it is necessary for formation of normal bone and for the calcification of rachitic bone. The mechanism of its action on bone is uncertain. In addition it promotes the absorption of calcium and phosphate from the gut, thus ensuring a sufficient supply of the minerals to the growing points of bones.

Therapeutic use. For prophylactic use cod liver oil is the best natural source. Not more than 10 ml should be taken daily. The therapeutic dose is 4,000 to 50,000 units daily; the vitamin is used in the treatment and prevention of rickets and osteomalacia. It is also useful in correcting low levels of serum calcium such as occur in the malabsorption syndrome and in hypoparathyroidism.

Side effects. As this vitamin is fat soluble it is not rapidly metabolised or excreted. If taken in excessive amounts it may accumulate in the body and produce toxic effects. The earliest toxic symptom in children is usually sudden loss of appetite. Nausea and vomiting are frequently associated. Thirst and polyuria soon follow. There may be severe constipation, alternating with bouts of diarrhoea. Headache and other pains are frequent. The child may become thin, wan, irritable, depressed and gradually fall into a stuporose condition which may suggest meningitis. In fatal cases metastatic calcification has been found at autopsy in the arteries, renal tubules, heart, lungs and elsewhere. The serum calcium may be elevated to 12 mg/100 ml or more, but it may remain normal.

Vitamin K (Menaphthon, *USA*)

Pharmacological action. The vitamin is necessary for the normal formation of prothrombin in the liver; the manner in which vitamin K participates in this process is not understood.

Therapeutic use. The vitamin is given to neonates in order to prevent bleeding in a newborn infant who has suffered from trauma at birth, or who shows signs of bleeding. In underdeveloped countries where haemorrhagic disease of the newborn is an important problem there is a strong case for prophylactic use of vitamin K_1 as a routine. The dose for a baby is 1 mg of vitamin K_1 (phytomenadione) intramuscularly, repeated in eight hours if necessary.

In cases of biliary obstruction and fistula, and in malabsorption, if surgery is contemplated, vitamin K_1 is essential pre-operatively for three days in a dose of 10 to 20 mg daily intramuscularly. When there is severe liver damage little or no improvement in the prothrombin level in the blood can be expected unless a blood transfusion is given.

In anticoagulant therapy with the phenindione group of drugs the 'prothrombin time' may increase to the point when bleeding results. In severe cases 20 mg of phytomenadione can be injected intravenously and repeated in four hours if the 'prothrombin time' has not returned to a safe level. In less severe cases the drug can be given by mouth (10–20 mg every eight hours).

Vitamin C (ascorbic acid)

Pharmacological action. Ascorbic acid maintains a healthy state of the capillary walls and the intercellular substance. It is a hydrogen transport agent in oxidation-reduction systems.

Therapeutic use. Ascorbic acid has specific effects in the treatment of scurvy. The aim should be to saturate the body with as little delay as possible; 250 mg by mouth four times daily should achieve this within a week.
Side effects. Synthetic ascorbic acid is harmless even in large doses.

Vitamin B_1 (thiamine)

Pharmacological action. The pyrophosphate of thiamine is the coenzyme of carboxylase, the enzyme concerned with the decarboxylation and oxidation of pyruvic acid. The normal function of nerve cells and the kidney is dependent on this vitamin.

Therapeutic use. Thiamine is life-saving in the treatment of cardio-vascular and infantile beriberi, and Wernicke's encephalopathy. It may be given, though without expectation of dramatic results, in cases of nutritional neuropathy. 25–100 mg daily for several weeks is required in the treatment of thiamine deficiency. Intramuscular injection may be efficacious where oral therapy fails.

Riboflavine (Vitamin B_2)

Pharmacological action. Riboflavine is present in the prosthetic groups of the flavo-proteins, essential for cellular oxidation.

Therapeutic use. There are no incontrovertible indications for the use of synthetic riboflavine; however there is probably an indication for its use in cases of malabsorption syndrome with angular stomatitis. The vitamin may be given orally or parenterally in doses of 5 mg three times daily.

Side effects. No side effects of treatment with riboflavine have been described.

Nicotinic acid (niacin)

Pharmacological action. Nicotinic acid amide is required for the action of NADH and NADPH (prosthetic groups in certain tissue oxidising enzymes).

Therapeutic use. Nicotinic acid and nicotinamide have specific and dramatic effects in pellagra and in secondary deficiency in malabsorption syndromes. The therapeutic dose is 50–250 mg daily (orally or by injection). Large doses produce a generalised and transient vasodilatation.

References

1. Davidson, S., and Passmore, R., *Human Nutrition and Dietetics* (1969), Livingstone, London.

This chapter was written by Dr P. I. Folb (Dept of Clinical Pharmacology, Guy's Hospital Medical School) and edited by Prof. J. R. Trounce.

Category 16

Vaccines and Sera

Smallpox vaccine

Pharmacological action. The vaccine is prepared from vaccinia (cowpox) virus. It is applied to the scarified skin, or by pressure inoculation of the skin, and it produces the local and general reactions of cowpox, and confers immunity for many years against smallpox.

Therapeutic use [1]. Ideally, vaccination might be carried out at four to six months of age depending on the infant immunisation programme and should be repeated on entering school, and at 5 to 10 year intervals thereafter, or at any time that exposure to smallpox is suspected. International travel requirements demand a three-year revaccination programme.

Three types of reaction to vaccination are recognised, depending on host susceptibility: (a) primary reaction, or 'take'; (b) an accelerated reaction, seen in partially immune individuals; (c) an immune reaction.

Failure to develop a reaction is not indicative of immunity and calls for revaccination with a fresh batch of vaccine.

Side effects and contraindications. 1. Generalised vaccinia. (It is not possible to know before vaccination which subjects will develop generalised vaccinia.)

2. Eczema vaccinatum. Vaccination is contraindicated in infants and others with eczema, and other forms of dermatitis; neither should these people be exposed to others who have recently been vaccinated.

3. Vaccinia gangrenosa (gangrenous vaccinia). This is an exceedingly rare complication of vaccination which is often fatal. It occurs in children with impaired mechanisms of antibody formation.

4. Congenital vaccinia may complicate vaccination during pregnancy and is possibly associated with an increased incidence of abortions. Vaccination during pregnancy is therefore contraindicated. The hazard is greater during the first and second trimester of pregnancy. (No teratogenic effect of vaccinia virus on the foetus has been demonstrated.)

5. Post-vaccinial encephalitis. The incidence of this complication in one study was 1:4,500. This incidence can be reduced by passive immunisation with antivaccinial gamma globulin at the time of primary vaccination.

Rabies vaccine

Pharmacological action. Vaccination with live, attenuated or inactivated rabies vaccine elicits antibody production in 10–14 days. This implies that vaccine therapy would be effective only where the incubation period exceeds that time. However, it is possible that antibody production is not the only mechanism of immunity and that the altered rabies virus serves to block receptor sites.

Therapeutic use [2, 3]. A course of 14 daily inoculations is usually given to an individual exposed to rabies.

Side effects and contraindications. The chief hazards of rabies vaccine are hypersensitivity reactions with severe local erythema, accompanied by fever and arthralgia in about 5 per cent of cases, and peripheral neuritis or allergic encephalomyelitis, caused by the rabbit brain tissue in which the virus is prepared, in 1 of 600 to 1 of 10,000 vaccinated individuals according to different reports. The neurological disability varies from transient neurological disturbance to permanent paralysis.

Poliomyelitis vaccine

Pharmacological action. The vaccine is prepared from strains of poliomyelitis virus. Two kinds are used; the living attenuated virus for oral administration (Sabin) and the killed vaccine (Salk). The living oral vaccine mimics the natural infection and confers the same quality of immunity; it produces local resistance to reinfection of the gut, probably a function of IgA antibodies. Circulating antibodies are also produced which limit the spread of the virus to the central nervous system. Killed virus vaccine produces high levels of circulating antibodies, initially IgM and later IgG. This probably blocks the spread of virus from the gut to the central nervous system.

Therapeutic use [4]. The three classified groups of poliomyelitis virus are given together orally as a trivalent virus, and three doses are given at intervals of about four to six weeks. Children are vaccinated at about six months of age, depending on the programme adopted. Killed vaccine is relatively little used at present.

Side effects and contraindications. Attenuated living vaccine is remarkably safe in practice. Occasionally poliomyelitis or neurovirulence of the attenuated virus have been reported.

Measles vaccine

Pharmacological action. As a rule, live attenuated measles virus is used. The antibody response after immunisation follows the same pattern as in natural measles. Protective amounts of the antibody are produced, and in general these amounts of antibody might be expected to remain protective permanently. Sero-conversion rates of 90–100 per cent have been obtained with vaccination of susceptible children. The occasional subject does not respond to measles vaccine, and therefore will remain susceptible to the natural disease.

Therapeutic use [5, 6]. The vaccine is used for prophylaxis. It is given in certain programmes by intramuscular injection followed by a subsequent injection 4–6 weeks later.

It is thought likely that the incidence of subacute sclerosing panencephalitis, a rare and chronically developing complication of natural measles, will be reduced by the vaccine. It is also likely that the acute encephalitic complications of measles will be reduced by the vaccine.

Side effects and complications. Few severe reactions are now encountered with the live attenuated vaccine. A mild illness, with fever, rash, malaise and upper respiratory discomfort occurs in approximately 5–10 per cent of vaccinations. Occasionally there may be a very high fever.

BCG vaccine (tuberculosis vaccine)

Pharmacological action. BCG is an attenuated live vaccine derived from a virulent strain of Mycobacterium tuberculosis var bovis; the assumption is that the artificial infection will enhance resistance to subsequent infection by pathogenic mycobacterial organisms, viz. Myco. tuberculosis, Myco. leprae and Myco. ulcerans. The reason for this protection is probably due to the wide range of common antigens shared by many species of mycobacterium.

Therapeutic use [7]. In subjects not previously infected with tubercle bacilli or other mycobacteria, BCG is capable of conferring 80 per cent protection against subsequent tuberculosis infection in all forms of the disease, and this protection lasts for more than 10 years. Ideally the first vaccination is given very early in life, again according to the programme adopted.

BCG vaccine has been shown to offer significant protection against the early indeterminate and tuberculoid forms of leprosy and to maintain its effect over a period of at least 44 months. There is no evidence yet that BCG vaccination protects against the lepromatous type of leprosy.

Protection against Buruli ulcer is given by BCG.

Side effects and contraindications. Modern preparations are safe and free of side effects.

Rubella vaccine

Pharmacological action [8]. Live, attenuated rubella virus is administered; a non-transmissible and inapparent infection is produced with satisfactory antibody production. There is a high rate (96–100 per cent) of seroconversion, but antibody titres are 4-fold to 16-fold lower than those following natural infection. The attenuated rubella virus is excreted into the throats of the vaccinees.

Therapeutic use [9]. Administration is by intravenous injection. The importance of the vaccine lies in its prevention of infection of the foetus following maternal infection in early pregnancy. An additional reason for vaccinating is that the disturbing symptoms of arthritis and arthralgia, which increase in severity with the age of the patient, are prevented or modified by the vaccine.

Details of the most suitable time for immunisation have still to be decided, but it is probably ideal that all young females should receive it before they reach reproductive age.

Side effects. Mild upper respiratory symptoms may occur following vaccination. Joint involvement with features in common with natural rubella has been noted; adult females are not frequently affected. It is not known whether or not the attenuated virus causes foetal damage.

Influenza vaccine

Pharmacological action. This is an aqueous suspension of inactivated but antigenic influenza virus. As a rule, the most recent strains of virus to cause epidemics and pandemics are included in the vaccine. Active immunisation is produced; protection develops in two to three weeks but is short-lived.

Therapeutic use [10]. The vaccine is administered prophylactically, as a single dose of 1 ml by deep subcutaneous injection, and aerosols are also being developed. It may be given during an epidemic, particularly to medical and nursing staff. In addition, it is given to patients at special risk, e.g. patients with chronic cardiac and pulmonary insufficiency. Vaccination must be yearly to maintain antibody levels. The limitation of the value of the vaccine is due to the multiple sero-types of the influenza viruses, and when a new serotype appears it frequently spreads to other countries before vaccine against it can be made.

Side effects and contraindications. A mild febrile reaction may be produced. The vaccine should not be given to subjects with a history of sensitivity or allergy.

Typhoid-paratyphoid vaccine

Pharmacological action. Vaccines containing killed Salmonella typhi with components of paratyphoid A and B are used. There is no doubt as to the effectiveness of the vaccines containing the salmonella typhi, but the value of the paratyphoid components is doubtful. With a potent vaccine immunity lasts for 3–5 years.

Therapeutic use. The vaccine is given by deep subcutaneous or intramuscular injection. The first dose is 0·25 ml, and the second dose given after an interval of 7 to 28 days is 0·5 ml depending on the manufacturer's instructions. In areas where the disease is prevalent reinforcing (booster) doses should be given every three years.

Side effects and contraindications. Reaction rates are high, with pain and/or swelling at the site of injection, chills and fever several hours after administration, myalgia, arthralgia, nausea and occasional vomiting.

Cholera vaccine

Pharmacological action [11]. The cholera vaccine employed at present in most areas of the world consists of a saline suspension of killed cells of cholera vibrio. The vaccines now available give significant protection, but this is of rather limited duration (3–6 months). Detailed requirements for cholera vaccine have been published by the World Health Organisation [12].

Therapeutic use. The vaccine is usually given subcutaneously or intramuscularly in two doses of 0·5 ml and 1·0 ml, 7–28 days apart. For mass immunisation, jet injector devices are very useful. Children under the age of 10 years are given reduced doses (0·1–0·3 ml). When mass immunisation is being carried out under epidemic conditions, it is often not possible to give two doses; in this case a single dose of 1·0 ml is preferred. Booster doses are generally given every six months.

Side effects [13]. Most people suffer a mild local reaction to the vaccine e.g. local tenderness, mild swelling and redness. A mild to moderate increase of temperature may occur. More severe reactions occur in a few individuals. Reactions usually persist for 2–3 days. These symptoms may respond to salicylates.

A previous florid sensitivity reaction to the vaccine is a contraindication to its repeated use. The safe use of the vaccine in pregnancy has not been established.

Diptheria toxoid

Pharmacological action. The toxoid is prepared from the toxin which appears in a culture of Corynebacterium diphtheriae. A very high degree of protection is provided.

Therapeutic use [14]. The toxoid is sometimes given together with tetanus toxoid. The basic course of immunisation comprises three injections, at intervals of 4 to 8 weeks between the first and second, and 6 to 12 months between the second and third. Booster doses of diphtheria toxoid are given only in certain armed forces and where there is a high risk of exposure to infection, e.g. among nurses in fever hospitals.

Side effects. Occasionally there is tenderness at the site of injection. Very rarely immunisation may be complicated by a general reaction (headache, vomiting, and malaise). These symptoms are transient.

The only serious hazard has been that of 'provocation poliomyelitis' developing in the limb into which the diphtheria antigen has been infected. This risk has been minimised by the general use of poliomyelitis vaccination.

References

1. Kaplan, C., *Brit. med. Bull.* (1969), **25**, 131.
2. Harrison, T. R., *Principles of Internal Medicine* (1966), McGraw-Hill, New York, 1720.
3. Turner, G. S., *Brit. med. Bull.* (1969), **25**, 136.
4. Beale, A. J. *ibid.*, 148.
5. Stokes, J. *Ann. Int. Med.*, (1970), **73**, 829.
6. Beale, A. J., *Brit. med. Bull.* (1969), **25**, 148.
7. Rees, R. J. W., *ibid*, 183.
8. Beale, A. J., *Brit. med. Bull.* (1969), **25**, 148.
9. Stokes, J., *Ann. Int. Med.*, (1970), **73**, 829.
10. Tyrrell, D. A. J., *ibid*, 165.
11. Feeley, J. C., *In: Principles and practice of cholera control;* pp. 87–93. World Health Organisation, Geneva.
12. Requirements for cholera vaccine (requirements for biological substances No. 4), revised 1968. *In: World Health Organisation Expert Committee on biological standardisation* (1969). Twenty-first report (Wld. Hlth. Org. tech. rep. ser., No. 413), Annex 1, pp. 27–44.
13. Gangarosa, E. J., and Faids, G. A., *Annals Int. Med.* (1971), **74**, 412–415.
14. Ellis, R. W. B., and Mitchell, R. G., *Disease in Infancy and childhood* (1968), 551, Livingstone, London.

This chapter was written by Dr P. I. Folb (Dept of Clinical Pharmacology, Guy's Hospital Medical School) and edited by Prof. J. R. Trounce.

Supplement A

DRUG INTERACTION

With ever-increasing numbers of potent agents available for prescription and simultaneous administration the problem of drug interaction is becoming a very serious one. And these interactions are not merely theoretical possibilities. Even now there is a large number of potentially dangerous effects that may be produced by the interaction of commonly used and necessary drugs [1, 2]. Interaction may occur at any site along the pathway from administration to excretion and occasionally even before the drugs are given. A classification of such interactions is appended (modified from Herxheimer, 1969 see [1]) with in addition a list of some of the more important drugs implicated.

1. *Before administration.* E.g. suxamethonium and thiopentone react chemically in solution.

2. *At the site of entry.* E.g. the chelating effect of oral tetracyclines on calcium and aluminium in the gut.

3. *Interaction during binding to blood or tissue proteins.* Many acidic drugs bind to plasma albumin, e.g. phenylbutazone, warfarin, clofibrate and sulphonamides and any two of these drugs may compete for this binding giving an abnormally high free plasma concentration of the drug which has the least affinity for the binding sites. A similar situation has been described for tissue proteins in relation to antimalarial therapy. Less often a drug will increase its binding to protein in the presence of another drug, e.g. pempidine and chlorothiazide [3].

4. *At the site of action.* E.g. isoprenaline and propranolol; folic acid and methotrexate, etc.

5. *During metabolism.* Here interactions are usually effected by inhibition or stimulation of drug metabolizing enzymes, e.g. barbiturates, antiepileptics and phenylbutazone are all potent stimulators of the liver microsomal enzymes which are responsible for the metabolism of these and other drugs, e.g. chloramphenicol, M.A.O. inhibitors and methylphenidate, see [4]. M.A.O. inhibitors, however, are better known for their inactivation of mono-amine oxidase and the potentiation of amines, such as tyramine, present in high quantities in certain foods.

6. *During excretion.* Competition may occur between drugs requiring the same pathway for excretion, e.g. probenicid and peni-

cillin. The excretion of weakly acidic or weakly basic drugs may be affected by agents that modify the urinary pH and therefore the degree of ionisation and tubular reabsorption.

Particular interactions to note

PHENYLBUTAZONE, SULPHONAMIDES, CLOFIBRATE and SALICYLATES may seriously potentiate the effect of oral anticoagulants, e.g. WARFARIN, due to its displacement from binding to serum albumin. Similarly, SALICYLATES may potentiate the effect of SULPHONAMIDES, SULPHONYL UREAS and METHOTREXATE. BARBITURATES reduce the effect of many drugs by stimulating the metabolising enzymes in the liver, and the drugs affected include, once again, the oral anticoagulants.

When the interaction produces a *reduced* effect the potentially serious consequences may not be realised until the inhibiting drug such as a barbiturate is stopped (e.g. on leaving hospital) and a previously well-controlled patient on an oral anticoagulant goes out of control. In addition to the barbiturates, glutethimide, dichloralphenazone and several other drugs also have this activity [5]. Chloral hydrate was thought to be free of this effect but instead it has now been shown that when metabolised it is able to displace warfarin from plasma albumin and can thus produce an effect similar to phenylbutazone [6], although it is unlikely to have serious clinical effects. Barbiturates potentiate the effects of alcohol on the central nervous system by quite a different mechanism.

M.A.O. INHIBITORS and METHYLPHENIDATE will increase the plasma concentration and effect of such drugs as BARBITURATES, most ANTIEPILEPTIC AGENTS and ORAL ANTICOAGULANTS by inhibiting drug metabolism.

It is obvious that therapeutic anticoagulation with oral agents (e.g. with warfarin or phenindione) may be disturbed by a variety of drug interactions. The mechanism of these is summarised in the table on the next page.

M.A.O. INHIBITORS will interact with AMINES of all kinds often with serious effects. TRICYCLIC antidepressants antagonise the hypotensive effects of ADRENERGIC blocking agents, see [10].

PROPRANOLOL may not only potentiate the hypoglycaemic effect of INSULIN but also masks the warning symptoms of sweating and tachycardia. PENTAZOCINE like other narcotic antagonists may precipitate a withdrawal syndrome in those physically dependent on other analgesics.

A comprehensive review of this subject is available [11] and an awareness of the general lines along which these interactions occur may help to reduce their incidence. Some drugs may interact by more than one mechanism, e.g. sulphonamides and sulphonyl ureas cause an effect both on plasma albumin binding and on drug metabolising enzymes. Nevertheless the basic point is that they interact and this is what should be remembered.

Drug Interaction and Anticoagulation

Mechanism	Examples of drugs implicated	Effect on Anticoagulation	References
1. Reduction in absorption of Vitamin K.	Oral liquid paraffin	Increased	[7]
2. Alteration of gut flora with reduced local synthesis of Vitamin K.	Broad spectrum antibiotics	Increased	[7]
3. Diarrhoea with increased loss of anticoagulant in the stools.	Broad spectrum antibiotics	Reduced	[7]
4. Decreased plasma albumin binding.	Phenylbutazone, salicylates, etc.	Increased	[8]
5. Increased drug metabolism.	Barbiturates, etc.	Reduced	[9]
6. Decreased drug metabolism.	M.A.O. inhibitors, methylphenidate, etc.	Increased	[4]

DRUGS AND RENAL FAILURE

A large number of drugs are excreted by the kidney and in renal failure accumulation of these drugs may occur. Under these circumstances smaller doses will be required. The dose can be determined (a) on an *ad hoc* basis, by observing the clinical response of the patient; (b) by repeated measurement of blood levels, if this is possible; or (c) by measuring the glomerular filtration rate and by calculation of the reduction in excretion which will occur. This latter method is only possible when the mode of excretion of the drug is known.

In general terms when a drug is largely excreted by glomerular filtration no reduction of dosage is required if the GFR is above 30 ml/min. If the GFR is between 15–30 ml/min, two-thirds of the dose is required and if it is below 15 ml/min, one-third of the dose is required.

Antibiotics [see 12]

1. The penicillins and cephaloridine are largely excreted by the kidney though in renal failure a certain amount is excreted by other routes, probably the liver.

2. Streptomycin, kanamycin, gentamycin. Great care is needed with these drugs as ototoxicity is a real risk. If possible blood levels should be estimated.

3. Tetracyclines are partially excreted via the kidneys and should be avoided in uraemia since they increase the blood urea.

4. Chloramphenicol is inactivated in the liver but accumulation of metabolities of possible toxicity can occur.

5. Fucidic acid and oleandomycin do not depend on renal clearance.

Narcotics – These are not excreted by the kidney.

Hypnotics and sedatives

Phenothiazines and barbiturates are partially excreted by the kidney. Long-acting barbiturates (such as phenobarbitone) are particularly likely to accumulate.

Diazepam and chlordiazepoxide are entirely metabolised and no reduced dose is required.

Cardiovascular drugs

Digoxin is partially excreted by the kidney and smaller doses are required.

Procainamide is about 50 per cent excreted in the urine and lignocaine largely excreted by the kidney.

Most blood pressure lowering drugs are partially or wholly excreted by the kidney with the possible exception of reserpine.

References

1. Herxheimer, A., *Prescribers' Journal* (1969), **9,** 62.
2. Launchbury, A. P., A table of some drug (and other) interactions. Initially published February 1966 in *J. Hosp. Pharm.*, **23,** 24, and later revised and published separately by Thomas Waide and Sons, Kirkstall Hall, Leeds, P.O. Box 140, England.
3. Dollery, C. T., Emslie-Smith, D., and Muggleton, P. G., *Proc. Roy. Soc. Med.* (1960), **53,** 592.
4. Garrettson, L. K., Perel, K. M., and Dayton, P. G., *J.A.M.A.* (1969), **207,** 2053.
5. Breckenridge, A., Orme, M. L'E., Davies, D. S., and Thorgeirsson, S., *Clin. Sci.* (1969), **37,** 565.
6. Editorial: Drugs altering anticoagulants. *Brit. Med. J.* (1971), **i,** 360.
7. Editors: Goodman, L. S. and Gilman, A. *The Pharmacological basis of therapeutics* (1970), Fourth Edition, pages 1453–4, Macmillan.
8. Aggeler, P. M., O'Reilly, R. A., Leong, L., and Kowitz, P. E., *New Eng. J. Med.* (1967), **276,** 496.
9. Burns, J. J., Cucinell, S. A., Koster, R., and Conney, A. H., *Ann. N.Y. Acad. Sci.* (1965), **123,** 273.
10. Skinner, C., Coull, D. C., and Johnston, A. W., *Lancet* (1969), **ii,** 564.
11. Prescott, L. F., *Lancet* (1969), **ii,** 1239.
12. Editorial: Antibacterial agents in renal failure, *Brit. med. J.* (1971), **i,** 621.

This section was written by Dr. Gordon Reeve (Department of Clinical Pharmacology, Guy's Hospital Medical School) and edited by Professor J. R. Trounce.

Supplement B

USE OF DRUGS IN PREGNANCY

Although it had been known since the beginning of this century that the administration of drugs during pregnancy could affect the offspring, it was only following the thalidomide disaster that physicians became aware that the teratogenic properties of drugs could be a real hazard to their patients. From experiments conducted in animals it is quite clear that most drugs can produce embryotoxic effects if given in adequate doses and at appropriate stages of pregnancy, so one must regard embryotoxicity as only one aspect of general toxicity. The important question is therefore; which drugs are likely to produce toxic effects on the embryo or foetus at dose levels which are non-toxic for the mother? The true answer is, unfortunately, that we do not know. Thalidomide was such a drug although the increasing awareness of its neurotoxicity was raising doubts about its value as a hypnotic. Some other drugs are known to affect the development of the foetus but before considering these, we should look at the types of toxic effect which drugs can produce. It is simplest to consider these in relation to the stage of pregnancy at which they are administered.

Effects of Drugs at Different Stages of Pregnancy

1. *Implantation Stage*. During the first two weeks or so following conception the blastocyst develops and implants. At this time drugs tend to exert all-or-none effects – they may have an anti-fertility action by preventing implantation or may cause abortion, but they are unlikely to produce any malformations at this time.
2. *Embryogenic Stage*. This is generally accepted to cover the period between the second or third and twelfth week of pregnancy during which time the embryo develops from a simple ball of cells to a clearly recognisable foetus. It is during this period that drugs may produce gross structural defects such as missing organs or limbs, anencephaly, exomphalos, cardiac defects, etc. Large doses of drugs may produce widespread effects which are incompatible with further development and so result in abortion, whereas lower doses may result in live but deformed babies.
3. *Foetogenic Stage*. This covers the period from the twelfth week to

term. It is mistakenly believed by many physicians that it is quite safe to use drugs in pregnant women during these last two trimesters since major congenital abnormalities will not be produced. While it is true that the major structures are already present by the twelfth week, a great deal of histological development continues through to term. In particular, cerebral cortical development occurs during this period and the time of maximum brain growth in man is in the last month before birth [1]. Drugs acting during the last two trimesters may result in functional defects, e.g. mental deficiency, which are not incompatible with life and are therefore in many respects more important.

It is clear from the above, that the possible dangers of drug therapy must be considered at *all* stages of pregnancy, and that due care must be taken before using drugs at any time in pregnant women.

Difficulty of recognising teratogenic drugs

The simplest drug to detect would be one which produced an easily recognised and unusual type of deformity in a high percentage of women exposed to risk. These requirements were met with thalidomide which affected about 20 per cent of women at risk, and yet it took six years and several thousand malformed babies before the association was recognised. With drugs producing more common types of abnormality the problem of recognition is even greater. For example in order to have a 95 per cent chance of detecting a drug which doubled the normal incidence of anencephaly, studies on 16,000 treated pregnant women would be required. It is obvious therefore that many more drugs than are at present known, may be embryotoxic.

Even greater difficulties arise when one considers possible delayed manifestations of embryotoxic activity. It has been known for some time that in animals, administration of a single dose of a carcinogen which was non-toxic for the mother, could result in death of all the progeny from CNS tumours [2]. These did not develop until one to two years after birth which was the middle of their expected life span. The possible relationship between the administration of drugs to pregnant women and the development of cancer subsequently in the offspring cannot be ignored. Vaginal adenocarcinoma which is very rare and then usually occurs in women over 50 years of age, has been reported [3] in 8 young women, aged 15–22 years. The most highly significant ($P < 0{\cdot}00001$) difference between these women and matched controls was that the mothers of seven of them had been treated during pregnancy with stilboestrol. It is possible that this altered the vaginal epithelium *in utero* in such a way as to predispose it to develop adenosis leading to adenocarcinoma when subjected to endogenous oestrogen at menarche.

Specific Recommendations

From all of this it is quite clear that since this is a relatively new and expanding field of study it is impossible to be dogmatic that any specific drugs are absolutely safe for use in pregnancy. On the other hand one should not be over pessimistic either and a nihilistic approach can be just as harmful if the pregnant patient is suffering from a condition which itself may lead to harm of the foetus.

It is impossible in a brief review to discuss all the evidence concerning individual drugs but the following summary gives an idea of the present state of knowledge in some of the fields which concern the general physician.

Analgesics

Narcotic Analgesics – Morphine and pethidine like all centrally acting drugs cross the placenta easily and can produce dependence *in utero* so that both the foetus and newborn infant may have a withdrawal syndrome which in the latter can be fatal. There is of course also a risk of respiratory depression in the newborn if these drugs are given within a few hours of delivery. There is no evidence concerning their effects in early pregnancy. Provided one is aware of these risks the drugs seem to be safe to use.

Minor Analgesics – There is no evidence in man that salicylates are harmful in early pregnancy. In the later stages however, they can cause foetal hypoprothrombinaemia and neonatal bleeding as well as other toxic effects. It might therefore be advisable to use paracetamol instead of aspirin where possible.

Antibiotics

It is known that infections – rubella, cytomegalic inclusion disease, syphilis, toxoplasmosis and possibly influenza and mumps as well as febrile and toxic states of the mother can all lead to foetal damage. Therefore it is never, in my opinion, justified to withhold antibiotics or chemotherapeutics in situations where the mother really requires them. On the other hand practically all of the antibiotics have been suspected of causing foetal damage and they should definitely not be used for trivial indications.

Penicillins including ampicillin seem to be the least toxic and where appropriate should be the first choice. In the early stages of pregnancy, short acting sulphonamides like sulphadimidine also appear to be safe though towards the end of pregnancy it may be better to use alternatives since sulphonamides can cause jaundice and kernicterus in the newborn. Tetracyclines are definitely known to be teratogenic. They cause dark staining of the teeth with hypoplasia of the enamel and increased susceptibility to caries. They may also cause some retardation of skeletal growth. Since the period of risk is from about the 18th week it is advisable to avoid the use of tetracycline after that time. If it is necessary to use a tetracycline then oxytetracycline should be used since this only causes a creamy coloured staining of the teeth which is barely detectable.

Streptomycin is known occasionally to cause 8th nerve damage in the foetus and this drug together with gentamycin, viomycin and kanamycin should be used only if absolutely necessary. Isoniazid appears to be safe in pregnancy. Chloramphenicol should be avoided in late pregnancy since the foetus and neonate are unable to metabolise it and its use can lead to circulatory collapse and the 'grey syndrome'.

Like the highly protein bound sulphonamides, novobiocin should be avoided in late pregnancy due to a risk of neonatal jaundice or kernicterus, and nitrofurantoin has been reported to cause neonatal haemolysis after maternal administration.

Anti-diabetics

Because of the higher than normal incidence of foetal abnormalities in diabetic women it is difficult to assess the effects of individual drugs. There is however a very clear general opinion that insulin is the hypoglycaemic of choice in the treatment of pregnant diabetics. The sulphonylureas, especially chlorpropamide and tolbutamide have been associated with multiple foetal malformations, foetal death and severe prolonged neonatal hypoglycaemia and are best avoided during pregnancy.

Anti-emetics

The usual 'morning sickness' can often be helped by reassurance and without the use of drugs. However severe nausea or vomiting or hyperemesis gravidarum may themselves lead to foetal damage and should be treated. A rather strange situation exists in this field since suspicion of teratogenesis was levelled at two of the most commonly used anti-emetics – meclozine and cyclizine. A detailed review of the evidence [4] failed to give a clear answer. However since more information on the use of these drugs in pregnancy exists than on any other anti-emetic, and since the risk with meclozine, if any, is certainly low, it would appear that meclozine should be the drug of choice for anti-emetic treatment. For very severe cases a phenothiazine, e.g. chlorpromazine should be used.

Hormones

Sex Hormones – The sex hormones – oestrogens, androgens and progestogens have been demonstrated to be teratogenic in man, resulting usually in masculinisation of female foetuses. There is in any case little evidence that these drugs are of value in treating threatened abortion and their use should be avoided. If however, it is necessary to use an oestrogen then for the reasons mentioned above concerning its possible carcinogenic action, stilboestrol should be avoided. Ethinyl oestradiol appears to be the safest oestrogen to use. The androgenic steroids and the synthetic progestogens ethisterone and norethisterone are most likely to cause masculinisation of females and should definitely be avoided. If a progestogen is required then progesterone itself or a 17 α-OH progesterone derivative (e.g. Delalutin or Provera) may be safer than the 19-nor progestogens.

Adrenocortical Hormones – Although ACTH and cortisone will regularly produce a high incidence of cleft palate in certain species and strains of animals, humans seem to be much less susceptible to this effect. Similarly, although there have been reported cases of infants with adreno-cortical failure due to steroid withdrawal after large doses of prednisolone to the mother, this is relatively rare and many women have been treated with large doses of cortisone or prednisone for Hodgkin's disease during pregnancy, and with a completely normal outcome. If therefore, it is necessary to use steroids during pregnancy for treatment of any serious condition, this can reasonably safely be done.

Thyroid Hormones – Anti-thyroid drugs and iodides may cause goitres in the foetus of such an extent as to prevent adequate respiration after birth. They may also result in hypo-or hyperthyroid states though cretinism is extremely rare. It is recommended [5] that minimum doses of antithyroid drugs should be used and that these should be tailed off with a view to ending treatment a month before the expected date of delivery. Radio-iodine should not be used since this may accumulate in and destroy the foetal thyroid.

Centrally Acting Drugs

Anti-epileptic drugs have been suspected of causing a higher than expected incidence of cleft palate in the offspring of epileptic mothers. Because multiple drug therapy is common in this situation, it is not possible to state which drugs are the most likely offenders. From animal studies, it seems likely that primidone and phenobarbitone may be causative factors. Coagulation defects resulting in neonatal haemorrhages have also been clearly demonstrated following phenytoin and phenobarbitone therapy. This can be treated by administration of vitamin K_1 to the mother during the last month of pregnancy. As there is little alternative but to use drugs in epileptic patients, it would seem advisable to continue with the lowest doses of the most effective drugs. This whole question is however at present under active review and these recommendations may change within the next year or so.

Hypnotics – The rational choice of a hypnotic for pregnant women is not at present possible because of the lack of adequate information. Because of the suspicions mentioned above about phenobarbitone, it may be advisable to use a non-barbiturate. Chloral hydrate seems to be harmless in early pregnancy as are the phenothiazines, e.g. promethazine (Phenergan), and these may seem a wiser choice than the newer and less well tested hypnotics.

Conclusions

All drugs must be considered as having a potential for foetal toxicity in the same way as they do for adult toxicity. This toxicity will not be seen in all women treated, nor even in all foetuses in one woman – it is known for only one of a pair of twins to be affected. Furthermore, whether the drug crosses the placenta or not is irrelevant since there are many ways in which teratogenic effects can be produced by an action on the mother or placenta [6]. Thus it is probable that drugs represent one factor in a multifactorial system leading to congenital defects.

No drug should be used in pregnant women (nor in anyone else) unless there is a real need for its use, and likewise no woman should be deprived of a drug who really needs it. The present evidence suggests that humans are relatively resistant to the teratogenic effects of drugs since despite wide differences in drug usage throughout the world, the incidence of congenital abnormalities is remarkably similar in different populations. However, with the increasing awareness of the possible long term effects that drug administration during pregnancy can have on the subsequent growth and physical and mental development of the offspring, it is well not to feel too complacent.

References

1. Dobbing, J., *Biol. Neonat.* (1965-66), **9,** 132.
2. Druckrey, H., Landschütz, S., C., and Ivankovic, S., *Z. Krebsforsch* (1970), **73,** 371.
3. Herbst, A. L., Ulfelder, H., and Poskanzer, D. C., *New Engl. J. Med.* (1971), **284,** 878.
4. Sadusk, J. F., and Palmisano, P. A., *J. Amer. Med. Ass.*, (1965), **194,** 987.
5. 'Today's Drugs', *Br. med. J.*, (1967), **3,** 220.
6. Sullivan, F. M., *Proc. roy. Soc. Med.*, (1970), **63,** 1252.

Other Useful References

Robson, J. M., Sullivan, F. M., and Smith, R. L., Eds., *Embryopathic Activity of Drugs*. Churchill: London (1965).

Lionel, N. D. W., 'Effect of Drugs on the Foetus and Newborn', *Ceylon Medical Journal* (1969), Sept., p. 19.

Brent, R. L., 'Medicolegal aspects of Teratology' *J. Pediat.* (1967), **71,** 288.

Meyler, L., and Herxheimer, A., Eds., 'Side Effects of Drugs', *Excerpta Med. Fdn.*, Amsterdam (1968).

This Section was written by F. M. Sullivan (Department of Pharmacology, Guy's Hospital Medical School) and edited by Professor J. R. Tounce.

In this section Professor Cranston and his team of experts have gathered together a guide to treatment of the commonest, most serious and most difficult problems in contemporary medical treatment. References to sources and further reading are given where appropriate.

A Guide to the Therapy of Common Diseases

by

W. I. Cranston

Professor of Medicine, St. Thomas's Hospital Medical School, London

Introduction

In this section we have tried to outline the principles of treatment of common illnesses. Very often decisions about treatment have to be made without all of the evidence upon which rational decisions can be made. This is particularly true in emergency situations, but it also applies to some extent in the management of almost all patients. We have attempted, so far as possible, to indicate the lines of treatment whose efficacy is supported by valid evidence, though it is impossible in a text of this size to quote the evidence, or to cover every speciality, *in extenso*. Where evidence is lacking or contradictory we have tried to indicate this.

With few exceptions, evidence of the benefit of treatment comes from controlled trials on groups of patients. This kind of evidence usually means that on average, a group of patients subjected to one kind of treatment does better than a similar group of patients subjected to another kind of treatment. The doctor is faced by a single patient, with individual quirks of behaviour and genetic structure. Though it is rational to treat the patient in the way suggested by the available evidence, this must be tempered with commonsense and the management tailored to fit the individual's needs, so far as possible. There is often a conflict between the ideal and the possible management and much of the art of treatment consists in compromise between theoretical ideals and practical actions.

The very act of prescribing treatment can cause considerable change in a patient's symptoms, whether the treatment is known to be effective or not. This type of placebo response is often helpful in therapy, and sometimes a hindrance. There is no reason why it should not be used, if it benefits the patient, provided that the doctor does not delude himself about the efficacy of the particular agent employed.

Category 1
The Gastrointestinal Tract

OESOPHAGUS

Hiatus hernia

Asymptomatic hiatus hernia is common and requires no treatment. Regurgitation of bitter gastric juice into the mouth occurs and is particularly related to bending, stooping and lying flat. Patients should be advised to avoid these positions. They should sleep propped up with pillows or with the head of the bed raised. In babies, specially constructed cradles are used. Reflux oesophagitis occurs when the acidic gastric contents repeatedly bathe the lower oesophagus and it is this that causes heartburn. It can be prevented by advice on posture, but, if the symptom persists and is troublesome, the patient should be treated with regular doses of alkalis. These are best given as a mixture after meals and as tablets 1–2 hourly between meals. Patients with symptoms from hiatus hernia are commonly obese and are often improved by being put on a reducing diet and losing weight.

Persistent reflux oesophagitis leads to an inflammatory narrowing of the lower oesophagus and this results in dysphagia. The narrowing is initially due to oedema and at this stage dysphagia is reversible by medical measures outlined above. At a later date a true fibrous stricture forms and surgical intervention will have to be considered. Whether or not this is necessary will depend on various clinical factors – such as the age and general health of the patient. If surgery is contraindicated patients may be kept relatively well by the medical measures outlined above and, if necessary, by mincing their food and avoiding solids that are prone to stick.

The surgical treatment of hiatus hernia is not generally satisfactory. This is probably because the surgeon cannot repair the dysfunctioning lower oesophageal sphincter, despite successful replacement of the stomach below the diaphragm. Surgery should therefore only be considered if medical treatment has been rigorously instituted and shown to be unsuccessful or if a fibrous stricture has formed. If it is undertaken its success is largely determined by the interest and expertise of the surgeon.

Achalasia

Achalasia is a neuromuscular disorder of the oesophagus which causes dysphagia, oesophageal regurgitation and oesophageal pain. These symptoms are best treated by a Heller's operation if a surgeon experienced in the operation is available. The operation consists in cutting the muscular layers of the lower two inches of the oesophagus. This allows food to pass through the previously narrow segment. Reflux oesophagitis may occur following the operation and will require treatment as indicated above. In some centres the muscle fibres of the lower oesophagus are forcibly split by inflating a ballon, (Mosher bag), placed in the lumen of the gastro-oesophageal junction under X-ray control. In experienced hands the procedure is successful and it has the advantage of avoiding a major surgical operation. It is usually done without general anaesthetic and is painful. If a Heller's operation is contraindicated, because of age or infirmity, it is sometimes possible to manage the patient with repeated dilations with Hurst bougies. These patients will also have to mince their food.

Scleroderma (diffuse systemic sclerosis.)

Scleroderma commonly affects the lower two thirds of the oesophagus. It causes progressive narrowing of the lumen and dysphagia. In this condition dysphagia is best treated by repeated dilations with a bougie which the patient can be taught to pass once or twice a day if necessary. Surgical resection of the stricture is contraindicated as the oesophageal wall is usually too diseased to allow for satisfactory anastomosis.

Diffuse oesophageal spasm

Diffuse oesophageal spasm is a neuromuscular disorder of the oesophagus in which the organ goes into intermittent episodes of spasm. It commonly presents with episodes of severe retrosternal pain that may mimic cardiac pain. The pain is not usually sufficiently frequent or troublesome to require a major surgical procedure, but, in selected cases, successful results have been achieved by oesophageal myotomy. In this operation the muscle coats are split over a long length of the oesophagus [1].

Belching

It is a normal physiological event for the lower oesophageal sphincter to relax from time to time and to allow gastric gas to pass into the oesophagus. This can be promoted by carminatives such as peppermint, which cause relaxation of the sphincter [2]. Once in the oesophagus the gas is usually expelled quietly. Noisy belching requires constriction of voluntary muscle and is thus under conscious control. This should be pointed out to patients who complain of noisy belching, and they should also be told not to swallow air. In a rare condition termed 'speaking oesophagus syndrome' the patient appears unable to prevent the noise which may be a considerable embarrassment to her.

STOMACH

Gastritis

Acute gastritis is a transient response of the stomach to ingestion of insulting substances. The gastric mucosa has remarkable recuperative abilities and therefore, although the mucosa can be shown to sustain damage from, for instance, a few soluble aspirin tablets, no significant clinical effect usually ensues. However ingestion of a large dose of a gastric irritant, such as staphylococcal endotoxin, corrosive poison or a bottle of whisky, will have significant clinical effects: vomiting, diarrhoea and, on occasion, gastrointestinal bleeding. An acute episode such as this is usually self-limiting within a few hours, but may require intravenous saline if loss of fluids is excessive. Repeated ingestion of alcohol causes early morning nausea and vomiting of mucus-rich fluid. This is best treated by reducing intake of alcohol but, if this is not possible, the patient should be advised to drink plenty of fluids and to use alkalis liberally. Because of the risk of precipitating gastric bleeding he should be advised not to take preparations that contain aspirin – even those that are advertised for 'hang-overs'.

Atrophic gastritis is common in persons over 50, particularly if they smoke, or drink alcohol. It does not cause pain and there is no specific treatment for it. Rarely patients with atrophic gastritis develop iron deficiency or frank gastric bleeding, and this will require appropriate treatment. Complete gastric atrophy in certain individuals leads to vitamin B_{12} deficiency and pernicious anaemia. This will require appropriate investigation and treatment with injections of vitamin B_{12}.

Peptic ulcer

The common sites for peptic ulcers are duodenum and stomach but they may also occur in the lower oesophagus, jejunum and in a Meckel's diverticulum. The management of gastric and duodenal ulcers that are causing pain as a predominant symptom will be discussed in this section. Bleeding and perforation are considered on page 7 of this Chapter.

Gastric ulcer

It is usually possible to decide on radiological or gastroscopic criteria that an ulcer in the stomach is benign, but it is important in terms of management to appreciate that malignancy is always a possibility. Benign gastric ulcers can, by appropriate medical management, be made to heal and it should be the aim of the physician to see that this occurs within three months. Failure to do this is an indication for surgery.

Removal of provoking factors. Alcohol, aspirin, indomethacin and phenylbutazone are known to damage gastric mucosa and can cause gastric ulcers [3]. Patients should be advised to avoid these substances. Those with chronic rheumatic disorders who require continuous administration of aspirin may be given this in the enteric coated form which does not harm the stomach. There is no proof that usual doses of steroids (i.e. prednisone 10–30 mg per day) are harmful to the human stomach although larger doses probably are. Smoking has been shown to delay healing of gastric ulcers and patients should therefore refrain from, or at least reduce, their tobacco consumption. Chronic diseases such as rheumatoid arthritis, cirrhosis and bronchitis and emphysema may well predispose to gastric ulceration. Patients' general health should be improved as much as possible by appropriate treatment of coexisting disease.

Alkalis. Frequent doses of alkalis are of known value in the treatment of pain due to gastric ulcers. They have not however been proved to heal the ulcers. They should be given regularly – half hourly if necessary – either as mixtures or in tablet form. Outpatients may find it convenient to take mixtures at meal times and to carry alkali tablets to suck in the intervals. Milk may be taken in lieu of alkalis between meals. Magnesium trisilicate causes diarrhoea in some patients and if this is troublesome, aluminium hydroxide, which tends to be constipating, can be used. The laxative effect of magnesium trisilicate is an advantage to bed-bound patients.

Bed rest. Hospitalisation and bed rest has been shown to improve the healing rate of gastric ulcers. It is common clinical experience that acute exacerbations of peptic ulcer settle within a week of the patient being admitted. Most gastric ulcers heal satisfactorily with conventional outpatient treatment but if the ulcer is very large or does not heal, inpatient treatment is indicated. Outpatients should be advised to get as much rest as possible and it may be necessary for them to have a period off work in order to do so.

Ulcer healing drugs. Carbenoxolone has been shown to enhance the rate of healing of gastric ulcers in both inpatients and outpatients [4]. In fact it is the only drug that has been shown to do so. Unfortunately it has two undesirable side effects – fluid retention and hypokalaemia. Patients are therefore at risk of being precipitated into cardiac failure. This can be prevented by the use of thiazide diuretics. In view of these problems carbenoxolone should only be used on those patients who have failed to respond satisfactorily to the above regime and they should be kept under careful supervision. Deglycyrrhizinated liquorice is claimed to improve healing of gastric ulcers without causing fluid retention but more experience with this drug is required.

Anticholinergics only produce a significant reduction in gastric acidity if given in sufficient amount to cause other unpleasant effects such as dry mouth, bladder dysfunction and blurred vision. As the symptoms of gastric ulcers can usually be controlled with regular meals and frequent ingestion of milk or alkalis, there is no indication to use anticholinergics.

Sedatives and tranquillizers may be required for patients with insomnia or anxiety states but there is no evidence that they have any therapeutic value in terms of ulcer healing.

'Bland' diets. There is no evidence that 'bland' diets improve the healing of gastric ulcers. Individual patients discover that particular foods upset them, and they should avoid these items. Patients should be advised to have meals at regular intervals and to have snacks or milk and biscuits between their main meals. Milk has a good buffering capacity and should be taken liberally during exacerbations of pain. Rigid 'bland' (uninteresting), foods are of no proven value. Patients should be advised to eat foods that suit them and that they like.

Duodenal ulcer

The essential of treating dyspepsia due to duodenal ulceration is to control the symptoms. It is not necessary, and is usually not possible, to show that the ulcer has healed. This is not important as the possibility of neoplasia does not arise and therefore the management does not rely on alterations in the radiological appearance. The symptoms can usually be controlled satisfactorily by frequent administration of alkalis and milk, regular meals, bed rest and hospitalisation if necessary. 'Bland' diets are not indicated [5]. Carbenoxolone or similar drugs are not proved to be effective for duodenal ulceration. If the pain persists and disrupts the patient's life, surgery should be advised.

Surgery for peptic ulcers

Perforation, possibility of carcinoma, and recurrent bleeding are absolute indications for surgery for gastric ulcers. Pyloric obstruction, perforation and repeated bleeding are absolute indications in the case of duodenal ulcers. Patients with repeated and incapacitating pain from gastric and duodenal ulcers may require surgery but the criteria for this decision will depend on many factors. In general it is best to operate on gastric ulcers if they fail to heal or if they recur after successful healing. For duodenal ulcers the decision about surgery depends mainly on an assessment of the patient's symptoms rather than the barium meal appearances. If the patient's life, and particularly his work, is being seriously disturbed by pain from the ulcer an operation should be advised. In general gastric surgery for peptic ulcers is very satisfactory and patients are relieved of distressing symptoms.

Haematemesis and melaena. Blood transfusion may be required immediately and a central venous pressure measurement is the best monitor of blood replacement. Once hypovolaemia has been corrected an attempt should be made to find the cause of the bleed. A history of recurrent dyspepsia suggests that bleeding is from a chronic peptic ulcer. Recent aspirin ingestion may indicate bleeding erosions. Examination of the patient may reveal important physical signs such as spleen and spider naevi (cirrhosis and varices), large hard liver (gastric carcinoma), telangectases in the mouth (Osler, Weber, Rendu disease) etc. If facilities are available barium meal or gastroscopy should be performed within twenty-four hours of admission to hospital.

The main problem in the management of acute haematemesis and melaena is to decide when to advise surgery. If the patient has a chronic peptic ulcer that has caused trouble for many years, surgery should be performed if there is bleeding after twenty-four hours. Difficulties arise when patients have had no previous gastric trouble. In this group, if the patient has taken aspirin or alcohol, it is likely that the bleeding is from an erosion and that it will stop spontaneously. In this situation medical measures (frequent small meals, regular doses of alkali and sedation) should be instituted. Occasionally bleeding may persist from multiple gastric erosions and radical gastric surgery will then be necessary. In general, surgery should be advised for any patient if bleeding continues for 48 hours, if it recurs after stopping, or if the patient has required 10 pints of blood.

Another clinical problem is the patient who has recurrent small bleeds causing repeated melaenae, with or without iron deficiency anaemia. This condition is particularly difficult to manage if the cause is not found by conventional radiological methods. 'Blind' laparotomy is usually unhelpful. In the elderly it is often best to manage the problem by iron replacement and intermittent blood transfusions. A laparotomy at the time of the bleed may reveal the source. These patients usually require the facilities and expertise of a specialised gastrointestinal unit.

SMALL INTESTINE

Coeliac syndrome

Coeliac syndrome is the adult equivalent of coeliac disease. It is malabsorption due to a primary abnormality of the small intestinal mucosa ('flat' mucosa). At least seventy-five per cent of adults with coeliac syndrome respond dramatically to gluten withdrawal. A gluten free diet imposes restrictions and inconvenience on the patient but there are two reasons for insisting that the patient should stick to it, even when clinically improved. Firstly, because he is likely to relapse if gluten is reintroduced. Secondly, because it is becoming increasingly appreciated that the coeliac mucosa is pre-malignant, and there is some evidence that gluten withdrawal reduces the risk of malignancy. Patients who respond well to gluten withdrawal do not require any other medicaments once their body stores of vitamins, iron etc. have been repleted. The Coeliac Society (116 Loudouin Road, London, N.W.8.), a patient's association, can advise and help those with this condition. A book giving useful recipes and advice on cooking with gluten free flour has recently been published [6].

During active phases of the disease patients may have deficiency of folic acid, iron, vitamin K, vitamin D and calcium and hypoproteinaemia. These substances should not be replaced before a firm diagnosis has been made by small intestinal biopsy. For three months after starting a gluten free diet, replacements of appropriate substances should be given. In the case of iron, vitamin K and vitamin D the drugs should be given initially by injection. Iron, folic acid and calcium should also be given by mouth. After three months patients do not require supplements if they have responded well to gluten withdrawal. They should however be kept under continuous observation.

A proportion – perhaps one quarter – of patients do not respond to gluten withdrawal. In these and also in patients who are severely ill, prednisone 10–20 mg thrice daily for two weeks, and reducing slowly to a maintenance dose of 5 to 15 mg per day should be given. Some patients are dramatically improved by this. The few that are not may have coexisting pancreatic failure which may need appropriate treatment. A course of antibiotics (e.g. tetracycline 250 mg four times daily, for two weeks) is sometimes worth trying in these individuals, as there is evidence that the small gut may become infected with pathogenic bacteria.

Other causes of malabsorption. Excess fat in the stool (steatorrhoea) is a common feature of many systemic disorders. For instance steatorrhoea may occur in diabetes, thyrotoxicosis. Addison's disease, cirrhosis and superior mesenteric artery occlusion. Treatment of the primary disorder (e.g. thyrotoxicosis or Addison's disease) will often reverse the disorder. In this section only intestinal causes of malabsorption will be considered and mainly those that have a precise and definite method of therapy.

Post-gastric surgery. Any operation for peptic ulceration (vagotomy, pyloroplasty, partial gastrectomy) may cause steatorrhoea. In most patients this is of no significance and can only be detected by biochemical measurement of stool fat. Patients who have had gastric surgery are at risk of developing clinically significant malabsorption, particularly those who have had a partial gastrectomy. Weight loss or failure to gain weight, may be due to malabsorption, although in many patients it is due to inadequate intake of calories. Iron deficiency anaemia is also common after gastric surgery. Women in their reproductive years are at particular risk and should be treated with parenteral and oral iron. Folic acid deficiency may cause megaloblastic anaemia and is usually due to inadequate diet. Megaloblastic anaemia due to vitamin B_{12} deficiency results from inadequate secretion of intrinsic factor from the gastric remnant. This will require treatment with injections of vitamin B_{12} (500 μg monthly). Osteomalacia occurs due to vitamin D malabsorption and loss of calcium in the stools. This requires treatment with injections of vitamin D (20,000 to 40,000 units weekly), until the bone lesions have healed. Calcium lactate in effervescent form should be given in a dose of 15 g. thrice daily.

The question of preventing overt iron deficiency and osteomalacia by prophylactic treatment with oral iron and oral calcium and vitamin D is a much disputed topic. In the writer's opinion it is best not to use these drugs prophylactically on patients who are clinically well, but to arrange annual visits so that the patients can be assessed, weighed and have haemoglobin estimations.

Short small intestine

Occasionally patients who have had intestinal surgery are left with an inadequate length of small intestine. These patients have to be carefully assessed to see that they do not have blind loops. Considerable improvement can be effected by the use of a low fat diet.

Bacterial invasion of the small intestine. Bacteria invade the small intestine if there is a stagnant segment of the gut. Blind loops of small intestine may result from gastro-intestinal surgery. These should be corrected surgically. If this is not possible broad spectrum antibiotics may be used (i.e. tetracycline 250 mg three or four times a day). *Fistulae* between segments of intestine may occur from Crohn's disease, carcinomas or after surgery and if possible these should be corrected surgically. *Jejunal diverticulosis* occurs in the elderly and is a not uncommon cause of diarrhoea, steatorrhoea and occasionally vitamin B_{12} deficiency. Intermittent courses of oral tetracycline (250 mg thrice daily for five to ten days) will control the symptoms in many of these patients and should be tried before subjecting the patient to surgery. It is often useful in these patients to give them a supply of the antibiotic and to advise them to take them for five days at the first sign of recurrence of diarrhoea. *Scleroderma* (diffuse systemic sclerosis) may affect the small intestine which dilates and becomes stagnant. Steatorrhoea can be improved in these patients by antibiotics.

Giardiasis

Infestation of the small intestine with Giardia lamblia causes diarrhoea and steatorrhoea with malabsorption. It is diagnosed by finding the organism in stools or the aspirate from small intestine. It is treated with mepacrine 100 mg three times daily for one week or metronidazole 200 mg three times daily for one week. Two or more courses may be required to eliminate the infection and if the infection is not eradicated larger doses of mepacrine can be used.

Crohn's disease

Crohn's disease affects predominantly the terminal small intestine but may involve any section of the gastrointestinal tract from stomach to anus. Crohn's colitis is becoming increasingly recognised and its treatment will be considered in the section dealing with colitis. In its usual form in the small intestine, the disease is a protracted one with relapses and remissions. Both medical measures and surgical intervention are valuable in its management so close co-operation is necessary between physician and surgeon. There is a form of acute localised small intestinal Crohn's disease which has a good prognosis. In one series 70 per cent of patients with this disorder had no recurrence after five years.

Medical measures. During acute exacerbations of the disease with pain, diarrhoea, steatorrhoea, fever and weight loss, patients will require admission to hospital. Bed rest is beneficial during these phases of the disease. Diarrhoea should be controlled with codeine phosphate or Lomotil (diphenoxylate hydrochloride and atropine sulphate). Cholestyramine is occasionally effective in stopping diarrhoea due to the cathartic effect of unabsorbed bile acids on the colon. Patients are commonly anaemic due to gastrointestinal bleeding and this should be corrected by parenteral iron or, if necessary, blood transfusion. Other deficiencies may be present because of malabsorption. Vitamin B_{12} deficiency occurs when there is considerable involvement of the ileum and should be treated by monthly injections of 500 μg of this vitamin. Hypoproteinaemia is due to loss of protein from the gut and requires a high protein diet. Weight loss may be helped by a diet containing medium chain triglycerides (MCT) rather than ordinary fats. MCT are more readily absorbed by diseased mucosa. MCT are obtained as an oil which may be used instead of fat for cooking and preparing food. A dietician's advice is required.

Corticosteroids are valuable in suppressing the inflammatory features of the disease. Prednisone should be given in doses of 45 mg per day for two weeks and then slowly reduced to a maintenance dose of 10–20 mg per day. They are particularly valuable in acute types of the disease when large portions of the small intestine are involved. There is some evidence that prednisone given on alternate days is as effective and avoids undesirable side effects. Some physicians prefer Inj ACTH (20 units per day for two weeks) for inpatients at the onset of treatment. Antibiotics do not usually help patients with Crohn's disease, but they are occasionally dramatically successful if the small intestine is infected through fistula formation or blind loops. Tetracycline 250 mg four times daily for ten days is recommended.

Surgical measures. Surgery is required if there is intestinal obstruction or fistulae between small intestine and large bowel or bladder. It is also useful in patients with chronic illness and debility due to a localised mass. Surgery may also be required for perianal abscess and anal fistula which commonly occur in this disorder. There is a high rate of recurrence (50–90 per cent) after surgery. The current trend is to resect the main segment of diseased gut but to be as conservative as possible. By-pass operations are felt, at present, to be less satisfactory. After surgery there is a good case for putting the patient on long term steroids (Prednisone 15 mg per day) for there is some evidence that this may reduce the recurrence rate.

There are many therapeutic possibilities for patients with Crohn's disease and it is uncommon not to be able to improve them even in the face of a severe relapse.

LARGE BOWEL

Proctitis

This is inflammation of the rectal mucosa without involvement of the colon. It may be caused by gonococcal infection in which case it will require treatment with a single injection of 300,000 units of procaine penicillin. Lymphogranuloma venereum causes proctitis that is usually associated with rectal stricture, fistula formation and inguinal lymphadenopathy. Tetracycline (2·0 g. daily for at least ten days) may prevent stricture formation in the early stages of this disease.

Non-specific proctitis is a condition analogous to ulcerative colitis but confined to the rectal mucosa. This is the commonest form of proctitis in the United Kingdom. Although a proportion of patients ultimately develop true ulcerative colitis, in many the disease remains localised to the rectum and in some it becomes quiescent after appropriate treatment. The symptoms of tenesmus and discharge of blood and mucus can often be considerably improved by the use of prednisolone (5 mg) suppositories. These should be given morning and night for three months and, if the symptoms are controlled and sigmoidoscopic appearance improved at the end of this, the frequency of administration should be gradually reduced over the succeeding three months. If the symptoms persist or become worse, ulcerative colitis should be suspected.

Ulcerative colitis

Patients with ulcerative colitis require the help and understanding of a sympathetic physician. Some physicians claim dramatic cures by unravelling the psychological background of these patients, but most rely on drugs. Tenesmus and frequent rectal discharge can often be improved by prednisolone suppositories twice daily which are worth trying initially. Even in its mild form the disease usually requires more energetic measures and it is advisable to admit the patient to hospital for a period of bed rest and asessment. Total withdrawal of milk and milk products is always worth trying, and is occasionally successful even in severe attacks. Persistent diarrhoea is an indication for prednisolone retention enemeta (20 mg prednisolone in 100 ml isotonic buffered solution), and while the patient is in hospital he can be taught to administer these himself. They should be given twice daily while in hospital but once the patient has been discharged it is preferable, if possible, for him to have them only at night just before retiring to bed. After instillation he should lie in bed for half an hour and should be encouraged to retain the enema for as long as possible. Salazopyrine (salicylazosulphapyridine) has been shown to reduce the incidence of relapse once a remission has been induced. It has no place in the treatment of the acute episode which can be better controlled by systemic steroids (vide infra). There is a good case for giving salazopyrine (0·5 g. four times daily for one year) after a remission has been induced. Most patients can tolerate this dose but those that develop nausea and vomiting should be given 0·5 g. thrice daily.

So far only mild attacks of ulcerative colitis have been considered. Patients may present initially with a severe 'fulminating' attack, or at any time a patient with the mild form may have a severe attack. These attacks require much more energetic measures for the patients are severely ill, dehydrated, anaemic and toxic. General measures include correction of fluid balance, administration of electrolytes – particularly potassium – and blood transfusion. Local corticosteroids in the form of prednisolone enemata may be tried. It is these patients that usually require systemic steroids. If the patient is having intravenous therapy, hydrocortisone hemisuccinate sodium 200–300 mg per day can be given in the drip. Otherwise oral prednisone (60 mg per day) can be used. Some physicians believe that a remission is more likely to be induced if ACTH is used and they recommend an initial dose of 80 units per day. There is some data to indicate that this clinical impression is valid [7]. Immunosuppressives have been used with apparent success and are at present under trial. At present their use should be confined to centres where their effectiveness can be properly evaluated. If the patient is severely ill an intravenous broad spectrum antibiotic such as ampicillin can be given after blood cultures have been taken. It is best to avoid oral antibiotics such as sulphonamides and tetracycline as these can provoke colitis. Anaemia is, in acute attacks, best treated by blood transfusion and body iron stores can be subsequently replenished by a course of parenteral iron. Lomotil (diphenoxylate hydrochloride and atropine sulphate) and codeine phosphate are usually useless in controlling the diarrhoea of severe attacks.

Surgery in ulcerative colitis. Total proctocolectomy cures ulcerative colitis. It is however a major surgical procedure with a significant mortality. It also leaves the patient with an ileostomy. The few patients who have the rectum spared of disease can be treated with total colectomy and ileorectal anastomosis. Total proctocolectomy has an important place in the management of ulcerative colitis and is indicated under the following circumstances:

(a) Toxic megacolon and failure to induce a remission in an acute fulminating episode of ulcerative colitis.

(b) Persistent illness and debility in patients with the chronic form of the disease.

(c) Risk of carcinoma occurring in a colitic colon. If there is total involvement of the colon with the disease, in a young patient who started with an acute attack, and if the patient has had the condition for ten years there are strong grounds for recommending prophylactic proctocolectomy because of the high risk of carcinoma.

Diverticular disease

Patients with uncomplicated diverticular disease (diverticulosis) may have some abdominal discomfort and altered bowel habits. The nature of the condition should be explained to them and they should be advised to report if their symptoms alter or they develop new ones. They should keep their bowel actions regular by means of a bulk forming medicament such as methyl cellulose or sterculia 1 teaspoonful daily, or a teaspoonful of bran with each meal. The amount of these substances should be increased until the patients are having daily actions. Acute episodes of constipation can be treated with standardised senna extract, or dioctyl sodium sulphosuccinate. Stronger purgatives, colonic lavage and enemata are dangerous and should not be used.

Low residue diet has no place in the management of this condition. These patients should be advised to avoid medicaments containing codeine.

Diverticulitis. Diverticulitis causes persistent left iliac fossa pain, tenderness and fever and malaise. It may progress to pericolic abscess. The patient should be treated in hospital. Initially no solid food should be allowed and fluids given orally, or intravenously. A broad spectrum antibiotic such as tetracycline is given by mouth, or if there is vomiting, intravenously. Pethidine, but not morphia, should be used to relieve the pain. Most cases of diverticulitis will respond to this regime and once the episode has subsided the patient should be advised to adhere to the medical regime described for diverticulosis. If the symptoms persist or become recurrent an operation may be necessary. Most surgeons advise resection but recently sigmoid myotomy has been used with apparent success [8]. Vesicocolic fistula is not uncommon in this condition and requires surgical treatment.

Chronic constipation

In a recent survey of bowel habit in a healthy population 98 per cent of 1500 people had between 3 bowel actions per day and 3 bowel actions per week. On this evidence the authors suggested that, in terms of frequency, constipation be defined as less than three bowel actions per week. Although only 1 per cent of subjects was constipated by these criteria 20 per cent took laxatives. It is clear that in healthy individuals there is considerable variation in the frequency of bowel action, and as long as an individual is having regular actions it is of no importance that he is having them only 3 or 4 times a week. The sensible management of ambulant healthy individuals who have occasional episodes of constipation is to increase the bulk of the stool by adding roughage to the diet or by using aperients for 1–2 weeks only.

The old, infirm and bed ridden are a considerable problem in regard to constipation and in them more energetic measures are required. In this group, in addition to foods and medicaments that increase the bulk of the stool, aperients are required. Senokot (standardised senna extract) should be given regularly in order to prevent severe constipation and faecal impaction. Senokot granules (1 to 2 teaspoonfuls every night) is recommended.

LIVER

Infective hepatitis

This is usually a mild illness from which the patient makes a spontaneous and complete recovery within a few weeks. During the prodromal phase anorexia, and fever occur before the patient is noticeably jaundiced, and hepatitis may not be suspected. During this phase the patient should be kept in bed and antipyretics should be used. There is some evidence that excessive physical exertion at the onset of the illness may cause fulminating hepatitis, so patients should be discouraged from taking exercise in order to 'work off' their symptoms. It is also a mistake to drink alcohol during the prodromal phase of hepatitis, but, as most patients lose their taste for alcohol early in the illness, this is not usually a clinical problem. Once the jaundice appears the patient often begins to feel better. He should be kept in bed while he is feeling ill and has a fever. The jaundice may take a few weeks to go and during this time he can be up and about, but he should not return to work until it has gone. If available, liver function tests will influence the management, and persistently abnormal biochemistry will result in a more cautious attitude. Once the patient has recovered he should be advised to avoid alcohol for six months.

A typical case of infective hepatitis occurring in a local epidemic is not difficult to diagnose correctly. It is important in any patient with jaundice to consider the differential diagnoses such as: serum hepatitis (hypodermic needles, tattooing, blood transfusions), drug induced hepatitis (monoamine oxidase inhibitors, halothane, chlorpromazine, anabolic steroids, oral contraceptives), Gilbert's disease (recurrent jaundice without bile in the urine and with normal liver function tests), ascending cholangitis (usually older patients with abdominal pain and fever), cirrhosis, alcoholic hepatitis and chronic active hepatitis. Most cases of jaundice can be diagnosed by the history, clinical examination and liver function tests, but a few cases will require admission to hospital for further investigation.

Fulminating hepatitis

Progressive jaundice and persistent fever after an attack of hepatitis signals the onset of fulminating hepatitis. This has a poor prognosis. Patients should be admitted to hospital immediately where full treatment for hepatic failure will be instituted. Exchange transfusion is successful in getting some of these patients out of coma, and in some centres is thought to be the treatment of choice for this condition. This view is not universally held and it is doubtful if exchange transfusion is justified, for it is expensive in terms of blood and has not been proved to be of value [9]. Corticosteroids sometimes improve the patient temporarily but it is doubtful if they materially affect the outcome. Procedures such as perfusing the patient's blood through a recently removed pig's liver can also improve the patient, but it has no effect on the progress of the hepatitis within the liver.

Chronic active hepatitis ('lupoid' hepatitis)

This condition often starts with an illness indistinguishable from infective hepatitis. However the illness persists, liver function tests remain abnormal, and the patient has recurrent bouts of jaundice and ill health. Further investigations show that the immuno-globulins are disturbed, L.E. cells may be found in the blood and liver biopsy shows the liver to be invaded by the lymphocytes and plasma cells. Some of these patients appear to go through an active phase of chronic active hepatitis and then make a clinically satisfactory recovery. Others have intermittent jaundice and ill health over months or years. Other organs may be involved during this illness including the joints and lungs. Corticosteroids improve the patient's symptoms, and in conjunction with immuno-suppressives may have some effect on controlling the progress of the inflammation in the liver.

Primary biliary cirrhosis

This is a condition that occurs in middle-aged women and is another form of diffuse hepatic disorder with an autoimmune background. An important clinical feature of this condition is itching due to failure of the liver to excrete bile salts. Jaundice is often mild or absent at the onset. The itching can be considerably improved in these patients with cholestyramine 1 g. four times daily which prevents the reabsorption of bile salts from the gut.

Cirrhosis

Treating the cause. In most patients with cirrhosis the pathological changes in the liver are irreversible. However in cirrhosis due to alcoholism and in haemochromatosis some improvement within the liver can be expected from appropriate treatment. Treatment of alcoholism is perhaps the most effective step in the management of the patient with alcoholic cirrhosis. The problems in stopping the individual drinking are considerable but, if the patient stops drinking, the prognosis is improved. Haemochromatosis is a rare cause of cirrhosis and one that is not uncommonly associated with alcoholism. It is an important one to diagnose as reduction of total body iron by repeated bleeding has been shown to reverse the cirrhotic process within the liver. In Wilson's disease (hepatolenticular degeneration) cirrhosis is due to copper overload. Methods of reducing body copper stores are being used.

Haematemesis and melaena. Oesophageal varices are an important cause of acute gastrointestinal bleeding associated with cirrhosis. However varices are by no means the only cause of bleeding in cirrhotic patients, particularly in the alcoholics. Chronic peptic ulcers are not uncommon in these patients, and multiple gastric erosions are also a significant cause of bleeding. It is important to diagnose in each patient the precise cause of the bleeding as this will affect the management of the case.

Prophylactic porta-caval anastomosis reduces the incidence of death from bleeding varices. Patients need to be carefully selected for this procedure, for those with poor hepatic function will develop portal systemic encephalopathy and hepatic failure. The group that appear to do best after prophylactic porta-caval shunt are young patients that have cryptogentic (post hepatitic) cirrhosis and good hepatic function, as assessed by liver function tests and serum albumin level.

The initial treatment of active bleeding varices should be blood replacement and pitressin. The latter is given intravenously in a dose of 20 units in 10 minutes. Side effects are pallor, abdominal colic and bowel evacuation. Pitressin reduces splanchnic and hepatic blood flow and thus allows the bleeding sites in the varix to become occluded. Unfortunately rebleeding is not uncommon. Oesophageal tamponade using a Sengstaken tube is a cumbersome and dangerous procedure which should not be used except by experienced physicians. Its only place would now appear to be in halting catastrophic haemorrhage while preparing for emergency surgery. Emergency surgery should be advised if the patient rebleeds, particularly if there is an experienced surgeon available. Apart from dealing with varices and portal hypertension the surgeon is able to deal with bleeding from an undiagnosed chronic peptic ulcer or erosion.

Portal systemic encephalopathy (*P.S.E.*). Hepatic precoma occurs when ammonia and amines absorbed from the gut have not been adequately detoxicated by the liver. These substances reach the brain and cause clouding of consciousness, neurological defects and coma. Failure of detoxication occurs both because of liver cell failure and because the absorbed materials from the gut are shunted past the liver via varices or portacaval anastomoses. Hepatic precoma is particularly likely to occur after a gastrointestinal bleed when there is protein in the gut. There are three measures that reverse this process:

1. Removal of protein from the gut lumen by enemata and aperients.
2. Neomycin 1 g. four times daily (to reduce bacteria which break down the proteins).
3. Reduce protein intake by placing the patient on a restricted protein diet.

In addition lactulose has recently been introduced for the treatment of P.S.E. [10]. This substance is metabolised by bacteria and converted to lactic acid which is thought to trap ammonia in the large bowel and remove it in the stools. It appears to be a useful measure in the management.

Oedema and ascites. Ascites in cirrhosis is usually due to a combination of raised intrahepatic pressure and reduced serum albumin in the blood. It is generally a mistake to treat it by paracentesis which will remove a large quantity of protein from the body. Rapid paracentesis can induce acute hepatic failure and should always be avoided. The patient should be treated with diuretics and potassium chloride. Spironolactone is of particular value. A double ended porta-caval shunt in which both ends of the cut portal vein are anastomosed to the inferior vena cava, has been used in an attempt to reduce the intra hepatic pressure. Although it is often successful in reducing ascites the patient may be made worse because of portal systemic encephalopathy. Once oedema and electrolyte disturbances develop in decompensated cirrhosis the prognosis is grave.

Amoebic hepatitis and amoebic abscess

Chloroquine is concentrated 500 times by the liver and is the drug of first choice for hepatic amoebiasis. It is usual to give 1 g. by mouth daily for two days followed by 0·5 g. daily for 19 days. If after 4 days there is no clinical improvement emetine hydrochloride, which is also concentrated in the liver, should be given. It is given by subcutaneous injection 60 mg daily for 10 days. Needle aspiration may be required to hasten resolution if an abscess is present, and open drainage may be required if there is secondary infection.

GALL BLADDER

Biliary colic

The pain of biliary colic is sufficiently severe to require potent analgesics. Morphia and pethidine are effective but both have the theoretical disadvantage that they cause spasm of smooth muscle. It is doubtful if this is relevant in relation to the disturbed motility of the duct caused by impaction of a biliary stone. Antispasmodics such as atropine (0·5 mg) or propantheline (15 mg) may be given 20 minutes before morphia or pethidine in order to prevent spasm. The new analgesics phenazocine and pentazocine are said not to affect smooth muscle and may be drugs of choice for bilary colic.

Acute cholecystitis

Acute cholecystitis is usually treated conservatively but early in the course of the disease it is possible to perform acute cholecystectomy. Some surgeons prefer to manage the condition this way. The orthodox management is to treat the patient with bed rest, fluids, restricted diet and antibiotics. Tetracycline is a good antibiotic to use as it is highly concentrated in bile and is usually effective against the infecting organisms. A new antibiotic, rifamide, which is given by intramuscular injection, is concentrated in bile to an even greater extent and appears to be the drug of choice for acute cholecystitis [11]. Once the attack has subsided the patient should have biliary tract radiology followed by elective cholecystectomy 2–3 months later.

Ascending cholangitis

In ascending cholangitis there is recurring fever (Charcot's intermittent fever), rigors, jaundice, abdominal pain and leucocytosis. There are three main causes: gall stone impacted in the common bile duct, stricture of the common bile duct and following surgical implantation of common bile duct into the upper small intestine. If the cause is a stone or stricture, symptoms will continue until the obstruction has been corrected surgically. The object of medical treatment of these patients should be to get them in as good condition as possible for surgery. The offending organism may be isolated by blood culture and the patient should then be given antibiotics. Patients who have had biliary tract surgery with reimplantation of the common bile duct (such as those who have had radical surgery for carcinoma of ampulla of Vater), may have recurrent attacks of ascending cholangitis which will require repeated courses of antibiotics. It is always worth performing an intravenous or percutaneous trans-hepatic cholangiogram to see if a stricture is present. This should be removed surgically. If the cause cannot be corrected surgically prophylactic antibiotics may be used in order to prevent organisms from invading the common bile duct.

HICCOUGH

Hiccough is spasmodic contraction of the diaphragm with simultaneous contracture of the glottis. It is commonly due to irritation of the stomach by alcohol, over-eating and highly spiced foods. Simple measures such as holding the breath, pulling the tongue, inducing sneezing by tickling the nose, sodium bicarbonate 0·6–1·2 g. in water or a carminative or 'gripe water' relieve most cases. Persistent hiccough is usually due to diaphragmatic irritation from peritonitis, paralytic ileus, subphrenic abscess, intrahepatic abscess, cholangitis and pancreatitis. It also occurs in uraemia and encephalitis. Occasionally hiccough lasting a few days occurs for no obvious cause, and epidemics of hiccough have been described. If hiccough is due to paralytic ileus gastric intubation may relieve it by releasing gas from the descended stomach. In other cases, treatment of the cause, (i.e. uraemia, subphrenic abscess), will stop the spasms. Injections of hyoscine, chlorpromazine or morphia will relieve hiccough in some cases. If it persists and the patient is becoming exhausted he should be admitted to hospital. Crushing one or both phrenic nerves and causing temporary diaphragmatic paralysis may be required in severe cases.

PANCREAS

Acute pancreatitis

This condition usually presents as an acute abdominal emergency with severe pain, paralytic ileus and shock. Occasionally patients present without pain but with severe shock. Diagnosis can be difficult and may only be made at laparotomy. Once the diagnosis has been firmly established most clinicians manage the condition conservatively.

Shock. During the acute phase the blood pressure may fall and this requires urgent treatment with intravenous blood and plasma. Intravenous electrolytes are needed to replace loss of intravascular fluids into the tissues. Released vasodepressive substances (i.e. kinins) may cause the low blood pressure and if hypotension persists intravenous steroids in large doses may be used. Intravenous vasopressor drugs may be used to raise the blood pressure.

Paralytic ileus. Many of these patients have some degree of paralytic ileus and it is therefore advisable to institute gastric suction. The removal of gastric acid may also inhibit a stimulus to pancreatic secretion.

Pain. Pain is severe and requires potent analgesics. Morphia causes spasm of the sphincter of Oddi and is best avoided. Pethidine is therefore probably the analgesic of choice and some recommend that atropine be given with it.

Hypocalcaemia. Hypocalcaemia is a feature of acute pancreatitis and may, on occasion, cause tetany. It is due to breakdown of fat by released pancreatic lipase and the subsequent formation of calcium soaps. If the serum calcium falls or tetany occurs intravenous calcium gluconate (20 ml of 10 per cent) should be given.

Antibiotics. Antibiotics do not influence the initial course of acute pancreatitis but should be used in an attempt to prevent the formation of abscess in the necrotic gland. Tetracycline or ampicillin should be given by mouth or intravenously.

Other measures. In severe cases other techniques have been claimed to be useful. Trasylol (a kallikrein inhibitor) has had enthusiastic supporters, but there is no evidence that it affects the outcome of acute pancreatitis in man, despite its efficiency in experimental pancreatitis in the dog. Trasylol is not recommended for this condition. Removal of pancreatic enzymes by peritoneal dialysis is worth considering [12]. It is not advisable to use this technique unless experience and facilities are available. Total pancreatectomy has been successfully used for fulminant pancreatitis but this should only be considered if an experienced surgeon is available for the operative risks are considerable. After the initial episode the patient may develop a pancreatic abscess of pancreatic pseudocyst. This will require drainage or appropriate surgical treatment.

Relapsing pancreatitis

Relapsing pancreatitis may be caused by chronic alcoholism. Some cases are associated with gallstones. The most distressing feature of this condition is the recurring episodes of severe epigastric pain. The bizarre features of the pain may make the diagnosis difficult. The simplest investigation is a straight X-ray of the abdomen, which may reveal pancreatic calcification. Secretin tests of pancreatic function are required to unravel the more difficult cases. All cases require biliary tract radiology.

Once the diagnosis has been made the essence of management is to relieve the pain surgically, before the patient becomes addicted to potent analgesics such as pethidine and morphia. Pancreatic surgery for relapsing painful pancreatitis is difficult and requires considerable experience. Many surgical manoeuvres have been recommended, the simplest being sphincterotomy. Some surgeons recommend localisation of the area of pancreatitis by pancreatic duct radiology at the time of surgery. They then relate the operative procedure to the radiological findings. Pancreatic drainage with removal of stones from the pancreatic duct, partial and total pancreatectomy are used to treat this condition.

Pancreatic insufficiency

Pancreatic failure may result from one attack of acute pancreatitis, or may be the end stage of recurring attacks of pancreatitis. Occasionally it develops with no preceding history of pancreatitis. Rarely it occurs in association with hyperparathyroidism, and a familial form of the condition has been described. Atrophy of the pancreas may also cause pancreatic failure, and this has been seen in severe long standing cases of coeliac syndrome. In pancreatic failure both exogenous and the endogenous secretions of the pancreas are not produced and patients develop both steatorrhoea and diabetes mellitus.

Pancreatic steatorrhoea. The amount of fat in the stools of patients with pancreatic steatorrhoea is very high – being usually more than 20 grams per 24 hours. The patients therefore commonly complain of diarrhoea. They may notice that they pass oil in the stools. This may be noticed as an 'oil slick' floating on the surface of the water. The excretion of this large amount of fat leads to weight loss despite a good or even increased appetite. In addition to fat, the stools may have a high nitrogen content. The diarrhoea and fattiness of the stools can be notably improved by placing the patient on a low fat diet. In addition the diet should be rich in protein. Pancreatic extract, such as pancreatin, can be used but it is often disappointing. It should be given well mixed with meals and patients should be advised to take an alkali beforehand to neutralize gastric acid which inactivates the enzyme. Many believe that the only clinical effect of pancreatic extract is to increase the protein intake and that it is clinically ineffective as a digestive enzyme. However it is worth trying and occasionally patients benefit from its use. Absorption of other constituents in pancreatic steatorrhoea is normal and it is uncommon for these patients to develop anaemia, osteomalacia or bleeding disorders.

Pancreatic diabetes. This occurs in pancreatic insufficiency due to both pancreatitis and pancreatic atrophy. It also occurs in haemochromatosis. It requires insulin but diabetic control is usually not difficult.

Fibrocystic disease

This condition affects children and leads to pancreatic steatorrhoea and recurrent chest infections. The principles of treating the steatorrhoea are as outlined above. These children also require antibiotics for their respiratory disease.

References

1. Gillies, M., Nicks, R., and Skyring, A., *Brit. med. J.* (1967), **2**, 527.
2. Editorial, *ibid*, (1969), **3**, 2.
3. Croft, D. N., *J. Pharm. Pharmac.* (1966), **18**, 354.
4. Langman, M. J. S., *Brit. med. J.* (1969), **4**, 100.
5. Editorial, *ibid*, 727–8.
6. Sheedy, C. B., and Keifetz, N., *Cooking for your Coeliac Child; Dietary Management in Malabsorption Disorders* (1969), The Dial Press Inc, New York.
7. Friedman, M., Hinton, J. M., and Lennard-Jones, J. E., *Gut* (1969), **10**, 194.
8. Reilly, M., *Proc. roy. Soc. Med.* (1969), **62**, 715.
9. Reynolds, T. B., *Gastroenterology* (1969), **56**, 170.
10. Elkington, S. G., Floch, M. H., and Conn, H. O., *New Eng. J. Med.* (1969), **281**, 408.
11. Acocella, G., Mattiussi, R., Nicolis, F. B., Pallanza, R., and Tenconi, L. T., *Gut* (1968), **9**, 536.
12. Editorial, *Brit. med. J.* (1965), **2**, 1448.

This chapter was written by Dr D. N. Croft (Consultant Physician, Isotope Department, St Thomas's Hospital) and edited by Professor W. I. Cranston.

Category 2
Renal Disease

Introduction

The chapter begins with four main sections dealing with the management of the major syndromes arising in renal disease: the acute nephritic syndrome, the nephrotic syndrome, and acute and chronic renal failure. It is no longer possible to consider the management of renal failure without placing this in the context of dialysis as a temporary or permanent replacement of renal function. The techniques of haemodialysis are beyond the scope of this book. Peritoneal dialysis may have to be carried out occasionally in any hospital and an outline of the technique is therefore included.

Increasingly, renal clinics will be backed by programmes for maintenance haemodialysis and transplantation. It is hoped that the fearful economic implications of providing facilities for treating terminal irreversible renal failure will stimulate a better understanding of the pathogenesis of renal diseases and eventually result in more specific and effective therapy to prevent their progression. Such measures as are at present available, are herein described.

THE MANAGEMENT OF THE ACUTE NEPHRITIC SYNDROME (Acute Nephritis)

In its fully developed form this is an acute illness with oedema, hypertension, raised jugular venous pressure, haematuria and proteinuria. Severe cases may be complicated by acute renal failure. There may be evidence of antecedent streptococcal infection. This syndrome may also occur in certain other diseases having in common inflammatory lesions of small blood vessels e.g. polyarteritis nodosa, anaphylactoid (Henoch-Schonlein) purpura or systemic lupus erythematosus. These possibilities must be considered in the management of any patient with this syndrome.

1. General management

Treatment of any antecedent infection. A swab should be taken from the throat or any other possible site of infection. The serum antistreptolysin

O (ASO) titre should also be determined. In practice many cases referred to hospital with acute nephritis have already received an antibiotic, thus reducing the chances of bacterial identification and decreasing the incidence of elevated ASO titres after streptococcal infections. It is customary to prescribe long term oral penicillin therapy for any patient with acute nephritis in whom there is evidence or suspicion of precipitating streptococcal infection. There is, however, no proof that such long term therapy influences the course of the renal disease.

Bed rest. The patient should be confined to bed while oedema, elevation of the jugular venous pressure, hypertension, oliguria or macroscopic haematuria persist. Microscopic haematuria may persist for many weeks and proteinuria of less than 1 g./day for many months. There is no good reason for keeping the patient in bed until these features disappear. If haematuria or proteinuria increase markedly when the patient gets up, some physicians would advise further bed rest.

Diet. Salt restriction is indicated while the jugular venous pressure remains elevated and oedema or hypertension persist. The sodium intake should then be less than 25 mEq/day if oedema is considerable. When the patient is oliguric (urine volume less than 400 ml per day), fluid intake should not exceed 500 ml/day plus the volume of urine passed on the previous day. The adequacy of fluid restriction should be monitored by weighing the patient daily.

Protein restriction is only indicated for azotaemic patients.

Diuretics. It is generally believed that these drugs are of little value but controlled observations on the use of the newer and more powerful diuretics (frusemide and ethacrynic acid) are as yet inadequate to assess their effects.

2. Management of complications

Severe Hypertension. Injections of pentolinium are suitable for urgent treatment; the initial dose is 2·5 mg I.M. and this can be doubled hourly until effective. The head of the bed must be raised. Reserpine (2·5–5·0 mg I.M.) is useful for less severe cases. Even in the absence of symptoms antihypertensive treatment should be started if the diastolic blood pressure rises to 105–110 mm Hg as serious further rises in pressure may then occur over a few hours. Alpha methyl dopa by mouth is a suitable drug for this situation.

Encephalopathy. If clouding of consciousness, focal neurological signs or fits occur, careful attention should be paid to control of hypertension and phenytoin sodium (100 mg b.d. I.M.) given. For fits or marked restlessness intravenous diazepam (2–10 mg given slowly), intravenous sodium amylobarbitone or intramuscular paraldehyde may be used.

Acute pulmonary oedema. Rarely, this may require emergency treatment by venesection before dialysis can be arranged. In this situation hypertension is usually severe and parenteral pentolinium may be used to control it.

Acute renal failure. When this complicates acute nephritis, it is treated as described below.

THE MANAGEMENT OF THE NEPHROTIC SYNDROME

1. Use of renal biopsy

Knowledge of the underlying renal lesion is necessary for correct management of the nephrotic syndrome, and a renal biopsy should be performed in any adult in whom this syndrome develops idiopathically. Renal biopsy is usually unnecessary when the nephrotic syndrome develops in a patient with long standing diabetes, established amyloidosis, or other disease likely to cause heavy proteinuria. In children the greater incidence of minimal change glomerular histology ('foot process' lesion only) which usually produces proteinuria that is highly selective, reduces the need for renal biopsy. In a child under five years with highly selective proteinuria it is reasonable to institute steroid therapy without renal biopsy.

2. Dietary and drug therapy

Treatment is aimed at ridding the patient of oedema and abolishing the proteinuria.

Diet. When the blood urea is normal a high protein intake of at least 2–3 g./kg. bodyweight should be encouraged. This may enable a patient with prolonged heavy proteinuria to achieve positive nitrogen balance. Modern diuretic therapy usually dispels oedema without strict restriction of sodium intake, but moderate salt restriction is sensible while oedema persists.

Diuretics. Mersalyl should no longer be used in the nephrotic syndrome. The thiazide diuretics, e.g. bendrofluazide 5–15 mg/day, are often effective and are cheap. Frusemide and ethacrynic acid are more powerful diuretics and may succeed where the thiazides fail. In resistant cases large doses of frusemide, 200 to 500 mg. or more, may be needed. If the blood urea level is markedly elevated (above 100 mg/100 ml) ethacrynic acid is probably better avoided in view of the risk of deafness.

With all the above diuretics potassium supplements are usually needed, the risk of hypokalaemia during diuresis in the nephrotic syndrome being considerable, presumably due to the associated aldosteronism. In this context aldosterone antagonists, e.g. spironolactone 25 mg four times daily, have a role and are best used with one of the above diuretics. Triamterene is also often a suitable diuretic, especially in the presence of hypokalaemia, but is better avoided if the blood urea is raised.

Albumin infusion. The intravenous infusion of salt-poor human serum albumin is expensive and its effect short-lived, the extra albumin being rapidly excreted by the kidney. Nonetheless it may occasionally permit diuretics to succeed where previously they had failed. Albumin, 1 g./kg bodyweight, is infused over several hours, a careful watch being kept on the jugular venous pressure, and the infusion slowed or stopped if the latter rises to 4 cm or more above the sternal angle.

Other plasma volume expanders, e.g. dextran, are less satisfactory but can be used in patients with diuretic resistant oedema when albumin is not available. Dextran or albumin infusion is occasionally needed for the nephrotic patient with severe hypotension associated with hypovolaemia. This complication is uncommon spontaneously but may arise for instance in the patient who has been over enthusiastically treated with diuretics.

Corticosteroids. It is now generally accepted that a trial of steroid therapy should be given to all patients with minimal glomerular changes on light microscopy ('foot process' lesion only on electron microscopy). Adult patients may respond initially only to large doses, e.g. prednisone 60 mg/day for 2 to 3 weeks. A smaller dose, e.g. 10–20 mg/day, may then be needed for 3 to 6 months to prevent or minimise proteinuria. In some patients the proteinuria returns whenever the steroid dose is reduced to this lower range. Long term steroid therapy using moderate doses, e.g. prednisone 20–40 mg/day for an adult, may then be successful but such doses carry correspondingly higher risks of serious complications. This problem is encountered most often in children and immunosuppressive drugs (vide infra) may prove of particular value in this group. Where steroid therapy is continued for many months or years an intermittent regime is recommended by some authorities, e.g. prednisone 20 mg/day for 4 consecutive days in each week, or on alternate days. There is however no unassailable evidence that such prolonged therapy with steroids, whether continuous or intermittent, improves the long term prognosis of patients with the minimal change lesion.

Steroid therapy is unlikely to succeed when the nephrotic syndrome is due to membranous glomerulonephritis. It has been claimed that prolonged therapy with steroids in low doses, e.g. prednisone 10 mg/day, delays deterioration in renal function in patients with membranous glomerulonephritis but this is not proven.

When the nephrotic syndrome is caused by proliferative glomerulonephritis in adults steroid-induced remissions are uncommon, even when the proteinuria is highly selective. Some patients, especially children, do appear to benefit and a trial of steroid therapy is reasonable. It is uncertain whether steroids affect the long term prognosis in this condition.

When systemic lupus erythematosus is complicated by nephrotic syndrome steroids are usually given in high doses (vide infra). Steroids are not beneficial in the nephrotic syndrome associated with diabetes, amyloidosis, or renal vein thrombosis. It has been claimed that steroids may hasten the deterioration in renal function in amyloidosis and their use in this condition is best avoided.

Immunosuppressive drugs. The use of these agents in treatment of the nephrotic syndrome is based on evidence that the glomerular damage may be mediated by immunological mechanisms. There have been several reports claiming success with azathioprine or cyclophosphamide, the early results of controlled trials suggest that the latter is more helpful, but it is not possible at present to define the role of these drugs with precision.

Encouraging results have been obtained with cyclophosphamide or azathioprine in children with steroid-resistant nephrotic syndrome associated with proliferative glomerulonephritis. Cyclophosphamide has been used in children without glomerular abnormalities on light microscopy who responded to steroids initially but then either became resistant or needed an unacceptably high dose to control proteinuria. It is not yet clear whether cyclophosphamide is more effective if given in doses sufficient to cause leucopenia, or whether it is advantageous to use prednisone in combination with it.

Within the limitations imposed by these uncertainties cyclophosphamide may be given in an initial dose of 3 mg/kg/day. In an oedematous child the weight to use in this calculation is the predicted mean weight for the height. Blood counts are performed 2 or 3 times each week for the first 2 or 3 weeks and weekly thereafter. This dose does not always produce leucopenia and if after 4 weeks the white count is still normal and no renal response has occurred the dose may be increased to 4 mg/kg/day, reducing to 2 or 3 mg/kg/day when leucopenia develops. Cyclophosphamide is given for a total period of 2 to 4 months and then withdrawn. Alopecia is common in adults with this regime, but the hair often grows again when the drug is stopped. Other side effects include chemical cystitis, nausea, vomiting and infections but these are all uncommon. Thrombocytopenia and anaemia are also uncommon but careful haematological supervision is mandatory.

3. Dialysis

Oliguric renal failure sometimes develops in a patient with the nephrotic syndrome. Hypovolaemia with renal circulatory insufficiency must then be considered and corrected if present by expansion of the plasma volume with albumin. If renal biopsy shows only minimal abnormalities steroid therapy is given and dialysis is performed as necessary, for such patients may not only recover from the renal failure, but may subsequently enter remission from the nephrotic syndrome. When renal biopsy shows membranous or proliferative glomerulonephritis oliguric renal failure is reputed to carry a very bad prognosis. However, some patients may recover useful renal function and maintenance dialysis should be given in this hope.

THE MANAGEMENT OF ACUTE RENAL FAILURE (A.R.F.)

1. The prevention of A.R.F.

The occurrence of A.R.F. can often be anticipated and possibly prevented if the wide variety of clinical contexts in which it may occur is appreciated. Timely resuscitative measures must then be applied to correct precipitating factors during the onset phase.

Hypovolaemia and hypotension. In the patient who is at risk of developing A.R.F. following battle or road traffic trauma, obstetric accidents or massive losses of fluid and electrolytes, the prompt replacement of blood and fluid losses is mandatory. Rapid replacement of intravascular volume and extracellular fluid is safer if the central venous pressure (C.V.P.) is monitored. In the management of burns the importance of fluid and electrolyte replacement must be stressed.

Septicaemia. Infection with gram negative organisms and septic abortions require urgent treatment with appropriate antibiotics, fluids and possibly other therapy relevant to septicaemia.

Intravascular haemolysis. When this threatens to cause A.R.F. low molecular weight dextran up to a maximum of 300 ml intravenously is advised.

Nephrotoxins. In any case of A.R.F. the possibility of exposure to nephrotoxic agent must be considered. Occasionally this may lead to the use of a specific antidote, e.g. BAL in mercury poisoning.

Urinary tract obstruction. Total anuria always suggests the possibility of urinary obstruction. Anuria alternating with polyuria and a history of renal colic are further pointers towards a postrenal cause of A.R.F. High dose infusion I.V.P. and radioactive renography may be helpful investigations in this context, but cystoscopy and ureterography may be needed to confirm or exclude obstruction with certainty. If obstruction cannot be removed, nephrostomy may be required.

Use of mannitol, diuretics and other measures. There is probably some final common pathway in the pathophysiology of acute tubular necrosis (A.T.N.), although it is not understood. Therefore, attempts to prevent the development of A.T.N. by interrupting the march of events at a later stage have been empirical. Paravertebral block, decapsulation of the kidneys and steriod therapy are all useless and increase the risk to the patient. Over expansion of the extracellular fluid space and the unrestrained 'pushing of fluids' in an attempt to 'force a diuresis' are also dangerous and ineffective.

Experimental and clinical studies indicate that the use of mannitol to induce an osmotic diuresis reduces the incidence of A.R.F. in certain situations. Therefore, mannitol (12·5 to 50 g.) is given prophylactically during cardiopulmonary bypass, certain vascular operations and surgery on jaundiced patients. There is less good evidence that mannitol is beneficial when given after the clinical insult has occurred. Nevertheless, since 50 ml of a 25 per cent solution of mannitol given I.V. over 3–5 minutes appears to be innocuous; it is probably worth a trial if A.R.F. has been diagnosed within a matter of hours of its onset. This dose may be repeated at 3 hourly intervals to a total of 50 g. unless there is any evidence of pulmonary oedema or water intoxication.

For similar reasons frusemide may also be tried: the minimum effective dose is not known, but 200 mg I.V. has been used.

2. The management of established A.R.F.

During the oliguric phase, the risks are those of overhydration, hyperkalaemia, uraemia, infection and those of the precipitating condition and its complications. Management therefore consists of appropriate monitoring of the patient, the institution of dietary and specific therapeutic measures, and, as early as possible, a decision as to whether or not to dialyse the patient.

If at all possible, the patient should be weighed daily, and weight should fall by 0·2–0·5 kg per day depending on the degree of catabolism occurring. The true weight at the time of onset of A.R.F. is that when all blood and fluid losses have been replaced so that the blood pressure and peripheral circulation are normal and when there is no rise in venous pressure or oedema. Records of fluid and electrolyte balance must be kept. A low reading thermometer should be available. An E.C.G. affords the quickest and most relevant information about the serum potassium level. Daily (or more frequent) electrolyte, blood urea and serum creatinine estimations help to follow the anticipated metabolic changes.

Superadded infections so often jeopardise the chances of survival in these patients that there will be few in whom bacteriological investigations are not required. Infection of the urinary tract is particularly hazardous and catheterisation should therefore be carried out only if essential (e.g. fractured pelvis) or to exclude obstruction. A wet bed or inaccurate fluid output figures are preferable to the risks of infection.

Emergency treatment of hyperkalaemia is indicated by advanced E.C.G. changes (loss of P waves, spread of QRS complex) and consists of intravenous calcium gluconate (20 ml of 10 per cent solution), dextrose (100 ml of 50 per cent solution) and insulin (10 units). Sodium bicarbonate (e.g. 100 ml of 8·4 per cent solution equalling 100 mEq) may be given if the sodium load is acceptable. If management is less urgent, exchange resins, preferably in the calcium phase (Calcium resonium either 15 g. orally up to three times daily or 30–60 g. as a retention enema) should be given.

It has been customary to prescribe a low protein (20 g.) high calorie (2,000 calories if possible) diet with restricted sodium intake (less than 25 mEq) and avoidance of all foods with a high potassium content. Supplementary vitamins should be given. Fluid intake is restricted to

300–500 ml plus any measured losses per day, subject to the overriding consideration of the weight change. However, the present tendency is for this regime to become more liberalised as the use of dialysis is extended. Intravenous feeding with high concentration glucose and lipids has its risks but may be of use for the occasional patient who cannot take foods by mouth.

Conservative management of A.R.F. will result in a successful outcome when the degree of catabolism is mild and the period of renal failure is a brief one, lasting for less than a week. In these cases, especially those following obstetric accidents, it is worthwhile administering an anabolic steroid; a single dose of nandrolone decanoate 50 mg I.M. lasts for two weeks. Conservative management should be carried out in collaboration with the team responsible for dialysis. In patients in whom the clinical context suggests that the rate of catabolism will be high dialysis is indicated. Once it has been decided that dialysis will be required it is best to commence this early, not waiting for some arbitrary biochemical indication. Any type of dialysis is not without risk and should be performed by a team regularly providing this service. Dialysis permits a liberalisation of the diet and fluid intake, the patient is kept fitter and not confined to bed. In severely catabolic cases and in some with abdominal injuries and surgery, haemodialysis is preferred; in the majority of patients peritoneal dialysis will suffice provided the period of acute renal failure is not too prolonged.

Frequently treatment by dialysis will have to be started in order to 'buy time' for diagnostic urological and radiological investigations to be performed. It is often necessary to combine renal biopsy with cystoscopy and ureterography. In the course of such a 'work-up' it will become apparent that many patients presenting as acute renal failure are, in fact, suffering from chronic renal disease. In these patients and in others with acute cortical necrosis a decision will be required as to whether to embark on a programme of maintenance haemodialysis and transplantation.

During the diuretic phase the loss of water and electrolytes because of large urinary volumes must be anticipated. Oral and intravenous replacement, particularly of potassium, may be necessary. Despite the dramatic increase in urinary volumes, renal function only recovers gradually and dialysis may still be required.

During the course of A.R.F. infections require prompt antibiotic therapy. It is important to remember that the dose regimes of many antibiotics require altering in the presence of renal failure. The importance of adequate expert nursing for patients with A.R.F. cannot be overemphasised.

THE MANAGEMENT OF CHRONIC RENAL FAILURE C.R.F.)

1. Making the most of existing renal function

This involves titrating dietary intake against the level of renal function which remains.

Fluid and electrolytes. Urea excretion is proportional to urine flow and advantage is sometimes gained by encouraging the patient to drink sufficient water to produce a daily urinary volume of 3 litres.

If a salt or water deficit develops in a patient with C.R.F. due to vomiting, diarrhoea, or inappropriate restriction of salt and water, renal perfusion is diminished with consequent reduction in G.F.R.* Patients should be weighed, their blood pressure measured and the state of hydration assessed at each outpatient visit. The importance of such monitoring cannot be overemphasised since a salt and water deficit may result in a permanent decrement in renal function.

Regular doses of exchange resins preferably in the calcium phase are sometimes needed to control hyperkalaemia.

Diet. Special diets, it must be emphasised, are palliative therapy and should be used only in order to prevent the dangers of hyperkalaemia, the effects of sodium overload, and the gastrointestinal symptoms associated with uraemia. In practice, it is usually necessary to restrict protein intake when the blood urea exceeds 150 mg/100 ml or at plasma creatinine levels greater than 7·0 mg/100 ml. The Giordano-Giovannetti diet (see references 2, 3 and 4) and its modifications has impressively altered the symptomatology of C.R.F., removing the distressing gastrointestinal symptoms and permitting life to continue, to a lower level of renal function.

However, some authorities advise a rather higher protein intake (0·5 g/kg/day) if a negative nitrogen balance and progressive loss of weight are to be avoided. The calorie intake should be as high as possible; Hycal (Beecham) contains approximately 244 calories per 100 ml. Vitamin supplements should be given to all patients and iron supplements may be necessary. Patients on the Giordano-Giovannetti regime should also receive methionine 0·5 g./day.

A programme of progressive reduction of protein intake in the face

*Glomerular filtration rate.

of worsening renal function requires planning in the light of the rate of progression of the renal disease, and of eventual plans for maintenance haemodialysis and renal grafting. The ability of the patient to maintain dietary discipline is reflected in a plasma urea; creatinine ratio of less than 20:1 (in mg per 100 ml). This may be a useful test of the cooperation which can be expected when regular dialysis becomes necessary.

Dialysis. Occasional peritoneal dialysis may be required when intercurrent infections or surgery increase the rate of catabolism. Some patients, notably those with polycystic disease, do surprisingly well with monthly or even less frequent dialyses.

2. Treating the complications of uraemia

Gastrointestinal symptoms. Nausea and vomiting may respond to diet alone or to a period of dialysis. Symptomatic relief can be obtained with thiethylperazine or chlorpromazine. Phenothiazines can also be used for the treatment of hiccough. Diarrhoea for which no other cause than uraemia can be found is of grave significance: dialysis is usually required.

Peptic ulceration is common in C.R.F. Antacids containing magnesium should be avoided and it will often not be possible to give those containing sodium.

Acidosis. No attempt need be made to raise the serum bicarbonate level with oral alkali, with the inevitable risk of sodium overload, unless the acidosis is symptomatic, i.e. causing dyspnoea and mental symptoms. Sodium bicarbonate 3–9 g. per day is effective if the patient can tolerate the sodium load; if not, calcium carbonate 6–10 g./day may be used.

Cardiovascular complications. Hypertension is considered later. If digoxin is used for cardiac failure, a reduced dose is necessary in the presence of renal failure. The effects of uraemia on myocardial function are cured by dialysis. A pericardial friction rub is common in the final stages of uraemia, not infrequently developing after dialysis has been commenced. There is no treatment other than dialysis.

Anaemia. Unless there has been blood loss and consequent iron deficiency the anaemia is unresponsive to all haematimics. Transfusion is rarely necessary, but is required to replace acute blood losses and sometimes in preparation for surgery. Because of the risks of producing cardiac failure, small transfusions of packed cells are best. The correction of the anaemia of C.R.F. by transfusion is a temporary phenomenon: it is likely to suppress the patient's marrow even further. Experience with dialysed patients has made it clear that a quite marked anaemia (P.C.V. of 15–20 per cent) is borne without undue symptoms.

Haemorrhagic complications. The haemorrhagic diathesis of uraemia has a complex basis and is only corrected by adequate dialysis. However, troublesome epistaxis may occur and the use of local cautery should not then be neglected.

Renal osteodystrophy. There are theoretical reasons for hoping that correction of acidosis and large supplements of calcium may retard the progression of this complication of long standing renal failure. Calcium carbonate (6–10 g. per day) achieves both purposes, but has not been widely adopted as a prophylactic measure.

Vitamin D (as calciferol 20,000–500,000 units per day) may dramatically heal the bone lesions of children and adolescents; in adults it should probably be reserved for those patients with bone pain or proximal myopathy. Vitamin D enhances the risks of vascular and other soft tissue calcification. The calcaemic effect of vitamin D may be delayed and the dose should not be increased more often than once a month. In adults a starting dose of 80,000 to 100,000 units per day is recommended. This should be doubled after a month if there is no clinical or biochemical improvement.

The risks of metastatic calcification are diminished if the calcium × phosphate product (when both are measured in mg/100 ml) is maintained at less than 70 by the administration of aluminium hydroxide gel B.P. (60–120 ml/day), in order to bind phosphate in the gut.

In a patient in whom any of these treatments is being given or contemplated frequent estimations of plasma calcium, phosphate and alkaline phosphatase must be performed.

It is becoming apparent that subtotal parathyroidectomy is needed more frequently, and may be carried out with less operative hazard in patients who have begun regular dialysis treatment. Severe bone disease may be an indication for earlier commencement of regular dialysis.

Uraemia neuropathy. Once this complication has appeared its progression can only be arrested by adequate dialysis and if maintenance dialysis is planned this must be commenced without delay.

Intercurrent infections. Infections of the urinary tract and other infections, e.g. pneumonia and septicaemia, are particularly likely in patients with renal failure who may also be receiving treatment with steroids and immunosuppressive drugs. Urgent therapy with an appropriate antibiotic regime (see section on the use of antibiotics in renal failure) must be instituted. Dialysis may be needed to cover the period of enhanced catabolism.

3. Planning the transfer to maintenance haemodialysis and transplantation

It is essential that plans are made well before the patient is moribund. If eventual dialysis and transplantation are decided upon the patient may be transferred earlier if there is evidence of bone disease or neuropathy, and more careful monitoring of these patients should be carried out to detect such complications. In patients on protein restriction the blood urea is a less useful parameter and it is necessary to follow the plasma creatinine also. Once the plasma creatinine has reached 15–20 mg/100 ml a sudden disaster (pericarditis, haemorrhage, fits etc.) is likely and it is usual to arrange for cannulation or formation of a fistula before this.

PREVENTION OF THE PROGRESSION OF CHRONIC RENAL DISEASE (C.R.D.)

This hinges on specific treatment of the underlying renal disease and on correction of factors which accelerate the deterioration in renal function.

1. Glomerulonephritis

There is no conclusive evidence from controlled trials that either steroids or immunosuppressive therapy alter the percentage of patients with glomerulonephritis in whom progression of renal disease occurs. Nevertheless, many units are prepared to try these agents in any patient with progressive glomerulonephritis. Recent reports suggest that indomethacin may suppress the inflammatory lesions in the glomeruli. It has also been claimed that heparin and dipyridamol may affect the renal arterial and capillary sclerosis seen in various forms of progressive renal disease. These agents await evaluation by controlled trials.

2. Renal infection (see also Management of U.T.I.).

In any type of renal disease, infections may result in a permanent decrement in renal function. Therefore bacteriological investigations and prompt therapy are important.

3. Urinary tract obstruction

It is rarely possible to disentangle the relative importance of obstruction and infection in the pathogenesis of renal damage. However, the importance of detecting and evaluating urinary tract obstruction must be fully realised, although its surgical correction is beyond the scope of this chapter.

4. Nephrotoxins

Recent awareness of the nephropathy associated with the consumption of large quantities of analgesics (often attributed particularly to phenacetin) means that it is now incumbent on the physician to take the appropriate history. This applies also to possible exposure to other nephrotoxins, e.g. heavy metals such as lead and cadmium.

5. Fluid and electrolyte abnormalities

The importance of adequate hydration and electrolyte balance in patients with C.R.F. has already been considered. Hypercalcaemia is a serious hazard and a correctable cause must be sought. Potassium deficiency also impairs renal function and must be corrected.

6. Hypertension

The need for an aggressive approach to anti-hypertensive therapy in patients with renal failure has become more widely recognised in the last few years. Previously it was generally believed that lowering the blood pressure in patients with advanced renal failure did little to prolong life and might even hasten death by further reducing the glomerular filtration rate (GFR). It is certainly desirable to avoid too precipitate a fall in blood pressure initially, but control of hypertension, particularly when in the malignant phase, is essential for the conservation of remaining renal function. Patients with essential hypertension in a malignant phase often present with poor renal function and may undergo periods of accelerated deterioration with very severe hypertension, florid retinopathy and rapid fall in renal function. In some patients in this group worthwhile improvement in renal function may follow control of the hypertension, and dialysis should be given when needed to allow time for healing of the arteriolar lesions. This policy should also be adopted for several weeks at least even when malignant hypertension complicates a primary renal disease such as proliferative glomerulonephritis.

There is no evidence that uraemic patients are especially prone to the side effects of any of the common antihypertensive drugs. Alpha-methyl dopa is a suitable drug for many patients, the required dose being judged by the blood pressure response as in non-uraemic patients. Hydralazine, guanethidine, debrisoquine or bethanidine may be used if control cannot be obtained with alpha-methyl-dopa.

Experience with regular haemodialysis has shown the vital importance of sodium and water in the control of hypertension. Most patients on regular dialysis become normotensive without drugs when sufficient salt and water have been removed from the body. This may eventually entail loss of up to 25 per cent of the weight at the start of dialysis.

When peritoneal dialysis is being used to control uraemia, while hypertension is treated, the removal of fluid and reduction in weight are an important part of antihypertensive therapy, and may rapidly lessen the need for drugs. During this phase a negative sodium balance is essential and hypernatraemia must be avoided. A dialysis solution containing 130 mEq Na/L is suitable for this purpose (available commercial solutions contain 141 mEq Na/L necessitating the addition of 80 ml sterile water or 5 per cent dextrose per litre). This solution is also more appropriate for patients with hyponatremia.

The recognition of the vital importance of sodium balance in control of hypertension also has important implications for the antihypertensive treatment of patients whose renal function is poor but adequate to avoid the need for dialysis. If good control of the blood pressure can be achieved with drugs such patients, when free of oedema, are probably best maintained in sodium balance by selecting a dietary sodium level to match their measured average daily sodium losses. An optimum weight is found for each patient at which the blood pressure is controlled. If blood pressure control cannot be achieved then negative sodium balance may be produced slowly while renal function and body-weight are followed carefully. Frusemide is a useful diuretic to achieve this, often being effective at low levels of renal function although large doses (500 mg or more) may be needed.

ANTIBIOTICS IN PATIENTS WITH RENAL FAILURE

The doses of antibiotics must be modified when they are prescribed for a patient with renal failure. Modification depends on the relationship of blood levels to renal function and on the levels at which toxic effects may occur.

General principles

The recommended dose schedule for commonly available drugs is shown in Table 1. This table should be used when blood level estimations of antibiotics are not available, but these are desirable wherever possible as considerable individual variation is encountered at all levels of renal function.

Fear of potential toxicity (Table 2) should not inhibit the choice of the best available antibiotic. Microscopic examination of infected material, bacteriological identification and *in vitro* sensitivity patterns should be used in making this choice.

It is always safe to give the usual loading dose of the antibiotic which is indicated. After this, if the antibiotic is one excreted through the kidney, the maintenance doses must be given less frequently to patients with renal failure than they would be to patients with normal renal function. The frequency of the maintenance dose depends, firstly, upon the proportion of the drugs usually removed from the blood by renal excretion, and, secondly, upon the degree of functional impairment in the individual patient. Antibiotics which are largely excreted by the kidney (e.g. streptomycin, tetracycline) have a prolonged half life in the serum of patients with renal failure and must therefore be administered less often. On the other hand, antibiotics which are excreted by extrarenal routes (e.g. chloramphenicol, erythromycin) can be given in normal doses even in the presence of severe renal failure.

If the patient is anuric or oliguric, has a glomerular filtration rate of less than 10 ml/min., or a serum creatinine concentration of more than 8 mg/100 ml the full modification of the dosage should be applied. If the serum creatinine is more than 3 mg/100 ml but less than 8 mg/100 ml, if the blood urea is raised but the glomerular filtration rate is more than 10 ml/min., or if the patient is in the diuretic phase of recovery from acute tubular necrosis the minor dose modification should be applied. If the glomerular filtration rate is reduced but neither the blood urea nor the serum creatinine is raised the full dose can be given.

Practical points

Combined pencillin and streptomycin. Because the excretion of these two drugs is affected unequally by renal failure, it is a dangerous combination to prescribe for any patient who may have renal disease.

Tetracycline. This antibiotic affects protein synthesis and in renal failure may cause a further elevation of the blood urea. Nausea, diarrhoea and vomiting may be particularly troublesome complications of tetracycline therapy. Chelates are formed with calcium and tetany may be precipitated. Care must therefore be taken to modify the dose of tetracycline in patients with renal failure. It is preferable to use an alternative drug.

Urinary infections in the presence of renal impairment. It is important to treat any infection of the urinary tract which may be causing further renal damage in a patient who already has renal failure. Unfortunately, nitrofurantoin and nalidixic acid take several days to achieve therapeutic concentrations in the urine of patients with renal failure. With high blood levels of nitrofurantoin peripheral neuropathy may occur and this drug is therefore contraindicated in this situation. Chloramphenicol is rapidly metabolised by extrarenal routes and does not reach the urine in therapeutic concentration in renal failure. Inactive metabolites accumulate in renal failure and may be responsible for the serious toxic effects of chloramphenicol. Ampicillin and cephaloridine reach the urine in good concentration even in the face of renal failure and are useful drugs for this problem. Unfortunately the cephalosporins have been associated with renal damage. This appears to be especially likely to occur if large doses are given to a patient with renal disease and if a diuretic is given at the same time. If any of the group I or group II drugs (Table 1) is chosen the dose must be modified according to the rules, and, because of the delay in renal excretion of the drug, the time taken to achieve satisfactory urinary concentrations will be longer than usual. The excretion rate of sulphadimidine is independent of glomerular filtration rate and in renal failure adequate urinary concentrations are achieved. Sulphonamides may prove especially effective when combined with trimethoprim.

Septicaemia with gram negative organisms. Ampicillin is often the first choice in these infections. Gentamicin and colistin in modified dosage can also be used especially if blood level estimations are available. If they are indicated potentially nephrotoxic drugs (e.g. kanamycin, polymyxin B) should not be withheld. Carbenicillin is useful against pseudomonas infections and lacks toxicity. Trimethoprim in combination with a sulphonamide adds a further weapon against these infections.

Tuberculosis. The treatment of tuberculosis in uraemic patients requires an appropriate reduction in the frequency of streptomycin injections but isoniazid can be given in full dosage. It is probably wise to add

Table 1 Recommended Dose of Antibiotics

		Renal Failure (a) Severe*	(b) Moderate†
Group I			
Marked reduction in dose	Streptomycin Tetracycline Polymyxin B Vancomycin Kanamycin	L.D. followed by M.D. every 3–4 days	L.D. followed by M.D. every 1–2 days
	Gentamicin Colistin Nitrofurantoin	M.D. 48 hourly	M.D. 24 hourly
Group II		L.D. followed by	L.D. followed by
Moderate reduction in dose	Carbenicillin	M.D. 8 hourly	
	Penicillin G	M.D. 8 hourly	M.D. 6 hourly
	Cephaloridine	M.D. 24 hourly	M.D. 12 hourly
	Cephalexin	M.D. 24 hourly	M.D. 12 hourly
	Trimethoprim	M.D. 24 hourly	M.D. 12 hourly
Group III			
No reduction in dose	Chloramphenicol Erythromycin Cloxacillin Sulphadimidine Isoniazid Fucidic Acid Cephalothin Rifampicin	as for normal renal function	as for normal renal function

L.D. = Loading Dose as for non-uraemic patients.
M.D. = Maintenance Dose (usually half the L.D.)

* (a) Oliguria; GFR < 10 ml/min; plasma creatinine > 8 mg/100 ml.
† (b) Plasma creatinine 3–8 mg/100 ml. Recovery phase of Acute Renal Failure.

pyridoxine to make the development of neuropathy less likely. No information is available concerning the use of thiacetazone in renal failure. Para-amino-salicylic acid (P.A.S.) appears to be excreted solely

Table 2 Antibiotics: Toxicity, Protein binding and Dialysance

	Potential Toxicity in Renal Failure	Protein Binding (per cent)	Dialysed
Group I			
Streptomycin	VIIIth nerve damage	34	+
Tetracycline	raised blood urea, tetany, D & V, nausea	25–75	±
Polymyxin B	Nephrotoxic	low	?
Kanamycin	Nephrotoxic, deafness	low	?
Colistin	Nephrotoxic, neuropathy	low	+
Nitrofurantoin	Peripheral neuropathy	25	?
Gentamicin	VIIIth nerve damage	25	+
Group II			
Carbenicillin	None reported	?	+
Penicillin G	Convulsions with v. high levels	50	±
Cephaloridine	? Nephrotoxic	Negligible	+++
Cephalexin	None established		
Trimethoprim	None reported	31	?
Group III			
Chloramphenicol	None peculiar to uraemia, but dangerous in neonate and jaundiced patients	25	+
Erythromycin	None reported	18	?
Cloxacillin	None reported	95	0
Ampicillin	Skin rashes common	22	±
Sulphadimidine	None reported	55	+
Isoniazid	None reported	?	+
Fucidic Acid	Nausea and vomiting		
Cephalothin	None reported		
Rifampicin	None reported		

by the kidney and its use in renal failure requires blood level estimations.

Antibiotics and dialysis. When patients are being treated by dialysis the dose of any antibiotic prescribed will require modification from the schedule given in Table 1 if it is removed appreciably by dialysis. The dialysance of drugs depends on their protein binding and other factors such as molecular size affecting transfer across the peritoneal membrane and the cellophane membranes of artificial kidneys (Table 2). For example, cephaloridine is only negligibly bound to serum proteins and is removed rapidly by dialysis; vancomycin which is a large molecule and is not removed by dialysis, persists in safe and therapeutic serum levels for 9–14 days after only a single injection of 1 g. in an oliguric or anuric patient.

THE MANAGEMENT OF URINARY TRACT INFECTIONS (U.T.I.)

Significant bacterial colonisation of the urine can only be diagnosed by quantitative cultures of a midstream specimen of urine (M.S.U.) or by culture of urine obtained by suprapubic aspiration.

Urine culture is required not only for the diagnosis of U.T.I., but also for confirmation of cure and during the follow up of the patient.

Acute lower U.T.I.

While awaiting bacteriological identification and sensitivity reports, treatment should be commenced by encouraging the patient to take a high fluid intake and by prescribing the antibiotic most likely to be appropriate.

The majority of domiciliary infections are due to E. Coli or P. mirabilis sensitive to most antibiotics. A week's course of sulphonamide results in a sterile urine in 80–90 per cent of these patients. If it fails to do so, the choice of a different antibiotic should be guided by sensitivity tests, but usually lies between ampicillin, nitrofurantoin, trimethoprim-sulphamethoxazole or tetracycline.

Infections arising in hospital are due to a wider range of organisms some of which may be resistant to many antibiotics. If symptoms necessitate treatment before the results of sensitivity testing are known, trimethoprim-sulphamethoxazole or ampicillin should be given

Alkalinisation of the urine enhances the effect of sulphonamides, penicillin, streptomycin, erythromycin, kanamycin and gentamycin. Potassium citrate introduces the danger of hyperkalaemia in a patient whose renal function is not known and, therefore, if the level of renal function is in doubt, sodium bicarbonate or sodium citrate should be used. The urine can be rendered acid by ammonium chloride or methionine. Acidification enhances the effect of tetracycline and cycloserine and is essential for the activity of the urinary antiseptic mandelamine. Ampicillin and nitrofurantoin are unaffected by urinary pH.

Asymptomatic bacteriuria

This is found in 5 per cent of women at their first attendances at antenatal clinics. In this group antibiotic treatment reduces the incidence of acute pyelonephritis which is otherwise high (25–40 per cent). Asymptomatic bacteriuria occurs in about 1 per cent of apparently healthy schoolgirls, but the prognostic implications of this are not yet established.

Acute pyelonephritis

If there are clinical reasons for considering that the infection involves the kidneys, the antibiotic used should be one which achieves good concentrations in the blood and tissues as well as in the urine. It is advised that treatment should be continued for two weeks after the urine is rendered sterile.

In domiciliary practice, where most of these infections are encountered, initial treatment with either ampicillin (which may be given intramuscularly) or trimethoprim-sulphamethoxazole is recommended.

The resistant organisms encountered in hospital frequently dictate a choice between parenteral gentamycin, kanamycin and colistin. If treatment must be started before sensitivities are available, gentamycin is probably the best choice because of its activity against P. aeruginosa. In patients with renal damage the dose of gentamycin and colistin must be adjusted to the level of renal failure, and it is advisable to monitor blood levels when possible. Carbenicillin is useful against infections with P. aeruginosa, but may need to be given in very high dosage (30–40 g. per day) if renal function is good. A synergistic action with gentamycin has been described.

Recurrent U.T.I.

In patients who have had an attack of acute pyelonephritis relapse (same organism) and reinfection (new organism) are common. Bacteriuria recurs within six months in 50 per cent of patients. Therefore, management should ideally continue with repeat of the urine culture at monthly intervals for six months. In this way it is hoped to detect bacteriuric recurrences and to treat them before they become symptomatic. If there is difficulty in achieving bacteriological cure despite the isolation of an apparently sensitive organism, or if a patient has recurrent U.T.I. it suggests that there is renal involvement. Such patients should be investigated in order to detect any structural abnormality or other factors affecting host resistance.

Relapses suggest a focus of infection in the urinary tract and there may be a surgically correctable structural abnormality. High dose antibiotic therapy is usually given. There is a difference of opinion as to whether this should be given for two or six weeks.

Reinfections can be managed by treating each recurrence, bacteriuric or symptomatic. In some cases it may prove most convenient to give the patient a week's supply of the antibiotic to be commenced as soon as symptoms recur. Alternatively, attempts may be made to keep the urine sterile by using long term prophylaxis with either single or rotating antibiotics. Long term low dose therapy (e.g. nitrofurantoin 100 mg each night) has been useful. Trimethoprim-sulphamethoxazole appears to be valuable for long term prophylaxis. In patients in whom a history relating recurrences to sexual intercourse is volunteered the prophylactic regime should be arranged accordingly.

SYSTEMIC DISEASES WHICH INVOLVE THE KIDNEY

This section will consider only therapy specific to the systemic disease concerned. The treatment of renal failure and the use of diuretics for oedema of renal origin in these diseases follow the principles already covered in previous sections unless stated otherwise.

Systemic Lupus Erythematosus (SLE)

Specific treatment for SLE with renal involvement consists of careful avoidance of precipitating factors (e.g. sunlight and some drugs) and the use of steroids or immunosuppressive agents. Although there have been no fully controlled trials there is much evidence that steroids are beneficial in some forms of this disease. A renal biopsy provides a guide to therapy although renal function and the urinary sediment must also be considered.

If the renal biopsy is normal or shows only minor focal proliferative changes in some glomeruli without tubular or interstitial abnormalities ('lupus glomerulitis') the choice lies between no therapy and steroids in moderate doses, e.g. prednisone 10–20 mg/day. When making this decision on purely renal grounds the GFR, the extent of proteinuria, abnormalities in the urinary sediment and any trend for better or worse in these features should all be considered. There is no evidence that the risks of prolonged high dose steroid therapy are warranted for this lesion, but the patient must be kept under review.

The renal biopsy may show uniform thickening of the basement membrane affecting all glomeruli with little or no evidence of cellular proliferation. This membranous lesion appears to have a slowly progressive course but there is no evidence yet that steroid therapy retards its progress. Nephrotic syndrome may complicate this lesion and it is reasonable then to undertake a trial of steroids in high dosage (prednisone 1 mg/kg/day) for 3 or 4 weeks, thereafter reducing to a smaller dose.

The most severe lesion which biopsy may reveal is termed "active lupus glomerulonephritis". Cellular proliferation in the glomeruli is prominent and focal areas of basement membrane thickening are often present. Local necrosis may be seen in some glomeruli together with haematoxyphil bodies, wire loop lesions and crescents. This appearance carries a bad prognosis, particularly if the blood urea is already elevated, and steroids should be given in high doses for 4 to 6 months or longer.

There are reports of improvement in renal lupus following the use of nitrogen mustard, 6-mercaptopurine, azathioprine cyclophosphamide and indomethacin, but the place of these drugs in therapy is not yet established.

Polyarteritis Nodosa (PAN)

A trial of steroids in high dosage (prednisone 45–60 mg/day or more) is justified in any case of PAN with evidence of renal involvement. If hypertension or renal failure are present the chances of improvement with steroids are slender, but there is little to be lost and an occasional patient responds even when acute renal failure has developed.

There have been claims of good results with azathioprine but controlled trials have not been reported.

When acute oliguric renal failure develops the outlook is very poor, but recovery of useful renal function may sometimes occur if life is preserved by dialysis for a period of a few weeks to give time for a trial of high dose steroid therapy.

Systemic Sclerosis

The kidney complications of this disease rarely dominate the clinical picture until renal failure develops. This may develop acutely or insidiously. There is no evidence that steroids are beneficial and some evidence that they may accelerate the renal failure. When proteinuria alone indicates renal involvement there is again little evidence that steroids are helpful and it seems reasonable on the information available not to use them. The effect of immunosuppressive therapy in this disease is unknown. Claims for other therapeutic agents, such as vasodilator drugs and chelating agents, have not been substantiated.

Haemolytic-Uraemic Syndromes

This includes a number of diseases probably with different aetiologies, but having in common a microangiopathy with occlusive lesions in small blood vessels, disseminated intravascular clotting, thrombocytopenia, haemolytic anaemia and frequently renal failure. This syndrome developed most frequently in two age groups: in children, where it is often preceded by a gastrointestinal disturbance; in young adults, where it is usually called Thrombotic Thrombocytopaenic Purpura (Moschowitz's Syndrome). A similar blood picture may complicate malignant hypertension, usually with renal failure, but such cases are distinguished by the sequence of events.

Steroids are usually given in large doses, but their usefulness is difficult to assess at present: in many reported cases they do not appear to have influenced the course of the disease, and one report concluded that they might be harmful. Anticoagulant therapy, usually with heparin, has been given with encouraging results. Dialysis has been used to control uraemia and subsequent improvement has been reported, although the mortality remains high when the disease is so severe. It seems reasonable at present to treat patients with this condition with heparin and dialysis as necessary. When this syndrome complicates malignant hypertension urgent antihypertensive therapy is imperative.

Henoch-Schönlein Purpura (Anaphylactoid Purpura)

Steroids do not affect the renal lesions of this condition but may be useful in management of the extrarenal lesions. Promising reports of the use of azathioprine or cyclophosphamide have appeared, but full evaluation of these drugs is not yet possible.

Goodpasture's Syndrome (Lung Purpura with Nephritis)
Steroids in large doses, e.g. prednisone 60–80 mg/day, should be given. If needed early in the cause of this illness dialysis should be performed to control uraemia as prolonged remissions can occur.

Diabetes
Proteinuria sometimes progressing to a nephrotic syndrome, chronic renal failure and urinary tract infection are the renal hazards of diabetes. It is not established that inadequate control of diabetes increases the incidence of these complications, but when they are present it seems prudent to pay careful attention to anti-diabetic therapy. In this context it should be realised that in patients with renal failure the degree of glycosuria may be a misleading guide to diabetic control. In advanced renal failure the insulin requirements may decrease.

The indications for restriction of salt, water and protein are similar to those in other renal diseases. When a nephrotic syndrome develops early in the course of diabetes a renal biopsy is indicated at least in children, in view of the report that in these circumstances, the biopsy may show only minimal abnormalities in the glomeruli and that steroids may then induce remission. Many diuretics impair carbohydrate tolerance and for the diabetic patient with oedema but without serious renal failure ethacrynic acid is the diuretic of choice as it does not have this side effect.

Urinary tract infection must be treated vigorously. Bladder catheterisation should be avoided whenever possible, particularly in diabetic coma, the management of which should be regulated by blood sugar determinations.

Hypophysectomy and adrenalectomy are not yet established in the management of diabetic nephropathy despite claims of improvement after these operations.

Gout
The treatment of acute attacks of both primary and secondary gout need not be modified by the presence of renal impairment. For long term treatment allopurinol (300–800 mg/day) is the drug of choice and avoids the risks of increased renal urate deposition and uric acid calculus formation carried by uricosuric drugs. The effective dosage of

allopurinol does not appear to be affected by renal failure and can be regulated by its effect on plasma urate levels as in non-uraemic patients.

Allopurinol increases the urinary excretion of xanthine but there is to date, no evidence that this is harmful.

Myelomatosis

A high fluid intake is advised as dehydration may accelerate cast formation within the renal tubules leading to intrarenal obstruction. Claims that intravenous pyelography may precipitate acute renal failure have been disputed, but certainly fluid restriction should be avoided prior to this investigation.

Hypercalcaemia should be treated urgently with steroids, and hyperuricaemia with allopurinol.

The development of acute renal failure is usually fatal, but where the patient's condition is otherwise acceptable and a precipitating cause for the renal failure can be defined (e.g. dehydration or hypercalcaemia) it is reasonable to perform dialysis as recovery from the renal failure in such circumstances has been recorded.

Amyloidosis

There is no specific therapy. In 'secondary' amyloidosis the finding of renal involvement makes radical treatment of the underlying disease imperative where this is possible. The use of steroids, e.g. in rheumatoid arthritis, poses a special problem in view of the evidence that steroids may increase amyloid formation. This latter contention is not proven and it is probably reasonable to continue steroid therapy if this is warranted on other grounds.

When renal amyloidosis is found without predisposing disease it is important to search for evidence of myeloma. Even when the latter diagnosis cannot be made analysis of plasma and urine proteins may disclose a monoclonal immunoglobulin proteinaemia. Treatment with melphalan can remove the evidence of dysproteinaemia in such patients but it is not known whether the further formation of amyloid is reduced by this treatment.

RENAL CALCULI

A high fluid intake is advisable for all patients with renal calculi. As the calcium content of tap water may be considerable (e.g. 6–12 mg/100 ml) this factor must be considered in patients with hypercalciuria, but it is generally believed that the benefits bestowed on stone-formers by urinary dilution outweigh this possible disadvantage.

Ureteric colic is treated with analgesics such as pethidine and the progress of the stone is monitored radiologically so that complete ureteric obstruction may be recognised and the stone removed surgically. Hippuran renography may also be used to detect ureteric obstruction.

Specific therapy depends on any demonstrable metabolic defect underlying stone formation.

Hypercalciuria

If hypercalciuria is due to hypercalcaemia the cause of the latter must be sought, paying particular attention to the diagnosis of hyperparathyroidism.

Hypercalciuria without hypercalcaemia may be part of a syndrome of renal tubular dysfunction needing treatment in its own right, e.g. renal tubular acidosis, when treatment with alkalis, sodium and potassium salts may be indicated.

Usually however hypercalciuria is an isolated finding in patients with renal calculi. Present day treatment is concentrated on dietary factors in this abnormality. Measures which lower urinary calcium excretion include (a) a low calcium diet, involving the use of softened water for cooking and drinking and often causing considerable domestic upheaval; (b) agents which reduce dietary calcium absorption, e.g. cellulose phosphate (15 g./day) or sodium phytate (6 g./day); (c) alkali therapy (sodium bicarbonate 8–10 g./day) when the urine is persistently acid; (d) a thiazide diuretic (e.g. bendrofluazide 5–10 mg/day) which decreases urinary calcium excretion without reducing calcium absorption from the gut or causing negative calcium balance.

Controlled observations on the long term effect of these measures on stone formation are lacking, although there are favourable short term reports particularly for the use of bendrofluazide.

Uric acid stones

These usually occur in a persistently acid urine and adequate alkali therapy is often successful at preventing their recurrence. Allopurinol is indicated for patients with increased urinary urate excretion or hyperuricaemia. It may be of particular value in preventing the complications of hyperuricaemia occurring in patients with leukaemias and reticuloses when urate excretion may be very high, especially during treatment with cytotoxic drugs or radiotherapy.

Cystine stones

Maintenance of urinary alkalinity (e.g. with sodium bicarbonate 10 g./day or more) and avoidance of urinary concentration are often successful in preventing stone formation in patients with cystinuria. However, this treatment involves attaining a urine output of at least 3 litres/day with the necessary production of large volumes of dilute urine at night. D-penicillamine forms a soluble complex with cystine, is effective at preventing stone formation and may even achieve the dissolution of existing stones. However, this treatment is expensive and potentially hazardous. It is best reserved for those patients not responding to the more simple measures given above.

PERITONEAL DIALYSIS

Requirements

Although peritoneal dialysis can be carried out in the general ward, the space and staff required makes the procedure more appropriately done in an intensive care ward or area. Modern sterile disposable peritoneal catheters with metal stylet and giving sets are usefully combined with a sterile disposable plastic bag for collection of effluent. The whole system then remains closed except for the moment when fresh bags (or bottles) of the dialysis solution are put up. Two solutions are required, one approximately isotonic and the other hypertonic, so that the rate of fluid removal can be controlled. It is usual to warm the solution to body temperature. Since tap water is likely to contain organisms it is preferable to warm the bags without wetting them; warming pads or a small incubator may be used. A chart is needed on which to plot hourly temperature, pulse, respirations and blood pressure recordings. Records must also be kept of the volumes of fluid run in and run out and of any additions to this fluid. It is customary to add heparin (500 units per litre) and potassium (4 mEq/L) after correction of hyperkalaemia. It is also useful to record the time taken to run the fluid in and out since this is a measure of the efficiency of the system.

Method

The bladder is emptied and the anterior abdominal wall prepared as for surgery. Using full asepsis the catheter is inserted under local anaesthesia through a small scalpel incision at a point one third of the distance from the umbilicus to the symphysis pubis in the midline. Other sites over the lower abdomen may also be used. If the patient can either tense or blow forward the anterior abdominal wall it improves the confidence of the operator. If not, some will advise running in two litres of fluid through a needle before inserting the catheter. This takes time. As soon as the catheter is definitely inside the peritoneum the stylet is withdrawn and the catheter is then passed down into the pelvis as far as it will comfortably go, avoiding pushing too hard because this may kink the catheter. The catheter is supplied with marks so that the direction of its curve is known. If more than 5 cm protrudes as in a small patient it may be convenient to cut this off before fitting the giving set. Only occasionally with the modern catheter is a purse string suture needed to retain the catheter and prevent leakage. In some units a gauze dressing with adhesive strapping is applied, and redressed after antiseptic washing once a day. Others suggest open techniques with frequent application of antiseptic lotion or antibiotic creams.

Most adults will be comfortable with two litre exchanges of dialysis fluid, but if this causes discomfort one litre exchanges should be used. The rate of exchange must then be doubled since the clearance achieved is related to the volume of dialysis fluid used per hour. The first three exchanges should be carried out as fast as the system will permit so as to flush out fibrin from the catheter and minimise the chances of an early blockage. The drainage period should be limited to a maximum of 40 minutes (20 minutes for one litre exchange) since it is usual for the volume of fluid to run out, to be less than that run in during the early stages. The inexperienced are worried by this if they have not been warned to expect it, and dialysis becomes less and less efficient as each exchange becomes more and more prolonged. It should be pointed out that to build up a residual volume so that dialysis is continual rather than intermittent is an advantage. With later exchanges, and as hypertonic solution is used, a negative fluid balance is readily achieved. When it is established that the system is working well, it is convenient to organise an hourly or half-hourly routine for the exchanges. The time taken for the fluid to run in and out then dictates the 'dwell' time when the exchange is left in the peritoneum.

The amount of dialysis required depends on the degree of uraemia when dialysis is begun and on the rate of catabolism. It is usual to commence with a 36 to 48 hour period. The catabolic patient with A.R.F.

will need continuous dialysis; stable patients with terminal renal failure have been managed for long periods of time on as little as 36 to 48 hours per week.

The dialysis effluent should be monitored for infection by daily cultures and microscopy for pus cells. Protein losses can exceed 100 g. per day and plasma may be needed to restore blood volume if the blood pressure falls. Routine physiotherapy should be instituted because pulmonary complications are common.

Bibliography

The reader is referred to the following text-books for general reading and further references.

1. *Diseases of the Kidney* (Ed. M. B. Strauss and L. G. Welt) (1963), London, Churchill.
2. *Renal Disease* (Ed. D. A. K. Black) (1967), Oxford, Blackwell, 2nd edition.
3. Wardener, H. E. de, *The Kidney* (1967), London, Churchill, 3rd edition.
4. Kerr, D. N. S., and Douglas, A. P., *A Short Text-book of Kidney Disease* (1968), London, Pitman.

This chapter was written by Dr N. F. Jones (Consultant Physician, St Thomas's Hospital) and Dr A. J. Wing (Consultant Physician, St Thomas's Hospital) and was edited by Professor W. I. Cranston.

Category 3
The Locomotor System

Introduction

Some of the methods of treatment useful in acute and chronic diseases of joints are non-specific, and are helpful as supportive treatment in a wide range of conditions. To avoid unnecessary repetition these methods will be described in more detail for the commonest inflammatory joint disease – rheumatoid arthritis, and for the commonest degenerative joint disease – osteoarthrosis. Where a disease has a specific method of treatment, it is usually used in conjunction with supportive measures.

INFLAMMATORY JOINT DISEASE

IDIOPATHIC

Rheumatoid arthritis

The cause of rheumatoid arthritis is not known. The disease has a familial incidence, is commoner in women, may be precipitated by many factors, and seems to be prolonged by an autoimmune process. Rheumatoid disease is a systemic disorder but in most patients synovitis dominates the clinical picture and leads to the features of arthritis – hot, swollen, painful, stiff joints. In children the systemic features often dominate with fever and weight loss, but this happens less often in adults. The local inflammation may affect any synovial joint, bursa, or tendon sheath in the body, and if sufficiently severe or prolonged may produce secondary mechanical changes such as joint instability and subluxation, or tendon rupture. The synovitis may affect one joint (monarticular) or many joints (polyarticular), and the onset may be gradual or sudden. It is impossible to predict accurately the course of the disease, but the following features are associated with a good prognosis: sudden onset; duration under one year; male sex; the absence of rheumatoid serum factor (Rose-Waaler and latex tests) or nodules. The diagnosis is suggested by the early appearance of radiological erosions, and confirmed by finding rheumatoid factor and nodules.

Treatment of rheumatoid arthritis may be directed at the inflammatory disease, whether systemic or local, or at the mechanical features, or both if appropriate.

Treatment

Early rheumatoid arthritis

It is often not possible to confirm the diagnosis as rheumatoid factor tests may be negative and nodules absent, and treatment must remain non-specific. In view of the widespread belief amongst the majority of patients that this disease is always progressive and is incurable, it is valuable to try to gain the confidence of the patient by explaining some relevant facts. In particular it should be stressed that the disease is crippling in only a minority, and that much can be done to help at all stages.

Rest. If the patient is systemically ill it is a great advantage to start treatment with a period of 2–3 weeks total bedrest. Whilst in bed the patient should have a good back support, a firm mattress, and a bed cradle. No special dietary, vitamin, or hormone supplements are of any value, but night sedatives should be given when necessary. If inflamed joints are painful at rest, they should be splinted in the position of optimum function. Splints may be made of plaster of paris or padded malleable wire, and are often needed for wrists and knees. The normal right-angle position of the ankle can be maintained with a board. Static muscle exercises should be given by a physiotherapist, and it may be an advantage to remove splints and move joints passively through their full range once or twice daily. Two spells each day lying prone help to prevent flexion contractures of the hips and knees. As the activity of the disease subsides, the patient should be encouraged to undertake more activity, and be gradually mobilised.

Local steroid injections. If only a small number of joints is affected they may be aspirated and hydrocortisone acetate injected, 0·5–2 ml (12·5–50 mg) according to the size of the joint. Occasionally hydrocortisone acetate produces a flare in the joint, probably an example of crystal synovitis. This may be avoided by using prednisolone trimethyl acetate (Ultracortenol) or methylprednisolone acetate (Depo-Medrone), and these may have a longer action. Steroids must not be injected if there is a possibility of joint infection.

Salicylates. Soluble aspirin is the drug of first choice but may cause indigestion or gastric ulceration and bleeding. A dose of up to 4 g. daily is given in divided doses. An enteric coated preparation may avoid gastric side effects.

Butazones. Phenylbutazone may be substituted for aspirin, or be added to it if extra effect is needed. As marrow suppression occasionally occurs, a preliminary blood count is essential to avoid confusion between blood dyscrasias caused by the disease and those due to treatment. Peptic and oral ulceration, fluid retention, and skin sensitivity, are other hazards. Phenylbutazone is usually taken orally, 100 mg t.d.s., but may be given as a suppository of 250 mg at night to relieve morning stiffness. Care must be taken not to exceed a total daily dose of 300 mg. An antacid coated preparation is also available for patients in whom indigestion is produced.

Oxyphenbutazone is an alternative preparation with similar indications, side effects and doses. However the same side effect is not always produced by the two preparations in the same patient, and it may be worth changing to avoid a minor complication.

Indomethacin. This is an alternative to butazones and carries no established risk of haematological side effects. However gastric ulceration and cerebral side effects (headache or muzziness) can occur by whichever route it is given. The usual oral starting dose is caps. indomethacin 25 mg t.d.s., and this may be increased to 50 mg t.d.s. A night time suppository of 100 mg is useful in combating morning stiffness, but care must be taken to avoid exceeding a total daily dose of 150 mg for long-term administration.

Fenamates. These drugs are useful alternatives which avoid both gastric and haematological side effects, but they sometimes cause severe diarrhoea. Caps. mefenamic acid 250 mg t.d.s., or caps. flufenamic acid 100 mg t.d.s. are prescribed.

Paracetamol is a mild analgesic which may also be useful for mild rheumatoid arthritis – dose 1 g. t.d.s. Morphine and its derivatives and mixtures containing phenacetin are not safe for long-term administration.

Continuing disease activity

If the disease activity continues the diagnosis is usually confirmed by the appearance of rheumatoid nodules or positive rheumatoid factor tests. When the diagnosis is certain, there is clinical or radiological evidence of disease progression (appearance of cortical bone erosions), the disease has failed to settle in one year, and the majority of symptoms are due to disease activity and not mechanical deformity, anti-rheumatoid therapy is indicated.

Sodium aurothiomalate (Myocrisin). The main toxic effects of gold salts are dermatitis, marrow suppression, and renal damage; therefore skin allergy, blood dyscrasias, and albuminuria are contraindications to their use. Treatment must be preceded by a blood count and each injection by an enquiry into skin symptoms (notably itching), and a urine test for albumin. Other marrow suppressant drugs (commonly phenylbutazone) must be stopped, and monthly blood counts arranged. Myocrisin is given by intra-muscular injection, test doses of 10 and 20 mg on separate days, then 50 mg weekly until a full course of 500 mg has been achieved. If remission has occurred, it may be worth continuing with 50 mg monthly until 1 gram has been given. Beneficial effects are not usually felt for two months.

Antimalarials. These also act slowly, and the recognition of irreversible retinitis has lead to decreased use. Rashes, bleaching of hair, corneal deposition, and exacerbation of psoriasis may occur. However, with expert ophthalmic supervision their use may occasionally be justified. Tabs. chloroquine phosphate 250 mg or hydroxychloroquine 200 mg are given once or twice daily for up to one year.

Steroids. These have a small but definite place in treatment. Extreme caution is needed in the use of steroids to suppress chronic diseases, as once started the drug can seldom be stopped. The aim should be not to exceed a dose which can be tolerated long term. Prednisone or prednisolone are used, are of identical potency, and are indicated in the following circumstances: 1. Severely active early disease if not controlled by the simpler measures described, may be partially suppressed by up to 10 mg of prednisone daily. It is better policy to start with a small dose of steroid and gradually increase it to the minimum needed, than to start with a large daily dose and attempt to reduce it to an acceptable level. The disease cannot be 'stamped-out' by large doses of steroids, and if a high dose is used early it is seldom possible to reduce it to a satisfactorily low dose. 2. Crippling early morning stiffness may occur in the absence of obvious disease activity. This stiffness is sometimes dramatically relieved by giving 5 mg prednisone at night (but it is worth trying the phenylbutazone or indomethacin suppositories first). This steroid dose is seldom the cause of major side effects. 3. Between these two extremes is the patient with chronic and progressive disease in whom social or economic pressures make it worth 'buying' a small number of years of relative freedom, and running the risk of steroid side effects later. 4. A special case for larger doses of prednisone exists when there are potentially lethal systemic features to the disease, often involving arteritis. Nail-fold vasculitis per se does not demand steroid treatment.

Immunosuppressive drugs. These have been used in rheumatoid arthritis, and azathioprine has been shown to have a steroid-sparing effect [1]. Azathioprine is used in a total daily dose of 2·5 mg per kg body-weight, and should be considered for those patients who are unable to tolerate the dose of steroids they need. Monthly blood counts are needed for control.

Chronic rheumatoid arthritis

A great deal can be done to match the patient and the environment to each other. Both can be modified.

Modification of patient. Weak muscles. These can be strengthened by intensive physiotherapy concentrating on static contraction of muscles to obtain maximum muscular effort with minimum joint stress. Faradic stimulation may help to initiate recovery of a severe and chronic weakness.

Contractures. It is possible for minor but disabling contractures of joint capsules to be corrected by manual stretching. Heat is useful as a preliminary local analgesic and may be applied by wax baths to the hands and feet, or via short wave diathermy or radiant heat to larger joints. More stubborn contractures may need correction by serial plasters, and a manipulation under anaesthetic (often with local steroid injection) is sometimes necessary for slowly responding contractures.

Supports. Stress may be diverted from unstable or painful joints. Polythene wrist splints, knee splints, walking aids, and surgical shoes are frequently of great help.

Surgery. The choice of operation is difficult as the pattern of progressive joint involvement cannot be predicted. Decisions must be taken with an orthopaedic surgeon. Early synovectomy may prevent damage to a diseased joint and is worth while if the disease is confined to a small number of joints. Ruptured tendons should be repaired. Late 'salvage' operations must be carefully chosen as an unsuccessful operation is demoralising. Synovectomy and debridement of a joint is a useful pain relieving procedure. Where joint stability is not essential excision arthroplasty is possible, and is often successful for painful metatarsal heads or a limited elbow. If stability must be maintained a replacement arthroplasty is preferable, and successful operations on hips and knees are currently being performed. Guaranteed lasting freedom from pain and permanent stability is achieved by arthrodesis, but this can seldom be recommended in a polyarthritic disease whose progress is uncertain.

Modification of environment. Despite all treatment this disease sometimes produces severe disability. When this occurs, the help of the occupational therapist, medical social worker, disablement resettlement officer, domiciliary services, local authorities, and voluntary organisations may be needed. The patient's ability to travel can be modified by a wheelchair or motor propelled vehicle, the home adapted to the disability, and work modified or the patient re-trained. Many of these modifications are most effective when initiated early.

Complications. The numerous non-articular features of rheumatoid disease usually need treatment along expectant lines; steroids are frequently not a sinecure and should be reserved for complications that are life-threatening.

Amyloid disease carries a poor prognosis and is not helped by steroids. Local nerve pressure should be surgically relieved, as in the carpal-tunnel syndrome. Septic joints are not rare in rheumatoid patients, especially if on steroids, and must be thought of in a monarticular 'flare'. 'Anaemia of inflammation' is common, and seldom responds to oral or parenteral iron. Iron-deficiency anaemia may be due to salicylate induced gastro-intestinal bleeding, and must be treated by stopping the offending drug and giving iron. The upper cervical spine is commonly affected by the disease with subsequent atlanto-axial subluxation[2]. During preparation for surgery special care must be taken to avoid abnormal or violent neck movements.

Psoriatic arthritis

This condition differs from rheumatoid disease in several important ways. There is seldom severe systemic upset, although an elevated E.S.R., anaemia, and weight loss may accompany the synovitis. The synovitis is usually less proliferative and destructive than that in rheumatoid arthritis, but fibrosis and ankylosis of joints are more common. Clinically the arthritis is often asymmetrical, may affect the terminal interphalangeal joints of the fingers and toes, sometimes affects the sacro-iliac joints and spine to give an atypical spondylitis, and is occasionally very destructive.

Psoriatic arthritis is not associated with rheumatoid nodules or serum factor, and with the rare exception of amyloid, it is not complicated by the many non-articular features of rheumatoid disease. The prognosis for both local joint destruction and systemic illness is therefore better.

TREATMENT

Rest. It is not often necessary to confine these patients to bed as there is seldom systemic illness. The affected joints may benefit from local splints and steroid injections.

Drugs. Those of use are the same as in early rheumatoid arthritis. Phenylbutazone in particular has a reputation for being most effective in psoriatic arthritis. Gold is not recommended for psoriatic arthritis since its effectiveness in this condition has not been demonstrated, and there may be more danger of severe skin reactions. Antimalarials should also be avoided as they too may provoke severe skin reactions. The indications for steroids are similar to those in rheumatoid arthritis but occur less often. Methotrexate has been claimed to be useful in severe combined skin and joint disease, but the danger of marrow suppression precludes its general use.

Surgery. Indications and techniques are similar to those in rheumatoid arthritis.

Reiter's disease

The syndrome of urethritis, conjunctivitis, and arthritis, is precipitated either by the urethritis or by dysentery. The patient is nearly always male and may be ill with fever, high E.S.R., and anaemia. The urethritis may be accompanied by prostatitis and cystitis, and recurrent bouts of iritis occur. Keratodermia blenorrhagica sometimes affects the soles of the feet, and mucous membrane lesions may occur in the mouth and on the glans penis. Occasionally the cardiovascular system is affected with heart block, pericarditis or aortic incompetence.

The locomotor features may involve 'soft tissues'; both plantar fasciitis and Achilles tendinitis are common. The arthritis is often asymmetrical usually affecting the legs. The knees, metatarsophalangeal joints, and the interphalangeal joints of the hallux and other toes are often involved.

Most initial attacks settle in a few months, but recurrence is common, and after several attacks severe foot deformities often remain. Occasionally the sacro-iliac and spinal joints are affected mimicking ankylosing spondylitis.

TREATMENT

The systemic illness is often sufficiently severe to justify admission to hospital. The venereologist should be consulted, and usually a 7 day course of a broad spectrum antibiotic is ordered to treat the urethritis. Where there are eye complications the ophthalmic surgeon should be consulted; chloramphenicol eyedrops are usually recommended to prevent secondary conjunctival infection, and atropine or steroid eyedrops may help the iritis. Skin and mucosal lesions should be treated with simple hygienic measures. No specific treatment is available.

Joints are often very acutely painful and swollen, and are helped by rest, local steroid injections and splints. Supervised static exercises are again valuable for maintaining muscle strength. Surgical footwear is often necessary to support deformed feet.

Drugs. Tabs. phenylbutazone 100 mg t.d.s., tabs, oxyphenbutazone 100 mg q.d.s., caps. indomethacin 25 mg t.d.s. are all probably more effective than salicylates. Systemic steroids may be needed if there is severe systemic disturbance which fails to settle with rest, but often their effect is disappointing.

Surgery. This may be helpful for the crippling foot deformities.

Prophylaxis. Contacts of the patient should be examined and treated as necessary. Exposure to repeated venereal infection may precipitate a relapse of the disease, and should be avoided.

Polymyalgia rheumatica

This syndrome of aching muscles in the elderly is not primarily a muscle disease but probably represents an inflammatory condition of central and proximal joints and bursae. There are many causes of the syndrome, amongst them myeloma, neoplasia, polymyositis and rheumatoid arthritis. Usually no underlying disease is found, and in these idiopathic cases there is a strong association with cranial giant cell arteritis, and occasionally with arteritis of major vessels elsewhere [3]. Thus it is important to make an attempt to uncover any sinister cause of the syndrome before embarking on suppressive treatment.

The idiopathic syndrome is commoner in women and may be diagnosed on the history of severe limb girdle stiffness in an elderly patient, the finding of limited central and proximal joint movement, and a high E.S.R. Unfortunately a very few patients with this syndrome have a normal E.S.R. even in the presence of cranial arteritis. Electromyographic findings and muscle biopsies are normal.

TREATMENT

If symptoms are relatively mild, and the E.S.R. only moderately raised (say up to 50 mm Westergren), phenylbutazone or indomethacin often relieve muscular symptoms. Arteritis will not be adequately suppressed, and it has been suggested that symptomatic improvement may lead to its being overlooked [4]. As cranial arteritis has been found occasionally in patients with no local symptoms or signs and even with a normal E.S.R. [5], a counsel of perfection includes routine temporal artery biopsy. Unfortunately the biopsy may not include a diseased segment of artery.

When the stiffness is 'crippling', or the E.S.R. markedly raised (say above 50 mm) steroids are often needed for control. Immediate steroid suppression is imperative when arteritis is suspected, as untreated involvement of retinal or cerebral arteries may lead to blindness or strokes. The suppressive action of steroids makes it desirable to complete investigations before these drugs are started, and investigations must now include a temporal artery biopsy. Failure to take this biopsy makes it more difficult to advise about long term management. Tabs. prednisone 30 mg daily is started and the dose titrated slowly down to the minimum needed to relieve symptoms and maintain a normal E.S.R. A maintenance dose of prednisone 5–15 mg daily may be needed for 1½–3 years, the natural history of the 'idiopathic' disease. The final steroid reduction is controlled by repeated E.S.R. estimations and observation of symptoms and signs.

An alternative school of opinion maintains that as no amount of investigation can absolutely exclude the possibility of cranial arteritis and its serious consequences, all patients with polymyalgia rheumatica should be treated with steroids. This opinion presupposes that the risk of treating a larger and miscellaneous group of disorders by steroid suppression is less than that of occasionally failing to detect and treat cranial arteritis, a hypothesis which has not been put to the test.

Ankylosing spondylitis

This is an inflammatory disease predominantly of the spine and usually affecting young men. The sacro-iliac joints are affected first, and the process classically ascends the spine. Occasionally the disease starts in a peripheral joint, and atypical forms occur in association with Reiter's disease, psoriasis, and chronic intestinal disorders. Iritis is a common complication; aortitis and amyloid disease are rare. The cervical spine may become rigid and fragile, and may be fatally fractured.

Pathological changes similar to those in rheumatoid disease may be found in synovial joints but usually there is a greater tendency to new bone formation and ankylosis. Vascular fibrous tissue invades intervertebral discs and vertebral bodies leading to calcification and ossification.

The early clinical features are recurrent low backache often with marked morning stiffness, and positive sacro-iliac tests. The E.S.R. is usually raised, and rheumatoid nodules and serum factor absent. X-rays may show erosion and sclerosis of the sacro-iliac joints early in the disease and ossification of intervertebral ligaments later.

Treatment

Preservation of mobility is the key to treatment. Comparatively short periods of enforced rest lead to marked stiffening. Normal active life should be encouraged, but violent sport or hobbies avoided. Breathing exercises are important, and there is a clinical impression that exercise regimes designed to counteract the kyphotic tendency help. Patients should use a firm mattress and should lie prone on a firm surface for fifteen minutes twice daily.

Drugs. In mild cases the anti-rheumatics used initially for rheumatoid arthritis will reduce symptoms. Phenylbutazone 100 mgm t.d.s., is so effective that it almost serves as a therapeutic test. If it is successful but cannot be tolerated, the antacid-coated version (Butazolidin-alka) may be used, or oxyphenbutazone substituted. Where side effects are produced by butazones, indomethacin 25 mg t.d.s. is next worth trial. Systemic steroids are rarely justified and then only for uncontrolled disease activity, but their effects are disappointing. Intra-articular steroids are helpful.

Radiotherapy. Deep X-ray therapy usually relieves the pain of spondylitis. As it does not influence the natural history, but increases the risk of leukaemia its use is reserved for special circumstances: 1. Patients unwilling or unable to take regular drugs under supervision. 2. Active disease uncontrolled by drugs. 3. A peripheral joint.

Surgery. Synovectomy and arthroplasty operations have similar indications to those in rheumatoid arthritis. A stiff hip is particularly disabling in a patient with a stiff back and invites arthroplasty. Where severe incapacitating kyphosis has developed, spinal osteotomy should be considered.

CRYSTAL SYNOVITIS

Gout

The arthritic features of gout are caused by the local deposition of urate crystals. This urate deposition results from persistently elevated blood uric acid levels, and these in turn are caused either by a genetically determined error of uric acid metabolism, or by an undue stress being placed upon normal uric acid metabolism. The additional stress may be due to high purine intake, abnormal turnover of nucleoprotein, or impaired renal urate handling. Frequently latent gout becomes overt when an undue stress is superimposed upon a covert metabolic error. Gout is commonest in adult males, less frequent in menopausal females, and rare in other groups.

Gouty arthritis should be suspected when arthritis of almost unrivalled acuteness occurs in the hallux metatarso-phalangeal joint, in the mid-tarsal joint, or less commonly in other peripheral joints. Gout rarely affects central joints and never in the first attack. Occasionally gout has a polyarticular onset and may resemble rheumatoid arthritis.

A suspected diagnosis of gout is sustained by finding repeatedly elevated blood uric acid levels. Caution in interpreting uric acid levels is necessary as they may be elevated by many drugs (notably thiazides and small doses of salicylates), and because normal values vary with the technique used by the laboratory. Confirmation of the diagnosis requires the identification of urate crystals in inflammatory joint fluid, synovial biopsy specimen, or the identification of a tophus. 'Punched-out' areas in bone X rays do not confirm the diagnosis as they may be confused with rheumatoid erosions.

Treatment

Acute attacks. The patient will spontaneously rest and protect the joint, and may find a cold compress or spray comforting. Adequate fluid intake is encouraged. Colchicine is the traditional, and effective, treatment. 1 mg is given at the first notion of an attack, followed by 0·5 mg 2-hourly until pain is relieved or nausea or diarrhoea supervene. Oral phenylbutazone is more effective. 200 mg should be given 6-hourly in the first day followed by 200 mg 8-hourly the second day, then 100 mg t.d.s. until the attack has settled. Intramuscular phenylbutazone 600 mg has no advantage in speed of action, but may be used in the presence of vomiting. Unfortunately if injected near a nerve it produces irrecoverable paralysis, so the placing of the injection must be made with great care. Oral indomethacin is a useful alternative and may be given 200 mg in the first day, reducing to 25 mg q.d.s. Intra-articular steroid injections are dramatically effective where feasible, but are often precluded by the technical difficulty of injecting an acutely painful, small joint. Intractable attacks may be relieved by A.C.T.H. gel 40 units or tabs. prednisone 25 mg daily, but relapses occur on withdrawal.

Interval treatment. Once started this type of treatment should be continued for life, as the metabolic disorder is not reversible. Therefore the diagnosis must be beyond reasonable doubt. Uric acid lowering drugs are given if: 1. acute attacks are occuring frequently; 2. the blood uric acid is repeatedly 2 mg per cent or more above the laboratory's upper limit of normal; or 3. bone tophi or clinical tophi are present. Uricosurics are the traditional first choice. Tabs. probenecid (Benemid) 0·5 g. is started once daily after food, working up to 1·5 or 2 g. daily. Should this dose be ineffective, or produce nausea, vomiting, or a rash, sulphinpyrazone should be substituted. Tabs, sulphinpyrazone 50 mg daily is given, gradually increasing to 50–100 mg t.d.s. If neither of these uricosuric drugs can be tolerated, or renal function is impaired or stones found, or gross uric acid overproduction and excretion is occurring, a xanthine oxidase inhibitor should be used. Tabs. allopurinol 100 mg daily should be started, and slowly increased to a therapeutic dose of 100–200 mg t.d.s. Rashes may occur but other side effects are rare, and this drug may eventually replace uricosurics as the drug of first choice [6]. Any drug which lowers the blood uric acid must be started in small doses as acute attacks of gout are induced by changes of blood level. During the first month and covering any increase in dose of these drugs, colchicine 0·5 mg b.d. or phenylbutazone 100 mg b.d. should be given prophylactically. Similar prophylactic cover for operations is necessary.

Surgery may be useful to remove mechanically disadvantageous or unsightly tophi. This is helpful in reducing the pool of uric acid to be cleared by the interval drugs.

Pseudogout

Crystals of calcium pyrophosphate may induce a synovitis resembling that of classical gout. Pseudogout tends to affect larger joints especially the knees, and seldom affect joints which are not the site of radiological chondrocalcinosis articularis. Chondrocalcinosis is sometimes associated with a chronic polyarthritis. In contrast with classical gout, the big toe is scarcely ever affected, there is no diagnostic blood test, and tophi do not occur. Pseudogout is one of two types of arthropathy associated with haemochromatosis.

The diagnosis is suspected when chondrocalcinosis is found in a patient with arthritis, and is confirmed by the identification of calcium pyrophosphate crystals in synovial joint fluid. These can be distinguished by polarised light techniques from urate crystals [7].

Treatment

Acute attacks are best treated by aspiration of the joint fluid and injection of steroid. Phenylbutazone, indomethacin and perhaps salicylates may help the chronic forms.

HAEMOPHILIC ARTHRITIS

Bleeding into joints occurs at some stage in most patients with factor VIII deficiency and causes acute arthritis of a severity matched only by crystal synovitis, infective arthritis, and rheumatic fever. The knee is the most commonly affected joint, followed by the ankle, elbow, shoulder and hip. Bleeds also occur into muscles and along tissue planes.

Following the haemarthrosis red cells are lysed within the joint, and the haemosiderin phagocytosed by synovial cells. Recurrent bleeds lead to capsular fibrosis, and in chronic arthropathy there may be contractures and enlargement of bone ends. Subcortical bleeds cause ischaemic lesions of bone ends and secondary degenerative changes follow. When there is a history of preceding trauma the bleed is often more severe.

Attacks may affect males of any age, and haemophilia should even be considered in adult males with painful joint swelling and haemorrhagic effusions. Constitutional disturbance is relatively mild, and rheumatoid factor tests negative.

Treatment

The acute arthritis needs immediate treatment to minimise the risk of permanent damage. Analgesics, ice packs, and splints relieve pain while the patient is sent to the nearest haemophilic centre. An intravenous infusion of anti-haemophilic globulin (A.H.G.) is given immediately. If there is obstruction to vessels or nerves near the joint, or if the joint is grossly distended, aspiration is indicated and should be carried out as the infusion starts. The skin and joint capsule are infiltrated with local anaesthetic through a fine bore needle, and the aspiration made through a wide bore needle. When the pain and swelling start to settle, static exercises to the muscles controlling the joint must be started to prevent the rapid muscular wasting .

Chronic arthritis often follows despite the best attempts at its prevention. When mild contractures occur, they may be corrected by gentle physiotherapeutic stretching, and the patient himself can often help with these manual procedures. If contractures are more severe, serial splints or manipulation under anaesthetic may be needed but the latter must be carried out under A.H.G. cover. Occasionally pathological fractures occur through porotic bone near chronically affected joints, and it may be difficult to differentiate the associated haemorrhage from an intra-articular bleed. It is possible to modify the load on a joint and reduce the incidence of bleeding, for example by providing a weight relieving caliper for the knee.

Reconstructive surgery can help in isolated cases and synovectomy is under trial in an attempt to prevent recurrent bleeds. It is sometimes necessary for these patients to live in a sheltered environment particularly during school and training years.

BONE INFECTIONS

Osteomyelitis – Acute Onset

This painful condition is an acute emergency. The staphylococcus is the commonest cause, and the infection enters the metaphysis of a bone via the blood stream. Occasionally the streptococcus, pneumococcus, salmonella, or brucella may be responsible. The organism multiplies in the bone marrow causing fever, tachycardia, leucocytosis, and severe pain. There is local tenderness of bone and later redness and swelling. The pus may isolate areas of bone which form sequestra, and nearly always causes periosteal elevation. X-ray changes are late, a patchy porosis appearing at about 2 weeks, followed by periosteal new bone, and later still dense sequestra.

Treatment

When possible blood cultures and aspiration should precede antibiotics, but if these investigations are not rapidly available antibiotics must not be delayed. Soluble penicillin in full doses is the treatment of choice. If there is a possibility of resistant organisms, a broad spectrum antibiotic, cloxacillin or fucidin should be added. If the response is slow the antibiotic cover should be changed.

Chronic Sequelae. Incomplete resolution may lead to recurrent flares, sinuses, or sequestra. These should be treated with antibiotics or by excision.

Osteomyelitis – Chronic Onset

Tuberculosis is the commonest cause of chronic bone infection; vertebrae are most commonly affected but occasionally flat bones (rib or skull), or a finger (dactylitis) may be involved. Spread is to adjacent vertebrae and the symptoms merely a dull ache and vague ill-health. Osteoporosis follows, and two infected vertebrae with the enclosed disc may collapse causing an angular kyphos. Abscess formation sometimes causes local spinal cord damage with paraplegia, and pus may track to point at a distance. The diagnosis is suspected from the general condition, the chronic history, loss of spinal movement, and the presence of a cold abscess. It is confirmed by the radiological appearance, and biopsy is rarely needed for confirmation.

Treatment

This consists basically of antituberculous drugs, and rest in a spinal bed. Surgery may be needed to remove necrotic tissue, to stabilise the spine, or to decompress the spinal cord.

DEGENERATIVE JOINT DISEASE

Osteoarthrosis

Degenerative disease of joints causes pain, deformity and limitation of joint movement, often in older people.

The basic pathology involves hyaline cartilage, whose status quo is normally maintained by the balance between wear and repair. There may be an unknown genetic fault in cartilage make-up which makes it wear more quickly (Primary O.A.), or there may be undue streses on the joint following inflammatory disease, obesity, malalignment or incongrous joint surfaces (Secondary O.A.). The earliest pathological change is dulling and softening of the cartilage surface accompanied by reduction in the staining of mucopolysaccharides. Later a tangential flaking of the cartilage is followed by the formation of deep fissures. Fragments of cartilage break off and lie in the cavity. Small fragments migrate into the synovium and are then phagocytosed. The ensuing reaction leads to fibrosis and to contracture of the joint capsule. Hyperaemia of the bone end ensues and stimulates formation of cartilage at the joint margin; some of this becomes calcified and ossified. These changes lead to the radiological changes of reduction in joint space (especially at the weight bearing area), and osteophyte formation. Cartilage may be worn away completely leaving a dense bony surface, a process called eburnation, and occasionally fragments of cartilage break off and form loose bodies in the joint. Pain is thought to arise either from hyperaemic bone or from capsular stretching, and it seems to be the latter mechanism which accounts for pain occurring frequently in joints whose extremes of range are used.

One or more joints may be affected. Swelling of the joint often feels bony hard, and fluid and soft tissue swelling are less obvious. There is no diagnostic test for this condition, and there are no systemic features. The E.S.R. is normal, and radiological changes including osteophyte formation often occur in symptomless joints. Therefore the diagnosis is clinical and rests upon finding symptoms and signs and later radiological changes in joints susceptible to osteoarthrosis. The pattern of joints affected varies with the cause. Primary O.A. often affects the terminal interphalangeal joints (Heberden's nodes), the carpo-metacarpal of the thumb, as well as weight bearing joints. Secondary O.A. affects the joints damaged by the predisposing cause, whether it be rheumatoid arthritis, gout, or an old fracture.

Treatment

This is influenced by the number, distribution and severity of the joints affected. As in other chronic painful diseases the patient's pain threshold must be assessed so that complex treatments are not ordered when gentle reassurance is required. Any underlying disorder should be treated, and whenever weight bearing joints are affected obesity reduced

Pain relief. Heat may be applied with wax baths, infra-red lamps, or short-wave diathermy, and unless accompanied by skilled physiotherapy is better provided by the patient using domestic methods. Hot water bottles, electric blankets, hot baths, and electric fires all provide temporary relief. The useful drugs are similar to those for early rheumatoid arthritis. Aspirin is often helpful, and codeine co. may add to its affect, but many patients prefer phenylbutazone or indomethacin. Sometimes acute 'flares' occur, possibly due to joint haemorrhage or damage to cartilage following minor trauma. An intra-articular steroid injection is then effective. Sometimes a few days bed rest relieves pain, and fortunately degenerative joints do not stiffen as quickly as inflammatory joints.

Improvement of range. Repetitive capsular strains are painful, and may be relieved by stretching the capsule. This stretching can be achieved gently by a physiotherapist using heat as an analgesic, or may be obtained more quickly by manipulation under anaesthetic.

Reduction of stress. Patients should be instructed not to "work off" their pain. Stress should be lessened by resting the affected joint when possible. In weight bearing joints this involves avoiding unnecessary standing, and the use of a walking stick.

Specific examples

Terminal interphalangeal joints. Wax baths, analgesics and exercises are useful. Steroids and surgery have no place.

Carpo-metacarpal of thumb. Recurrent pain is occasionally relieved by a suitable splint, and a local steroid injection may help. Excision arthroplasty or arthrodesis is needed when pain is severe.

Wrist. This usually follows rheumatoid arthritis or injury. A polythene splint or steroid injection may help, but arthrodesis is occasionally required.

Elbow. This frequently does not cause symptoms as extremes of range are rarely required. Splints are helpful, and arthrodesis and arthroplasty occasionally useful. Stretching is rarely possible and attempts may be harmful. Tendon lesions are frequent near the elbow, and must be distinguished from joint disease. Tendon lesions respond to hydrocortisone acetate infiltration or local frictions.

Shoulder. This is rarely the site of primary O.A., and pain is more often caused by a capsulitis. Local steroids often relieve pain, and stretching may hasten recovery of range. Tendon lesions are common and again must be differentiated clinically from joint capsule pathology. After accurate localisation they are effectively treated by steroid injections or frictions.

Hip. Short-wave diathermy, stretching and analgesics suffice for mild degrees. A walking stick is frequently helpful, and should have a rubber tip. Osteotomy is sometimes used to relax the joint capsule, but when severe, arthrodesis or arthroplasty may be needed.

Knee. If analgesics fail, a polythene splint may help. The quadriceps muscle wastes quickly and should have intensive static exercises.

Arthrodesis, osteotomy, and arthroplasty all have a place. If the main disease is of the patello-femoral joint, patellectomy should be considered.

Hallux metatarso-phalangeal. A rockered sole often eases pain, but occasionally arthroplasty or arthrodesis is necessary.

Disc prolapse and spondylosis

These degenerative or traumatic disorders of the spinal column may give bouts of pain and limitation of movement, usually affecting the low lumbar or low cervical regions.

Minor injuries to the posterior longitudinal ligament sometimes combined with degenerative changes in disc material allow postero-lateral or posterior bulging of the intervertebral disc.

1. A small protrusion disturbs the symmetry of the articulations between vertebrae and leads to asymmetrical limitation of spinal movement. Impingement on the pain sensitive dura mater leads to pain of rather vague and apparently extra-segmental reference. With cervical protrusions pain is referred to the shoulder, interscapular region, or the head; from lumbar protrusions it is referred to the low back, sacro-iliac region or buttock. Dural irritation is usually accompanied by dural signs – limitation of femoral or sciatic stretch tests.

2. If the protrusion is larger nerve root pain may follow. Commonly this is C7 distribution from a cervical lesion, and L5 or S1 (sciatica) from a lumbar disc protrusion. Motor, reflex, or sensory deficits may occur.

3. A very large cervical protrusion may damage the spinal cord, causing spastic paraparesis, and in the lumbar region the cauda equina may be damaged leading to bladder symptoms. These features can occur in the absence of gross radiological changes, but diminution of intervertebral joint space and osteophyte formation are often seen.

Apophyseal and neurocentral joints also undergo degenerative changes which may cause pain and limitation of movement. It is difficult to know how frequently these joints are the cause of symptoms, or how often radiological changes which are found reflect the disturbed anatomy at the disc joints. Occasionally a large osteophyte will cause a root palsy by obstructing a cervical intervertebral foramen.

These mechanical disorders of the spine are suggested by an episodic history, relief by rest, and the complete absence of systemic upset. A slowly progressive onset, unremitting pain, symmetrical limitation of movements, neurological signs, or involvement of more than one nerve root should raise the suspicion of a more serious pathology. Sacro-iliac tests are negative.

TREATMENT

Conservative. As pain from these lesions is often self-limiting, active intervention is seldom essential. Analgesics and rest are the foundations of treatment and should be matched to the severity of pain. Salicylates, compound codeine, dihydrocodeine, pethidine or morphine may be needed. Rest is most effectively achieved in bed, as only in the horizontal position is no bodyweight being transmitted through the discs. The cervical spine should be maintained in a neutral position by adjustment of pillows, and the lumbar spine supported by boards beneath the mattress. Lesser degrees of rest may be obtained whilst ambulant by supplying a semi-rigid collar, or a lumbo-sacral belt with steel supports, or a plaster of paris or polythene corset. When bedrest has allowed almost complete relief of pain, gradual mobilisation should be encouraged.

Accessory treatments. Manipulation may hasten reduction [8] of either cervical or lumbar disc prolapse and is indicated in acute lesions causing limitation of movement and dural pain. Manipulation is contraindicated in the presence of severe pain, root pain, neurological deficit, disturbance of micturition, vascular disease, or when there is any doubt about the diagnosis. Cervical manipulations are performed with manual traction, and most manoeuvres involve rotation away from the side of maximum pain.

Traction seems to hasten relief of root pain, presumably by reducing the extent of disc protrusion [9]. The main indication is root pain in the absence of neurological deficit, and traction may also be tried if manipulation has failed. Traction is best given daily. Cervical traction of 20 lbs should be applied with the patient supine, but stronger and more effective traction may be given with the patient sitting, lumbar thoracic harness, and a force of up to 120 lbs (45 kilograms) applied through a harness pulling on the pelvis.

Epidural analgesia gives temporary relief from severe sciatica or lumbago. This is particularly useful for the few days of intense pain which accompany root interruption. 40–50 ml of ½ per cent procaine in normal saline (with no preservative or adrenaline) is injected through the sacral hiatus, and usually produces several hours of analgesia; sometimes pain does not return completely. Most uni-radicular palsies recover in one year, [10] but supportive measures (e.g. a toe-spring) may be needed meantime.

Prophylaxis. Indoctrination of the patient into habits which spare the lumbar spine stresses while flexed are helpful, and these habits can be re-inforced by supplying a correctly fitted lumbo-sacral belt. It may be necessary for the patient to change his occupation to avoid harmful stresses.

Operative. Laminectomy and disc removal, or spinal fusion should be considered in conjunction with an orthopaedic or neuro-surgeon for several clinical situations. 1. Frequent incapacitating recurrences not prevented by simpler measures. 2. Insufficient relief by other methods. 3. Serious neurological features (long tract signs from cervical protrusions, progressive or multiple root involvement, or bladder symptoms in lumbar protrusions).

References

General

Apley, A. Graham, *A system of Orthopaedics and Fractures* (1968), 3rd edition, Butterworths, London.

Copeman, W. S. C., *Textbook of the Rheumatic Diseases* (1969), 4th edition, Edinburgh, Livingstone.

Cyriax, James, *Textbook of Orthopaedic Medicine*, volume 1 (1969), 5th edition, Bailliere, Tindall & Cassell, London.

Specific

1. Mason, M., Currey, H. L. F., Barnes, C. G., Dunne, J. F., Hazelman, B. L., and Strickland, I. D., *Brit. med. J.* (1969), **1**, 420.
2. Mathews, J. A., *Annals of the Rheumatic Diseases* (1969), **28**, 260.
3. Hamrin, B., Jonsson, N., and Hellston, S., *ibid.* (1968), **27**, 397.
4. Wadman, B., and Werner, I., *Lancet* (1967), **i**, 597.
5. Bruk, M. I., *Annals of the Rheumatic Diseases* (1967), **26**, 103.
6. Scott, J. T., Hall, A. P., and Grahame, R., *Brit. med. J.* (1966), **2**, 321.
7. Currey, H. L. F., *Proc. roy. Soc. Med.* (1968), **61**, 969.
8. Mathews, J. A., and Yates, D. A. H., *Brit. med. J.* (1969), **3**, 669.
9. Mathews, J. A., *Annals of Physical Medicine* (1968), **9**, 275.
10. Yates, D. A. H., *ibid.* (1964), **7**, 169.

This chapter was written by Dr J. A. Mathews, (Consultant Physician, Department of Rheumatology and Physical Medicine, St Thomas's Hospital) and edited by Professor W. I. Cranston.

Category 4

Dermatology

Introduction

In this short account of dermatological treatment attention will be given to general principles rather than detail. In particular, the numerous local applications available will not be listed as their effect is better learnt by practice. Further, all dermatologists have their own collection of favourite local applications and there would seem to be no particular merit in listing the author's rather than those of another dermatologist. Proprietary blends of active chemicals, such as steroids and antibacterial agents, are constantly changing, and any list is likely to be out of date before it is published. The principles of treatment, however, and the active drugs available in dermatological practice change more slowly. Local applications should be kept to a simple regimen and sensitisers avoided.

The first essential in treatment is accurate diagnosis. A large proportion of dermatological conditions are exogenously determined and appropriate modification of the environmental factors may play a major part in treatment. This is particularly so in eczema. It is not sufficient to diagnose eczema and then apply a potent combined steroid-antibacterial cream. Every effort must be made by careful history taking to determine the skin sites first involved and the pattern of spread. Only in this way is it possible to suspect and diagnose an allergic contact or a primary irritant eczema. Once such an eczema has become widespread the original pattern may be forgotten by the patient, and no longer able to be discovered by the doctor. If the cause is not identified and removed in an exogenous eczema, then the condition is likely to persist indefinitely in spite of the most vigorous local treatment. It may be possible to suppress temporarily a primary irritant eczema with locally applied steroids, but it is the realisation by the patient of the environmental factors involved and their avoidance which will determine the long term success or failure of treatment. A further example of the importance of accurate diagnosis is in the treatment of intertrigo when infection with yeasts and fungi must be distinguished from seborrhoeic eczema or flexural psoriasis, and the importance of accurate diagnosis and its influence on effective treatment cannot be sufficiently stressed.

ECZEMA

Exogenous

After the cause of the eczema has been removed the most essential part of treatment is to obtain complete mental and physical rest for the patient. The patients who most persistently assert that rest is impossible are usually most in need of it, and if the patient is leading a busy life the only way in which the necessary relaxation may be found is by admission to hospital. Quite frequently mild sedation is necessary and an antihistamine by mouth such as promethazine hydrochloride or chlorpheniramine seems to accomplish this and reduce the skin irritation.

In the acute stage the skin may be cleansed and cooled by sponging with physiological saline or a dilute solution of potassium permanganate. This may be followed by the local application of calamine containing 0·25 per cent Mild Silver Protein or a steroid lotion. If there is secondary infection a steroid lotion containing the appropriate antibiotic or possibly one of the hydroxyquinoline derivatives is often helpful. As the skin heals and dries then the lotions may be replaced by the same ingredients in a cream base. With further improvement an ointment base may be tolerated as a vehicle for the active ingredients. At this stage tar is sometimes more effective than local steroids, and may be used in gradually increasing concentrations from 2–6 per cent. If scratching is playing a part in perpetuating the skin changes, then occlusive dressings with bandages impregnated with hydrocortisone or tar may be extremely useful. It is exceptional for the use of systemic steroids to be justifiable. If at any stage secondary infection is severe, then a systemic antibiotic may be necessary. The following should always be avoided in local applications due to the risk of sensitisation: penicillin, sulphonamides, antihistamines and local anaesthetics.

Bathing, which must be prohibited during the initial stages, may be gradually introduced using Emulsifying Ointment in place of soap for cleansing purposes; an important practical point is to warn the patient that this will make the bath extremely slippery. When the eczema has settled then patch testing may be undertaken if an allergic contact eczema is suspected.

Before the patient returns home it is important that a full and careful explanation be given of the ways in which his life must be modified. Too many patients return home without realising that after an attack of primary irritant eczema it is necessary to protect their skin against irritants for an indefinite period, nor may patients with allergic contact eczema realise that the allergy will persist for the rest of their lives.

After returning home the patient should, whenever possible, have a period of convalescence before a gradual return to full activity.

Atopic eczema

The course of this disorder is usually one of periodic exacerbations and remissions throughout childhood, fortunately with a tendency to improve, in the majority of patients, as puberty approaches. The exacerbations may be related to climatic factors, or periods of emotional stress but there may be no obvious precipitating factors. Diet has no effect on the disease. Treatment is directed at helping the child and the parents through the difficult periods by sedation, local therapy and encouragement. Sedation at night with antihistamines is helpful as these children are often extremely wakeful and seem to be able to endure long periods without sleep. If the family becomes demoralised by lack of sleep or the patient's skin is deteriorating, a period of in-patient treatment may be helpful. Local applications containing tar or steroids are the most useful. Some patients show a strong preference for either cream or ointment bases. The newer potent steroids should be used with caution as they may easily cause dermal atrophy. Recurrent boils sometimes complicate the situation and an antibacterial cream combined with a steroid may be employed such as 1 per cent hydrocortisone acetate in chlorhexidine cream BPC; occasionally ultraviolet light baths seem to be helpful. The skin is often very dry and Emulsifying Ointment may be used for cleansing purposes. Systemic steroids may, on very rare occasions, be justified. Vaccination for the patient and the whole family must be avoided because of the danger of eczema vaccinatum[1].

Seborrhoeic eczema

This variety of constitutional eczema is sufficiently different from the varieties of eczema already discussed to warrant a separate description of the treatment. Mild dandruff may be treated by rubbing into the scalp at night Aqueous Cream containing 1–2 per cent of salicylic acid and 1–2 per cent precipitated sulphur. This should be left on overnight and removed in the morning with a medicated shampoo containing coal tar and hexachlorophane. The process may be repeated twice weekly. If there is a great deal of irritation and erythema a steroid lotion or cream may be used or, even better, a steroid in a non-greasy base specially formulated for the scalp. If there is infection and crusting a combined steroid-antibacterial cream may be used. Aqueous Cream with sulphur and salicylic acid may also be used for eczematous patches over the sternum.

The generalised eruptive petaloid seborrhoeids which trouble these patients should be treated by bed rest and mild sedation with an antihistamine by mouth in the acute phase together with the local application of calamine with 1–2 per cent coal tar solution or a weak steroid lotion or cream.

The intertriginous eczema and fissuring in the groins, perineum and axillae and retro-auricular areas usually respond very well to a steroid-antibacterial cream. This is also very helpful for the frequently associated pruritus ani and Aqueous Cream should be used for cleansing purposes in place of soap when bathing and should also be used after defaecation.

Napkin rash

This is due to the irritant effect of wet alkaline napkins on the skin, together with infection by yeasts and bacteria. An important part of treatment is the correct laundering of napkins. After washing they should be carefully rinsed to remove all traces of soap or detergent and should then be soaked in an antiseptic such as 1:8000 benzalkonium chloride to kill urea-splitting organisms which make them alkaline and extremely irritating to the skin. Frequent changing of the napkins is essential to keep the skin as dry as possible. A steroid lotion or cream containing one of the hydroxyquinoline derivatives may be used in the acute stage and nystatin ointment should be used if there is infection with Candida albicans. Zinc and Castor Oil Ointment is a helpful protective local application when the rash is healing.

PSORIASIS

This is one of the commonest and most persistent eruptions. It is almost always possible to obtain a good measure of control but the time taken by different patients to do this varies a great deal. As relapse is unfortunately very common after cessation of treatment then each patient must be encouraged to decide how much time to devote to his eruption; this will depend upon the severity of the psoriasis and how much it worries the individual patient. Treatment consists almost entirely of local applications and these vary with the type of psoriasis.

Guttate psoriasis

This widespread eruption of small psoriatic lesions, which may be precipitated by a streptococcal throat infection, usually tends to improve spontaneously. The speed of improvement sometimes seems to be increased by local applications such as Oily Cream containing 2–4 per cent coal tar solution. An alternative is ultra violet light baths but these should not be given in the early acute phase. Quite frequently the clearing is not complete and then local applications are required as described under chronic psoriasis below.

Chronic psoriasis

If the psoriasis is of limited extent, then treatment may be carried out by the patient at home. If however, it is widespread, a period of inpatient treatment will be needed. Local applications containing tar or dithranol are usually very effective. These should be applied after a bath when the scales may be removed by gently scrubbing. After drying, the preparation should be applied accurately to the lesions and covered with a light dressing. Suitable applications are an ointment containing salicylic acid and strong coal tar solution* and Lassar's Paste with 0·25 per cent dithranol which may gradually be increased to 1 per cent and occasionally even stronger, if well tolerated. The effect of these applications is enhanced by ultra violet light. The newer potent steroid applications such as fluocinolone acetonide and betamethasone valerate are sometimes very helpful. Their effect is increased by occluding the area with plastic film and sealing the edges to the skin with cellulose tape. Their effect may also sometimes be enhanced by the addition of coal tar solution in a concentration of 2 to 8 per cent. Tar baths may be helpful particularly when a patient with widespread psoriasis is being treated at home: 30–60 ml of coal tar solution should be added to a bath.

Flexural psoriasis

This may occur in the perineum, axillae and under the breasts. The most effective treatment is the local application of fluocinolone ace-

* Salicylic Acid 2.g., Strong Coal Tar Solution 6.g., Emulsifying Ointment ad 100.g.

tonide or betamethasone valerate cream or ointment and these may be more effective when combined with one of the hydroxyquinoline derivatives. If these are used for any length of time in the flexures, dermal atrophy and striae are unfortunately quite common. Fungi and yeasts may flourish in the flexural lesions and may need appropriate treatment.

Psoriasis of the scalp

This usually responds quite well to oil of cade cream*. This should be massaged into the scalp at night, usually twice weekly is sufficient, and shampooed out in the morning with a medicated shampoo containing coal tar and hexachlorophane. If the patient finds this régime very troublesome then the newer potent steroids may be acceptable when formulated specially for the scalp. Occasionally betamethasone valerate cream with 0·1 per cent dithranol is very effective.

There is no treatment which is safe and effective for psoriasis of the nails.

Systemic treatment

Oral triamcinolone often produces a dramatic clearing of lesions. Control is only maintained, however, by increasing the dose with the risk of unpleasant side effects. Often when the dose is reduced this causes a severe rebound effect which may be pustular [2]. This can be a very serious complication.

When psoriasis is of such severity as to incapacitate a patient or to prevent him from working then it may be justifiable to administer the folic acid antagonist, methotrexate [3, 4]. This is a treatment which carries considerable risk and should only be done under circumstances where the necessary biochemical investigations may be routinely performed. It is rarely justifiable during the reproductive period of life. However, under special circumstances, it may produce well worth while improvement.

Diet

At the moment there is no evidence that special diets have any part to play in the treatment of psoriasis.

* Oil of Cade 6.g., Precipitated Sulphur 3.g., Salicylic Acid 2.g., Coconut Oil 20.g., Emulsifying Ointment 69.g.

ACNE

Complete control of this troublesome and disfiguring condition is often difficult but it is usually possible to obtain sufficient improvement to make the rather time-consuming treatment worth-while. In more severe cases treatment is important in that it will prevent or reduce scarring. Treatment will have to be continued until spontaneous remission of the disease occurs. These facts should be kindly but firmly explained to patients to avoid misunderstanding and disappointment.

Local treatment is aimed at the removal of blackheads and excess sebum and causing a mild desquamation. Blackheads should be removed carefully and completely by the patient with a proper expressor, a few being done each day; the help of a parent is valuable for difficult or inaccessible ones. Removal of sebum should be carried out, before going to bed, with a detergent solution such as Cetrimide Solution BPC. A detergent washing tablet is often helpful and may be applied with a shaving brush which is used to massage the skin at the same time. The cleansing agent should be removed by thoroughly rinsing the skin with water and after drying, one of the following local applications should be applied: Calamine lotion with 4–8 per cent precipitated sulphur for the face, back and chest; a cream containing 10 per cent benzoyl peroxide for the face; Resorcinol and Sulphur Paste BPC – full or half strength – for the chest and back. A wide range of other local applications is available but control is generally possible with simple measures if these are carried out carefully and regularly. The local applications should be left on overnight and then removed with the usual toilet soap in the morning. If this regimen produces too much erythema and a sore skin the sebum removal should be limited to alternate nights.

Cystic acne is particularly persistent and may cause severe scarring. It sometimes responds very well to tetracycline by mouth starting at 250 mg four times a day for a week and gradually reducing to 250 mg twice daily; courses should last 4–6 weeks but may be repeated. Persistent cysts may respond well to freezing with carbon dioxide snow for 10–15 seconds; some may require surgical drainage or diathermy puncture.

Courses of ultra-violet light may be helpful for all types of acne but should be carried out under medical supervision. Occasionally dietary factors are important but the patient is usually well aware of these and avoids the offending things. Hormone therapy and superficial X-rays are better avoided.

An endocrine cause for acne should be borne in mind and menstrual irregularities enquired about and hirsutism noted.

Acne rosacea

These patients should try and avoid the factors which they know produce flushing of the face, but this is often difficult. Forbidding alcohol would seem too severe a restriction for many patients and mild sedation may be more effective. Tetracycline by mouth in a dose of 250 mg once or twice daily may be dramatic in its effect. Helpful local applications are 1 or 2 per cent precipitated sulphur in Aqueous Cream applied with massage at night and Hydrocortisone Cream BPC in the morning. The potent steroid applications should not be used.

SKIN INFECTIONS

The skin is susceptible to attack by a wide range of organisms both bacterial and fungal. In many of these conditions there exist constitutional factors which predispose the patient to such attacks. Only the common infections are here described.

Impetigo

This is the most superficial of the bacterial infections and is most often the result of staphylococcal infection but may be a combined staphylococcal and streptococcal infection. It is almost always susceptible to local antibacterial agents and only rarely are systemic antibiotics needed. In impetigo of the scalp the possibility of pediculosis must be borne in mind.

A swab should be taken at the first attendance for bacterial culture and sensitivities to be performed. Treatment need not await the results but may be modified at the next attendance if the clinical response has been disappointing. All lesions should be gently cleaned three or four times daily with Cetrimide Solution BPC; if this is poorly tolerated then physiological saline may be used. This should be followed by the local application of an antibacterial agent; Chlortetracycline Ointment BPC is one of the most effective of these and sensitivity reactions are rare; its use, however, should be limited to outpatients because of the risk of bacterial resistance developing. Another very effective agent is a mixture of 0·25 per cent neomycin and 0·025 per cent gramicidin in an ointment base. It is usually possible to eliminate the infection in 1–2 weeks. Children should be kept away from school and each child should use his own towel in the home.

Recurrent boils and carbuncles

This is a frequently encountered problem and very often the underlying cause remains obscure. Eczema is a common background and diabetes must be excluded. The object of treatment is to reduce the staphylococcal population of the skin and eliminate the staphylococci carried in the nose and perineum. Cultures and sensitivities should be carried out from a boil and also from the nose and perineum; in family outbreaks the whole family should be investigated in this way and carriers of staphylococci should be treated. Chlorhexidine 0·1 per cent-neomycin 0·5 per cent cream should be applied to the nasal vestibuli twice daily. Chlorhexidine Cream BPC should be applied to the perineum twice daily and also to the skin round the boils. Hexachlorophane soap helps to reduce the skin population of staphylococci. Systemic antibiotics may be needed if the boils are large and localising poorly and surgical drainage should be carried out when appropriate.

Chronic paronychia

The predisposing factors are wet work and a poor peripheral circulation in this chronic infection of the nail fold with bacteria and yeasts – usually Staph. albus and Candida albicans.

The only effective remedy is to keep the appropriate fingers completely dry for a period of 3–6 months. This should be done by wearing cotton gloves for all housework to reduce the necessity for frequent hand washing. All wet work should be done in rubber gloves with cotton gloves underneath; the rubber gloves should not be worn for longer than five minutes at a time. Essential personal washing should be done with waterproof finger stalls on the appropriate fingers with an elastic band round the base of the finger. A great deal of encouragement to follow this regimen is needed by most patients. Local applications are only of secondary importance but Magenta Paint BPC or 3 per cent clioquinol cream may be useful.

Fungal

The diagnosis of all suspected fungal infections should be confirmed by microscopical examination and, where facilities allow, should be identified by culture.

Acute and severe tinea of the feet or groins is usually better treated with the patient resting in bed. If there is secondary bacterial infection and cellulitis then systemic antibiotics may be needed. Local treatment initially should be limited to sponging or soaking in physiological saline or aqueous 1:8000 potassium permanganate. This may be followed by the application of calamine with 0·25 per cent Mild Silver Protein or possibly a steroid-hydroxyquinoline mixture. As the local inflammatory reaction settles then more potent anti-fungal agents may be applied as in chronic infections.

Chronic tinea of the feet may be treated as follows: local application of Compound Benzoic Acid Ointment BPC (Whitfield's Ointment) at night and light cotton socks should be worn in bed. The feet should be washed in the morning and the feet powdered with Zinc Undecenoate Dusting Powder BPC. Nylon socks should be worn during the day and sandals have an advantage over shoes.

Chronic tinea of the groins may be treated with half strength Compound Benzoic Acid Ointment BPC or Zinc Undecenoate Ointment BPC.

The anti-fungal antibiotic griseofulvin is effective against a wide range of fungi and is particularly useful in widespread fungal infections, in fungal infection of the nails and in ringworm of the scalp. It is fungistatic and probably works by being incorporated into the new keratin being formed and thereby preventing invasion by the fungus; it therefore takes time in which to work, and for example in ringworm of the scalp, treatment must continue until non-infected hair has grown out – a period of 6–8 weeks. The infected portions of the hairs should then be removed with clippers. Tinea of the nails may require griseofulvin therapy for 6–12 months or even longer. It is not effective against Candida albicans. The drug is given in a dose of 125 mg four times a day for an adult and two or three times a day for a child.

Pityriasis versicolor may be treated by the local application of a 10 per cent aqueous solution of sodium thiosulphate twice daily. In all superficial fungal infections relapses are common.

INFESTATIONS

Scabies

The acaricide most usually employed is Benzyl Benzoate Application BP which is the 25 per cent emulsion. Equally satisfactory is gamma benzene hexachloride – usually the 1 per cent cream. The latter preparation is rather less irritating to the skin and is as effective as Benzyl Benzoate.

The method of using either is the same. The application is creamed on after a bath, to the whole body surface except the face and scalp. The process is repeated on the second day without bathing. On the third day the patient is instructed to bath, to dress in clean clothing and to change the bed linen. Clothing should be laundered, cleaned or left to hang for a week. The whole family must be treated in this way even if symptom free, as itching may not occur for several weeks after infestation and its absence must not be taken to mean freedom from infestation. Irritation may persist for 2–3 weeks and does not necessarily imply failure of cure. When treatment does fail it is usually due to faulty technique in applying the acaricide or failure to treat other members of the household.

Pediculosis

The drugs employed are either dicophane (DDT) or gamma benzene hexachloride (Gamma B.H.C.). These are available in a range of preparations as powder, cream, lotion and shampoo. Their use is described fully elsewhere [5].

SKIN TUMOURS

Virus warts

Before starting treatment the diagnosis must be verified by seeing the presence of a papillary structure within the lesion. To do this it may be necessary to pare away the superficial keratin with a sharp scalpel.

A large proportion of warts disappear without treatment within a year or so. For this reason treatment should not be too energetically pursued if it involves the production of scarring or upsetting a child. Simple remedies consist of paring the lesion daily and painting with 6 per cent Formalin or Salicylic Acid Collodin BPC. The effect of these may be enhanced by prior maceration either with 40 per cent salicylic acid plaster or zinc oxide self-adhesive plaster. This treatment may be carried out by the patient. More resistant lesions may require treatment by freezing with carbon dioxide 'slush' – a mixture of solid carbon dioxide and acetone; this may be applied accurately to the wart with a fine brush for 3–4 minutes. Plantar warts may be frozen with carbon dioxide snow in a wooden holder applied with firm pressure until a white rim of frozen skin appears around the periphery of the applicator – this usually takes about five minutes. Occasionally warts have to be curetted under local or general anaesthesia and the base treated with electrocautery or a silver nitrate stick. Even with great care the recurrence rate is about 10 per cent and another disadvantage is the production of scarring. It is often difficult to be sure when there is a recurrence of warty tissue in a scarred area on the sole and this may lead to further curettage and scarring. If a large number of warts is present it is wise to treat only a few at a time, whatever method is employed, as treatment of warts in one area not infrequently leads to involution of them all.

Genital warts should be treated by painting the lesions accurately with 25 per cent podophyllin in alcohol or acetone, followed by powdering with talc. The patient is instructed to bath and wash off the podophyllin after about six hours. Local reactions may be severe and for this reason if the warts are extensive a trial area only should be treated initially. If the treatment is well tolerated it may be repeated on alternate days.

Seborrhoeic warts

These are conveniently treated by curettage under local anaesthesia. They may be very numerous and as the sole reason for their removal is a cosmetic one, only the ones on exposed skin need be dealt with.

Basal cell carcinomata

It is always desirable to ascertain the histology of these lesions as mistakes in diagnosis can occur even when the clinical picture does not seem in doubt. This may be done by biopsy before embarking on treatment, or, if the lesion is small, excision biopsy may be carried out. Treatment is by excision, curettage or radiotherapy. The choice of treatment will depend upon the histological type of lesion, its site and size and to some extent on the local facilities available. Curettage is probably better avoided unless the operator is experienced in this method of treatment. There should be adequate follow-up of patients.

Keratoses and Squamous cell carcinomata

Although keratoses are common in the middle-aged and elderly only a very small proportion progress to squamous cell carcinomata which are capable of metastasising. Such a transition is heralded by a period of rapid growth in the size of the keratosis. Keratoses may be dealt with by freezing with carbon dioxide snow or 'slush' or by curettage. Where malignant change is suspected the lesion should be excised and examined histologically. The management and follow-up of patients with multiple keratoses is probably better left in the hands of people experienced in this field.

Cellular naevi and Melanomata

A patient usually seeks advice about a mole either for cosmetic reasons or because the lesion has changed in some way. If treatment is asked for on cosmetic grounds the only method which should be employed is complete excision followed by histological examination of the lesion. The decision whether or not to do this is a question of balancing the patient's dislike of the mole against his dislike of the appearance of the scar which is likely to result. Factors to consider are the size and site of the mole and the skill of the operator and should be discussed frankly with the patient before a decision is taken. Moles may sometimes require removal when they are being rubbed by clothing.

Change in a mole may consist of an increase in size, a change in the amount of distribution of pigment, inflammation, ulceration and bleeding or even itching. Any such change in a mole should be followed by its complete excision as soon as possible and by histological examination. The extent of the operation required is often a difficult decision at the time of the primary excision. If the histological examination shows the lesion to be malignant and invading, further surgery may be necessary. The degree of malignancy and hence the extent of the surgery required should not be decided by quick smear techniques but should be based on the appearance of paraffin sections. Endolymphatic injection of radio-active substances following excision seems to be a promising method of increasing the survival rate; the incidence of complications is much less than following a block dissection of regional glands [6].

References

1. Copeman, P. W. M., and Wallace, H. J., *Brit. med. J.* (1964), **2**, 906.
2. Baker, H., and Ryan T. J., *Brit. J. Derm.* (1968), **80**, 771.
3. Rees, R. B., Bennett, J. H., Maibach, H. J., and Arnold, H. L., *Archiv. Dermatol.* (1967), **95**, 2.
4. Ryan, T. J., and Baker, H., *Brit. J. Derm.* (1969), **80**, 134.
5. Warin, R. P., *Prescribers Journal* (1968), **7**, 138.
6. Edwards, J. M., and Kinmonth, J. B., *Brit. med. J.* (1968), **1**, 18.

This chapter was written by Dr P. F. D. Naylor, (Reader in Dermatology, Honorary Consultant, St Thomas's Hospital) and edited by Professor W. I. Cranston.

Category 5

Hypothermia and Exposure

Hypothermia is arbitrarily defined as a rectal or oesophageal temperature below 35°C. There is progressive mental slowing, confusion and unconsciousness as the body temperature falls from this level, but vital functions are seriously affected only when the temperature falls below 28–30°C. There is then a danger of sudden death from ventricular fibrillation. Below 18–25°C the heart is incapable of maintaining an effective circulation even if it remains in normal rhythm. On rewarming the main hazard is that blood volume will have fallen progressively during hypothermia, so that vasodilatation produced by warming can lead to a failure of venous return to the heart and a serious fall in arterial blood pressure.

Prevention or reversal of these hazards is the main object of the management of both accidental hypothermia, which causes most of the deaths of healthy people exposed to cold water or air, and of secondary hypothermia in which body cooling results from drugs or disease. Before considering the management of the various forms of hypothermia in more detail it is useful to have some general principles in mind.

Survival in accidental hypothermia depends most on whether the victim himself takes effective steps to retard body cooling and on the immediate actions taken by his rescuers. These steps are often the reverse of what common sense dictates. Even when they are not, neither victims nor rescuers normally take the right actions unless they know clearly what to do in advance so that it is a major medical responsibility to advise potential victims, aquatic and open air clubs, and rescue organisations. What happens in hospital, both with accidental and secondary hypothermia, is of lesser importance but still influences the chances of survival considerably. The most important general principle at this stage is that it is easier to kill a viable patient by well intentioned but ill-considered treatment than it is to save a patient who would otherwise have died. When in doubt it is better at this stage to expect spontaneous recovery than to attempt resuscitative treatment before full information is available.

PREVENTIVE AND EMERGENCY TREATMENT

Immersion hypothermia

Because of the high thermal conductivity and specific heat of water, body temperature falls rapidly during immersion and most shipwreck victims die of hypothermia rather than drowning. Thin men can cool to dangerous levels within 30 minutes in water at 0°C; they ultimately die of hypothermia in water as warm as 23°C, and without protection even fat men die in water colder than 12°C.

Before entering the water after a shipwreck survivors should be advised to put on thick clothing as well as the usual lifejacket, since even conventional non-waterproof clothing greatly retards body cooling in cold water. If the water is colder than 12°C the clothing should include gloves and footwear, since cold vasodilatation will otherwise greatly increase heat loss from the extremities, and since the extremities can otherwise freeze in sea-water that is near its freezing point of −1·9°C. Since exercise increases the rate at which body temperature falls in cold water, survivors should be advised to float still with their lifejacket or wreckage while they wait for rescue, and not to swim about if they can avoid it.

Confusion or unconsciousness after rescue suggests a dangerous degree of hypothermia. A heart rate below 50/min, which must be counted by palpation of the heart as peripheral arteries are constricted in hypothermia, will provide sufficient confirmation if no thermometer is available. People with this degree of cooling are liable to die after rescue from hypothermic arrest of the heart, because of continued loss of heat from the body core to the cold skin. The only effective way of preventing this and of restoring cardiac action if hypothermic arrest does occur is to put the patient into a bath of water at 40–44°C. If no thermometer is available the water should be as hot as the rescuer's hand can stand. The limbs should be left out of the water to minimise ischaemic damage from heating them before circulation is restored. Even if the victim is apparently dead every effort should be made to locate a bath quickly; one patient has been revived after as long as 60 minutes of hypothermic cardiac arrest, but cerebral damage is probably inevitable if the delay is much longer than this. While cardiac arrest persists cardiac massage and mouth-to-mouth artificial respiration may help to preserve life if trained people are available to give them. They should be given at not more than half the usual rate, in view of the reduced metabolism in hypothermia.

If the patient has a regular and improving heart beat and respiration after 20 minutes in the hot bath he should be removed from it, dried, and lain flat under blankets to finish rewarming slowly. In cases of hypothermic cardiac arrest nothing is lost by continuing the bath for longer, and giving cardiac massage and artificial respiration until the patient shows signs of life or is clearly dead. It is in any case important to remove the patient from the bath as soon as the risk of hypothermic cardiac arrest is over as this minimises the risk of sudden vasodilatation with a dangerous fall in blood pressure.

Hypothermia in walkers and climbers

The obvious preventive advice, that people should not undertake walking or climbing expeditions that they lack the physical fitness or the expertise to complete, is more readily given than received. One important and more acceptable piece of practical advice is that once it becomes clear that shelter cannot be reached by dark it is better to stop and prepare a bivouac in good time than to continue and collapse from exhaustion without one.

Since cooling in air is relatively slow the victim is seldom undergoing rapid chilling of the body core, and so is seldom in danger of death from cardiac arrest, at the time of rescue. For the same reason victims of cold air exposure have usually been hypothermic for longer than immersion cases so that a hot bath carries a greater risk of producing a serious fall in arterial pressure. Unless hypothermic cardiac arrest or extreme slowing of the heart and respiration demand a hot bath, cold air exposure cases should simply be lain flat under blankets in a sheltered, and preferably a warm, room and allowed to rewarm slowly.

People exposed to cold air have frostbite more often than immersion victims. If tissues are still frozen when the patient is seen they should be treated by plunging the affected part into hot water (40–44°C). The limb should then be dried, exposed to air and protected from injury.

Hypothermia in infancy and old age

The high ratio of surface to mass in infants, particularly in premature infants, makes them susceptible to falls of body temperature in cool environments that present no problem to adults. No general susceptibility to hypothermia is produced by old age, but a few old people have defective metabolic responses to cold and readily become hypothermic in poorly heated houses. Infants show a similar but temporary and special susceptibility to cold after a period of cold exposure, perhaps because of depletion of the brown fat that is known to be the source of many newborn animals' metabolic response to cold.

The most important measures in these conditions are preventive ones, to advise parents that too much fresh air in winter without adequate clothing can mean a dead baby, and to ensure that old people's houses have adequate heating. As regards treatment, the victims should be placed in a room or incubator at 32–34°C, since their defective capacity for temperature regulation may be unable to restore a normal temperature if they are simply wrapped in blankets. After recovery they continue to need special protection from cold; an infant will remain highly susceptible to hypothermia for a week or two, and an old person may remain so indefinitely.

Hypothermia due to drugs or disease

Narcotic agents, diabetic coma or insulin-induced hypoglycaemia, myxoedema, or lesions of the hypothalamus can all induce hypothermia by impairing one or more of the mechanisms for maintaining body temperature. Since moderate hypothermia helps to preserve life in most of these conditions no active warming should be undertaken until an accurate diagnosis can be made, and preferably not until the patient is in hospital where the underlying condition can be effectively treated. The same is true to a lesser extent in hypothermia due to catastrophic illness such as massive cerebrovascular accidents or infection, although hypothermia is then often little more than a part of the process of dying. In all these cases the safest emergency action is to do no more than to lie the patient flat and wrap him in blankets to prevent further cooling until he is transported to hospital.

HOSPITAL TREATMENT

By the time that a patient reaches hospital or a room equipped for resuscitation body temperature has almost invariably stabilised or started to rise, so provided the patient is alive the danger of subsequent death from progressive cooling of the heart and brain is over. Most victims of hypothermia who are not suffering from some other fatal condition recover from this point if left alone, and the most important points about management at this stage are negative ones. Ventricular fibrillation can be precipitated by unnecessary insertion of an airway or an oesophageal temperature probe during hypothermia, because of the reflex bradycardia that irritation of the throat produces. It can also be precipitated by vigorous cardiac massage and artificial ventilation, which causes a profound fall in pCO_2 in hypothermic patients.

If an airway is unavoidable it should be inserted with great care.

Otherwise the patient should be lain flat and covered with blankets. E.C.G. should be recorded, blood pressure measured by a sphygmomanometer, and body temperature followed by a rectal thermistor while the patient is unconscious, and by a low-reading oral mercury thermometer which follows changes in cardiac temperature more closely when consciousness returns. Facilities for positive pressure respiration, cardiac massage and electrical defibrillation should be kept close by but used only if ventricular fibrillation appears. Atrial fibrillation is common in hypothermia; it does not require treatment. Antifibrillatory drugs should not be given prophylactically to chilled patients, as many of these drugs have been shown actually to produce ventricular fibrillation or cardiac arrest in hypothermic animals. If repeated ventricular fibrillation demands an attempt to reduce ventricular irritability, cautious administration of 0·1–0·8 mg/kg of lignocaine hydrochloride intravenously, in 1·5 per cent solution, is probably the safest course. Hydrocortisone is often given in hypothermia but there is no clear evidence that it is beneficial.

In patients with hypothermia secondary to disease, the underlying condition must be diagnosed at this stage. This is often difficult while body temperature remains low, but enough signs of the causal condition are usually present to allow a diagnosis provided it is kept in mind that hypothermia itself produces cardiac slowing and arrythmias, clouded consciousness, high blood glucose and slow utilisation of any injected glucose. Any blood samples required to confirm a clinical diagnosis must be taken from an artery, or from a vein in an arm that has been in water at 40°C for 10 minutes to restore blood flow. Casual peripheral venous samples taken from an ischaemic limb in hypothermia can be highly misleading.

After the diagnosis is made it may be necessary to accelerate rewarming if the patient is obese, as spontaneous rewarming in such people is often inconveniently slow. The most satisfactory way to do this is to immerse one arm in water at 40–44°C. Such acceleration of rewarming is needed particularly for patients in diabetic coma, as they are resistant to insulin while body temperature remains low. If arterial pressure falls below 70 mm Hg as body temperature rises it can usually be restored by raising the foot of the bed and discontinuing any active rewarming. If hypotension persists intravenous dextran solution can be given to expand the blood volume.

When the patient's body temperature has risen above 35°C it is advisable to measure blood pH and blood glucose, particularly if the patient fails to recover full consciousness and normal respiration by this stage. Severe metabolic acidosis has been reported on rewarming following prolonged hypothermia. A blood pH below 7·2 calls for up to 200 mEq of sodium bicarbonate intravenously, and a blood dextrose below 50 mg/100 ml calls for 20–50 ml of 50 per cent dextrose intravenously. It is generally unwise to try to correct blood pH earlier while the patient is still severely hypothermic. Dangerous acidosis is very unusual while body temperature remains low, and inaccuracies in correcting standard laboratory estimations of pH at 37°C for blood taken from a hypothermic patient can lead to erroneous 'treatment' of non-existent disturbances.

After body temperature has returned to normal any non-freezing cold injury of the limbs will show itself as persistent hyperaemia, pain – and if severe by distal anaesthesia and weakness – and later contractures of muscle. Injury by frostbite will again show itself as hyperaemia, pain, and anaesthesia, but also with later gangrene affecting mainly the skin. Both conditions are best treated simply by elevating the affected limbs to reduce oedema, keeping them dry, and giving the patient analgesics to relieve pain. Intravenous heparin and dextran, and hyperbaric oxygen, have all been used in frostbite but as they are not of proven value and carry some risk they are not advisable in routine treatment. Surgery has no place, at least until any dead skin has sloughed; it can do great harm at an earlier stage by damaging viable tissue. Months later sympathectomy can be useful in relieving the excessive sweating and sensitivity to heat and cold that are a frequent late result of severe immersion injury.

Further Reading

Hey, E. N., and Katz, G., *Arch. Dis. Childh.* (1969), **44**, 323.

Hockaday, T. D. R., Cranston, W. I., Cooper, K. E., and Mottram, R. F., *Lancet* (1962), **ii**, 428.

Keatinge, W. R., *Survival in Cold Water. The physiology and treatment of immersion hypothermia and of drowning* (1969), Blackwell Scientific Publications.

Laufman, H., *J. Amer. med. Ass.* (1951), **147**, 1201.

MacMillan, A. L., Corbett, J. L., Johnson, R. H., Crampton Smith, A., Spalding, J. M. K., and Wollner, L., *Lancet* (1967), **ii**, 165.

Niazi, S. A., and Lewis, F. J., *Ann. Surg.* (1958), **147**, 264.

Pugh, L. G. C., *Lancet* (1964), **i**, 1210.

This chapter was written by Dr W. R. Keatinge (Reader in Physiology, The London Hospital Medical College) and edited by Professor W. I. Cranston.

Category 6

Common Endocrinological and Metabolic Diseases

NUTRITIONAL OBESITY [1]

The immediate aim of treatment is to achieve weight reduction. However, it is equally important to re-educate the patient into more normal dietary habits. The first of these objectives is much more easily attained than the second.

Dieting

In order to produce weight loss in obesity it is necessary to reduce the calorie intake of the patient.

In mild obesity (10–20 per cent above predicted weight) it is enough to prescribe a free diet except for a number of specified foodstuffs of high carbohydrate content.

A recent schedule based on this principle is shown in Section C.

Should the general advice contained in the free diet sheet prove inadequate then it may be necessary to spell out in more detail what the patient should be eating. Since it is impracticable for the home dieter to weigh every item another diet has been devised to give advice on amounts to be eaten (see Section C).

If all other methods fail, the excessively obese patient (>30 per cent of desirable weight) may be taken into hospital for total starvation. Although this has been carried out for periods up to four months it is more usual to totally withdraw food for only approximately two weeks. Prolonged treatment of this sort has caused death through heart failure and should not be prescribed for the elderly or for any patient who might have a cardiac abnormality; there is also a suggestion that even the young and previously healthy myocardium might be at risk. However, if total starvation is indicated, vitamin and potassium supplements should be given together with allopurinol. This last drug is used to prevent the symptomatic hyperuricaemia that might otherwise complicate the fast.

A liquid diet such as 'Complan' or 'Metercal' provides approximately 900 calories a day and may be the only way some patients can be persuaded to reduce their dietary intake.

Another way a 'packaged diet' can be provided is by a variety of commercially available biscuits containing protein, vitamins and methyl cellulose. These are usually supplemented with milk and are particularly useful for inducing weight loss in those who are minimally obese and who do not wish to adhere to a complex dietary regime.

Dietary aids. Artificial sweeteners such as saccharin allow the dieter to enjoy a sweet taste from a non-carbohydrate, a-caloric source.

Starch reduced bread allows the patient to have bread with a low carbohydrate content. When eating this, it is necessary to limit the amount ingested.

Appetite suppressants. Although the treatment of obesity depends on reducing the food intake of the patient it may on occasion be necessary to administer a substance that reduces the appetite. This aid to dieting should be prescribed reluctantly, as an important factor in the long-term success of a dietary regime is that the patient should become tolerant of the hunger initially produced by reducing the intake. If hunger is removed by a drug then the patient cannot recognise and conquer it. This leads to difficulty in inducing a permanent change in eating habits. For this reason, and also for the sake of cost, it may be preferable to prescribe courses of an anorectic agent alternating each month with a placebo.

The indications for drug treatment are:

1. Patients who have great difficulty in keeping to a diet.
2. Depression, either preceding or following weight loss.

The drugs most useful in the suppression of appetite are:

Phenmetrazine: 50–75 mg day in divided doses or as slow release capsules.

Diethylpropion: 75–100 mg day in divided doses or as slow release tablets.

Phentermine: 15–30 mg daily.

Fenfluramine: 20 mg–40 mg twice daily.

Since phenmetrazine and phentermine produce restlessness and insomnia, they should be administered early in the day. Fenfluramine is said to have a sedative effect and is given at 10 a.m. and 4.00 p.m. Only fenfluramine should be given to patients with hypertension or heart disease or to a depressed patient within two weeks of stopping antidepressive therapy with monoamine oxidase inhibitors. Because of the risk of addiction and as there are more effective drugs, amphetamines should not be prescribed.

Another class of drugs that has been found to depress appetite are the biguanides, oral hypoglycaemic agents used in some cases of diabetes.

It has also been suggested that bulk, taken as methyl cellulose granules or biscuits, reduces appetite. However, the evidence obtained from controlled trials is that this approach to appetite reduction is ineffective.

Other methods for weight reduction that are either ineffective or dangerous include laxatives, thyroxine or triiodo-thyronine tablets, chorionic gonadotrophin injections and jejuno-colic shunt operations.

Exercise. Walking three miles a day utilises about 300 calories. This exercise, additional to that normally taken by the patient, will result in weight loss of 2–4 lbs a month. If the subject is young and fit, he will lose an equal amount of weight if he plays tennis or swims for 30 minutes a day or bicycles for 45 minutes a day.

Any patient, who is on a weight reducing programme, should be seen at least monthly, or preferably weekly, by their attending physicians in order that they may be encouraged, sympathised with or cajoled into adhering to their diet. The closer the supervision of the patient, the more likely the success of the treatment.

ANOREXIA NERVOSA [2]

The first aim of treatment requires that the patient's nutritional status is restored to normal. This normally necessitates admission to hospital in order that the intake of food can be closely supervised and the patient separated from her parents. The diet is gradually increased from 1500–5000 calories in the course of two weeks. At the start of treatment the patient is kept in bed and given 100–300 mg/day of chlorpromazine which can be increased by 150 mg/day to the limit of tolerance; this helps overcome the patient's fear of food. Pari passu with this, one hour after breakfast insulin is begun, first 10 u; the dose is then increased until mild hypoglycaemia results. As soon as this appears a large meal is given; in this way food is seen by the patient to be beneficial. Once the patient is gaining weight psychotherapy can be given; indeed patients suffering from this condition, which has a high relapse rate, require the prolonged supervision of a skilled psychiatrist [2].

DIABETES MELLITUS [3, 4, 5]

The management of each individual case is a continuing process of trial and error. It is therefore not possible to provide detailed instructions, only guide lines.

Aims of therapy. Before detailing the types of treatment available for diabetes, it is necessary to state the objectives to be accomplished.

Reasoning from the known biochemical abnormalities in the disease would suggest that a practical index of successful treatment would be to restore the blood glucose level to normal. However, this accomplishment, even if it were universally possible, may result in considerably more disruption to the patient's life than if the blood glucose remained relatively uncontrolled. Although there is some evidence to show that in insulin-requiring diabetics the better the control the fewer the complications, it is not apparent whether this is because better control leads to fewer complications or because patients with a milder disease, who have a tendency to develop fewer complications, are more easy to control. Until this problem can be resolved the aim of treatment should be, to maintain the patient in good health by:

1. Correcting diabetic symptoms.
2. Avoiding the complications of treatment, particularly hypoglycaemia.

The agents used in the treatment of diabetes mellitus are:

1. Diet.
2. Insulin.
3. Sulphonylureas.
4. Biguanides.

Diet. There are two reasons for dieting the diabetic:

1. Weight reduction.
2. Control of carbohydrate intake.

Dieting is valuable in the elderly obese patient in whom weight reduction is indicated.

In the young, besides as a means to weight loss, where indicated, it is necessary to prescribe a diet in order to control the carbohydrate intake. The advantage of the patient eating a measured amount of carbohydrate is that the effect of other treatments, such as insulin or oral hypoglycaemic agents are less variable when the carbohydrate intake is held relatively constant. There is, moreover, evidence to suggest that patients who have an entirely unrestricted intake develop more complications than those whose diet is controlled. The patient may be given a list of portions of various foods containing a fixed amount, normally 10 g. of carbohydrate. Using such a list as a guide it is relatively simple to have a daily intake approximating to the general amount advised by the physician.

The acutal amount of carbohydrate to be recommended varies from patient to patient; those taking insulin tend to require more than those treated by other means. An adult of normal weight will need a daily intake of 120–250 g. taken at such times that the dietary tendency to hyperglycaemia is countered by, and itself counters, the maximal hypoglycaemic action of the administered insulin. If insulin is not required then the carbohydrate load should be spread out over the day so that the patient is at no time excessively hyperglycaemic.

If the diabetic is obese, then the carbohydrate intake should be limited to 100 g. or less. However, it must be remembered that severe carbohydrate restriction is itself a cause of ketonuria.

Although it has been suggested that animal fat might contribute to the atherosclerosis of the diabetic, not enough evidence has yet accumulated to justify the prescription of a diet low in animal fat and high in unsaturated fat as a useful therapeutic measure in the prevention of diabetic vascular disease.

Insulin. The indications for insulin therapy are:

1. Ketosis, when not due to starvation.
2. In childhood, adolescence and young adulthood.
3. Temporarily, to cover an illness or surgical operation in some patients taking oral hypoglycaemic agents.

The reasons for choosing a particular insulin are given below.

Insulin	*Indications*
Soluble	Ketosis. Coma when large amounts (>80 u) per day are required. Where requirement is rapidly changing. (e.g. Childhood diabetes.)
Actrapid	As for soluble. Allergy or resistance to bovine insulin.
Isophane	Used in preference to protamine zinc as action begins earlier, lasts a shorter time – thus reducing risk of nocturnal hypoglycaemia – and is more consistent.

Rapitard	As for isophane.
Insulin zinc suspension (Lente)	This may provide control with one injection a day in the insulin-requiring patient with a relatively mild form of the disease.
Protamine zinc.	Occasionally mixed with soluble to provide control with one injection a day.

Sulphonylureas. These drugs are used extensively in the treatment of maturity onset diabetes and are effective in controlling the disease in a large proportion of this group of patients.

There are however a number of contraindications to the use of sulphonylureas:

1. Ketosis, not due to over restriction of carbohydrate.
2. Total pancreatectomy.

The obese diabetic who can be controlled by diet alone should, in the first instance, be encouraged to lose weight rather than be prescribed a sulphonylurea. If the patient, despite exhortation, remains obese or if weight loss does not control symptoms and blood glucose, then a biguanide or sulphonylurea can be given.

The drugs most frequently used are chlorpropamide, tolbutamide, acetohexamide, tolazamide and glibencleride. Side effects are rare.

If the diabetes is not controlled by a sulphonylurea and diet then either a biguanide can be added to the regime or the patient will require insulin.

Biguanides. Although the mechanism of action of this group of drugs remains unclear they may be used:

1. With sulphonylureas to achieve control in some maturity onset diabetics, thereby avoiding the need for insulin.

2. In some obese maturity onset diabetics the anorexia produced may reduce the food intake with consequent weight loss; this, in turn, leads to control of the blood glucose.

Unfortunately, however, there is a high incidence of side effects which may necessitate stopping the drug.

Transfer from insulin to oral hypoglycaemic agents. If there is no history of ketosis and if the insulin requirement does not exceed 40 u/day, it may be possible to replace insulin with a sulphonylurea, perhaps combined with a biguanide.

If tolbutamide is used the insulin may be stopped as the tablets are started. With chlorpropamide the insulin is withdrawn gradually over five days once the oral treatment has been begun. Throughout the period of changeover daily measurements of urine sugar and ketones must be made together, if possible, with daily blood glucose estimations. If there is any sign of developing ketosis insulin should be reinstituted.

Exercise. The diabetic should take a moderate amount of physical exercise. Any unusual increase in physical activity introduces instability into the therapeutic regimen with a requirement for either more carbohydrate in the diet (and sugar for emergencies) or less insulin.

Choosing the treatment. Possible schemes for deciding the optimum treatment for the individual diabetic are shown in tables I and II.

Table I

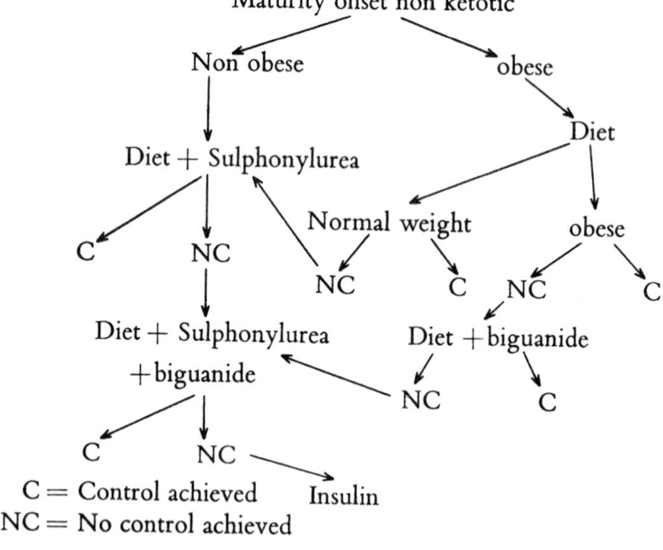

Table II

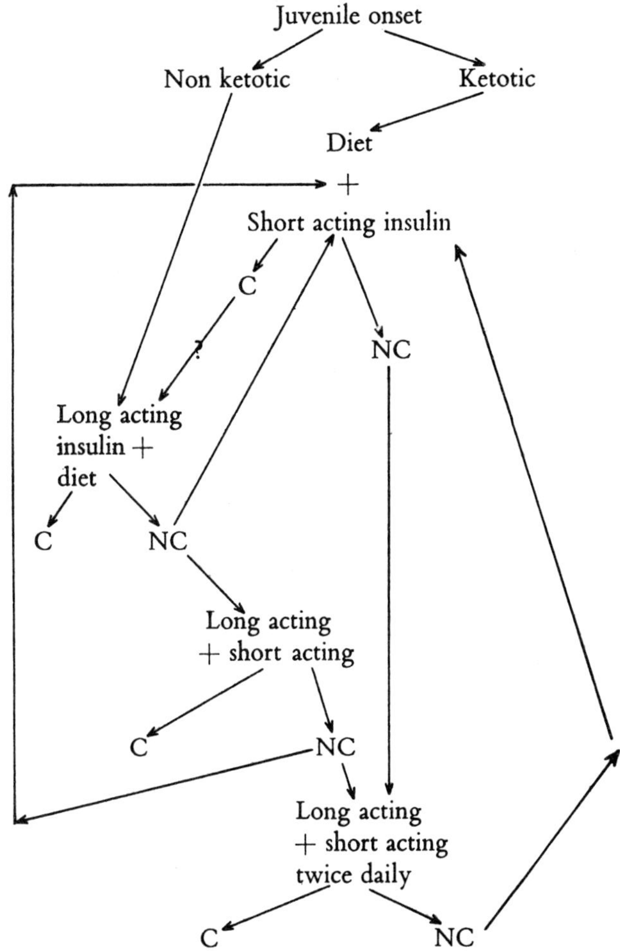

C = Control achieved
NC = No control achieved

Control may be defined as a blood glucose normal or near normal throughout the 24 hours. Since it is usually impossible to obtain frequent blood specimens, preprandial venous blood glucoses <110 mg/per cent may be taken to indicate good control. A urine collected over this period should be glucose and ketone free.

The diabetes is not controlled if the preprandial blood glucose exceeds 150 mg/per cent, if the urine consistently contains more than ½ per cent glucose or if there is any ketonuria.

Between these two extremes lies a degree of chemical control that may be acceptable, given the patient's individual circumstances.

It is however essential that, apart from restoring the chemistry towards normal, the treatment removes the symptoms of the disease.

Urine testing and control of treatment. In the long-term management of the disease it is desirable to have the patient test his own urine. The urine should at all times be ketone free. Apart from an occasional trace ($<\frac{1}{2}$ per cent) the urine should remain glucose free when the patient is dieted and/or receiving oral agents.

During stabilisation and at times of unsatisfactory control the urine should be tested immediately before all meals.

For day-to-day adjustments of dose the urine should be tested before the injection and when the insulin is exerting its maximal effect.

Insulin should be given initially as soluble insulin (SI) or Rapitard 20 u. twice daily in the more severe cases or, in milder subjects as Isophane or Lente 20 u. daily. Treatment may then be modified by blood sugar measurement and by following the urine glucose (Clinitest) providing the patient has a normal threshold.

Insulin resistance. If this occurs the patient should be changed to porcine insulin (Actrapid). If this is ineffective steroid therapy (prednisone 10 mg thrice daily may reduce the insulin requirement. In a minority of patients large doses of SI are inevitably required (using insulin 320 u/ml).

Childhood diabetes. Diabetic children almost invariably require insulin. For psychological reasons an attempt should be made to control the disease with one injection a day of a long acting preparation, although, if the child presents with ketoacidosis, the initial stabilisation must be performed with frequent doses of SI. As soon as possible the child should be taught self-injection. The diet must be adequate in calories but moderately restricted in carbohydrate. Care is needed to balance the carbohydrate intake against the exercise/insulin requirements to avoid excessively frequent hypoglycaemic reactions.

The pregnant diabetic. Carbohydrate intake should be 150–250 g./day. From the second trimester onwards there is usually a rise in insulin requirements as indicated by blood glucose changes. Ketosis must be avoided for its effect on the foetus. From thirty-two weeks the patient should be admitted to hospital. The blood sugar should be monitored during labour to anticipate hypoglycaemia. The obstetric problems that arise are best managed by a specialist obstetrician.

Intercurrent illness. Even if the patient becomes anorectic, there will be a temporary rise in insulin requirement. The dose should be increased early in order to prevent ketoacidosis.

Surgery. Apart from the very mild case the surgical diabetic will require insulin. The occasional well-controlled maturity onset patient need only change his normal regime by omitting treatment on the day of operation.

It is wise to stabilise the patient on soluble insulin 2–3 days preoperatively. For an elective procedure under general anaesthesia, it is preferable to schedule the operation for the morning. If the urine is sugar free then 10–20 g. of glucose should be given intravenously – oral glucose should not be given within 8 hours of surgery owing to the risks of vomiting and inhalation of the vomit. If ketosis is present the operation must be delayed until the condition is brought under control. During a long operation the patient should be watched for signs of hypoglycaemia – tachycardia and sweating. Also, the blood sugar should be estimated with Dextrostix. If hypoglycaemia develops, I.V. glucose must be given. Postoperatively a blood sugar should be taken to assess the need for insulin; if it is required then it should be accompanied by glucose given by a suitable route. Because of the heightened risks of infection, catheterisation should be avoided as a means of obtaining urine samples.

When the patient has passed through the immediate postoperative period the normal regimen of insulin administration can be resumed, accompanied by a normal carbohydrate load given in an appropriate manner.

For emergency surgery every case must be managed individually. The best guide to treatment comes from measurement of the blood glucose and bicarbonate. If the patient is ketotic, this becomes the therapeutic priority unless the emergency is so dire as to require immediate operation.

The complications. There is no specific treatment for diabetic neuropathy, nephropathy or angiopathy. Because of the risk of hypoglycaemia in the diabetic under treatment, the use of propranolol is contraindicated for the relief of angina pectoris in this group of patients.

The onset of diabetic gangrene can be delayed by careful attention to hygiene of the feet.

A vascular surgeon should be consulted on the management of circulatory insufficiency.

The rare specific diabetic cataract can be reversed if found early and the diabetes controlled. Control of blood glucose may induce refractive errors that disappear spontaneously after a few weeks. Some patients with diabetic retinopathy are benefited by pituitary destruction. However, the criteria for employing such a procedure are very strict and only a limited number of candidates are suitable.

Coma and pre-coma

Ketoacidosis. The seriousness of this condition demands that the patient should be treated in hospital. Initially a blood glucose estimation should be carried out and repeated every two hours until the physician is satisfied that the glucose is falling at an adequate rate.

Insulin is the basis of treatment. When the diagnosis has been made soluble insulin should be injected 50–100 u. I.V. and 50–100 u. I.M. If the fall in blood glucose is only slight after two hours the initial dose should be repeated. If the patient's clinical and biochemical condition remains unchanged or worsens the insulin dose should be doubled. If the blood glucose fall is adequate the two hour dose of insulin is withheld and a four hourly regime established. As the blood glucose level approaches the renal threshold, treatment can be based on urine testing. The risk of hypoglycaemia is in this way reduced – as a further precaution blood glucose measurements can be carried out.

Fluid and electrolytes. An intravenous infusion should be started when the first dose of insulin is given. Total fluids given should be approximately:

1 litre in first 1 hour.
4 litres in first 12 hours.
6 litres in first 24 hours.

The fluid should be basically 0·9 per cent sodium chloride, containing approximately 30 mEq of sodium bicarbonate in each of the first 3 litres. Alternatively, the total amount of bicarbonate needed can be roughly estimated from the sum: (25-Plasma bicarb. (mEq/1)) × 10 milliequivalents.

A wise precaution is to insert a long catheter into a central vein for the measurement of venous pressure and thereby to control the rate of fluid administration.

Since hypokalaemia may develop in the course of treatment it is essential to monitor the plasma K^+ 2–4 hourly at the same time as blood glucose and other electrolytes are measured. Providing the urine output is adequate, potassium chloride 25 mEq/hour is given in the intravenous drip after four hours of a satisfactory response to insulin. The potassium deficit that will eventually require correction is approximately 200 mEq.

When treatment is begun the stomach contents should be aspirated through a tube and nothing given by mouth. After 24 hours of satisfactory treatment it is usually possible to begin feeding by mouth with carbohydrate drinks.

The treatment of diabetic ketoacidosis is not complete until the cause has been located and treated appropriately.

Hyperosmolar coma. This should be treated with moderate amounts of insulin – smaller than those required for ketoacidosis – and 0·45 per cent sodium chloride I.V. Fluid requirements may be large, and the venous pressure should be monitored. Not all patients with this condition will require permanent insulin treatment.

Lactic acidosis. This is treated with intravenous sodium bicarbonate and, if possible, by removal of the cause of the lactate accumulation.

Hypoglycaemia. If possible the patient should immediately ingest carbohydrate-containing food or drink at the onset of symptoms.

When stupor or coma is present 10 g. of glucose should be given I.V.; some patients, however, may require up to 100 g. before the blood glucose is restored to normal. This should be done as quickly as possible to prevent permanent brain damage.

An alternative but less rapidly effective treatment, is to administer glucagon 0·5–1·0 mg I.M.

Soon after recovery the patient should be given a carbohydrate load by mouth to prevent relapse. The cause of the hypoglycaemia should be sought and the treatment regime modified if necessary.

In prolonged hypoglycaemia coma the patient should be tube fed and the blood glucose maintained at approximately 200 mg per cent. Cases of 'irreversible' coma should also receive intravenous hydrocortisone.

HYPOGLYCAEMIA [6]

This should be treated according to the cause.

Insulin-induced hypoglycaemia in the diabetic has already been discussed (q.v.).

A pancreatic islet-cell tumour should be removed. When this course is impossible hypoglycaemia can be treated with diazoxide, glucocorticoids and glucagon.

Reactive hypoglycaemia may be difficult to treat. Measures that have been advocated include a low carbohydrate diet, frequent small feeds rather than a few large meals, and prohibition of tobacco.

Neonatal hypoglycaemia is treated with intravenous glucose using the blood glucose as a yardstick. Treatment is normally necessary for only the first week of life.

Idiopathic hypoglycaemia in childhood may be treated with corticosteroids, diazoxide or by long-acting zinc glucagon. In the acute attacks intravenous or oral glucose should be given.

Leucine sensitivity should be managed in the same way as idiopathic hypoglycaemia, since it is impracticable to prescribe a leucine-free diet.

THYROID

Hyperthyroidism [7]

There are three ways of suppressing thyroid overactivity:

1. Antithyroid drugs.
2. Radioactive iodine.
3. Surgery.

Drugs. The indications for this form of treatment are:

(i) A small diffuse goitre.
(ii) Gross hyperthyroidism with cardiac involvement (vide infra).
(iii) Pregnancy.
(iv) Childhood.
(v) The patient is being treated for the first time.
(vi) The preparation of a patient for radioactive iodine or surgery.

The disadvantages are:

(i) The goitrogenic effects. Thus, antithyroid drugs should not be used as the definitive treatment in patients with retrosternal prolongation of the goitre.

(ii) The recurrence of the hyperthyroidism in 40 per cent of the patients when therapy is eventually stopped.

(iii) Side effects, of which the most important is agranulocytosis. These are unusual with the drugs currently in use.

The drugs most frequently used are:

Carbimazole or Methimazole.

Starting dose: 15–20 mg three times a day.

Maintenance dose: 5 mg once daily–5 mg three times a day.

Methylthiouracil or propylthyrouracil starting dose: 150–200 mg thrice daily. Maintenance dose 50 mg one to three times daily. In order to prevent the onset of iatrogenic hypothyroidism it is wise to maintain the starting dose no longer than two months and then to reduce the treatment at monthly intervals approximating to a schedule which, for carbimazole, is:

1st month 60 mg/day in divided doses.
2nd month 45 mg/day in divided doses.
3rd month 30 mg/day in divided doses.
4th month 20 mg/day in divided doses.
5th month 15 mg/day in divided doses.

The therapy should be altered according to the patient's condition; if he shows signs of relapsing the dose should be increased, if hypothyroidism appears, the drug should be decreased. Treatment should be maintained for at least six months after the patient has become euthyroid. If hyperthyroidism recurs when treatment is stopped, either radioactive iodine or surgery should be employed.

It may be possible to prevent enlargement of the gland that occurs when anti-thyroid drugs are given by simultaneously administering trioiodothyronine.

Radioactive Iodine (^{131}I). This is indicated when the thyrotoxic patient

(i) is over 40 years old;
(ii) has heart disease (vide infra);
(iii) has intercurrent disease;
(iv) is mentally ill.

It is contraindicated in:

(i) Patients under 40, because of the possible risk of inducing thyroid cancer or leukaemia.

(ii) Pregnancy.

(iii) Toxic nodular goitre in areas where goitre is endemic and there is thus a heightened risk of thyroid cancer.

The important complications of radio-iodine therapy are:

(i) Hypothyroidism, which occurs at a rate of 10 per cent per annum and remains a recurrent risk throughout the patient's life.

(ii) Thyroid storm, a rare event, but particularly serious in the cardiac patient. This occurs 1–2 weeks after therapy.

(iii) A transient tracheitis or thyroiditis.

Since radioiodine is very slow in exerting an effect, it is sometimes wise to make the patient euthyroid with drugs before giving the radioactive material.

Surgery. This should be performed:

1. When the patient has a large goitre.
2. When the patient has a solitary nodule that might be cancerous.
3. When drug treatment fails in a person under 40 years old.
4. In retrosternal goitre.
5. Pregnancy, during the second trimester, as an alternative to drugs.

It is contraindicated in the old, the ill and the mentally unstable.

Preparation for surgery

(i) Render the patient euthyroid with anti-thyroid drugs.

(ii) Admit to hospital. Stop drugs.

(iii) Administer either potassium iodide 100 mg/day in milk or Lugol's iodine 1·0 ml/day for approximately 2 weeks. This manoeuvre decreases the increased vascularity of the gland produced by the anti-thyroid drug.

Alternatively:

Administer propranolol (vide infra) for 2–3 weeks then (iii) as above.

Propranolol. There is evidence that this drug, used in a dose of 40 mg four times daily rapidly controls some of the clinical features of hyperthyroidism. In particular it induces a diminution of malaise, palpitations, sweating and nervousness, with a concomitant reduction in pulse rate and tremor. It should not, however, be employed in the presence of heart failure.

It has also been given instead of the antithyroid drugs to patients receiving ^{131}I or being prepared for surgery.

Ophthalmic manifestations. If the exophthalmos warrants treatment, simple measures such as padding the eye or the wearing of dark glasses may be tried.

Should the condition increase in severity tarsorrhaphy may be necessary to prevent corneal ulceration.

Orbital decompression is the ultimate in surgical treatment for malignant exophthalmos where sight is threatened.

There is no medical way of managing exophthalmos that is universally accepted. Some claim that triiodothyronine 125 μgm/day given with the antithyroid therapy reduces the incidence and severity of exophthalmos.

There is a suggestion that the instillation of guanethidine eye drops (2 drops twice daily, of a 10 per cent solution) may lessen exophthalmos. However, if this treatment is continued for 2 months or so, punctate keratitis may appear. Should this happen a 5 per cent solution should be substituted; this allows the keratitis to heal but maintains the improvement in the exophthalmos.

Finally, some patients with malignant exophthalmos show an improvement with very large doses of corticosteroids – up to 150 mg/day of prednisone. Unfortunately, however, steroid dosage at this level inevitably leads to side effects, so the dose should be gradually reduced as soon as the eye signs allow.

Pretibial myxoedema. This is best treated with occlusive dressings of topical corticosteroids.

Myxoedema

In this condition the secretion of the thyroid gland can be replaced either with L-thyroxine (T_4) or L-triodothyronine (T_3). There is no longer any place for desiccated thyroid in the drug cupboard.

T_4 0·1 mg is approximately equivalent to T_3 0·02 mg. Unless the patient is receiving immediate replacement therapy after total thyroidectomy it is usual to increase the treatment very slowly until maintenance levels are reached. This is because the myocardium may not recover at a rate fast enough to permit it to cope with the demands made on it during the period of recovery of the rest of the body. If the patient has angina pectoris it is better to use T_3 than T_4 as the shorter duration of action of the former enables the effects of overtreatment to be rapidly stopped.

The usual course is to begin at a T_4 dose of 0·05–0·1 mg/day and then to increase the dose in weekly stages of 0·05 or 0·1 mg until a maintenance dose of 0·2–0·3 mg/day is reached. If an equivalent dose of T_3 is given it should be divided so that it is taken 2 or 3 times a day.

In many cases it is possible to make the patient euthyroid. However, in those with severe underlying heart disease, it may be preferable to undertreat so that some degree of hypothyroidism remains.

Hashimoto's thyroiditis

This is treated with T_4. This will reduce the size of the gland and make the patient euthyroid.

ADRENAL [8]

Cushing's syndrome

The choice of treatment for this condition is contingent on the underlying pathology.

If, as is most likely, the patient is suffering from adrenal hyperplasia due to an abnormality of the hypothalamico – pituitary – adrenal axis, the choice of therapy lies between destruction of the pituitary gland or total removal of the adrenal glands.

The pituitary gland may be destroyed by surgical removal, cryosurgery or local implantation of radioactive seeds.

This is currently the treatment of choice providing that:

(a) Adrenal hyperplasia due to pituitary hyperactivity has been diagnosed with certainty.

(b) The treatment is carried out at a specialist centre.

(c) The patient does not wish to remain fertile.

(d) The patient is no longer growing.

If any one of these criteria is not satisfied adrenalectomy is indicated. The drawbacks to this operation are:

(a) The technical difficulty.

(b) The occurrence of a pituitary tumour, that may not become manifest until after adrenalectomy, in approximately 10 per cent of patients with Cushing's syndrome.

The main disadvantage to hypophysectomy is the ensuing panhypopituitarism.

Following either operation the patient must be managed as for adrenalectomy (q.v.). However, the hypophysectomised patient does not require mineralocorticoid but will need substitution of thyroid (q.v.) and, possibly, also sex hormones. Diabetes insipidus following hypophysectomy is usually transient and may be controlled by intramuscular injections of pitressin tannate in oil 1 i.u., once or twice daily.

Adrenal hyperplasia due to corticotrophin (ACTH) originating from a non-endocrine tumour may, if indicated, be treated by total adrenalectomy or removal of the source of ACTH if this is surgically feasible. In Cushing's syndrome due to adrenocortical adenoma or carcinoma the appropriate gland should be totally removed under steroid cover. The drug treatment of inoperable adrenal carcinoma with metyrapone, or aminoglutethimide is generally unsatisfactory although remissions with these agents have, on occasion, been reported.

Addison's disease

The treatment of this condition requires the administration of a glucocorticoid and a mineralocorticoid.

Apart from the situations detailed below, the following are normally given:

Glucocorticoid. Tabs. cortisone acetate 25–50 mg/day by mouth in divided doses. The optimum dose is usually 37·5 mg/day (i.e. 12·5 mg three times daily.

Mineralocorticoid. Tablets fludrocortisone 0·05–0·2 mg/day (usually 0·1 mg/day) in a single dose. If the patient cannot be relied upon, or if he should become ill and be unable to take his tablets, the risk of the rapid development of a severe Addisonian crisis can be reduced by the intramuscular administration of Deoxycorticosterone trimethyl acetate (DOCTMA) 50–75 mg once a month, instead of the oral mineralocorticoid.

In hot climates, it may be necessary to administer sodium chloride tablets since, even in treated Addison's disease, it may not be possible to achieve maximal sodium conservation.

Intercurrent illness will require an increase in the dose of cortisone to 100 mg day. If there is doubt that the steroid is being absorbed it may be given parenterally; however, it is important to note that intramuscular cortisone acetate does not act until approximately 12 hours after injection.

Addisonian crisis requires the repeated I.V. injection of 200 mg. hydrocortisone sodium succinate in an intravenous saline and, if the patient is hypoglycaemic, glucose infusion. Before treatment is begun, blood should be sampled for cortisol, glucose and electrolyte measurements. Treatment should be begun without waiting for the result.

Corticosteroid cover for surgery

1. *Adrenalectomy*: the following drugs should all be given.

(*a*) Cortisone acetate intramuscularly.

100 mg daily; day before operation, day of operation, days 1–3 post operatively.

75 mg daily, days 4–6.

50 mg daily, days 7–9.

Then 37·5 mg a day permanently.

If the postoperative recovery is not uneventful, it may be temporarily necessary to continue the cortisone at the higher dosage.

As soon as the patient can be treated by mouth the same dose may be given in tablet form in divided doses 2–3 times a day.

(b) Hydrocortisone sodium succinate.

Day of operation: 100 mg intramuscularly with premedication, or 100 mg intravenously at the time of induction of the anaesthetic. Ampoules of the preparation should be available in the operating theatre; this will avoid unnecessary delay in the administration of the hormone should it be required urgently. Further doses of 50–100 mg I.V. may be given if there is a fall in systolic blood pressure to below

90 mg Hg.; it should be noted that post-operative hypotension however is more often due to haemorrhage than to steroid deficiency.

(c) Mineralocorticoid.

This should be instituted as soon as the cortisone therapy has been reduced to 50 mg daily. (For details vide management of Addison's disease).

2. *Patients already receiving steroid therapy*. The regime is the same as for adrenalectomy, except that if the patient is taking more than 75 mg a day or cortisone or its equivalent (15 mg of prednisone) they will require to continue this in addition to the amounts recommended for adrenalectomy.

Patients coming to operation within six months of receiving steroid therapy should be managed according to the schedule set out for adrenalectomy except that they can finally be weaned from the steroid at the end of the convalescent phase.

HYPOPITUITARISM

The cause of this should be found, and if possible, remedied. If there is secondary hypofunction of the adrenals, thyroid and gonads, it is important that the adrenal deficiency is treated first, as the prior administration of thyroid hormone may precipitate an Addisonian crisis. The target gland deficiencies should be treated as for myxoedema and Addison's disease, except that mineralocorticoid substitution is usually unnecessary.

The gonadal deficiency can be managed with continuous androgen therapy in the male. In the female, cyclical oestrogens are given for three weeks in every month. Infertility can sometimes be overcome by the injection of human gonadotrophin preparations administered under specialist supervision.

It is possible to treat pituitary dwarfism in children with human growth hormone; this treatment requires close clinical and metabolic control, as the supply of this hormone preparation is severely limited.

DIABETES INSIPIDUS

This may be controlled by pitressin tannate in oil I.M., lysine vasopressin nose drops, chlorothiazide or chlorpropamide tablets. It is possible to overdose with the antidiuretic hormone preparation thereby inducing water intoxication. Diabetes insipidus is usually transient following hypophysectomy and does not require treatment for longer than a week or two.

METABOLIC BONE DISEASE [9]

This requires calciferol and, in the initial stages of treatment, calcium supplements. If tetany occurs, it may be necessary to give intravenous calcium.

If the cause of the rickets is dietary, the deficiency should be rectified either by public health measures or by permanent supplementation with small amounts (400 u/day) of vitamin D. If the rickets is secondary to other diseases, then these should be treated; when this is impossible the vitamin D therapy will have to be continued and the treatment monitored with plasma calcium, phosphorous and alkaline phosphatase estimations. Some patients may require very large doses (50,000–500,000 u/day) to restore the calcium and bone to normal.

References and further reading

1. D. Craddock, *Obesity and its Management*, Livingstone, Edinburgh, 1969.
2. P. Dally, *Anorexia Nervosa*, Wm. Heinemann Medical books, London, 1969.
3. *Diabetes Mellitus: Diagnosis and Treatment*, ed G. J. Hamli and T. S. Danowski, American Diabetes Association, New York, 1967.
4. J. Malins, *Clinical Diabetes Mellitus*, Eyre and Spottiswoode, London, 1968.
5. W. G. Oakley, D. A. Pyke, and K. W. Taylor, *Clinical Diabetes and its Biochemical Basis*, Blackwell, Oxford and Edinburgh, 1968.
6. V. Marks, and F. C. Rose, *Hypoglycaemia*, Blackwell, Oxford, 1965.
7. *The Thyroid Gland* by S. H. Ingbar and K. A. Woeber in Textbook of Endocrinology, ed R. H. Williams, 4th ed., Saunders, Philadelphia, 1968.
8. I. H. Mills, *Clinical Aspects of Adrenal Function*, Blackwell, Oxford 1964.
9. *Calcium metabolism and the bone*, 2nd edition, By P. Fourman and P. Royer, Blackwell, Oxford and Edinburgh, 1968.

This chapter was written by Dr D. R. London (Senior Lecturer in Chemical Pathology and Honorary Consultant Physician, St Thomas's Hospital) and edited by Professor W. I. Cranston.

Category 7
Sexually Transmitted Infections

It is essential to obtain the patient's maximum co-operation and as far as possible to prevent default, as many patients when symptoms have disappeared feel that further treatment is unnecessary. A full explanation of the reasons for treatment should always be given according to the patient's intelligence. It is wise also to treat the patients' families as well and to consider the whole as a unit. For every infected patient there must always be another and far better results will be obtained if both partners can be treated, if not together in confidence, at least under the same roof. For example it is no good telling a husband that he is cured and may resume a normal sexual life if it is not noticed that on the preceding day, his wife had a positive culture returned for gonorrhoea! Reinfection and further trouble would only follow. Indirectly this also helps to inculcate a sense of responsibility into patients towards others, the lack of which is so important a factor in the spread of this type of infection.

SYPHILIS

There is an enormous amount of literature about the treatment of syphilis and numerous different treatment schedules have been used. Those described here have the merit of simplicity and of being generally applicable. The important principle of treatment is that there should be a continuously maintained low concentration of penicillin in the blood stream for a minimum period of 8 days. In order to preserve an adequate margin of safety somewhat longer periods of treatment are recommended. The best form of penicillin to use is procaine penicillin G. by itself, or suspended in aluminium monostearate to delay absorption. A daily injection of 600,000 or 900,000 units of either preparation will provide adequate blood levels. In cases of sero-negative primary syphilis when Treponema pallidum has been recovered from the sores but the blood tests are all negative, a course of ten such injections is adequate, but in late primary syphilis with positive serology and in all cases of secondary syphilis and early latency within the first year of infection, fifteen such injections should be given. When daily attendance is not possible, or is unlikely to be secured, a single dose of 2·4 megaunits of benzathene penicillin is likely to give an effective blood level for about two weeks. This type of injection is rather painful and may very well cause the patient to default. Follow up is required for two years. Blood tests should be done two weeks after the end of treatment, and thereafter monthly for three months, and then three monthly until two years have passed. During the second year the cerebrospinal fluid should be examined. In just under 1 per cent of cases it will be found to be abnormal. In such an event re-treatment will be required as otherwise the patient may develop neurosyphilis. In sero-positive cases it may take up to six months before all the blood tests have reverted to negative, but such slow reversion is not an indication for further treatment. Infectious relapse occurs in under 2 per cent of sero-negative primary cases and in just over 4 per cent of all other cases of early syphilis. It is usually preceded by serological relapse which can be detected if adequate follow up was maintained, before the occurrence of actual lesions which are often fleeting and superficial but are likely to be infectious. If such relapse occurs the disease will continue into the latent phase. All the available evidence suggests that after two years the disease is in fact permanently cured and the patients may be discharged. Exceptions are so few that any further follow-up with consequent anxieties for the patient, is not justified, and indeed the great majority of relapses occur during the first year.

The Jarisch-Herxheimer reaction

This is a focal and generalised exacerbation of symptoms which follows treatment with almost any reagent except perhaps bismuth or mercury. It is believed to be due to the liberation of endotoxins consequent upon the death of large numbers of treponemes but this explanation is purely theoretical. The reactions varies from a transient feeling of malaise to a severe exacerbation of all the symptoms coupled with generalised aching in the limbs, headache and high pyrexia occasionally with rigors. It is essential to warn the patients that this may occur – which it does in over 50 per cent of cases. It does no harm at this stage of the disease. Alcohol should be forbidden while treatment is actually being given. Most text books suggest that sexual intercourse should be banned for two years but it is doubtful if many authorities insist upon this now. If a couple living together are both infected provided that observation is maintained there seems no valid reason why intercourse should not be permitted with each other after treatment of both has been finished. When one of the pair is uninfected at least three months observation of both should elapse and the uninfected partner should know all the facts. Intercourse with others should be avoided for at least six months, preferably for one year. Where these conditions are not fulfilled somewhat more frequent blood testing may reveal an incipient relapse before any damage has been done. When patients are allergic to penicillin the treatment of choice is with tetracycline or erythromycin 500 mg four times a day for ten or fourteen days respectively. The follow-up should be for at least two years. This treatment is less satisfactory partly because there is no guarantee that the patients will always remember to take the tablets. There are no indications today for the use of arsenicals nor is there evidence that the addition of bismuth to penicillin produces superior results. In latent and late syphilis the general principles of treatment are similar. At least 15 injections of penicillin should be given and in the more severe form of tertiary syphilis, as many as 20 to 30 in the first course. Opinions differ as to whether further maintenance courses of treatment are required. Many maintain that one long course is adequate. Some physicians, however, prefer to add maintenance courses of penicillin, usually consisting of 10 injections each, although larger doses of 1·2 or 2·4 megaunits may be given at weekly intervals for 6–8 weeks. At the very most four such courses should be given and if it is intended to give more than one course the patients should be informed at the beginning, as otherwise the apparently haphazard administration of further courses may be very demoralizing. It is probable that patients with very early cardio-vascular or neurological lesions, for example in early tabes or general paresis, may benefit from further courses as it is obviously important to prevent any spread of the syphilitic process – but there is no evidence that patients with cardiac failure or in the late stages of neurosyphilis really benefit from prolonged treatment. The Jarisch-Herxheimer reaction may occur in both cardio-vascular and neurological cases. It is, however, rare in the former and may consist of attacks of anginal pain or exceptionally, an actual coronary thrombosis. In neurological cases, particularly in general paresis, convulsions may occur and rare instances of death have been reported. There is some evidence that the severity of these reactions may be reduced by the prior administration of steroids, for example prednisone 20–30 mg daily for three days – with commencement of penicillin on the third day, Graciansky and Grupper (1961). Prior administration of bismuth for three weeks has sometimes been used but in cases of general paresis is inadvisable as the sooner treatment is begun the better the results. The fallacy that 10 injections is all that is required to cure any stage of syphilis must be exploded. The writer had three examples when such treatment led to disaster. A patient of 36 with general paresis was given 10 injections of penicillin and no follow up. Six months later a fatal exacerbation occurred. Another patient with early tabes was given 10 injections. An X-ray examination of the aorta at that time disclosed no abnormality – four years later he had an aortic aneurysm. Another patient with latent syphilis had pneumonia and was given the equivalent of 10 injections. Four years later he had marked tabes dorsalis.

Apart from their use for the prevention of Jarisch-Herxheimer reactions, in late cases of syphilis steroids are generally contraindicated except in interstitial keratitis where they are valuable locally; in some cases of 'Charcot joints' and in cases of nerve deafness. In some cases of gumma formation too rapid treatment with penicillin is believed to result in excessive scar formation with the so-called therapeutic paradox and it is believed that an initial course of bismuth for 3 weeks 0·2 g. twice weekly intramuscularly, coupled with oral potassium iodide (1 g. three times a day for two weeks) may prevent this.

Maternal syphilis

The infection reaches the foetus across the placenta. Treatment with penicillin will prevent this and a course of 10 injections is all that is required to ensure a normal child. Follow up of the child should be at one month and at six months. Cord bloods are unreliable owing to the mixture of maternal reagin or treponemal antibodies. Passive transfer of such antibodies may take place in the infant and positive results at one month, provided that the child is fit, should be disregarded and the tests repeated. At six months they should all be negative.

Some authorities assert that it is only necessary to treat the first pregnancy but Moore (1949) found that after treatment had been withheld in 390 pregnancies, 3 syphilitic infants were born. The writer had a case of a patient who, 22 years after her initial infection and after 8 normal pregnancies in every one of which she had received anti-syphilitic teatment, produced a child with active congenital syphilis. It would therefore seem wise to treat all such pregnancies, except possibly those in women who have had only sero-negative primary syphilis, and have been discharged as cured. Active congenital syphilis at birth is very rare in the United Kingdom but when it does occur the infant may be acutely ill and the sooner penicillin treatment is given the better. The suggested dosage is 450,000–600,000 units/kg over a period of from 10–15 days. The mortality rate may be quite high and there is some evidence that Jarisch-Herxheimer reaction may be contributory so that the administration of steroids may be advisable, at any rate for the first two or three days.

GONORRHOEA

In uncomplicated gonorrhoea, so far as penicillin is concerned, one injection to provide an adequate blood level for 24 hours is all that is required. In the early days of penicillin treatment 300,000 units of procaine penicillin G was adequate but owing to the fact that numerous strains of gonococci have acquired varying degrees of insensitivity it is usual to begin with considerably larger dosages ranging from 900,000 units up to 1·8 megaunits. If treatment is effective by the third day in the male the discharge should have ceased and the urine should be clear without haze or shreds. Further tests should be done at the end of one week, two weeks and four weeks, at which stage prostatic massage should be carried out. The prostatic bead should not contain any pus, still less, of course, gonococci. Some authorities urethroscope every case but this is not always practicable, and essential only in certain instances discussed below. Blood tests for syphilis should be done at the beginning and at the end and in certain cases if there is any risk of previous exposure to syphilis, or in districts where the latter disease is prevalent, further blood tests should be done at the end of three and even six months. In practice this is not often possible because very few patients will attend for that length of time.

In women urethral and cervical smears and cultures should be performed on the third day, at the end of a week, two weeks and four weeks but with special emphasis on the time immediately following the first period after treatment. Similar considerations apply with regard to blood tests. Sexual intercourse should be avoided for at least a month and alcohol, which, because it is excreted in the urine, tends to aggravate this type of infection, for ten days.

In uncomplicated cases, with the exception of ampicillin which may be given orally in a dose of 250 mg followed by a second one after six hours, oral penicillins should be avoided as they are far less effective. In cases of penicillin allergy a single injection only of streptomycin

1 g. intramuscularly may be given, or a three or four day course of tetracycline or oxytetracycline 250 mg four times a day. But in general these treatments are less effective than penicillin. The difficulty arises with strains of organism that are insensitive to penicillin. When the sensitivity is 0·03 units per millilitre almost every case will be cured. As it decreases to 0·06 a failure rate of approximately 20 per cent may be expected and at 0·25 units per millilitre of minimum inhibitory concentration the failure rate may exceed 90 per cent, with the standard dosage. It may therefore, be necessary to give as much as 3·6 or even 4·8 megaunits which is about the maximum dose that can be tolerated by ambulant patients. The writer and his colleagues tried the effect of giving a large oral dose of ampicillin, 2 or 3 g., at the same time as an intramuscular injection of 3·6 megaunits of procaine penicillin and succeeded in curing 54 out of 60 cases where standard treatment had failed. Fluker and Hewitt (1969). It is no good giving multiple small injections of penicillin, say of less than a megaunit, over a period of several days as the infection simply will not be cured. Unfortunately, cases of penicillin insensitivity almost invariably show complete resistance to streptomycin and if an infection fails to respond to a single gram of streptomycin then it is no good proceeding with the antibiotic. Tetracyclines sometimes succeed, and also erythromycin, but again there seems to be some linkage in resistance to these antibiotics. Spiromycin may be tried – 250 mg four times a day for three or four days or in the form of one dose of 2·5 g. at once. Siboulet and Durel (1961) obtained cure in 764 (97 per cent) of 784 males so treated but it is doubtful if such an excellent response would be obtained today. Sulphonamides in their original form are practically useless but when combined with trimethoprim as in the tablets Septrin or Bactrim which contains 80 mg of trimethoprim and 400 mg of sulphamethoxazole, cure rates in excess of 90 per cent are being obtained. Two tablets are given in the morning and two in the evening for from 5 to 7 days. Injection of Kanamycin – 2 g. – is also effective but the ototoxicity (affecting the cochlea) of this antibiotic should be very much borne in mind. The latter is particularly effective for rectal gonorrhoea and cure rates of over 90 per cent have been reported from many sources. The writer and colleagues obtained cure in 88 out of 100 patients, using Kanamycin and in only 68 out of 100 patients using 1·8 megaunits of procaine penicillin. This form of gonorrhoea is always much more obstinate. At least three negative rectal smears and cultures taken through a proctoscope, should be obtained after treatment of

rectal gonorrhoea on the third day, and after one, two and four weeks. Treatment of complications will be dealt with under non-gonococcal urethritis, in the male, and in the female, Bartholinitis and salpingitis are the commonest. The former must be treated by daily injections of penicillin of at least 2·0 megaunits daily or possibly with a tetracycline or Bactrim. This, if given soon enough, may prevent pus formation but if an abscess forms it must be drained, preferably by aspiration. Bed rest may be required. If a permanent cyst results, marsupialisation may subsequently be required. In cases of salpingitis, bed rest is advisable and antibiotic treatment should be conducted on similar lines. If there is pus formation then operation may be required with drainage. Sterility is a not uncommon sequel owing to the blockage of the Fallopian tubes.

Gonococcal ophthalmia neonatorum which in the United Kingdom is a notifiable condition, is also potentially a very dangerous one in which the eyes may be destroyed completely within 48 hours. Parenteral injection of penicillin is required but local treatment is the more important with douching of the eyes and the instillation of penicillin eye drops at the rate of 1 per minute into each eye until the discharge has ceased. The manoeuvre may be repeated if the discharge subsequently recurs. Chloramphenicol eye drops may also be used, preferably in alternation with or as an adjuvant to penicillin.

NON-GONOCOCCAL URETHRITIS

Those cases of urethritis secondary to some general medical or surgical conditions will depend upon treatment of that particular condition and do not concern us here. This leaves three types of urethritis. Firstly the non-specific urethritis of unknown aetiology, secondly, urethritis due to trichomonas and thirdly that due to Candida albicans. The first type is by far the most common. The least unsatisfactory treatment is with tetracycline, either oxytetracycline or tetracycline usually given as 250 mg 4 times a day for 5 days. The cure rate is probably about 80 per cent. Patients should be seen either on the third day or at the end of the course; at the end of one, two and four weeks. The discharge disappears and the urine clears much more slowly than in gonorrhoea, but by the end of a week or ten days there should be no symptoms. Unfortunately, relapse is very common during the first month though it rarely happens thereafter, and no patient should be guaranteed a cure in a shorter period. About 70–75 per cent of patients are in fact cured but the remainder will need further treatment. A second line of defence is an injection of streptomycin associated with a sulphonamide for 5 days. All the evidence suggests that this combination is three times as effective as either alone, but the cure rate which used to be claimed as approaching 80 per cent does not now seem to be much more than 60–65 per cent. It is customary to use long acting sulphonamides. The writer showed, in a paper as yet unpublished, that the long acting sulphonamide, sulphamethoxydiazine was statistically superior to sulphamethoxypyridazine. Thirdly, if both the other methods fail, a course of urethral irrigations for from 10 to 14 days using either 1 in 10,000 oxycyanide of mercury or 1 in 10,000 potassium permanganate may effect a cure.

In certain relapsing cases that initially respond to tetracycline, it may be worth restarting the tetracycline at full dosage for 5 days, followed by half dosage, that is to say 250 mg twice a day, for a further 10 or 14 days, and a prolonged period of 3–6 weeks or more on 250 mg daily. This seems to prevent relapse in a limited number of cases. Many leading physicians in London in recent months seem to have come independently to the conclusion that considerably larger dosages of oxytetracycline are indicated than ever before, the schedules employed ranging from oxytetracycline 500 mg four times daily for at least one week and in some instances for as long as three weeks. No doubt a number of papers will be published in due course. Other antibiotics are usually much less effective and the least effective of all is penicillin. Those patients whose infection persists or recurs after three weeks or so should invariably have the prostate examined and this in any case should be done at the end of four weeks before the patient is discharged. If the trouble persists for more than six weeks urethroscopy and the passage of a sound is essential to exclude a pre-existing urethral stricture.

PROSTATITIS

Treatment is unsatisfactory but the best method seems to be a prolonged course of tetracycline accompanied by weekly or even biweekly prostatic massage for about 6 or 8 weeks. Some cases seem to respond after a holiday. Alcohol and sexual activity should be eschewed as long as there is any evidence of active infection.

REITER'S DISEASE

Reiter's disease which consists of urethritis, arthritis and eye manifestations sometimes associated with skin and buccal eruptions presents a difficult problem. The urethritis must be treated on the lines already indicated. Bed rest is advisable and where acute arthritis is present, immobilisation is advisable often using a pillow in the early stages. Later on a bi-valved plaster may be helpful. Nevertheless complete immobilisation is inadvisable as this over a period may lead to a stiff joint. If the joint is very distended with fluid, especially the knee, aspiration with steroid replacement may be helpful or delayed resolution over a period exceeding a month is another indication for this treatment. Phenylbutazone in a minimum dosage of 400 mg daily (100 mg four times daily) seems to have a slightly specific effect and to be better than other analgesics but the occurrence of blood dyscrazias must be remembered. Steroid therapy seems to be disappointing but in acute cases that persist for more than a month it may be tried in a dosage equivalent to 40 mg of prednisone daily. If the eye is involved, irrigation may be required with bland drops for a simple conjunctivitis, but if an anterior uveitis is found, mydriatics and steroid therapy will be required and an ophthalmologist's advice should be sought. It should be remembered that Reiter's disease is not gonococcal arthritis. This latter is a rare suppurative arthritis and gonococci will be found in the joint fluid.

TRICHOMONIASIS

Trichomoniasis in both male and female is best treated with metronidazole (Flagyl) 200 mg 3 times a day for a week. Results are excellent and at least 85 per cent of patients are cured. In the event of failure the dosage may be doubled. In the female, failure is often due to reinfection from the male consort and although a few males show evidence of urethritis from this cause, the majority who are infected are symptomless carriers. If both partners are treated, sexual intercourse should be avoided until treatment is complete. In the event of complete failure, acetarsol pessaries, two morning and evening, may be employed in the female. In the male, only urethral irrigations will be effective, though nifuratel 200 mg 3 times a day by mouth may be tried first in the male – and also in the female together with pessaries. There is slight, as yet unpublished, evidence that Amphotericin B pessaries may have some effect against Trichomonas vaginalis but so far no treatment is the equal of metronidazole.

CANDIDIASIS

Candidiasis in both sexes is very troublesome. The most satisfactory treatment in the female is either with nystatin pessaries 1 morning and evening for at least two weeks – there is some evidence that reinfection may occur from the rectum. If this is confirmed by the isolation of Candida albicans from the stools or from rectal swabs, or where such investigations are impracticable, when it is suspected, oral nystatin, 1 tablet four times a day for a week, is a useful adjuvant. Amphotericin B pessaries, 1 at night for 14 days, may also be effective as well as Candicidin. Sometimes it may be necessary to continue treatment for at least two months and to use any or all of these remedies in quick succession. In the male, urethral irrigations used to be required as nystatin which is not absorbed from the alimentary tract, is ineffective but it appears that nifuratel given by mouth may be effective in some of the few cases of male urethritis due to this cause.

When there is local inflammation, either vulvitis in the female or balanoposthitis in the male, then nystatin cream may be helpful. In those rare cases when the male develops a hypersensitivity of the skin to an infection in the female partner, this may be suppressed by local steroid treatment but obviously elimination of the trouble in the female genital tract is the only permanent answer.

FEMALE CONTACTS OF MALE PATIENTS WITH NON-GONOCOCCAL URETHRITIS

Females should always be examined and if any lesion is found it should be treated on its merits. If only a cervicitis is found or nothing else, the particular treatment which has cured the male partner – usually a tetracycline – is the only logical step to take in the female. This may prevent reinfection of the male. Very often when recurrence occurs in the male it is due to an overlooked focus of infection – for example, a prostatitis or developing stricture.

CHANCROID

Chancroid or soft sore is not very common in the United Kingdom except in certain port clinics. The important thing here is to remember that the condition may coexist with syphilis and that syphilis cannot be excluded without three months observation following treatment, with repetition of blood tests to exclude it. Sulphonamides are usually effective in a course of five days or alternatively a daily injection of streptomycin, either alone or with sulphonamides for five days is curative. Tetracyclines may be used but these are better avoided on account of the possible masking of syphilis. If a bubo forms it will have to be drained and aspiration is the best treatment. Phagoedena, once so destructive, is never seen today, at least in the United Kingdom. It used to result in partial or complete gangrene of the penis.

LYMPHOGRANULOMA VENEREUM

This again is seen only in the major ports of the United Kingdom, but is common in many sub-tropical areas. Once the diagnosis has been established, treatment is required for a minimum of from 10 to 14 days. Sulphonamides may be used, full dosage for a week dropping to half dosage for the second week. Tetracyclines are also useful, 500 mg four times a day for from 10 to 14 days, or more recently triactyloleandamycin (Evramycin) in a similar dosage and in a certain series 11 out of 13 cases were permanently cured (Fluker 1963). If a bubo forms then aspiration will be required. Rectal stricture is sometimes seen in females and dilatation of this may be required, together of course, with the appropriate chemotherapy or antibiotic treatment. If one of the above remedies fails, then another should be tried and it will be extremely unlikely to meet a case resistant to all three.

GRANULOMA INGUINALAE

Antimony, once used, no longer has a place in treatment. Streptomycin intramuscularly is effective. A total of 20 g. is adequate in most cases, given over a period of 5 days. If a smaller and somewhat safer dosage is used, this is effective but slower. Tetracyclines are also effective – a dosage of 500 mg daily for 10 to 20 days being curative and probably safer than streptomycin but syphilis must be excluded before their use.

YAWS

Yaws does not occur in the United Kingdom in its natural form but latent cases are sometimes seen, in whom the diagnosis from syphilis is often extremely difficult. Normally this condition requires less penicillin than syphilis, but if treatment schedules similar to those of syphilis are given cure can be guaranteed and this amount of treatment is an additional safeguard in the event of an error of differential diagnosis between the two conditions.

CONDYLOMATOSIS OR GENITAL WARTS

The term 'venereal warts' is undesirable. These lesions are very common and are frequently transmitted by sexual intercourse. Consequently peri-anal lesions are common in male homosexuals. Treatment in both sexes in early cases is with the resin podophyllin which should be applied to the warts usually as a 25 per cent solution in spirit. Care should be taken to prevent the solution from burning the surrounding skin, and it should always be washed off after six hours. The warts turn white and usually after three or four reapplications will separate. Lesions on mucous membranes sometimes do better from the application of trichloracetic acid. If, however, the warts are particularly hard or very deep seated, local applications are ineffective and diathermy is required – usually under a local anaesthetic. Intravaginal or cervical warts in the female are better dealt with under general anaesthesia. Peri-anal or intra-rectal warts usually respond poorly to local applications and become exceedingly sore and tender. Much the best treatment is with repeated diathermy, preferably under a local anaesthetic. These lesions have a tendency to recur and although surgery under a general anaesthetic with admission to hospital may temporarily get rid of them, the limited follow up possible in the ordinary surgical outpatients is insufficient to prevent generalised recurrence, whereas, if they are dealt with a few at a time under local anaesthesia, the end results are often much superior. All predisposing causes such as trichomoniasis or candidiasis in the female should of course be removed.

References

Fluker, J. L., Hewitt, A. B., *Brit. J. Vener. Dis.* (1969), **45**, 317.
Fluker, J. L., *ibid.* (1963), **39**, 24.
Graciansky, P. de, and Grupper, U., *ibid.* (1961), **37**.
Moore, J. E., *ibid.* (1949), **25**, 169.
Siboulet, A., and Durel, P., *ibid.* (1961), **37**, 240.

This chapter was written by Dr J. L. Fluker (Consultant in Charge, Department of Sexually Transmitted Infection, Charing Cross Hospital Group. Consultant to the Home Office) and edited by Professor W. I. Cranston.

Category 8

The Nervous System

PARKINSON'S DISEASE

Drug treatment

The belladona alkaloids used for treating Parkinson's disease have now been replaced by a number of synthetic compounds with anticholinergic and antihistamine action. Benzhexol, orphenadrine, benztropine or methixene have a more specific central action and fewer peripheral atropine-like side effects. Benzhexol is a suitable initial treatment in a dose of 4 mg per day, increasing slowly to 24 mg until maximum benefit is reached or side effects become troublesome (dry mouth, urinary retention, constipation, vertigo, confusion, hallucinations). There is usually a substantial relief of rigidity although tremor and akinesia are less affected. Tolerance varies greatly and if side effects are severe, the drug may be replaced wholly or partly by one of the above alternatives. Anticholinergic drugs should be given with caution in the presence of glaucoma or prostatic enlargement and sudden withdrawal of drugs should be avoided because it may provoke a Parkinsonian crisis. When tremor is the principal symptom, methixene 15–60 mg/day may be more effective than benzhexol.

Tremor is made worse by nervous tension and a simple sedative, phenobarbitone 60 mg per day or chlordiazepoxide 10 mg per day may be used in times of stress. The beta-adrenergic blocking agent proppanolol (90 mg per day) also has a beneficial effect on tremor in some patients, although the majority are little helped.

L-Dopa has received much recent attention and is still being evaluated. It has an undoubted beneficial effect in many patients, including severe cases, and those unresponsive to other drugs. Akinesia, dysphonia, dysphagia and oculogyric crises, which respond poorly to other treatments, may be dramatically relieved. Mental confusion and dementia are not helped and may be aggravated. The dose is 2–10 g. daily. Post-encephalitic cases respond to, and tolerate, a smaller dose. Nausea and vomiting are frequent side effects. Others include choreoathetosis and postural hypotension. L-Dopa may be used in combination with other drugs except methixine which is contraindicated because of its monoamine oxidase inhibitor action.

The dose of hypotensive drugs may need to be reduced.

Surgical treatment. Stereotaxic lesions in the thalamus may abolish or lessen Parkinsonian tremor in the contralateral limbs without loss of voluntary power and is the treatment of choice in patients with disabling unilateral tremor. Substantial improvement is usually obtained although the tremor may reappear again in a mild form after some months and the disease appears to progress as before. Elderly patients with bilateral disease, dysphagia, dysphonia, dementia or severe disturbances of equilibrium respond poorly to operation. The operative morbidity and mortality is considerably increased in hypertensive patients.

General measures. Immobility, tremor, excessive salivation and difficulty with speech often give a false impression of dementia. Every effort should be made to keep the patient mobile and at work, though writing and tasks involving manual dexterity become increasingly difficult. Physiotherapy can be most useful in treating patients with disturbances of equilibrium and gait and in those with a progressive flexion dystonia.

Although many patients with Parkinson's disease become moderately or severely incapacitated within 5 years of onset, sometimes the disorder remains static and well controlled for many years. Patients often become depressed soon after diagnosis and require reassurance that neither mental deterioration nor rapidly progressive invalidism need ensue. Additional drug treatment for depression may be required.

OTHER INVOLUNTARY MOVEMENTS

Familial tremor responds best to alcohol but there is a considerable hazard of addiction. Mephenesin 0.5–2 g. per day or diazepam 5–20 mg/day may also give some relief.

Sydenham's chorea is often adequately controlled with phenobarbitone but chlorpromazine hydrochloride 50–150 mg/day may be used if the movements are more violent.

Chlorpromazine is also used in larger dose (100–300 mg/day) in the treatment of the early stages of hemiballismus. The dose can be reduced as the involuntary movements become less. Hemiballismus also responds, sometimes dramatically, to tetrabenazine 150 mg/day. Tetrabenazine 50–150 mg/day is becoming increasingly used to control the movements of choreoathetosis and Huntington's chorea and in the treatment of dystonic states such as blepharospasm, torsion dystonia, phenothiazine induced dystonia and writer's cramp.

EPILEPSY

General management

Epilepsy may occur in a structurally normal brain or be secondary to brain damage. In both groups suppression of epileptic activity is necessary, combined in the latter group with removal of the primary cause if possible. In constitutional epilepsy seizures usually begin in early childhood or adolescence, occasionally in adult life. Fever or intercurrent illness often provoke seizures in predisposed children. There is a tendency for epileptic seizures to disappear as the child matures but about one third of childhood epileptics continue to have seizures in adult life.

Seizures vary greatly in type and frequency and in the ease with which they may be controlled. In many severe cases, abolition of seizures is not practical short of a dose of anticonvulsants which would render the patient continuously drowsy or ataxic. Many epileptics become aware of factors which provoke attacks, such as drowsiness, lack of sleep, fever, visual flicker, nervous tension, premenstrual fluid-retention and alcohol. Others recognize abnormalities of mood, headache or involuntary myoclonic jerking as a prelude to an attack. Mental deterioration when it occurs is due to coincident brain disease or to the effects of head injury, asphyxia and drug overdose.

Grand mal

Anticonvulsant treatment should be initiated in patients having repeated seizures. A start is made with a small dose increasing slowly to the limit of tolerance or until seizures are controlled. It is unprofitable to change the drug régime too frequently. Anticonvulsant treatment should be continued at full dose for at least two years after cessation of seizures. It may then be gradually withdrawn. Sudden withdrawal of anticonvulsant or addictive drugs may provoke status epilepticus. Phenobarbitone is the initial drug of choice for most types of epilepsy. The dose is 30 to 150 mg per day in divided doses according to age. If control is unsatisfactory sodium phenytoin 50 mg to 300 mg per day is added. Primidone 250 mg to 1500 mg per day may be used as a substitute for phenobarbitone and in combination with sodium phenytoin. The combination of primidone and phenobarbitone is apt to lead to excessive drowsiness.

Temporal lobe seizures of psychomotor type may respond poorly to phenobarbitone; the combination of sodium phenytoin with a tranquillizing drug such as diazepam or chlordiazepoxide may be effective. Sulthiame is a sulphonamide derivative advocated for psychomotor seizures or for resistant grand mal; the dose is 100 to 600 mg daily and it may be combined with other anticonvulsants. Phenuride (dose 200–1000 mg daily) is an acetylurea derivative which is usually reserved for grand mal or temporal lobe seizures resistant to other drugs and it is most effective when combined with other anticonvulsants. Carbamazepine is another drug with anticonvulsant properties which may be used alone or in combination in cases of unresponsive fits in a dose of 400 to 1000 mg a day.

Petit mal

In this common variety of childhood epilepsy, the drug of choice is ethosuximide, given initially in a dose of 500 mg per day, increasingly slowly to 1·5 g. Since suxinimide drugs alone may increase the tendency to convulsive seizures it is best combined with phenytoin.

Surgical treatment of epilepsy

Surgical excision of a localised cortical epileptogenic focus in the temporal lobe may be considered when seizures are poorly controlled by medication and when repeated E.E.G. examinations show a persistent epileptic focus in a localised and accessible part of a temporal lobe, preferably in the non-dominant hemisphere.

Status epilepticus

Failure to recover consciousness between seizures adds considerably to the dangers of epilepsy and immediate hospital treatment is required. Special attention is directed at maintaining a clear air way, at stopping seizures and at preventing hyperpyrexia and cerebral oedema. For first aid treatment, an immediate injection of a soluble barbiturate (sodium phenobarbitone 400 mg intramuscularly), may be given but is often ineffective. Continued use of barbiturates runs the risk of respiratory depression and one or more of the following drugs are to be preferred.

(a) Slow intravenous injection of diazepam, 10 mg repeated every 15 mins up to 400 mg. Increasing tolerance and a reversible leucopenia may occur if the drug is continued for more than a few days at high dose.

(b) Intramuscular injection of paraldehyde 10 ml.

(c) Intravenous infusion of paraldehyde, 5 ml in 500 ml saline by slow drip.

(d) Intravenous injection of diphenylhydantoin 250–500 mg (not exceeding 50 mg/minute).

Should seizures continue, the patient may be anaesthetised for a short time using an intravenous barbiturate anaesthetic agent such as thiopentone and maintaining adequate oxygenation. Raised intracranial pressure is treated by lumbar puncture and cerebral oedema by the injection of dexamethasone 4 mg I.M. Although status epilepticus may continue for some days, the condition is self limiting and eventual recovery occurs provided brain damage does not occur as a complication of coma. For this reason in intractable cases, muscular paralysis may be induced with curare while artificial positive pressure respiration is maintained. Treatment may be continued for some days while anticonvulsants are administered in the usual dose. An E.E.G. is used to monitor cerebral epileptic activity. Continuous minor or focal epilepsy may be more difficult to control but does not present the same danger to life and the dose of anticonvulsants may in these cases be increased more slowly.

CEREBRAL VASCULAR DISEASE

Indications for treatment. The arterial disorder underlying most common types of vascular disease is atheroma, a process causing fibrous and fatty change in the intima of large and medium sized arteries. These changes may be aggravated by hypertension, which in addition causes thickening and degeneration of small arteries and arterioles. Deposition of platelets on roughened arterial surface initiates thrombosis and the resultant mixed thrombus may occlude the vessel or become organised and incorporated into an atheromatous lesion.

By the time symptoms of cerebral ischaemia develop, atheromatous degeneration is usually widespread and probably irreversible by medical treatment, although it might possibly have been prevented by treatment early in life. In occlusive vascular disease treatment may be directed at prevention of fibrin formation and of hypertension. Fibrinolytic therapy is not used at present in the cerebral circulation due to the risk of allergic reactions and of haemorrhage, and drugs acting on platelet aggregation are now being evaluated.

Transient cerebral ischaemia

This common symptom has a number of causes including recurrent embolism from heart or arterial wall, systemic hypotension or diminished cardiac output, diversion of blood to extracerebral tissues, or hypertensive vascular spasm. Either anaemia or polycythaemia may also predispose to its occurrence. Since attacks are rarely observed, it is often impossible to be certain of the aetiology. Assessment of treatment is also difficult, since attacks often cease spontaneously. Only about 50 per cent of patients develop a completed 'stroke'. Prognosis is better in the vertebrobasilar territory than in the carotid territory.

Arteriography is recommended for recurrent ischaemic attacks within the carotid territory, unless there is severe hypertension, widespread vascular disease or advanced age.

If a localised accessible carotid stenosis is found, endarterectomy abolishes attacks in the great majority of patients. Visualisation of the other carotid artery or of all the other extracranial arteries is advisable before operation. Arteriography is not routinely undertaken for vertebrobasilar ischaemia unless there is clinical evidence of common carotid, innominate or subclavian occlusion.

Anticoagulant treatment with coumarin drugs (dose controlled by regular prothrombin estimations) effectively abolishes or reduces transient attacks although the incidence of completed or fatal stroke is not materially altered. Anticoagulant treatment for a period of 12 months is recommended for all patients with transient ischaemia who are unsuitable for surgery and who have no medical contraindications (peptic ulcer, liver disease). Many common drugs (e.g. aspirin) may change the required dose of anticoagulants.

Patients having transient ischaemic attacks from bland embolism in association with chronic rheumatic carditis require continuous anticoagulant treatment indefinitely unless the cardiac lesion is surgically corrected, when this treatment may, sometimes be discontinued.

Attacks associated with transient hypertension or hypotension should be treated by appropriate regulation of blood pressure. Iatrogenic postural hypotension is commonly due to sedative or psychotropic drugs. Successful treatment of anaemia, dysproteinaemia or cardiac failure may also result in the cessation of attacks of cerebral ischaemia.

Major stroke

Stroke in evolution. In some patients the neurological deficit produced by ischaemia may evolve slowly over hours or days. The cause is usually an extension of arterial thrombosis, often in the carotid artery, or the development of cerebral oedema. Rapid and early anticoagulant treatment should be given and continued for 6 months as this has been shown to improve prognosis. If brain swelling or raised intracranial pressure is suspected, dexamethasone 2–4 mg intramuscularly may be given in the acute stage. A stroke in evolution may be difficult to distinguish from subdural or intracerebral haematoma or from cerebral tumour, all of which require surgical treatment. Arteriography and C.S.F. examination may be necessary to exclude other non-vascular lesions but the results of surgery on the carotid artery during the acute phase are poor.

Completed stroke. In most patients, the onset of cerebral infarction is rapid and the condition has stabilised before admission to hospital. Nothing can be done at present to restore ischaemic cerebral damage or the patency of occluded intracerebral arteries. Treatment is aimed at prevention of complications, by ensuring adequate air-way, oxygen therapy (if cyanosis is present) prophylactic antibiotics and physiotherapy for chest infection. Vasodilators, such as 5 per cent CO_2 inhalation, increase blood flow to normal brain but probably not to infarcted areas. There is no evidence that they are beneficial. If consciousness is depressed attention to hyperpyrexia, water and electrolyte balance, nutrition, and the care of the skin and bladder are necessary. Anticoagulants are of no value in preventing further strokes except in cases of embolism from the left atrium, when treatment should be started one week after the stroke and continued indefinitely. Anticoagulants may however, decrease the incidence of venous thromboembolism in bedridden patients during the acute phase. In all patients surviving a completed stroke, early ambulation and physiotherapy are encouraged.

Hypertensive vascular disease

Patients with chronic hypertension tend to suffer multiple minor strokes, often mistaken for transient ischaemic attacks. Unlike the latter, the effect is cumulative and the end result is a state of dementia, pseudobulbar palsy, with bilateral pyramidal and extrapyramidal signs. Early treatment of severe hypertension is recommended in the hope of arresting the underlying arteriolar degeneration. Severe episodes of hypotension should be avoided since cerebral ischaemia may be aggravated but in general the dangers of treating high blood pressure in the presence of cerebral vascular disease appear to have been overestimated. Although vasodilator drugs such as cyclandelate may cause short term increase in cerebral blood flow, they are of doubtful value in the treatment of chronic cerebrovascular disease.

Subarachnoid haemorrhage

Subarachnoid haemorrhage usually arises from rupture of an aneurysm near the Circle of Willis. Less common causes are leakage of a cerebral arteriovenous malformation, subarachnoid extension of intracerebral haemorrhage, rupture of a small hypertensive artery, paroxysmal hypertension (which may be drug induced) or head trauma. In some cases no causes can be found. In aneurysm cases, there is a large initial mortality (approximately 40 per cent) due to cerebral compression and oedema. Such patients die within 6–48 hours and no treatment is available beyond routine care of coma. Conscious patients and those whose condition is stable or improving after 48 hours require full arteriographic investigation to identify the bleeding aneurysm. A number of surgical techniques are available, such as ligation of the carotid or parent intracerebral artery, trapping, clipping or wrapping the aneurysm and evacuation of intracerebral haematoma. All procedures carry some risk and this must be weighed against the dangers of re-bleeding. The incidence of death from a second haemorrhage is considerable during the first two weeks, thereafter diminishes rapidly and is relatively small after six weeks. In general, in patients seen within two weeks and having aneurysm of the distal carotid or posterior communicating artery, treatment is by carotid ligation or by direct surgical treatment of the aneurysm. Middle cerebral aneurysms are treated by direct surgery and anterior communicating aneurysms by proximal clip or by wrapping. In patients surviving for two weeks after bleeding and in patients with no demonstrable aneurysm, conservative treatment is indicated. This entails at least one month of strict bed rest with hypotensive therapy if chronic hypertension is present.

Subdural haemorrhage

The chronic evolution of a subdural haematoma is thought to result from venous bleeding following minor head trauma and is commonest in elderly patients. Treatment is by surgical evacuation with removal of the surrounding membrane.

Intracerebral haemorrhage

Spontaneous intracerebral haemorrhage occurs almost only in hypertensive patients and arises from rupture of small intracerebral arteries in the basal ganglia, cerebellum, pons or hemisphere white matter. Bleeding is less rapid than in subarachnoid haemorrhage. Some haemorrhages remain small and localised but the majority extend into the subarachnoid space.

Immediate treatment. In hemisphere or pontine bleeding, death in 6–48 hours is frequent. There is no indication for early surgical treatment; supportive care of comatose patients is instituted. In patients who show no further deterioration after 72 hours arteriography is undertaken to find the size and situation of haematoma. If no spontaneous improvement occurs or if signs of raised intracranial pressure develop, surgical evacuation of the haematoma may be indicated if in an accessible situation (e.g. subcortical white matter). In suspected cerebellar haemorrhage, radiological investigation is recommended, since early surgical evacuation improves prognosis.

Cranial Arteritis

In this variety of vascular disease the external rather than the internal carotid branches are affected. The disorder is painful but usually recovers completely; involvement of the arteries to the optic nerve or retina (arising from the ophthalmic artery) may, however, lead to permanent visual impairment. It is always desirable to confirm the diagnosis by biopsy of a temporal artery but treatment should be given immediately since in some patients visual complications may be prevented. Prednisone is started at high dose, 40 mg per day, and the dose is reduced at weekly intervals by 5 mg. Relief of headache and muscle pain is rapid. The maintenance dose should be the smallest dose which adequately controls symptoms and keeps the sedimentation rate within normal limits. It may be necessary to continue treatment for many months and sometimes for years. Proximal muscle pain and weakness may be caused both by giant cell arteritis (polymyalgia rheumatica) and by corticosteroid treatment, so that it may be difficult to know whether to increase or decrease the dose should these symptoms develop.

MIGRAINE

General management. It is helpful to explain to the patient with migraine that the pain originates in over-reactive blood vessels and that liability to attacks will continue throughout life, although becoming less pronounced after middle age. Many patients discover provoking factors such as nervous tension, physical exertion, pre-menstrual fluid retention, ingestion of alcohol or certain foods such as cheese or chocolate, and learn to avoid them. Oral contraceptive drugs may produce migraine for the first time, or may provoke attacks in a migrainous subject.

Migraine usually disappears during pregnancy. Migraine is essentially a paroxysmal condition, and seldom causes continuous or daily headaches. When such headaches occur in a migrainous subject, there is usually a super-imposed anxiety or depressive reaction, requiring separate treatment. Migraine sufferers are often intelligent and conscientious; they are also suggestible and a placebo effect is common with any new remedy.

Treatment of the attack. Mild attacks respond to simple analgesics, such as soluble aspirin. Attacks of moderate severity may often be terminated by an ergotamine preparation, ergotamine tartrate, 2–4 mg sublingually, or a compound tablet (of ergotamine, 1 mg, caffeine 100 mg) by mouth. If severe nausea is present, a combination of ergotamine with an antihistamine is indicated; ergotamine tartrate 2 mg, caffeine 100 mg, cyclizine HCL 50 mg. In a severe attack an injection of ergotamine tartrate, 1 mg subcutaneously or a suppository containing ergotamine may be effective. All preparations are much more efficacious if taken early in an attack. Prostration, faintness, nausea and photophobia and drowsiness are features of some migraine attacks, and necessitate the patient lying down in a dark room. Sleep should be encouraged in severe attacks since the pain usually disappears on waking.

Prevention of attacks. Frequent attacks are best prevented by regular administration of a small dose of ergotamine combined with a sedative. A suitable preparation is ergotamine 0·3 mg, belladonna alkaloids 0·1 mg, phenobarbitone 20 mg. When headaches wake the patient from sleep the drug should be taken on retiring. Long term daily treatment with ergotamine requires careful supervision but small quantities are taken daily without ill effect by large numbers of patients. Some patients are sensitive to the drug and any suggestion of digital artery spasm is a contraindication to its use.

Methysergide, a potent antagonist of serotonin, has recently been introduced as a preventative drug in patients suffering frequent disabling attacks. The drug may relieve headache unresponsive to ergotamine preparation, but general or long-term use is not recommended because of side effects. These occur in about 20 per cent of patients and can be severe (arterial occlusions, retro-peritoneal or retro-pleural fibrosis, vertigo, vomiting). Sudden withdrawal may provoke severe headache. The dose is 1–2 mg daily up to a maximum of 6 mg, and it may be used in combination with ergotamine.

Migrainous neuralgia

Attacks of migrainous neuralgia often occur in groups separated by long intervals of freedom. The most effective treatment is preventative, using a compound ergotamine preparation as for migraine. Most attacks are nocturnal and the drug is effective taken in the evening by mouth or by suppository. About every week or so the drug is stopped to ascertain whether treatment is still necessary. Methysergide may also be prescribed for resistant cases (dose 2–4 mg taken at night).

HERPETIC NEURALGIA

Root pain and hyperaesthesia commonly occur at the time of the skin eruption in herpes zoster. There is evidence that corticotrophin 40 units/day for 5 days not only eases these symptoms but may lessen the incidence of post herpetic neuralgia.

Severe constant, spontaneous pain and cutaneous hyperaesthesia are features of this intractable condition. Non-narcotic analgesics such as aspirin, paracetamol (1,000 mg per day), dextropropoxyphene (250 mg per day), mefenamic acid (1,000 mg per day) may give relief. The narcotic analgesics are best avoided, because of the risk of addiction. Local peripheral nerve block with procaine or phenol is sometimes helpful for a limited period. Cutaneous vibratory treatment which has a temporary anaesthetising effect on nerve endings may alleviate hyperaesthesia. Patients with post-herpetic neuralgia are often obsessional and depressed, and may be helped more by anti-depressive than by analgesic treatment. Phenelzine 30–45 mg/day with chlordiazepoxide 20 mg per day (and with the appropriate dietary restrictions) is recommended. Herpes zoster may be symptomatic of an underlying neoplastic or lymphomatous lesion.

TRIGEMINAL NEURALGIA

In this condition which occurs almost always in the elderly, attacks of severe lancinating pain occur in one or more divisions of the trigeminal nerve on one side; pain is provoked by touching the skin, eating and by cold. Attacks are episodic and long periods of freedom occur. In repeated attacks the pain remains unilateral but may spread to affect other divisions of the nerve. General measures include the avoidance of precipitating factors and the treatment of super-added affective disorder. Mild attacks may be helped by simple analgesics but in most cases the specific remedy, carbamazepine, is still required. This is given orally 200 mg per day in divided doses, increasing if necessary slowly to 1,000 mg per day, or until toxic effects occur (ataxia, drowsiness, nausea, skin rashes). Rapid suppression of severe pain occurs although a mild sensation may continue. The dose is maintained at the minimum level which will suppress symptoms; it is unwise to continue treatment for longer than six months because of the danger of granulopenia. The drug does not prevent future relapses.

If no relief occurs, surgical treatment may be necessary. This consists of alcoholic injection of the trigeminal ganglion or division of its sensory root. This produces a permanent cure, but the patient should be warned of loss of facial sensation which ensues.

POLYNEURITIS

Symmetrical lesions of motor and sensory peripheral nerve fibres, the maximum damage falling on the longest fibres, comprise a common syndrome of multiple aetiology. In general terms the prognosis is favourable if the underlying cause can be remedied, since in many cases axons survive, the blocking of conduction being due to segmental demyelination. Remaining fibres may slowly regenerate and peripheral sprouting may re-inervate denervated muscles.

The metabolic peripheral neuropathies of diabetes, polyarteritis nodosa or rheumatoid disease, uraemia or porphyria improve with control of the underlying disease.

Toxic peripheral neuropathy caused by drugs usually responds to prompt withdrawal of the drug, but the neural damage may be permanent (as in thalidomide neuropathy). Drugs interfering with metabolic pathways and producing an induced deficiency may require supplementary treatment (e.g. pyridoxin in isoniazid neuropathy). Neuropathy from heavy metal poisoning may require specific treatment with penicillamine.

In deficiency states neuropathy can in theory be due to lack of a number of B vitamins (thiamine, nicotinamide, pantothenic acid) alone or in combination with alcoholism. In practice, multiple deficiency is always present and large doses of a multiple vitamin preparation are recommended, with parenteral therapy in acute cases. In genetically determined neuropathy (peroneal muscular atrophy, hereditary sensory neuropathy, Dejerine-Sottas neuropathy) the course is usually slowly progressive and unresponsive to treatment. A possible exception is Refsum's disease where the accumulation of an abnormal metabolite (phytanic acid) may possibly be improved by dietary means.

Acute infective polyneuritis

Acute infective polyneuritis is a self-limiting, rapidly progressive, predominantly motor neuropathy which may complicate a number of infectious fevers, immune reactions, or may occur in isolation. A major advance in treatment has been the management of respiratory complication by mechanically assisted ventilation and by preventing the inhalation of pooled pharyngeal secretions. Establishment of an adequate airway is the first requirement. Involvement of the respiratory or pharyngeal nerves may necessitate tube feeding, tracheostomy and assisted respiration and regular chest physiotherapy and bronchial aspiration for adequate ventilation and to prevent pulmonary collapse and infection. A vital capacity of less than one litre, the recurrence of restlessness or cyanosis due to hypercapnia or hypoxia are indications for tracheostomy. Pooled pharyngeal secretions are aspirated regularly and a cuffed tracheostomy tube is a further safeguard against inhalation.

There is some evidence that steroids (prednisone 40 mg a day) or corticotrophin (A.C.T.H. 40 units per day) may improve the prognosis. A short two week course of treatment is recommended. Although the majority even of severe cases recover, and assisted respiration should be continued for months if necessary, a few patients show irreversible denervation. The disease may also follow a chronic relapsing course.

General measures in severe polyneuritis

1. Paralysis and sensory loss necessitate careful positioning and frequent turning to prevent pressure sores.
2. Urinary retention may require an in-dwelling catheter and continuous drainage, combined with a high fluid intake and sulphonamide treatment to minimise urinary infection and stone formation.
3. Loss of weight and muscle wasting is often severe; a high-caloric and protein diet is required during recovery.
4. Limb pain in early stages is often severe and may require pethidine (50 mg I.M.). It should be used with caution because of the dangers of respiratory depression.
5. Electrolyte disturbances, especially potassium deficiency, may complicate steroid therapy.
6. Daily passive exercises and light splinting may be needed to prevent contractures, especially of the tendo-achilles.
7. Hallucinations and affective disturbances may be due to paralysis and sensory deprivation, to drugs and to the environment of the intensive care unit.

8. Autonomic disturbances such as absent sweating and baroceptor reflexes occur frequently. Orthostatic hypotension and syncope are preventable by appropriate positioning of the patient and by leg bandages.

VITAMIN B_{12} DEFICIENCY

The neurological damage produced by deficient vitamin B_{12} affects peripheral nerves, spinal cord, optic nerves and cerebral hemispheres. Cases presenting with neurological involvement frequently have no anaemia although the bone marrow is megaloblastic. Treatment is begun urgently as soon as the diagnosis is established since spinal cord damage may progress rapidly, and is often irreversible. A daily injection of 1,000 μg hydroxocobalamin is given for two weeks. The same dose is then given twice weekly and continued until no further improvement occurs. The dose is then gradually reduced. For maintenance therapy, a single injection of 1,000 μg every three to four weeks is adequate.

There is usually an immediate improvement in general well-being and mental symptoms. Distal sensory loss, paraesthesiae and optic nerve symptoms improve more slowly. Symptoms indicative of cord damage such as sphincter disturbance may show little change. Occasional patients show sensitivity to hydroxocobalamin and cyanocobalamin may be substituted. A high-protein diet with supplements of other vitamins is advisable. In cases of optic neuropathy, tobacco and excess of alcohol are contraindicated.

MULTIPLE SCLEROSIS AND PARAPLEGIA

Only supportive and palliative treatment is available for multiple sclerosis but the acute episodes of focal demyelination, e.g. retrobulbar neuritis, and partial spinal cord lesions, show a strong tendency to full symptomatic recovery. No treatment may be necessary if the patient already shows evidence of improvement, but if the condition is deteriorating or showing no spontaneous resolution, within a few days, corticotrophin in high dose (60 units per day for 1 week; 30 units per day for 1 week) may accelerate recovery, although prognosis and future relapses are probably unaffected. Cases with cerebellar or vestibular disorder respond poorly to treatment. There is no evidence that long-term corticotrophin treatment is of value.

Treatment of chronic multiple sclerosis. Paraplegia with ataxia and variable sensory loss is a common end result of many types of pathology in the spinal cord. Treatment aims at reducing spasticity and flexor spasms, preventing contractures, pressure sores and urinary complications.

Spasticity. This results from heightened reflex activity of spinal fusimotor neurones following removal of the inhibitory influences of pyramidal and extra-pyramidal pathways. Drugs having a depressant effect on synaptic activity at cord or brain stem level such as diazepam 5–20 mg per day, mephenesin 0·5 g. to 2 g. per day, meprobamate 800–1600 mg per day, and tigloidine hydrobromide 1,000–2,000 mg per day may be used. In general, the effects are slight and disappear on continued treatment. Drowsiness and ataxia are troublesome side effects. Best results are obtained with diazepam and by temporarily substituting another drug when this loses its initial effectiveness.

In cases retaining moderate voluntary power but disabled by spasticity or flexor spasms reduction of reflex activity by chemical damage to sensory and motor roots may improve motility. Cases with unilateral spasticity are most suitable. 1 ml of phenol 5 per cent in glycerine is injected intrathecally in the appropriate region with careful positioning of the patient. Some cutaneous sensory loss may result but is seldom severe. Sphincter disturbance may be aggravated if lower sacral segments are damaged.

Contractures are best prevented by frequent passive movements, by measures to combat spasticity and by suitable positioning in bed; avoiding flexion at the hip and knee and extension at the ankle; established contractures may require surgical treatment. Active muscle exercises are of great value at all stages; standing and walking between bars encourages the development of tone in anti-gravity muscles, and discourages a tendency to flexion. Patients may also develop useful movement by employing muscles above the level of the lesion.

Avoidance of urinary infection largely determines the length of survival of the paraplegic patient. Aseptic catheterisation, (e.g. by 'no-touch' technique) in the early stages is essential. Spastic or mechanical outflow obstruction renders the infection of residual urine almost inevitable, and may be relieved by surgical treatment in suitable cases.

MUSCLE DISEASES

Myasthenia Gravis

The intermittent course of the disorder makes the assessment of treatment difficult. The aim is to give sufficient anticholinesterase drugs to enable the patient to lead a normal life, though it is seldom possible to restore full muscle power. Excessive dose of anticholinesterase may itself cause muscle weakness and muscles in different parts of the body may show varying degrees of responsiveness. Relapses are often caused by intercurrent infection. Hyperthyroidism is frequently associated with myasthenia gravis and requires separate treatment. A myasthenic syndrome usually responding poorly to anticholinesterase may occur with oat-cell carcinoma of the bronchus.

The most widely used drug is Neostigmine bromide 15 mg by mouth 2 to 12 times daily. The period of action is up to 4 hours and if necessary the longer acting Pyridostigmine 60–120 mg, one to four times daily may be added. Abdominal colic if troublesome may be relieved by oral Atropine 0.6 mg. In some cases a potentiating effect is found by adding Ephedrine 15 mg to each dose of Neostigmine. Good results sometimes follow the use of Corticotrophin or Corticosteroids given either as a 2-week course to induce a remission or on long term daily or on alternate days. Temporary deterioration may occur in the first few days of Corticotrophin treatment.

Assisted positive pressure respiration may be necessary in severe myasthenia, especially if a chest infection develops. If muscle weakness is due to over-treatment, a period of assisted respiration may restore responsiveness. Weakness in the limbs responds best to anticholinesterase drugs and the effect on ocular, facial and bulbar weakness is less satisfactory. If disability remains severe on full doses of anticholinesterase drugs after some months, or if increasing muscle weakness especially in respiratory or swallowing muscles becomes evident, a thymectomy should be considered. Response to the operation is best in young females with a short history of myasthenia. Purely ocular myasthenia may be little affected, and patients with malignant thymic tumours respond poorly to all forms of treatment.

Myositis

Suppression of the inflammatory process, relief of muscle pain and tenderness, and improvement of muscle power is usually possible with Corticosteroids. Treatment should begin at a large dose 40–60 mg/day, reducing over a few weeks to the smallest maintenance dose which gives relief of symptoms. Treatment may have to be continued for many months and side effects (peptic ulceration, vertebral collapse) are frequent. Skin lesions are little affected. A remission may occur, especially in children.

Muscle cramps, myotonia

An effective treatment for most types of nocturnal muscle cramp, irrespective of the cause, and for all types of myotonia, is Quinine Bisulphate 300–600 mg at night or t.i.d.

BACTERIAL MENINGITIS

Specific therapy is available for many of the varieties of bacterial meningitis and the isolation of the causative organism from C.S.F. or blood is the first objective. Early treatment is imperative and should be given as soon as cultures have been set up. Acute bacterial meningitis is most commonly caused by N. meningitidis, Str. pneumoniae or H. influenzae. Less common organisms are Group A streptococci, staphylococcus pyogenes, E. coli and Pseudomonas. In many cases no organisms can be isolated due to previous antibiotic treatment.

Pyogenic meningitis

In all types of pyogenic meningitis, the C.S.F. is turbid and under increased pressure. Hundreds or thousands of polymorphs are usually present (cell count is very variable) and protein content is moderately raised (100 to 600 mg); sugar is markedly reduced or absent.*

If the C.S.F. is turbid or purulent, it is reasonable to inject 10,000 units of benzyl penicillin intrathecally at the time of lumbar puncture. If organisms can be identified on the stained C.S.F. smear, appropriate antibiotic treatment should be commenced without delay. If no organisms are seen, the patient should be given either:

(a) Chloramphenicol 1–2 g. daily by mouth or intramuscularly, together with sulphadiazine 1–1·5 g. 4 hourly, or

(b) Ampicillin 16 g. daily I.V., and sulphadiazine 1–1·5 g. 4 hourly. When the results of C.S.F. culture are known, it may be necessary to change the regime. If no organisms are obtained on culture, but clinical improvement is seen, treatment should be continued for 7 days after clinical signs have settled. Once bacteria have been identified, the following dose schedules are appropriate for adults.

* Microscopic examination of the spun deposit of C.S.F. for organisms, which may be intracellular or extracellular, should always be carried out.

N. Meningitidis. Sulphadiazine 1–1·5 g. 4 hourly and penicillin 1 mega unit 6 hourly. Lumbar puncture will be required to check progress after about 48 hours, but in the uncomplicated case it is usually unnecessary to repeat it thereafter. Treatment should continue for 8–10 days.

Str. Pneumoniae. Either:

(a) Penicillin 4 mega units I.M. every 4 hours or;

(b) Penicillin 10–15,000 units intrathecally each day until 24 hours after the C.S.F. is sterile, and penicillin I.M., 1 mega unit 4 times daily. This infection is often associated with otitis media, sinusitis or acquired or congenital bone defects. These will require treatment. Frequent lumbar punctures will be required whichever treatment is used, to check the response to treatment and to detect relapses, which are relatively common. Treatment should in any event be continued for twenty-one days, or until all signs have settled for at least one week. Response to treatment is usually slow and cerebral abscess occurs more frequently than in other forms of meningitis.

H. Influenzae. Either:

(a) Chloramphenicol – 1·2 g. daily I.M. with sulphadiazine as above or

(b) Ampicillin 16 g. daily I.V. with sulphadiazine as above.

Treatment is continued for 14 days as fever responds more slowly to treatment than in meningococcal meningitis and a lymphocytic pleocytosis in the C.S.F. may also persist.

Other organisms. The treatment of meningitis due to other organisms will depend upon sensitivity tests; cooperation with the bacteriologist is essential. It may be necessary to employ cephaloridine, cloxacillin, gentamycin or carbenicillin in certain cases, particularly those following head injury or neurosurgery.

Other treatment. If vomiting and dehydration are severe, especially in infants, parenteral fluids may be required. Hypotension, coma or an extensive purpuric rash are indications for intravenous hydrocortisone 100 mg 3-hourly, supplemented by oral treatment. Young children and all patients with a history of epileptic seizures should be given phenobarbitone.

Tuberculous Meningitis

In all cases of meningitis with a lymphocytic cellular reaction, the C.S.F. should be examined and cultured for acid-fast bacilli. The cell count is variable (usually 25 to 500 per cubic mm), and C.S.F. sugar is in the range 20–40 mg per cent. Culture of tubercle bacilli takes several weeks and treatment cannot await the results of sensitivity tests. Bacilli may show a primary resistance to standard drugs or resistance may be acquired during treatment (secondary resistance).

This chapter was written by Dr R. W. Ross Russell (Consultant Neurologist, St Thomas's Hospital and The National Hospital for Nervous Diseases) and edited by Professor W. I. Cranston.

Category 9
Blood Disorders

Introduction

In this section no attempt has been made to consider all possible régimes of treatment for all recognised blood disorders. The principles of treatment of common or important conditions have been discussed and lines of treatment, based on these principles, have been suggested. Where appropriate key references have been given and these will give a lead into the more detailed or controversial aspects of therapy.

IRON DEFICIENCY

The background to treatment

Iron deficiency, though common, is easily mismanaged and treatment is perhaps most effectively based on an understanding of iron balance.

In the normal adult the body iron is distributed between the red cells (2,500 mg), the respiratory enzymes of somatic cells (600 mg) and the available iron store (800 mg). The normal daily loss (1·5 mg in men and 2·5 mg in menstruating women) is easily balanced by absorption from a normal diet which, in the United Kingdom for example, contains approximately 15 mg of iron.

The iron deficient patient certainly cannot absorb more than 10 mg of iron from such a diet and, since 20 ml of blood contains about 10 mg of iron, an average loss of more than 20 ml per day will establish negative iron balance with progressive store depletion and subsequent anaemia. Somatic cellular iron depletion with epithelial changes may be associated with the anaemia but, in a few patients, may precede it.

In iron deficiency absorption is enhanced and, although many variables alter the proportion of orally administered iron which is absorbed, the dose is, in the present context, the most important. With, for example, oral ferrous sulphate the compromise between maximal absorption and minimal intolerance is achieved with approximately 200 mg given three times daily. This will induce a net absorption of about 50–60 mg of elemental iron. Although these figures are only very approximate it can be calculated that absorption of this order will not only meet the demands of maximal possible erythropoiesis but will also balance iron depletion caused by any rate of blood loss which could be accepted as chronic rather than acute.

Against this background certain principles of treatment can be suggested.

Principles of treatment

Diagnosis. Except in situations where facilities for precise diagnosis are not available empirical administration of iron to anaemic patients should be avoided. In the absence of iron deficiency it is ineffective and in certain conditions, such as thalassaemia and sideroblastic anaemia, it may be harmful. It is perhaps even more important to emphasise that iron deficiency is inevitably the by-product of some primary disorder, such as chronic blood loss or malabsorption, and that recognition and treatment of the primary condition is often of more importance to the patient than treatment of the iron deficiency itself.

Management. In the anaemic iron-deficient patient effectively administered iron will be preferentially used for haemoglobin synthesis, the haemoglobin level will revert to normal and there may, therefore, be complete symptomatic improvement while the iron stores are still depleted. At this stage, in the absence of clear explanation and firm encouragement, there is a natural tendency for the patient to discontinue iron. In the patient in whom the cause of the iron deficiency has been removed this is of little importance since a state of positive iron balance will exist and the store and somatic cellular iron will be gradually repleted and maintained by normal absorption from a normal diet. In the patient who must continue in negative iron balance – for example the young woman with dysfunctional menorrhagia – discontinuation of therapy as the haemoglobin level returns to normal, with reversion to negative iron balance, is the commonest cause of recurrent iron deficiency. Such patients *must* be maintained on a continued iron supplement.

Since symptoms are probably not a valid index of marginal iron deficiency (Wood and Elwood, 1966) the effectiveness of maintenance should be checked by measurement of haemoglobin level and, if somatic iron deficiency without anaemia is suspected, by determination of serum iron and binding capacity after withdrawal of therapy for one week.

Failure to respond to adequate therapy in true deficiency is most commonly due to failure to take the iron but an associated infection or deficiency of B_{12} or folate should be excluded.

Choice of preparation

A very large number of effective iron preparations are available and only the principles of their use will be discussed.

1. Provided the dose is adequate the rate of response to any effective iron preparation is determined by the erythropoietic capacity of the marrow and not by the route of administration. Providing the patient does not suffer from a malabsorption syndrome oral therapy will produce as rapid a rise in haemoglobin as parenteral therapy.

2. There is little to support the view that sophisticated oral preparations reduce intolerance or that in practice additives, such as ascorbic acid, significantly increase absorption.

3. Combined preparations of iron and other haematinics have no place in therapy, except possibly in pregnancy where a combination of iron and folic acid is not illogical and may be convenient.

4. The vast majority of iron deficient patients can be effectively and inexpensively treated with oral ferrous sulphate (200 mg t.d.s.). Parenteral therapy, using iron dextran or iron sorbitol complexes intermittently or as total dose infusion (iron dextran), is relatively expensive, not without risk and should be reserved for patients who either cannot absorb oral iron, cannot be relied upon to take it or have genuine intolerance for oral preparations.

The whole subject is well reviewed by Bothwell and Finch (1962).

MEGALOBLASTIC ANAEMIA

Megaloblastic anaemias are almost invariably due to deficiency of vitamin B_{12} or folic acid or both. Adequate management requires an understanding of how these deficiencies can arise and also of the principles upon which diagnosis is based.

Causes of vitamin B_{12} or folic acid deficiency

Vitamin B_{12} is absorbed from the terminal ileum in the presence of intrinsic factor which is secreted by the gastric mucosa. Deficiency of this vitamin is almost always the result of impaired absorption; only rarely is it due to inadequate dietary intake. Defective absorption can arise because of:

1. Lack of intrinsic factor, as in pernicious anaemia.

2. Reduced absorptive capacity of ileal mucosa due to resection or mucosal disease (as in 'malabsorption syndromes').

3. Competition for vitamin B_{12} by intestinal parasites or bacteria (as in 'blind loop' syndromes).

Folic acid is absorbed from the duodenum and jejunum. Inadequate dietary intake is probably not uncommon (especially with prolonged cooking of foods) and will contribute to deficiency due to:

1. Increased demand for folic acid when cellular turnover is rapid, as in physiological states (e.g. pregnancy) or pathological conditions (e.g. chronic blood loss or malignancies).

2. Malabsorption syndromes (as above).

3. Administration of drugs (e.g. anticonvulsants or folic acid antagonists).

Diagnosis

Diagnosis depends first, on confirming that erythropoiesis is unequivocally megaloblastic, by examining the bone marrow, and secondly on establishing the nature and cause of the vitamin deficiency. The latter may be suggested by the clinical features but confirmation usually requires special investigations e.g. tests of vitamin B_{12} absorption, assay of serum B_{12} and folate, etc. (See Chanarin, 1969). The nature of the deficiency is confirmed by adequate clinical and haematological response to administration of the deficient vitamin.

Management

1. The cause of a deficiency should be eliminated if possible.

2. The deficiency should be corrected by administering the appropriate vitamin(s).

(a) *Vitamin B_{12}*, preferably in the form of hydroxocobalamin, is given by intramuscular injection. To replenish body stores and to obtain an optimal response 1,000 μg may be given on alternate days for four doses. Thereafter 500 to 1,000 μg should be injected weekly until the haemoglobin concentration becomes normal. Maintenance doses (e.g. 1,000 μg every two months) must be continued *for life* when the cause of the deficiency is irreversible, as in pernicious anaemia. There is no good evidence that neurological damage is more rapidly reversed by giving more vitamin B_{12} than is required to maintain full haematological remission.

(b) *Folic acid* is usually given orally (daily dose of 5 mg to 15 mg) but may be given intramuscularly to patients who are vomiting or for initiating treatment in malabsorptive states. Prophylactic administration in pregnancy is desirable, especially during the last trimester. The optimal dose in pregnancy is debatable but probably should not be less than the minimal daily requirement of 300 μg. Higher doses may be necessary in the presence of iron deficiency, intercurrent infections or multiple pregnancy.

3. *Choice of preparation.* 'Long-acting' preparations of vitamin B_{12} for maintenance therapy have no advantages over hydroxocobalamin, nor have expensive oral combinations of vitamin B_{12} and intrinsic factor which usually lose their effect. Folic acid may usefully be combined with iron for prophylactic treatment in pregnancy but indiscriminate use of multivitamin preparations containing folic acid is to be deplored since this may delay the diagnosis of vitamin B_{12} deficiency until irreversible neurological damage has occurred.

THE REFRACTORY ANAEMIAS

This is a heterogenous group of conditions which have in common an anaemia which, in the vast majority of patients, fails to respond to any specific therapy. The haemoglobin must therefore be maintained, often for long periods, by blood transfusion. A central part of effective treatment is the proper management of these repeated transfusions. The importance of non-traumatic infusion, preservation of veins, the selection and preparation of blood and the management of iron overload should be studied carefully (see references).

The treatment of anaemia of infection, chronic disease and renal failure is considered later and here it is only necessary to consider some specific points in the management of thalassaemia, sideroblastic anaemia and the aplastic anaemias.

Thalassaemia

Patients with thalassaemia 'minor' rarely need more than a correct diagnosis and the avoidance of transfusion and iron therapy.

While there are a few children with thalassaemia 'major' who can maintain haemoglobin levels between 6 and 7 g. per cent with infrequent transfusions the majority require regular transfusion from the age of six months. For well being and normal growth the haemoglobin should be kept above 8 g. per cent (Wolman, 1964) but the more transfusion is required to achieve this the more rapidly will the lethal effects of iron overload develop. Chelating agents should be used, but are disappointing (Sephton Smith, 1964). Splenectomy, which may produce a slight but valuable reduction in the transfusion requirement, should only be considered when some association of considerable splenomegaly, inadequate response to transfusion and symptomless thrombocytopenia indicate a hypersplenic state.

Folic acid deficiency is common and prophylactic folic acid (300 μg daily) should be given.

The sideroblastic anaemias

This is a heterogenous group (Mollin and Hoffbrand, 1968) and, while in many patients repeated transfusion becomes the only effective treatment, a proportion of patients respond to specific therapy. In the primary acquired group some, generally younger, patients will make complete and sustained response to continuous small doses of pyridoxine (1–50 mg daily). In others, larger doses of pyridoxine (100–600 mg daily) may, sometimes after many months, usefully modify transfusion requirements. Even in the absence of folate deficiency folic acid (5–10 mg daily) should be given and in all patients adequate trials of pyridoxine, folic acid, crude liver extract, ascorbic acid and niacin – singly or in combinations, should precede the acceptance of transfusion as the only effective treatment.

Among the secondary sideroblastic anaemias those due to drugs, such as PAS, isoniazid, cycloserine, pyrazinamide, phenacetin and paracetamol should respond to withdrawal of the drug or treatment with pyridoxine.

Acellular marrow failure (aplastic anaemia)

For obvious reasons a drug or environmental aetiology should be sought and excluded. Remission is rare and only occurs either spontaneously, as in some children at puberty, or in a small proportion of patients treated with anabolic steroids. Of these oxymethalone seems at present the most useful, having produced good responses in some cases (Sanchez Medal, 1964. Allen, Fine, Necheles and Damashek, 1968). Doses used have been between 2 and 6 mg/kg daily for up to two months. Therapy is continued at a lower dose if there is remission, for there is inevitably some virilisation.

In this group in particular the management of transfusion, infection and thrombocytopenia is important.

Pure red cell aplasia

Prednisone may be useful and the dose should be 40 to 60 mg daily in adults and approximately 2 mg/kg/day in children. The dose should be cut down rapidly after three or four weeks, although smaller maintenance doses may be needed if there is a response.

THE ANAEMIA OF INFECTION AND CHRONIC DISEASE

A considerable proportion of patients with prolonged, severe chronic infection or with chronic non-infective processes such as rheumatoid arthritis develop an anaemia. In most cases the anaemia is of production failure type with occasionally a mild haemolytic component. There is often an associated abnormality of iron metabolism which may prompt iron therapy (Cartwright, 1966). In fact, these anaemias are refractory to all specific therapy and even when there is a co-incidental cause of anaemia, such as true iron or folate deficiency, response to specific therapy will, in the presence of continued infection or chronic disease, be considerably or completely inhibited.

The treatment of this type of anaemia is the treatment of the primary disease and resolution of the chronic disease or infection is usually followed by a spontaneous rise in haemoglobin.

In certain situations, for example as a preparation for surgery or when anaemia is severe, transfusion may be necessary. In general, however, if a patient can, unaided, maintain a haemoglobin level around 9 g. per cent, attempts should not be made to maintain a transient normal haemoglobin level by repeated transfusion as this adds risk without conferring significant benefit.

HAEMOLYTIC ANAEMIA

Haemolytic anaemia may be due to intrinsic defects of the red cell, usually congenital, or to extrinsic causes, usually acquired. Most patients with chronic haemolytic anaemias establish an equilibrium whereby a satisfactory haemoglobin level is maintained by increased erythropoietic activity. Decompensation may occur if marrow activity is suppressed by infection and, therefore, all infections in patients with haemolytic anaemia should be treated vigorously. Folate depletion is likely to occur, especially if demands are increased, as by pregnancy, and although routine folate supplements are not indicated careful observation is needed to anticipate potential deficiencies. Iron is rarely required in haemolytic states, as increased erythropoietic activity stimulates iron absorption, and it should never be given without laboratory proof of iron deficiency because of the danger of iron overload. Blood transfusion should be avoided in chronic haemolytic anaemia unless decompensation occurs, because it disturbs the established equilibrium and may contribute to haemosiderosis.

INTRINSIC RED CELL DEFECTS

Congenital (excluding the haemoglobinopathies)

Of the many known congenital defects of the red cell, only two are of importance clinically, hereditary spherocytosis and glucose-6-phosphate dehydrogenase (G6PD) deficiency.

Hereditary spherocytosis

Most patients maintain acceptable haemoglobin levels in the absence of infection or pregnancy, but in occasional patients the condition may be either so severe that haemolysis is present at birth or so mild that it is discovered as an incidental finding in middle age. A frequent complication is biliary obstruction and cholangitis due to pigment stones. The only effective treatment is splenectomy which, although not curing the red cell defect, prevents their premature destruction. Elective splenectomy should be recommended in all patients but especially in those who are anaemic or who have had an aplastic crisis or who have pigment stones. The results are usually excellent, although the operation should, if possible, be deferred until after childhood as there is evidence of an increased rate of late septicaemia in splenectomised children.

Glucose-6-phosphate dehydrogenase (G6PD) deficiency

This disorder affects principally Negroes and the Mediterranean races but most subjects have no haemolysis unless treated with oxidant drugs; a list of the most important drugs is given in Table 1. Before a potentially G6PD deficient patient is given a high-risk drug, screening tests should, ideally, be performed on his red cells to exclude this defect (see Dacie, 1967a for details). If haemolysis occurs, it is usually self-limiting as only the older cell population is susceptible. No treatment is

Table 1

DRUGS IN CURRENT USE WHICH HAVE CAUSED HAEMOLYSIS IN G6PD DEFICIENT SUBJECTS

Antimalarials. Primaquine, chloroquine, dapsone.

Sulphonamides. Sulphadiazine, sulphadimidine, sulphamethoxypridazine, salicylazosulphapyridine.

Antibiotics etc. Chloramphenicol, nitrofurantoin.

Antipyretics. Phenacetin, aspirin.

Antituberculous drugs. Para-aminosalicylic acid, sodium salt (PAS).

Synthetic analogues. Synkavit (especially in newborn infants).

available apart from withdrawal of the drug and blood transfusion if indicated.

ACQUIRED

Paroxysmal nocturnal haemoglobinuria (PNH)

This rare disorder is the only known example of an acquired intrinsic red cell defect. At the present time, there is no specific treatment other than blood transfusion. Patients are often sensitive to transfused plasma which may accelerate haemolysis and in such cases red cells washed in saline should be used. Iron is rarely needed in patients receiving regular transfusions, and it should never be given without demonstration of iron deficiency as there is evidence that it exacerbates haemolysis. Splenectomy is of no value and the place of steroids has not been established, but if marrow aplasia is a feature the use of androgens is reasonable (see review by Dacie, 1967b).

Acquired haemolytic anaemia due to extrinsic causes

Haemolysis may be a complicating feature of many diseases, but as a rule, no specific treatment is indicated apart from treatment of the primary condition or blood transfusion. Only the treatment of the autoimmune and microangiopathic haemolytic anaemias will be discussed in detail here.

Autoimmune haemolytic anaemia (AIHA)

The AIHA's may be divided into 'warm' and 'cold' antibody types depending on the nature of the antibody. As the treatment is different in each case serological studies are essential. Either type may be primary and idiopathic or secondary to infectious disease, lymphoma, chronic lymphatic leukaemia, collagen disease, carcinoma or drugs. A thorough search for a primary cause should be made as the anaemia often responds to treatment of this condition.

'Warm' antibody type. The first line of treatment is corticosteroids. Prednisone, or equivalent, should be given in doses of up to 60 mg daily, depending on the severity of haemolysis. This dose should be reduced as rapidly as possible to a level which adequately controls the haemolysis. Most patients respond, although the antiglobulin test may remain positive. Some patients seem to benefit from the use of ACTH, although they fail to show improvement with synthetic steroids.

Blood transfusion should be avoided if possible as the donor cells are usually rapidly destroyed but blood should not be withheld if anaemia is endangering life. Serological investigations may reveal that the antibody has specificity, usually within the rhesus system, in which case it may be possible to select appropriate blood for transfusion.

If steroids fail to control the haemolysis, or if side effects limit their use, splenectomy should be considered. If significant splenic sequestration can be demonstrated by the use of Cr^{51} labelled red cells, splenectomy should certainly be recommended, but in severe cases it should be performed even in the absence of this evidence as most patients seem to benefit to some extent.

If the above measures fail to control the disease, immunosuppressive drugs should be tried. The data available at present on the use of these drugs in AIHA is inconclusive, but some patients with warm antibodies have undoubtedly improved. Most experience has been gained with azathioprine (Imuran) given in a dose of between 100–200 mgs daily. The present evidence suggests that these drugs should be used only after more conventional therapy has failed (Dacie and Worrledge, 1969).

'Cold' antibody type. AIHA of this type may complicate infections or may occur as a chronic disease in elderly people. The former are usually transitory and do not require treatment. Similarly, most patients with the chronic cold haemagglutinin disease need no treatment beyond protection from the cold. Cortico-steroids and splenectomy are of little value and are not recommended. Blood transfusion should be restricted as far as possible because donor cells are usually destroyed more readily than the patient's own cells. More success has been claimed for the use of immunosuppressive drugs in this condition,

and these drugs are probably the treatment of choice. Chlorambucil is the most widely used drug, the dose being from 2 to 4 mg per day.

Microangiopathic haemolytic anaemias

These anaemias are found in such conditions as the haemolytic-uraemic syndrome in children, malignant hypertension, eclampsia, thrombotic thrombocytopenic purpura, abruptio placentae and disseminated carcinoma. Haemolysis is the result of red cell fragmentation which is probably secondary to intravascular coagulation occurring in the small blood vessels. Treatment initially should be directed to the primary cause. The effective control of blood pressure and renal failure is particularly important. Anaemia should be corrected by blood transfusion. Cortico-steroids are of doubtful use, and may be contraindicated in intravascular coagulation. Recent evidence suggests that in severe cases the outlook is improved by heparin therapy which blocks further intravascular coagulation. Sufficient heparin must be given to produce a significant lengthening of the whole blood clotting time and the dose may need to be of the order of 10,000–20,000 units daily. (See reviews by Brain *et al.*, 1968, and Brain 1969.)

SICKLE-CELL DISEASE, HAEMOGLOBIN C DISEASE AND HAEMOGLOBIN E DISEASE

The collective term sickle-cell disease covers a number of related haematological states of widely varying clinical severity. All these conditions have in common the possession of sickle haemoglobin (Hb.S). Of these disorders sickle-cell anaemia is the most severe and results in about 80,000 deaths, often in childhood, per annum. Sickle-cell thalassaemia and sickle-cell haemoglobin C disease are rarer and although capable of causing death, are usually less severe. The sickle-cell trait, the common carrier state, is virtually benign although there may be sickling crises during severe anoxia, such as can occur in a badly delivered anaesthetic.

Sickle-cell disease is different from haemoglobin C disease and haemoglobin E disease, the other common abnormal haemoglobin diseases. This is because sickle haemoglobin is unique in being insoluble when deoxygenated and therefore, during a period of anoxia, it will crystallise out within the red blood cell. As a result, the red cell changes into its characteristic sickle form. These sickle-cells entwine in small blood vessels and give rise to scattered infarcts, the unique and often lethal feature of this group of inherited haemolytic diseases.

The ease with which sickling occurs *in vivo* depends upon the concentration of sickle haemoglobin within the red cell – circulating misshapen sickle-cells are commonly present in sickle-cell anaemia, the homozygous sickling state, whereas they are not present in the heterozygous carrier state, the sickle-cell trait. All red cells containing Hb.S will sickle under conditions of severe anoxia and therefore even the virtually harmless sickle-cell trait will give a positive *in vitro* 'sickle test'.

The severity of sickle-cell anaemia appears related to its geographical situation. In Central Africa most cases die in early childhood whereas sickle-cell anaemia is relatively benign in the West Indies, where women with this disease not uncommonly bear children. In other parts of the world, for example in North American Negroes, the condition is of intermediate severity.

General therapeutic care

The maintenance of good nutrition and prompt treatment of infection are important in the management of any child with a chronic haemolytic anaemia and probably account for the increased survival of such children born into families of high social status. To ensure medical supervision, early diagnosis is important and, because sickling infarcts may mimic surgical catastrophies, prior diagnosis may prevent unnecessary operations, since operative procedures are always poorly tolerated by patients with sickling disorders.

Treatment of anaemia

Without complications, such as can occur in infections and pregnancy, Hb.C disease and Hb.E disease are comparatively mild chronic haemolytic anaemias. In sickle-cell anaemia, the haemoglobin level is commonly between 5–10 g. per cent but despite this, the patients are often well compensated, because their red cells release oxygen more readily than normal. Frequent transfusions are not practical and would in any case result in iron overload. Transfusions should be reserved for haemolytic or aplastic crises which may well prove fatal, especially during pregnancy or infections. Young children may also become anaemic as a result of massive sequestration of red cells into the spleen. All patients with chronic haemolytic disorders may require prophylactic folic acid and this is particularly important when such a patient becomes pregnant. Patients with chonic haemolytic disorders over-absorb iron and iron therapy should therefore be avoided unless iron deficiency has been proved.

Treatment of the infarctive crisis

The infarctive crisis is unique to sickle-cell disease and does not occur without the presence of Hb.S within the red cell. Such crises may be extremely painful and present difficult surgical diagnostic problems.

The patient should be given analgesics, bearing in mind that addiction may become a problem. Dehydration should be prevented as this increases the risk of further sickling.

Although many drugs have been claimed to be helpful in both preventing and treating sickling, anti-sickling reagents are often not beneficial. Heparin has been used to diminish the risk of massive marrow embolism, which may follow an attack of bone pain. This has been especially advocated during pregnancy. Magnesium sulphate (1 to 2 ml 50 per cent aqueous solution given slowly intravenously) acts as a vasodilator and some success has followed the use of this reagent in a sickling crisis. The long term administration of sodium bicarbonate by mouth (sufficient to keep the urine alkaline to litmus) may reduce the number of painful crises.

Treatment of leg ulcers

Chronic leg ulcers may render a patient unemployable. The results of an operative approach to this problem may be disappointing and conservative treatment, limited to cleaning and regular dressings with a bland antiseptic such as Eusol, often proves rewarding.

Hypersplenism

Classical sickle-cell anaemia is characterised by a scarred impalpable spleen, which has undergone 'autosplenectomy' as a result of recurrent infarcts. Patients with haemoglobin C disease, haemoglobin E disease, sickle-cell thalassaemia and sickle-cell haemoglobin C disease often have large spleens and on occasions may suffer from hypersplenism, which should be suspected when the anaemia is unduly severe, when the immediate response to transfusion is poor or if an unexplained thrombocytopenia develops. In these situations splenectomy may be helpful.

Genetic counselling

It must be remembered that apart from very rare examples of a recent mutation the haemoglobinopathies are inherited disorders. If both parents carry the sickle-cell gene there is a one in four chance that the child will have sickle-cell anaemia. Marriage guidance and selection of a suitable partner is being increasingly sought in areas where the haemoglobinopathies are a clinical problem.

Suitable references for general reading are Lehmann and Huntsman (1966); Nechelef, Allen and Finkel (1969).

THE LEUKAEMIAS

Treatment of leukaemias is based on the concept that these disorders may be curable if the self-renewing population of abnormal leukaemic cells can be completely eliminated from the body. While this goal is not yet attainable, the recent exploitation of specific nutritional and antigenic differences between normal and leukaemic cells has increased the hope that it may eventually be reached. At present, treatment depends mainly upon the use of cytotoxic drugs to suppress, or control, the leukaemic process (chemotherapy) together with meticulous supportive care.

In *acute leukaemias*, the aim of chemotherapy is, first, to produce the greatest possible reduction of the leukaemic cell mass as rapidly as possible so that a complete clinical and haematological *remission* is obtained, and second, to maintain this remission for as long as possible. In *chronic leukaemias*, especially the chronic myeloid form, chemotherapy at present aims at restraining the abnormal cellular proliferation. The pharmacology of the drugs in current use has been reviewed earlier in this book. In all myeloproliferative disorders, uric acid turnover may be high, and increased by treatment. This may need to be controlled with allopurinol, in a dose of 200–400 mg daily.

Acute leukaemias

As far as response to treatment is concerned, acute leukaemias are usually divided into two cytological categories, 'lymphoblastic' and 'myeloid' forms. The latter group, which includes the myeloblastic, myelomonocytic and histiocytic varieties, remit much less frequently than the 'lymphoblastic' type. Since over 90 per cent of acute leukaemias in children appear to be 'lymphoblastic', whereas this form is rare in adults, it is convenient to consider treatment of children and of adults separately.

Treatment in children. 1. *Current conventional régimes* for treating acute lymphoblastic leukamia in children are based upon the observations that:

(a) Some drugs, e.g. prednisone and vincristine, are more effective for *inducing* a remission, whereas others, e.g. 6-mercaptopurine and methotrexate, are better used for *maintaining* remissions.

(b) Remissions are more frequently induced and better maintained if drugs are used in combination although, for maintaining remissions, it is not yet clear whether drugs are best used simultaneously, sequentially or cyclically.

Thus to induce a remission, the combination of prednisone (e.g. 40 mg/m^2/day by mouth) and vincristine (e.g. 2 mg/m^2/week by intravenous injection) is effective in about 90 per cent of cases.

For maintaining a remission, treatment with 6-mercaptopurine (e.g. 90 mg/m^2/day by mouth) and/or methotrexate (e.g. 20 mg/m^2 twice weekly, orally or parenterally) may be continued until there is evidence of relapse or significant depression of normal bone marrow function.

2. More recent *experimental régimes* attempt to obliterate leukaemic cell populations during the maintenance period by using combinations of drugs in massive dosage over short periods, sometimes followed by *immunotherapy*. It is not yet clear to what extent such methods may be superior to more conventional forms of treatment.

Treatment in adults. Acute 'lymphoblastic' leukaemia in adults is treated on the same basis as the disease in children but remissions are less frequently obtained.

Acute myeloid leukaemias have proved particularly resistant to chemotherapy. Cytosine arabinoside and rubidomycin are probably the agents of choice at present (remission rates of 20 to 30 per cent) but their use should probably be reserved for centres able to cope with the profound myelosuppression they can cause. A less satisfactory alternative is the combination of prednisone and 6-mercaptopurine which may also be used for maintenance if a remission is obtained.

Leukaemic meningitis

This complication is not uncommon, especially in children in maintained haematological remission. It generally responds to methotrexate injected intrathecally at a dose of 5 mg to 10 mg twice weekly until the blast count in the cerebrospinal fluid is less than 10 per cu. mm.

Referring patients

Patients with leukaemia should be referred if possible to a centre which has appropriate facilities for proper management and supervision of treatment. However the evidence at present available suggests that the marginal advantages in survival which derive from treatment in highly specialised units may not necessarily outweigh the disadvantages arising from disruption of family life or removal of a child far from the home environment.

Chronic myeloid leukaemia

Patients with chronic myeloid leukaemia can be kept in good health for long periods if the abnormal proliferation of granulocytes is carefully controlled.

Busulphan is the chemotherapeutic agent of choice. It is started orally at a daily dose of 0·065 mg/kg body weight and continued until the leukocyte count has fallen to 15,000 to 20,000/cu. mm. The drug should then be stopped (because the count generally continues falling for a few weeks) but resumed as required, on a long term, continuous or intermittent basis to maintain the leukocyte count within normal limits.

In 60 to 70 per cent of cases, the disease progresses to a terminal 'blastic' phase for which there is no effective definitive treatment but which may respond briefly to prednisone and 6-mercaptopurine or vincristine. In other patients, intractable bone marrow failure, probably the result of prolonged or excessive chemotherapy, develops and death usually results from anaemia, infection or uncontrollable haemorrhage. In a few patients there is transition to a myelofibrotic state and the treatment of this is discussed later. In some patients prolonged busulphan therapy may produce skin pigmentation or, occasionally, pulmonary fibrotic changes – the so-called 'busulphan lung'.

Even when there is an obvious hypersplenic component splenectomy should be avoided as the effect is often disastrous.

Chronic lymphatic leukaemia

In this condition a gradual accumulation of abnormal lymphocytes in blood, bone marrow and lymphoid tissue may be associated with neutropenia and defective synthesis of immunoglobulins. Patients are therefore particularly vulnerable to infection and vigorous treatment with antibiotics and with γ-globulin is at least as important as chemotherapy.

The leukaemic process may remain static for long periods in some patients, particularly the elderly, and treatment is then probably unnecessary. In most cases however, the presence, or recrudescence, of active disease demands control and intermittent courses, or long term low dose régimes of chemotherapy may be required. Chlorambucil is probably the drug of choice although other alkylating agents, especially cyclophosphamide, may occasionally be more effective. Chlorambucil is given by mouth, the recommended initial daily dose being 0·15 mg/kg body weight, reducing to lower maintenance levels.

Chlorambucil should not be used in the presence of significant depression of the bone marrow. In such cases treatment should be started with prednisone (e.g. 40 mg daily by mouth) and continued until adequate haemopoietic function is restored. The steroid may then be tailed off and treatment begun with chlorambucil. Prednisone is also of value for treating the acquired haemolytic anaemias which can occur. Long courses of steroids should however be avoided because of the risk of infection although, if there is slow response to adequate chemotherapy, a short course combined with chemotherapy may induce a more rapid resolution.

Some patients develop troublesome local enlargements of lymph nodes but without any indication for systemic chemotherapy. In such cases external irradiation of the affected glands may give considerable relief.

General symptomatic and supportive therapy in the leukaemias
Supportive measures to control morbidity are important and particularly so when normal bone marrow function is impaired. Anaemic patients may require blood transfusion and acute haemorrhage due to thrombocytopenia may be controlled by transfusion of platelets.

The presence of an unresponsive auto-immune haemolytic anaemia or a hypersplenic syndrome may be an indication for splenectomy and in chronic lymphatic leukaemia, in contrast to chronic myeloid leukaemia, excellent results may be obtained in very carefully selected patients. Infections must be promptly and energetically treated with appropriate antibiotics used in effective doses. Finally, the importance of careful psychological management of the patient and his relatives cannot be emphasised too strongly.

Some recent general reviews are those by Boesen and Davis (1969), Galton (1969), Silver (1969) and Henderson (1969).

POLYCYTHAEMIA, THROMBOCYTHAEMIA AND MYELOFIBROSIS

Proliferative polycythaemia (primary polycythaemia, polycythaemia vera), thrombocythaemia and myelofibrosis are, clinically at least, closely related conditions and although a proportion of patients presenting with one of these conditions will at some time undergo transition to another they are, in the present context, best considered separately. Although the treatment of the other forms of polycythaemia – renal, anoxic, and relative – is usually the treatment of the primary condition, some specific aspects of their therapy need discussion here.

Renal polycythaemia

In general no patient with polycythaemia should be treated until a renal cause has been excluded. If a relevant renal lesion is established surgical removal, after reduction of the venous haematocrit by venesection, is the treatment of choice and will be followed by a fall in the plasma erythropoietin and reversion of the red cell mass to normal. Venesection is a poor substitute but, if surgery is contraindicated, may relieve polycythaemic symptoms.

Anoxic polycythaemia

Since this is a compensatory phenomenon there is, in the vast majority of patients an absolute contraindication to treatment of the polycythaemia. In occasional patients abnormally high haematocrit levels (70–80 per cent) may represent a disadvantageous over-compensation. In such patients some reduction in red cell mass may produce symptomatic improvement with an increase in arterial PO^2. The approach should be cautious and the venesections small since reduction in red cell mass or blood volume below a critical level may be disastrous.

Relative polycythaemia

The apparent polycythaemia associated with burns and severe dehydration demands restoration of normal plasma volume. In the Gaisbock, 'stress' polycythaemia syndromes differential diagnosis from the true polycythaemias by demonstration of a normal red cell mass will establish that modification of the red cell mass is unnecessary.

Proliferative polycythaemia (Polycythaemia vera)

In terms of treatment patients with this condition fall into two main groups. In the first the increases in venous haematocrit (<55 per cent) and red cell mass (<250 ml) are marginal and there are no apparent symptoms. These patients require observation rather than immediate treatment. The second group comprises patients with symptoms and greater increases in haematocrit and red cell mass. In these patients it is essential to reduce the red cell mass, not only to produce subjective relief but also to eliminate the considerable risk of thrombotic episodes.

Venesection, chemotherapy and irradiation may be used to achieve this but there is not universal agreement on the treatment of choice. Irradiation, using ^{32}P, is simple and usually effective but it is now widely accepted that it produces an increased incidence of acute leukaemic transformation in polycythaemics. Venesection is also effective and carries no radiation hazard but its therapeutic effect is partly, but not entirely, dependent on the induction of iron deficiency and in some, but surprisingly few, patients this may produce its own signs and symptoms.

In practice it seems sensible to rely on venesection as the first line of therapy. The haematocrit should be reduced to between 45 per cent and 50 per cent as rapidly as possible and venesections of 500 ml two to three times a week will achieve this in two to three weeks. The majority of patients will then only require single venesections of 500 ml every 3 to 4 months to maintain an acceptable haematocrit. If a faster rate of relapse requires venesection at more frequent intervals or if symptoms of iron deficiency preclude treatment by venesection alone chemotherapy may be used to depress erythropoiesis. In the average adult busulphan 2–6 mg/day, with dose and duration of therapy controlled by response and monitoring of leukocyte and platelet counts, will usually reduce the need for venesection. If iron is administered at this stage it should be used sparingly or there may be reversion to the polycythaemic state.

The last line of approach in the few patients whom venesection and chemotherapy fail is ^{32}P administered, usually after venesection, in a single initial dose of approximately 5 mCi. Subsequent dosage will be determined by response and rate of relapse.

Thrombocythaemia

The mechanisms by which the high abnormal platelet counts found in this condition produce haemorrhage or microvascular occlusive lesions are complex and not clearly understood. Empirical chemotherapy with reduction of the platelet count to the normal range is, however, extremely effective. Busulphan is the drug of choice and the régime is identical with that used in the treatment of chronic myeloid leukaemia. Although the initial rate of response is often slow continued maintenance therapy is usually unnecessary since the platelet count once reduced, may remain at a normal level for many months without treatment. The slowly rising platelet count of relapse precedes the recurrence of symptoms and is easily controlled by a short course of busulphan.

In occasional patients who present with a severe bleeding syndrome, transfusion may be necessary but a short course of corticosteroids (Prednisone 20 mg t.d.s. for 7–10 days) may be surprisingly effective.

Myelofibrosis

This is one of the few myeloproliferative disorders in which diagnosis is not necessarily an indication for treatment. The natural progression of the disease, commonly presenting in the 5th and 6th decades, is slow. The elderly patient with a modest anaemia and considerable splenomegaly will often remain in a steady state, well and working for a number of years if spared the complications of enthusiastic therapy. At some stage an unacceptable degree of anaemia, unmanageable by transfusion and often associated with gross splenomegaly will make treatment necessary. In the vast majority of patients irradiation, chemotherapy and corticosteroids are quite ineffective. There is a strong case for splenectomy at this stage since the anaemia, transfusion requirements and thrombocytopenia may be considerably modified by elimination of the non-specific hypersplenic component. This operation should not be undertaken as a prophylactic measure in the well, steady state myelofibrotic, should not be postponed until the operative risk is unacceptable and should not be rejected on the invalid grounds that the spleen in myelofibrosis is a useful site of haemopoiesis.

HODGKIN'S DISEASE

It is now realistic to talk of cure for patients with early Hodgkin's disease (Stages I and II). Since treatment and prognosis are largely determined by the distribution of disease on presentation, accurate staging, using lymphangiography if necessary, is essential, (Rosenberg, 1966). Prognosis is indirectly related to histology for, although all histological types seem equally radio-sensitive the more malignant types usually present at a later stage.

With the possibility of cure the interests of the patient, who may require both radiotherapy and chemotherapy during the course of the disease, are best served by a close co-operation between radiotherapist and chemotherapist, preferably working in a combined clinic and effectively interchanging information with the family doctor.

Indications for radiotherapy and chemotherapy. Stages I and II should be treated with radical radiotherapy and cure should be the objective (Easson, and Russell, 1963; Prosnit *et al.*, 1969). In Stage III radical radiotherapy should be considered but, in both Stage III and Stage IV, systemic symptoms are common and these require treatment by chemotherapy. Focal lesions are still best treated with local radiotherapy and, particularly with mediastinal lesions, the relative timing of radiotherapy and chemotherapy is important. In acute cord compression initial neuro-surgery may be essential while chemotherapy or radiotherapy may be equally effective in patients with slower onset.

Choice of chemotherapeutic agents. The choice of drug will largely depend on the systemic symptoms. If these are mild one of the oral alkylating agents, such as chlorambucil or cyclophosphamide, is indicated. If they are severe or lesions are extensive intravenous therapy, with vinblastine for example, is likely to be more rapidly effective. The most rapid responses, for urgent relief of pressure symptoms, may be produced by intravenous mustine hydrochloride. Both mustine and cyclophosphamide may be given intrapleurally or intraperitoneally in the management of pleural and peritoneal lesions (Boesen and Davis, 1969).

Dosage, duration and control of chemotherapy

General. Treatment with the tolerated dose of a single agent for short periods, with interval periods for marrow recovery, is now considered preferable to continuous low dose therapy. Although very intensive treatment with combinations of drugs may produce a higher remission rate there is yet no clear evidence that length of remission or survival is prolonged (Boesen and Davis, 1969).

Specific. The general pharmacology and dosimetry of chemotherapeutic drugs is considered earlier in this book but some specific aspects of their use in Hodgkin's disease must be considered here.

The alkylating agents. With the short course, high dose régime the oral dose of chlorambucil is 0·2–0·4 mg/kg daily for 10–14 days. Cyclophosphamide may be given orally (100–200 mg/daily) or intravenously in a dose of 100–400 mg/daily for 5 days. It produces less thrombocytopenia than chlorambucil or mustine but chemical cystitis occurs in 3 per cent of cases and alopecia in 20 per cent when the total dose exceeds 3 to 4 g. Mustine (0·4 mg/kg in one total dose or in three daily divided doses) must be given intravenously over a period of 1–2 minutes, into a fast running saline or 5 per cent dextrose infusion since paravenous leaks produce tissue necrosis. Premedication with chlorpromazine (50 mg) and phenobarbitone (100 mg) will diminish or prevent the nausea and vomiting, which may follow this therapy.

Vinblastine. 0·1 mg/kg I.V. weekly, increasing the dose by 0·05 mg/kg to a maximum of 15 mg per injection until leukopenia (less than 4000/cu mm) occurs. After this a dose is given just below the leukopenic dose weekly or every 2 weeks. After remission the lowest dose necessary to maintain remission should be used. Side effects are negligible at this dosage but watch must be kept for neurotoxicity; tissue damage occurs with paravenous injection.

Procarbazine. 50 mg increasing to 150–300 mg orally daily. Gradual increase usually avoids the otherwise common complaint of nausea. If necessary the same dose can be given intravenously. After 2–3 weeks on this dose a lower maintenance dose can be used or the drug used intermittently at higher dose. This drug is a methyl hydrazine derivative and may cause haemolysis with prolonged use, the action of phenothiazines may be potentiated and it should not be given at the same time as other monoamine oxidase inhibitors. Hot flushes may occur when alcohol is taken.

Vincristine. 2 mg/M^2 at weekly intervals for 2 to 3 weeks. A single dose must not exceed 3·5 mg. This drug may be useful if bone marrow depression limits treatment, but it should mainly be used in combination with other drugs (Boesen and Davis, 1969). Neurotoxicity is related to total dose but constipation and paraesthesiae with areflexia are not uncommon. Constipation can be avoided by using a mixture containing dioctyl sodium sulphosuccinate and methyl cellulose.

Prednisone. The indications for this drug are first, an autoimmune haemolytic anaemia (rare in Hodgkin's disease). Secondly in conjunction with cytotoxic drugs as part of 'multiple drug therapy' (Boesen and Davis, 1969). Thirdly, when bone marrow depression is marked and continued chemotherapy or radiotherapy are necessary in the face of advancing disease. Except in the multiple drug régimes the useful dose rarely exceeds 40 to 60 mg daily, and the usual disadvantages of long continued administration apply.

Supportive treatment

Infections. Patients with Hodgkin's disease are subject to unusual and repeated infections (e.g. Torula meningitis). Meticulous investigation in the appropriate clinical context is part of management. Oral or more extensive moniliasis is a frequent complication and should be prevented if possible by giving nystatin or amphotericin B to suck if oral antibiotics are prescribed.

Symptomatic. Systemic symptoms of itching, fever and sweats should regress quickly if the disease is responding to treatment. Valium (diazepam) or Phenergan (promethazine hydrochloride) with, if necessary, heavy sedation at night, are useful for itching. Phenylbutazone 400–600 mg on one day followed by a few days on lower dosage may be useful to stop fever but should not be continued for longer. Blood or platelet transfusions may be needed at some stage if severe marrow depression occurs. Antiemetics may be needed during radiotherapy or intensive chemotherapy. Appropriate and sufficient analgesic drugs must be used when indicated.

The other malignant lymphomas

These present too wide a clinical and histological spectrum to be dealt with in detail here. Suitable references are suggested. (Boesen and Davis, 1969, Hope-Stone, 1969, Hilton and Sutton, 1962).

The significance of staging, prognosis and indications for a particular form of treatment are less certain than in Hodgkin's disease. Generally speaking, localised disease is treated by radical radiotherapy – in some cases following surgical removal of the 'tumour' (e.g. primary lymphoma of tonsil or bowel). Even in generalised disease radiotherapy is the treatment of choice for local symptoms of pain, pressure on vital organs and to decrease large tumour masses.

Alkylating agents, prednisone, and vincristine, are the most useful drugs singly or in combination. Auto-immune haemolytic anaemia is not uncommon and prednisone is particularly indicated in this complication. Other cytotoxic drugs may be effective but less so than in Hodgkin's disease. Repeated bacterial infections may be a problem because of abnormalities in immunoglobulin synthesis. Carefully used therapeutic and prophylactic antibiotics, anti-fungal agents and possibly gamma globulin injections, are important adjuncts to treatment.

MYELOMA AND MACROGLOBULINAEMIA

Myelomatosis

This disease is due to an abnormal proliferation of plasma cells which causes both local and generalised symptoms, and treatment must be aimed at reducing the plasma cell mass. Few of the symptoms are caused directly by the myeloma protein, but its level is related to the mass of tumour and does enable the response to treatment to be assessed.

Recent evidence suggests that two cytotoxic drugs, cyclophosphamide and melphalan are equally effective, and that their use results in improvement in both the length and quality of survival. Treatment should be continuous and some marrow suppression should be produced if maximum therapeutic effect is to be achieved. An initial course of 80–100 mg melphalan should be given over a period of 20–25 days, the total dose being controlled by twice weekly leukocyte and platelet counts. Treatment is stopped for 10 days and restarted on recovery of the platelet count to at least 100,000 per cu mm and the white count to at least 2,000 per cu mm. A maintenance dose of between 1 and 4 mg melphalan daily is given. Intermittent courses lasting 7–10 days with a break of a similar time between each course may be needed to maintain acceptable counts, but treatment should not be stopped entirely. Cyclophosphamide is used in a similar way, the initial dose being 100–150 mg daily, followed by 50–100 mg daily. If severe thrombocytopenia or leucopenia occurs, either from bone marrow replacement or from cytotoxic therapy, corticosteroids, e.g. prednisone 20 mg daily, should be given. Anaemia should be corrected by blood transfusion. Relief of pain from bone lesions is often striking, although healing of fractures seldom occurs. The best results are associated with a slow reduction in the myeloma protein level but a rapid fall in serum or urinary protein is a poor prognostic sign as these patients usually relapse quickly (Hobbs, 1969a and b). If relapse occurs a change of treatment is unlikely to be successful.

Radiotherapy has no influence on the long-term prognosis, but is of great value in the treatment of local bone lesions which are causing pain or disability.

Hypercalcaemia is a serious and frequent complication, often unrelated to the extent of bone involvement, and can cause coma and renal failure. The first essential is to ensure that the patient is fully hydrated, using intravenous fluids if necessary. Melphalan may produce a dramatic fall in serum calcium levels, but most patients respond to steroids in high dose, e.g. prednisone 40 mg daily.

The other serious complication and bad prognostic sign is renal failure which may be due to hypercalcaemia, Bence Jones proteinuria, myeloma kidney, or amyloid. Hydration and correction of hypercalcaemia are imperative. Uraemia is not a contraindication to the use of cytotoxic agents but a smaller dose should be given and the blood count must be watched carefully.

Exceptionally high levels of myeloma globulin, usually in excess of 10 g/100 ml serum, may produce hyperviscosity symptoms, and plasmapheresis may be indicated (see below). Similar symptoms may occur if the myeloma protein is a cryoglobulin, and in this case exposure to cold must be avoided.

Macroglobulinaemia

The clinical picture of macroglobulinaemia differs from myeloma in that hyperviscosity and bleeding symptoms predominate and bone lesions are infrequent. These symptoms are directly related to the increased levels of macroglobulin and the prime aim of treatment must be to reduce the level of this protein. Two methods of treatment are available, cytotoxic drugs and plasmapheresis.

Cytotoxic drugs have been less successful in the treatment of macroglobulinaemia than of myeloma. Chlorambucil is the most widely used drug and as for myeloma, treatment should be continuous as long as the blood count permits. The usual dose is 4–10 mg daily initially, and 2–4 mg daily thereafter for maintenance. Cyclophosphamide 50–100 mg daily is an acceptable alternative.

Plasmapheresis is a useful method of treatment of acute symptoms due to increased viscosity. In patients with chronic symptoms, intermittent plasmapheresis may be combined with chemotherapy but it is impossible to achieve a lasting reduction in macroglobulin levels by this method alone. The indications for plasmapheresis should be clinical and not biochemical as individual patient and protein variation affects the relationship between macroglobulin level and viscosity symptoms. Intensive plasmapheresis is distressing to the patient and can result in loss of normal plasma proteins, including clotting factors, immunoglobulins, and platelets. A reasonable method is to remove between 500 and 600 ml of plasma daily for about 10 days or until symptoms are relieved. This is best achieved by removing a unit of blood from the patient, centrifuging it, separating cells and plasma, and then returning the red cells to the patient. This process is then repeated until sufficient plasma has been removed. The retransfusion of the patient's own red cells eliminates the risk of transmitting serum hepatitis or of mismatching. Not more than one unit of blood should be removed from the patient without some form of replacement. If special plastic units are used throughout, the whole process can be completed in a closed system, so reducing the risk of contamination.

Steroids are relatively ineffective in the treatment of macroglobulinemia, although they should be given if bleeding is a prominent feature. Penicillamine has been used to try and depolymerise the macroglobulin molecules and so reduce viscosity. It is an expensive form of treatment which is not justified by the results obtained.

BLEEDING DISORDERS

1. MANAGEMENT OF THE LIFE-LONG BLEEDING DISORDERS

The haemostatic defect in the life-long bleeding disorders is nearly always due to a congenital deficiency of a single clotting factor. Bleeding episodes are treated by the intravenous infusion of the appropriate blood product to supply the missing factor. For any but the most routine situations it must be possible to control treatment by monitoring the level of the factor in the patient's blood.

Haemophilia (Factor–VIII deficiency)

Therapeutic materials. With fresh normal *plasma* the patient's factor-VIII level may be raised from zero to about 20 per cent of normal but to avoid circulatory overload higher doses must be given as concentrates. *Concentrates of human factor VIII*, e.g. 'cryoprecipitate' (Pool and Shannon, 1965), are available through Blood Transfusion Services and commercially; and concentrates from bovine and porcine blood may be obtained commercially in Britain.

Management of bleeding episodes. The characteristic bleeding into *joints* and *muscles* and *spreading haematomata* deserve urgent antihaemophilic treatment if pain is severe enough to require analgesia or to interfere significantly with function. Human factor VIII from one of the above sources should be given in sufficient quantity to maintain the patient's plasma level above about 10 per cent for a few hours. Adequate immediate analgesia must also be provided, but the ultimate relief of pain depends on the control of bleeding. Further doses of factor VIII at *c.* 6–12 hour intervals should be given until it is apparent that the pain is not returning and function is improving, but a single treatment applied within a few hours of onset, on an outpatient basis, will often suffice. There is good evidence that the provision of an emergency treatment service for haemarthrosis materially reduces the long-term incidence of crippling (Ali *et al.*, 1967).

A tight effusion of the knee may be aspirated to relieve pain, after generous antihaemophilic cover, and with the utmost gentleness.

In *haematuria* the blood loss is usually less than would appear and the mere presence of blood in the urine can be ignored for a week or two. Factor VIII should, however, be given generously if the passage of clots is causing ureteric colic, if the urine is infected or if the patient is becoming anaemic. Repeated attacks should be investigated, but cystoscopy requires antihaemophilic cover. In *epistaxis*, antihaemophilic infusion should be combined with local treatment, e.g. limited electro-cautery of a bleeding point, or covering a diffusely bleeding area with a small piece of absorbable dressing. Ordinary packing may provoke further bleeding when it is removed. *Intra-abdominal bleeding* (e.g. the 'psoas syndrome') or bleeding into the *central nervous system* require more vigorous antihaemophilic treatment and should be managed in hospital.

If the patient does not respond to antihaemophilic treatment for a particular incident, the factor VIII level in the patient's plasma after infusion should be monitored and the dose adjusted to give a sufficient level. If the level obtained is disproportionately low his plasma should be tested for inactivation of factor VIII. If this is demonstrated, factor VIII must either be withheld entirely, in the hope that the antibody will die away, or given in massive doses temporarily to saturate circulating antibody and leave some residual therapeutic activity, after which a further rise in antibody titre may unfortunately be expected in a few days. Immunosuppressive drugs have not so far proved helpful.

Management of post-traumatic bleeding. Following major trauma, the minimum haemostatic level of factor VIII is about 30 per cent, which must be maintained by divided or continuous infusion until the wound is reasonably consolidated. There is some evidence that antihaemophilic cover may be reduced if the patient's fibrinolytic mechanism is concommitantly blocked by the administration of Epsilon-aminocaproic acid, at least following dental extraction (Reid *et al.*, 1964; Cooksey *et al.*, 1966) and orthopaedic operations (Storti *et al.*, 1969). The management of elective surgery in haemophiliacs is best carried out in a Haemophilia Centre.

Other clotting factor deficiencies

Christmas disease (*factor IX deficiency*) is managed on the same lines as haemophilia. Factor IX may be given as whole fresh plasma, or as a concentrate containing prothrombin and factors VII, IX and X, which is becoming available from various centres. *Von Willebrand's disease* may be treated by whole fresh plasma which shortens the bleeding time for a few hours and allows the patient to synthesise factor VIII normally for a day or two. This may initially be supplemented by factor VIII concentrate, if an immediate increase in factor VIII is required. The bleeding in *congenital afibrinogenaemia* responds well to infusions of purified fibrinogen. *Congenital deficiencies of other clotting factors* may be treated by infusions of whole plasma or of the concentrate of prothrombin and factors VII, IX and X, as appropriate, along the same lines as haemophilia.

II. MANAGEMENT OF BLEEDING IN DISORDERS KNOWN TO BE ASSOCIATED WITH PARTICULAR CLOTTING DEFECTS

Deficiencies of clotting factors

In *liver disease* deficient clotting factors may be replaced before traumatic assaults, including liver biopsy, on the lines suggested for haemophilia. Overdose with *oral anticoagulants* may be treated with vitamin K_1 or, more rapidly, by replacement of the relevant factors on the lines suggested for haemophilia. *Haemorrhagic disease of the newborn and prematurity* (Cade *et al.*, 1969) may be treated on the same lines with whole plasma.

III. MANAGEMENT OF THE DEFIBRINATION SYNDROME

Principles of management

The defibrination syndrome is usually the result of continuous intravascular coagulation with secondary activation of fibrinolysis, although sometimes fibrinolysis may predominate. Management may be on three lines: first, to resolve the underlying disorder; second, to support the haemostatic reserve by intravenous infusion of those components which have been seriously depleted; and third, to block defibrination in the blood.

Indications for treatment

The need for treatment depends on the expected duration of the provocative underlying condition, the likelihood and danger of bleeding in the given situation (wounds, etc.) and the degree of depletion of the haemostatic reserve. In a rapidly resolving situation, such as the later stages of labour, no haematological treatment may be required because defibrination may be expected to remit spontaneously when the uterus contracts after delivery. If the patient is bleeding abnormally, where there is special risk of bleeding, or if bleeding would be serious if it occurred, the haemostatic reserve should be maintained above the critical level. *Fibrinogen* can be given as a concentrate in a dose of about 6 g.; *factor VIII and fibrinogen* can be given together as cryoprecipitate, as in the treatment of haemophilia, if available; *other factors* are best given as whole fresh plasma; *platelets* may also be given as platelet-rich plasma or platelet concentrates, although it is probably more important to replace the clotting factors first. The fate of infused materials should be monitored because the rate at which they disappear from the circulation will indicate the activity of the defibrination process. Replacement alone should not be continued for more than about twenty-four hours since the continuous deposition of fibrin may lead to serious micro-embolisation (Graham *et al.*, 1957). Intravascular coagulation may be rapidly blocked by heparin (Merskey *et al.*, 1964) or over the longer term with oral anticoagulants (Mannucci *et al.*, 1968). At the beginning of anti-coagulant treatment it may be wise also to restore haemostatic components which are seriously depleted, to prevent bleeding from anticoagulation; when the intravascular consumption of haemostatic factors is blocked by the anticoagulant the patient's own synthesis may be expected to restore normal levels in about twenty-four hours. Antifibrinolytic drugs should only be given if intravascular clotting can be excluded or blocked, or else the embolic component of the syndrome may be seriously aggravated, (Naeye, 1962).

THROMBOCYTOPENIA

Thrombocytopenia is a common cause of a generalised tendency to bleed spontaneously from small vessels, especially in the skin and mucous membranes (purpura). In the majority of cases, some more or less easily recognised cause is responsible for the reduction in the platelet count (secondary thrombocytopenias) but in a few patients no cause can be demonstrated by the usual methods of investigation (idiopathic thrombocytopenic purpura or ITP). Management of thrombocytopenia therefore requires not only an understanding of the methods of treatment, which are discussed below, but also an appreciation of the principles underlying differential diagnosis between the numerous causes of purpura (see Hardisty and Ingram, 1965).

Management of ITP

Treatment of ITP is based largely upon the administration of corticosteroids (usually prednisone) and splenectomy together with local haemostatic measures and supportive therapy, particularly transfusion of blood or of platelets. The use of these measures depends upon the age of the patient and the severity and duration of the symptoms.

Treatment in children. Most cases of ITP in children run an acute, self-limiting course and the aim of treatment is to tide the patient over the acute phase in the hope that a spontaneous remission will occur. In mild cases no active treatment may be necessary but in more severe cases, prednisone may be required in high doses (e.g. 2 mg/kg body weight/day), together with transfusion, to control bleeding. Because of the risk of side-effects, prednisone should not be continued at high dosage for more than a few weeks by which time either a remission will have occurred or there will usually have been sufficient improvement to justify gradual withdrawal of the steroid. In a few cases, haemorrhagic manifestations may remain sufficiently severe to require continuing treatment with prednisone at the lowest effective dose and if troublesome bleeding persists for more than about six months, splenectomy may have to be considered.

Treatment in adults. ITP in adults commonly follows a chronic course with recurrent remissions and relapses and long lasting spontaneous remissions are rare. If bleeding is more than trivial, an attempt should be made to obtain a remission by using steroids as described above. If, after an adequate trial of prednisone, patients have failed to remit, or need a high maintenance dose to control bleeding, splenectomy is indicated. A sustained remission follows splenectomy in about two thirds of patients but in the remainder the operation has either no effect or a temporary response is followed by a relapse.

In such cases a further course of steroids may produce a remission or a small maintenance dose of prednisone may control symptoms. Immunosuppressive agents, e.g. azathioprine, have also been used since in such circumstances it is possible that an abnormal immunological mechanism is operating (Baldini, 1966). Remissions have occasionally been obtained but this approach requires further evaluation. When a relapse follows some months or years after splenectomy, the possibility that some functional splenic tissue (e.g. a splenunculus) may remain should always be investigated and laparotomy undertaken for its removal if necessary.

The treatment of ITP during pregnancy requires special consideration which is beyond the scope of the present discussion (see Hardisty and Ingram, 1965).

Management of secondary thrombocytopenias

Treatment should be aimed at alleviating or eliminating the underlying cause. Steroids and transfusion of blood and platelets may be required to control severe bleeding but splenectomy is generally not indicated.

BLOOD TRANSFUSION AND THE USE OF BLOOD PRODUCTS

The administration of blood or blood products carries appreciable risks and should never be undertaken without weighing carefully the possible benefits against the potential hazards.

The whole subject is very fully covered by Mollison (1967). The use and preparation of specific blood products is discussed by Greenhalt and Perry (1969).

Indications for the Specific Use of Blood and Blood Products

Acute Blood Loss

This is the main indication for the use of *whole stored blood.* The decision to transfuse can usually be based on clinical judgement and observation of systolic pressure but in complex situations measurement of central venous pressure may be necessary. Since the immediate requirement is the correction of hypovolaemia rather than anaemia initial infusion of a blood substitute is as effective as and considerably less dangerous than inadequately cross matched blood. A *dextran* with a molecular weight of about 70,000 (e.g. Macrodex, Pharmacia Ltd.,) is the most satisfactory preparation. It is contra-indicated in patients who have a bleeding diathesis. *Freeze dried plasma* is not recommended for, although it is an efficient blood volume expander, there is an appreciable risk of serum hepatitis.

Whole fresh blood is only indicated when it is necessary to transfuse both red cells and factors lost on storage, such as platelets and Factors V, VIII and X. This may occur when a primary bleeding disorder causes considerable blood loss or when haemostatic defects follow massive haemorrhage treated by massive transfusion. With *massive transfusion* (rapid infusion of more than 2 litres of stored blood) there are additional problems, for hypocalcaemia, hyperkalaemia and hypothermia may lead to cardiac arrest (Churchill Davidson, 1968). Hypocalcaemia can be prevented by administration of 10 ml. of 10% calcium gluconate per 500 ml. of blood given. Hypothermia, perhaps the most important factor, can be prevented by warming of blood immediately before transfusion but it is essential that special equipment is used for this (Bennett, 1968).

Chronic Anaemia

When anaemia can be corrected by specific therapy (iron, B_{12}, folate) transfusion should be avoided and is unnecessary even in the severely anaemic patient. All patients with severe anaemia are especially liable to *circulatory overload* and when transfusion is essential, as in marrow failure, *packed red cells* should be given at not more than 70 ml. per hour. A rapidly acting diuretic, such as frusemide (20 mg. i.v.) should also be given.

Thrombocytopenia

Platelet transfusions may produce temporary but useful arrest of spontaneous or post-traumatic thrombocytopenic bleeding. In the absence of bleeding they have no prophylactic value except as immediate cover for surgery in thrombocytopenic patients. Platelets from at least six units of blood are required for effect in adults. They may be given as platelet rich plasma (volume 1250 ml.) or, less effectively, as a platelet concentrate (volume c. 50 ml.) and the preparations must be used within six hours of collection.

Hypoproteinaemia

Substantially *salt free, freeze dried albumin* preparations are available but should only be used for the treatment of specific episodes since long term maintenance of protein equilibrium by albumin infusion is impracticable.

Hypogammaglobulinaemia

Pooled adult human *gamma globulin* provides a source of antibodies against the common infective diseases. It is used in prophylaxis against certain infectious diseases and in the treatment of hypogammaglobulinaemia.

There is evidence that in congenital hypogammablobulinaemia the incidence of infections is reduced if the gamma globulin level is kept above 150 mg. per 100 ml. (M.R.C. 1969). The preparations available contain almost pure IgG and are unsuitable therefore for the treatment of IgA or IgM defects. The indication for gamma globulin therapy is that the serum IgG level should be below 200 mg. per 100 ml. The recommended dosage is an initial loading dose of 0·05 g. /kg. daily for five days followed by 0·025 g./kg. weekly. The injections are given intramuscularly and are painful. Intravenous administration may lead to severe allergic reactions and should be avoided. Gamma globulin will not replace defective cellular immunity.

Hypogammaglobulinaemia may complicate other diseases, particularly chronic lymphatic leukaemia and myelomatosis. If recurrent infections occur in these diseases gamma globulin replacement therapy should be tried using the dosage schedule already laid down. If the patient can tolerate the injections it is worth persisting as some patients are benefited considerably.

There is also a place for gamma globulin in the treatment of acute infections in hypogammaglobulinaemic patients who are not receiving regular replacement therapy. A short intensive course, as for the loading dose, should be given together with appropriate antibiotic cover. Severe infections in infants during the period of transient hypogammaglobulinaemia, which accompanies the decline of maternal antibodies, are another indication for gamma globulin therapy.

Coagulation Defects

The use of special fractions such as *cryoprecipitate*, *fresh frozen plasma* and *fibrinogen* has been considered elsewhere.

THE SELECTION OF BLOOD FOR TRANSFUSION

Whenever possible blood of the same ABO and rhesus group should be used. Group O cells may, in emergency, be given to recipients of other ABO groups but large quantities of group O plasma should not be transfused because of the danger of a haemolytic reaction due to the destruction of the recipients red cells by isoagglutinins in the transfused plasma. The same restriction applies to the use of group A or B blood for group AB recipients.

Rhesus positive blood may be given to rhesus negative recipients who have never previously been exposed to the rhesus antigen by transfusion or pregnancy but, as sensitisation may result, it should be given in exceptional circumstances only and never to pre-menopausal women. It must be emphasised that whenever blood of a different ABO or rhesus group is used it must be fully cross matched. If, in an emergency, the clinical situation is judged to be so desperate that cells must be given and transfusion cannot be deferred until properly cross matched blood is available then blood of the same ABO and rhesus group of the patient should be given rather than group O rhesus negative blood.

The Management of Some Complications of Transfusion

The prevention of circulatory overload and the management of massive transfusion have already been considered.

Haemolytic Transfusion Reactions

If a haemolytic reaction is suspected the transfusion should be stopped immediately and the blood bottle and the giving set should be sent to the laboratory immediately with two specimens of blood, one clotted and one heparinised, taken from a vein well away from the infusion site. There is no specific treatment but the patient's blood pressure must be maintained by the use of vasopressor agents and intravenous hydrocortisone. Maintenance of blood volume is of cardinal importance and a suitable volume expander should be given until more blood can be cross matched. Careful observation of fluid balance should be made and all urine passed should be sent to the laboratory. If renal failure does supervene appropriate treatment should be instituted.

If bleeding develops the possibility of an induced defibrination or fibrinolytic syndrome should be considered.

Febrile Reactions

These are frequent in multiple-transfused patients and can often be prevented by the use of an antihistamine, e.g. chlorpheniramine, 10 mg. i.m. or promethazine hydrochloride, 25 mg. I.M. at the start of a transfusion.

Iron Overload

Transfusion of twenty 500 ml. units of whole blood gives an increase in body iron load of 4000—5000 mg. Patients who must be maintained by repeated transfusion for long periods may therefore develop transfusional siderosis. In such patients the removal of body iron by chelation should be attempted. Infusion of 4 gm. of desferrioxamine in 200 ml. saline at each transfusion will only produce a urinary iron excretion of around 30 mg. in the iron loaded patient. Increased dose does not give significantly increased excretion and more frequent intravenous or intramuscular chelation usually proves impracticable or intolerable. At present, therefore, chelation is inadequate but worthwhile.

Thrombophlebitis

The care of veins, particularly in repeated or prolonged infusions, is of paramount importance. The most effective single precaution that can be taken is to ensure that, in high risk situations such as haemophilia and the refractory anaemias, infusions are only set up by the most experienced operator available. Other points are:

1. In small or frightened children light general anaesthetic will often save trauma to vein, child and operator.

2. Dextrose solutions are irritant and should not be administered through the same giving set as blood or sludging and thrombophlebitis will occur.

3. A small cannula, preferably of plastic type, is less traumatic than a needle and should be used, particularly for prolonged infusions.

References

Ali, A. M., Gandy, R. H., Britten, M. I., and Dormandy, K. M., *Brit. med. J.* (1967), **3**, 828.

Allen, D. M., Fine, M. H., Necheles, T. F., and Damaschek, W., *Blood* (1968), **32**, 83.

Baldini, M., *New Eng. J. Med.* (1966), **274**, 1245.

Bennett, P. S., *Proc. Roy. Soc. Med.* (1968), **61**, 687.

Boesen, E., and Davis, W., *Cytotoxic Drugs in the Treatment of Cancer* (1969), Edward Arnold Ltd., London.

Bothwell, T. H., and Finch, C. A., *Iron Metabolism* (1962), J. & A. Churchill, London.

Brain, M. C., Baker, L. R. I., McBride, J. A., Rudenberg, M. L., and Dacie, J. V., *Brit. J. Haemat.* (1968), **15**, 603.

Brain, M. C., *Seminars in Haematology* (1969), **6**, 2, 162.

Cade, J. F., Hirsh, J., and Martin, M., *Brit. med. J.* (1969), **2**, 281.

Cartwright, G. E., *Seminars in Haematology* (1966), **3**, 351.

Chanarin, I., *The Megaloblastic Anaemias* (1969), Blackwell Scientific Publications, Oxford.

Churchill Davidson, H. C., *Proc. Roy. Soc. Med.* (1968), **61**, 681.

Cooksey, M. W., Perry, C. B., and Raper, A. B., *Brit. med. J.* (1966), **2**, 1633.

Dacie, J. V., *The Haemolytic Anaemias Congenital and Acquired. Part IV* (1967a), Drug-induced haemolysis. 2nd ed. J. & A. Churchill, London.

Dacie, J. V., *ibid.* (1967b), Paroxysmal nocturnal haemoglobinuria.

Dacie, J. V., and Worrledge, S. M. (1969). Auto-immune haemolytic anaemia. In Brown, E. B., and Moore, C. V. (eds.). *Progress in Haematology*, Vol. vi. Grune & Stratton, New York.

Easson, E. C., and Russell, M. H., *Brit. med. J.* (1963), **i**, 1704.

Galton, D. A. G., *Seminars in Haematology* (1969), **6**, 323.

Graham, J. H., Emerson, C. P., and Anglem, T. J., *New Eng. J. Med.* (1957), **257**, 101.

Greenwalt, T. S., and Perry, S. (1969). Preservation and utilization of the components of human blood. p. 148–181 in *Progress in Haematology. Volume VI.* Ed. Brown, E. B., and Moore, C. V.,Wm. Heinemann, London.

Hardisty, R. M., and Ingram, G. I. C., *Bleeding Disorders: Investigation and Management* (1965), Blackwell Scientific Publications, Oxford.

Henderson, E. S., *Seminars in Haematology* (1969), **6**, 271.

Hilton, G., and Sutton, P. M., *Lancet* (1962), **i**, 283.

Hobbs, J. R., *Brit. J. Haemat.*, (1969a), **16**, 599.

Hobbs, J. R., *ibid* (1969b), **16**, 607.

Hope-Stone, H. F., *Brit. J. Radiol.* (1969), **42**, 770.

Lehman, H., and Huntsman, R. G., *Man's Haemoglobins.* (1966), North-Holland Publishing Company, Amsterdam.

Mannucci, P. M., Lobina, G. F., and Dioguardi, N., *Coagulation* (1968), **1**, 305.

Medical Research Council Working Party, *Lancet* (1969), **i**, 163.

Merskey, C., Johnson, A. J., Pert, J. H., and Wohl, H., *Blood* (1964), **24**, 701.

Mollin, D. L., and Hoffbrand, A. V., Chapter on Sideroblastic Anaemia in *Recent Advances in Clinical Pathology* (1968), Editor S. C. Dyke. J. & A. Churchill Ltd., London.

Mollison, P. L., *Blood Transfusion in Clinical Medicine* (1967), 4th edition. Blackwell Scientific Publications, Oxford.

Naeye, R. L., *Blood* (1962), **19**, 694.

Nechelef, T. F., Allen, D. M., and Finkel, H. E., *Clinical Disorders of Hemoglobin Structure and Synthesis* (1969), Appleton-Century-Crofts, New York.

Pool, J. G., and Shannon, A. E., *New Eng. J. Med.*, (1965), **273**, 1443.

Prosnit, L. R., Hellman, S., Von Essen, C. F., Kligerman, M. M., *Am. J. Roentg.* (1969), **105**, 618.

Reid,W. O., Lucas, O. N., Francisco, J., Geisler, P. H. and Erslev, A. J., *Am. J. med. Sci.* (1964), **248**, 184.

Rosenberg, S. (1966). Report of the committee on the staging of Hodgkin's disease. *Cancer Research*, **26**, (i), 1310.
Sanchez-Medal, L., Pizzuto, J., Torre-Lopez, E., and Derby, R., *Arch. Intern. Med.* (1964), **113**, 721.
Silver, R. T., *Seminars in Haematology* (1969), **6**, 344.
Storti, E., Traldi, A., Tosatti, E., and Davoli, G., *Gazzetta Sanitaria* (1969), **40**, 229.
Sephton-Smith, R., *Ann. New York Acad. Sci.* (1964), **119**, 776.
Wolman, I. J., *ibid*, **119**, 736.
Wood, M. M., and Elwood, P. C., *Brit. J. prev. Soc. Med.* (1966), **20**, 117.

This article was written by the following members of the Department of Haematology, St Thomas's Hospital Medical School and edited by Professor W. I. Cranston.

J. V. Allison	*Lecturer in Haematology* Megaloblastic anaemias The leukaemias Thrombocytopenia
D. Collins	*Consultant Radiotherapist* Hodgkin's disease and other lymphomas (Jointly)
R. G. Huntsman	*Reader in Haematology and Consultant Haematologist* Sickle cell disease Haemoglobin C disease Haemoglobin E disease
G. I. C. Ingram	*Reader in Experimental Haematology,* *Honorary Consultant Haematologist* The bleeding disorders
G. L. Scott	*Honorary Consultant Haematologist* The haemolytic anaemias Myeloma and macroglobulinaemia Blood transfusion and the use of blood products
T. M. Vanier	*Consultant Haematologist,* *Senior Lecturer in Haematology* The refractory anaemias Hodgkin's disease and other lymphomas (Jointly)
G. Wetherley-Mein	*Professor of Haematology,* *Honorary Consultant Haematologist* Iron deficiency Anaemia of infection and chronic disease Polycythaemia, thrombocythaemia, myelofibrosis

Category 10

The Cardiovascular System

CARDIAC FAILURE

Cardiac failure may be predominantly left sided, predominantly right sided, or a mixture of the two. Strictly speaking, cardiac failure is present when the ventricular function curve is flattened, i.e. when a given increment of filling pressure gives an abnormally small increment of stroke volume. An elevated venous pressure may also be present when the ventricular function curve is normal, but cardiac output is high. This is found in anaemia, thyrotoxicosis, beri-beri, acute nephritis and cor pulmonale.

It is impossible to decide clinically whether the ventricular function curve is abnormal in these conditions; in general, peripheral vasodilation suggests a more or less normal function curve, and vasoconstriction suggests an impaired one.

Left Ventricular Failure

This occurs when the function curve of the left side of the heart is significantly flatter than that on the right. Thus, to maintain the same stroke output from each ventricle, a very much higher filling pressure is necessary in the left atrium and ventricle. This high pressure requires an equal, or greater pressure rise in the pulmonary veins and capillaries. Consequently, there is an increased transinduction of fluid within the lungs. Lymphatic flow will increase, and will to some extent counteract this effect, but the net result is the development of pulmonary oedema. There is a decrease in lung compliance, and usually a marked interference with normal ventilation – perfusion relationships, resulting in arterial hypoxia, which may be of severe degree. Severe dyspnoea and orthopnoea are observed, and some relief is usually obtained if the patient sits up. This is probably because of some pooling of blood in the legs, resulting in a reduced right sided filling pressure and stroke output. Left sided filling pressure and stroke output also fall, until the stroke outputs from the two sides are balanced. Because the left sided function curve is flatter than that of the right, the fall in left sided filling pressure is much greater than the fall in right sided filling pressure, and in this way relief is obtained.

Left ventricular failure may be due to a sudden impairment of left ventricular function, as following a myocardial infarct. Function is more gradually impaired in patients with hypertension, left sided valvular lesions, or ischaemic heart disease. There is some evidence to indicate that attacks of angina may be associated with transient impairment of left ventricular function. Not uncommonly, episodes of left ventricular failure may be induced, in patients with compromised ventricular function, by the onset of rapid arrhythmias or by over-transfusion.

Management

Many attacks of left ventricular failure are spontaneously self-limiting, especially in patients with insidious progression of left ventricular impairment.

If the patient is seen in an acute attack, morphine should be administered (15 mg I.M. or 10 mg slowly I.V.). Intravenous frusemide (20–40 mg) is of value in preventing subsequent attacks, but the duration of individual attacks of failure is usually so short that a diuretic action has little influence upon the attack in progress.

Oxygen is of value if it can be given, but the distressed and very dyspnoeic patient will often not tolerate its administration until the effects of posture or morphine have become apparent. These measures will control the attack of left ventricular failure in most patients, except some of those with extensive myocardial infarcts who may require treatment with digitalis. The desperately ill patient, and the patient who has been over-transfused, may require venesection, of 500–1000 ml of blood, or even more, in the latter case.

Management thereafter depends upon the cause of the attack. Hypertension should be treated. Patients with valvular lesions will require treatment with digitalis and diuretics and investigation to determine the appropriateness of surgery.

Congestive Cardial Failure

Right sided cardiac failure or congestive cardiac failure may be due to an increased work load on the right ventricle, to impairment of the capacity of ventricular muscle to cope with a normal load, or to a combination of the two. Congestive failure may follow impairment of left sided function, without a preceding history of left ventricular failure.

An increased right ventricular work load may be due to valvular abnormalities or to an increased pulmonary vascular resistance, possibly with a high cardiac output, as in cor pulmonale. Impaired functional capacity of the ventricular muscle may be due to ischaemia, or to any kind of cardiomyopathy; congestive cardiac failure may follow any sustained tachycardia, though this is usually associated with impaired cardiac muscle function.

Congestive cardiac failure usually presents with breathlessness, oedema, raised central venous pressure, and hepatic enlargement. Management can be considered in two parts:

(a) The general management of patients with cardiac failure.
(b) Treatment directed toward influencing the cause of cardiac failure.

The general management of congestive cardiac failure

The initial aim of treatment is to rest the myocardium; this means resting the patient. Patients with severe cardiac failure should be at rest in bed. They should be propped up, with the legs either horizontal or hanging down. If the legs are horizontal, it is usually easier to remove oedema from the legs, but in severe cardiac failure, especially if left ventricular failure is present, it may be necessary, for the patient's comfort, to have the legs dependent. In this position there is theoretically a greater risk of development of deep vein thrombosis, so it is probably better avoided unless it is dictated by the patient's comfort. Many of these patients have lost their appetites and the diet should be light, and so far as possible, tailored to the patient's appetite rather than to any arbitrary scheme. Added salt should be avoided, but strict salt restriction is usually an unnecessary penance to impose upon the patient, at least until other treatments have failed. A commode is preferable to a bed-pan, because its use involves the expenditure of less energy.

The obese patient with cardiac failure will require weight reduction, but this is something which takes time and is a second order aim of treatment.

The mainstays of drug treatment are digitalis preparations and diuretics. Digoxin is given unless;

(a) there is evidence of recent digitalis treatment or,
(b) there is evidence of hypokalaemia.

Some patients in chronic cardiac failure are depleted of potassium, particularly if diurectics have been given; though serum potassium is a poor guide to total body potassium, a low serum level indicates a need for caution in the use of digitalis.

For a rapid effect, adult patients may be given an initial dose of 1.0–1.5 mg digoxin, followed by 0.25 mg 6 hourly until an adequate response is obtained or evidence of toxicity appears. Toxicity may be manifest by gastro-intestinal disturbances, particularly nausea, or by the development of ectopic beats or other arlythmias. Maintenance doses of digoxin usually lie between 0.25 mg once daily and 0.25 mg three times daily. Digoxin may be given intravenously, as a slow injection of 0.5–1.0 mg, if the patient has not previously received this drug; this method of administration may be particularly valuable in patients with left ventricular failure. Other digitalis preparations may sometimes succeed in patients who develop toxic effects with digoxin; daily maintenance doses of digitoxin usually lie between 0.05–0.2 mg, and of Lanataside C between 0.25 and 0.75 mg.

If possible, the patient should be weighed each day, since body weight usually provides a better index of response to treatment than fluid balance charts. The response to treatment is assessed, by falling body weight and disappearance of oedema, reduction in central venous pressure and diuresis. In patients with atrial fibrillation, an additional guide is provided by the heart rate (not the pulse rate); it is usual to aim at a heart rate of 65–80/min. at rest, in this condition. The development of toxic effects or a heart rate below 55/min is an indication for reducing the dose. It is commonly necessary to titrate the dose of the drug almost to the limit of tolerance, in order to obtain an adequate effect. After recovery from an episode of congestive cardiac failure, it may be necessary for the patient to continue to take a maintenance dose of digitalis, the size of which must be determined for the individual patient by trial and error. If the primary cause of the cardiac failure is remediable, the patient may not require such maintenance treatment.

Many different diuretics are available, and it is better for the practitioner to familiarise himself with one drug, and to use this as the drug of first choice, moving to other agents only if a definite indication exists. A rapid diuresis can be induced by intravenous frusemide (20–40 mg), or by intramuscular injection of 2 ml of mercuramide; the former will usually produce a more rapid, but shorter lasting diuresis than the latter. If there is less urgency, any of the benzthiazide diuretics, may be used, with due attention to potassium supplements. In general, it is better to employ potassium chloride preparations than those which do not contain chloride. Once the patient's dry weight has been attained, continuous treatment with diuretics may be necessary. At this stage, there is no advantage in using one of the more rapidly acting diuretics. Some have advocated the use of diuretics and potassium supplements on alternate days, but there is no convincing evidence that this kind of regime results in fewer side effects than continuous treatment with both agents.

When a stable situation has been reached, it is necessary to consider the patient's future activities in relation to his capacities, and, as in all chronic diseases, it may be necessary to alter his mode of life.

Intractable congestive failure

Few heart diseases are completely curable, and thus, as patients become older, heart failure tends to become more and more difficult to treat. If the above measures have failed, complete rest is imperative. It is often possible to reduce oedema in patients who are resistant to full digitalisation and the use of single diuretics, by a combination of diuretics. The object is to try to increase glomerular filtration rate at a time when the renal tubules are being influenced at a number of different levels. Several combinations are possible, but one which is usually effective is:

at time 0	Triamterene 100 mg orally.
0 + 30 mins.	Mercuramide 2 ml intramuscularly (it is better to inject this into the upper limb, which is usually less oedematous than the lower.)
0 + 60 mins.	Frusemide 40 mg I.V.
0 + 90 mins.	Aminophylline 250 mg (slowly) I.V.

Combinations of this type may succeed in mobilising fluid after less drastic measures have failed. If these combinations are used frequently, and particularly if dietary sodium intake is severely restricted, there is a risk of decreasing glomerular filtration and the production of azotaemia. If a diuresis cannot be established, reduction of dietary sodium below 10 m.Eq daily may be required. With marked reduction of sodium intake, there is usually a further increase in aldosterone secretion, and a tendency for increasing urinary potassium loss, particularly if benzthiazide diuretics are being given. The dangers of potassium depletion are exaggerated by the digitalis which such patients should be receiving, and adequate potassium supplements must be maintained. In the late states of intractable cardiac failure, hyponatraemia is commonly found, and is of grave prognostic significance.

These patients have an excess of total body sodium but an even greater excess of total body water, for reasons that are as yet uncertain. The addition of hypertonic saline is harmful, and the only measure that may help, is the restriction of fluid intake to less than 800 ml/day.

Nausea and vomiting are not uncommon in untreated cardiac failure, and are also common side-effects of digitalis preparations and of some potassium preparations. These symptoms can sometimes be difficult to assess and to treat. If no digitalis effect is evident upon the E.C.G., and in the absence of any arrhythmias which might be due to digitalis, it is reasonable to continue the drug, unless nausea is clearly related to the consumption of the tablets. In this case the dose may need to be reduced, or alternatively a different preparation of digitalis may be substituted.

Treatment of the underlying cause of cardiac failure

(a) *Valvular and structural lesions.* The development of cardiac failure in patients with valvular lesions may be an indication for surgical treatment of the underlying abnormality; this decision will require cardiological investigation. Cardiac failure may be precipitated by subacute bacteral endocarditis in such patients.

(b) *Hypertension.* If a patient with hypertension shows signs of cardiac failure, this is an indication for treatment of the hypertension.

(c) *Pulmonary heart disease.* Cor pulmonale, usually secondary to obstructive airways disease, is a common cause of elevated venous pressure and oedema. As previously indicated, this is not necessarily evidence of impaired right ventricular function, and the cardiac output is often high; a warm skin is often present. Episodes of apparent cardiac failure are commonly precipitated by acute respiratory infections, sometimes manifest only by a change of sputum from mucoid to purulent. The most important aspect of management is to treat these infections energetically with antibiotics, appropriate oxygen therapy and physiotherapy. The use of digitalis and diuretics in this condition is controversial. There is a theoretical argument that the reduction of venous pressure by diuresis, might be followed by a fall of cardiac output and hence an increase in tissue hypoxia. There is, however, no convincing evidence that harm is produced by the use of digitalis and diuretics, and most physicians employ these agents in this condition. Patients with chronic respiratory disease, usually have high plasma bicarbonate concentrations, and sometimes carbonic anhydrase inhibitors (acetazoleamide 500 mg daily, dichlorphenamide 50 mg daily) will induce a diuresis in patients who are relatively refractory to other agents.

Heart failure secondary to pulmonary emboli is also common, and may present in two says. Firstly, there is acute failure due to recurrent massive (and usually multiple) pulmonary emboli, and secondly the insidious onset of predominantly right-sided cardiac failure in patients with no history to suggest thrombophlebitis. Diagnosis can be particularly difficult in the second group, and hangs upon the exclusion of significant airway obstruction in patients with pulmonary hypertension, but without other cause for cardiac failure. Treatment is as for cardiac failure generally, together with the use of anticoagulants.

(d) *Beri beri.* This condition is uncommon, but its importance lies in the fact that it can be cured. Warm extremities, a bounding pulse, tender leg muscles and a dietary history of deficiency suggest the diagnosis. Treatment is by the oral or intra-muscular administration of 50 mg thiamine, followed by dietary supervision.

(e) *Myocardial ischaemia.* Cardiac failure may arise insidiously, in patients with myocardial ischaemia. In this situation, it should be treated as indicated above. If propranolol has been used to control anginal pain, it will have to be withdrawn when cardiac failure develops, as it will further impair the function of the failing ventricle.

Cardiac failure may also arise acutely, following myocardial infarction. The common association of ventricular arrhythmias may make treatment difficult in these circumstances. If numerous ventricular extrasystoles are present, they may be controlled by intravenous lignocaine in a dose of 75–100 mg, followed by a continuous infusion at a rate of 1–2 mg/minute. If the extrasystoles are controlled in this way, digoxin should not be withheld, and diuretics should be given, though the heart rate and rhythm should be frequently observed and the serum potassium regularly checked. In really severe heart muscle failure, with peripheral vasoconstriction, low blood pressure and oliguria, intravenous isoprenaline may be used as a continuous infusion at a rate of 0·1–2 μgm/minute. This procedure requires continuous monitoring, and facilities for defibrillation. The object is to control the infusion rate in such a way as to increase myocardial function without inducing serious arrhythmias, and the balance may be difficult to sustain. Concomitant administration of lignocaine may prevent or control ventricular arrhythmias, but it must be stressed that this kind of procedure should only be carried out where facilities for intensive care are available.

(f) *Arrhythmias*. Sustained high heart rates may cause many of the signs of cardiac failure, particularly in hearts already diseased. Treatment of the arrhythmia will often control the cardiac failure. If atrial fibrillation cannot be converted to sinus rhythm in patients with rheumatic heart disease, long term anticoagulant treatment should be instituted, as there is evidence that this decreases the risk of embolisation.

(g) *Anaemia*. Patients with severe anaemia frequently have raised jugular venous pressures, commonly with a high cardiac output. This state, like that in thyrotoxicosis, does not necessarily indicate impairment of cardiac muscle function and the signs usually regress when the underlying cause is treated.

(h) *Thyrotoxicosis*. Patients with thyrotoxicosis have a high cardiac output, and not infrequently a modest elevation of venous pressure, which does not indicate cardiac failure. True cardiac failure may arise, however, usually due to rapid atrial fibrillation in older patients. This should be treated by conventional methods, (though it may sometimes be difficult to control the heart rate with digitalis), while the thyrotoxicosis is controlled, usually with carbimazole or an equivalent preparation. Propranolol will suppress many of the manifestations of thyrotoxicosis, but it is unwise to use this in patients with cardiac failure. Rapid atrial fibrillation in the thyrotoxic patient can often be slowed with practolol, 100 mg thrice daily. This agent is less likely than propranolol to impair ventricular function. Once the patient is euthyroid, the atrial fibrillation should be corrected with cardioversion.

MYOCARDIAL ISCHAEMIA

The progressive narrowing of the coronary arteries by atheroma, common in many societies, results in two varieties of symptom complexes – angina pectoris and myocardial infarction. These descriptions of symptoms correlate only to a rough extent with pathological changes; most patients with angina pectoris have occlusion of at least one coronary artery, and many have areas of myocardial necrosis. The management of these conditions may be considered under two headings the treatment of the symptom complex, and the prevention or retardation of the underlying advancing process of atheroma.

Management of the symptom complex

(a) *Angina pectoris*. Attacks of pain are brought on, when the supply of blood to the myocardium is insufficient to meet its needs. Thus rational treatment requires an increase of blood supply, a decrease of requirements, or both. An increase in the effective availability of oxygen can be achieved by the treatment of severe anaemia, if this exists, but there are no other non-surgical methods of increasing effective blood flow in patients with coronary artery disease. Surgical treatment may include the implantation of the internal mammary artery into the myocardium, or replacement of a diseased aortic valve, but these are specialised procedures and will not be further considered here.

The most important aspects of treatment concern the reduction of myocardial work. Myocardial oxygen consumption is roughly proportional to the work done by the heart; a simplified, but reasonably effective index of this work is given by the product of systolic blood pressure and heart rate. Thus either hypertension or tachycardia merits treatment. During or just before the attack, the sublingual administration of glyceryl trinitrate (0·5 mg) reduces the left ventricular work load by a peripheral vaso-dilator action. It transiently reduces arterial pressure, and, by dilating veins, causes a decrease in atrial filling pressure and thus cardiac output. It therefore reduces myocardial blood flow requirements in two ways, and it is the only drug, with the exception of amyl nitrite, which can be used during the acute anginal attack. Its use may be limited by faintness, headache, flushing, or a feeling of fullness in the head. Frequency of dosage is limited only by side effects of this kind.

Prevention of attacks of angina can be achieved in several ways. Reduction of weight will indirectly reduce the myocardial work load, and this should always be undertaken in patients who are obese. The long-acting nitrates have little or no demonstrable superiority to inert tablets, and there is little point in using them. Propranolol does have a demonstrable effect, and in many patients it will increase exercise tolerance considerably. It reduces the myocardial work load by slowing the heart rate, reducing cardiac output and decreasing the velocity of ejection of blood with each ventricular contraction. It also has a modest effect in reducing arterial blood pressure. It should be used with great caution in patients at risk of heart failure, as it decreases the effectiveness of ventricular contraction. An initial dose of 10 mg thrice daily may be used, but frequently the patient requires larger doses of up to 240 mg thrice daily. A history of asthma should always be sought before using propranolol, as this agent may exacerbate or induce attacks in susceptible patients. Such patients may be treated with practolol or oxprenalol. Diabetics on insulin may require careful observation if given propranolol, as it may render hypoglycaemic attacks more severe.

In general, the patient with angina must live within his exercise tolerance, and this may require modification of his employment and his home circumstances. This is an exercise in compromise.

(b) *Myocardial infarction*. The acute problems of myocardial infarction are discussed in the next chapter and will not be further mentioned here.

Influencing the course of coronary artery disease

Many attempts have been made and are being made, to influence the progression of occlusive arterial disease in all parts of the circulation, but particularly in the coronary arteries. It is difficult to do this in a rational way, because the pathogenesis of arterial disease is not clearly understood. It is clear that there is a relationship between various serum lipids and arterial disease, and a probably independent relationship between arterial pressure and arterial disease. The striking variation in the prevalence and incidence of occlusive vascular disease in different populations and the indications that this difference is almost certainly in part due to environmental factors, encourages the view that it ought to be possible to influence the progress of this condition. Several approaches have been tried, based upon empirical findings. Almost all of these approaches require long-term dietary or drug manipulation, and the major problem that arises, as with all chronic diseases, is the difficulty of getting asymptomatic persons to accept modification of their way of life for a nebulous future benefit. The small effect of the known risk of bronchial carcinoma on cigarette consumption is an example of this sociological, rather than medical, problem. There is no reason to doubt that similar problems will arise with other prophylactic regimes.

(a) *Smoking*. There is reasonably good evidence that abstention from cigarettes will reduce the risk of myocardial infarction.

(b) *Anticoagulants*. Numerous trials of anticoagulants have been carried out, both in the acute phase following myocardial infarction, and in the prevention of subsequent infarcts. Most of these studies have some defects of design or control, and it is extremely difficult to carry out ideal clinical trials. The defects of these trials have been pointed out by Gifford and Feinstein (1969).

It is probably reasonable to employ anticoagulants to prevent pulmonary emboli after an acute myocardial infarction, if the patient is likely to remain in bed for more than two weeks.

The evidence that long term anticoagulant treatment influences prognosis in patients who have had myocardial infarcts is conflicting, but it is probably safe to say that if the use of these drugs confers any benefit, it is a very small one, and it is very doubtful whether their long-term use is justified. There is also some rather conflicting evidence that the sudden cessation of long-term anticoagulants may be followed by a transiently increased risk of vascular occlusive episodes.

(c) *Influencing serum lipid patterns.* Two general approaches have been used:

(i) Altering the diet, either by reducing lipid intake, or by giving unsaturated fatty acids.

(ii) Altering the lipid pattern by drugs, such as clofibrate or cholestyramine.

There is good evidence that the pattern of serum lipids may be modified by these means, but the evidence that this affects the progress of vascular disease is still scanty and conflicting. As with anticoagulants, the evidence suggests that any benefit conferred is a small one, and the decision whether to use these methods is an individual one. It can, of course, be argued that these methods might be very effective if started early enough in life, but there is no evidence at all on this score.

(d) *Influencing fibrinolysis.* There is some evidence of impairment of fibrinolysis in patients with myocardial infarction, and evidence that this abnormality may be corrected by the administration of phenformin (50 mg daily) and ethylestrenol (4 mg daily). This regime also reduces platelet adhesiveness. As with all the other preventive regimes there is no conclusive evidence that this treatment influences survival, and it is not free of side-effects.

SUBACUTE BACTERIAL ENDOCARDITIS

Prevention

Patients known to have rheumatic valvular disease should be given prophylactic antibiotics *immediately* before, and for 48 hours after dental surgery or minor surgical procedures. Ideally, the gingival margin should be swabbed within three days of the proposed treatment; if penicillin-resistant organisms are found, the appropriate antibiotic should be given. Otherwise benzyl penicillin in a dose of 2 mega units daily should be employed.

Treatment

If the organism is known, its antibiotic sensitivity should be established, and the appropriate antibiotic given in adequate dose for six weeks. It is of considerable importance to establish, after treatment has been instituted, that the patient's own serum is bactericidal to his own organism, obtained before treatment.

It is becoming much more common to fail to isolate a micro-organism from patients who clinically have subacute bacterial endocarditis. The possibility of Q fever should always be considered, and if type I antibodies are detected the patients should be treated with tetracycline and/or lincomycin. In other patients with negative blood cultures, the choice of antibiotic can be difficult. It is usual to start with penicillin and streptomycin, the former given in large doses of up to 100 mega-units daily, depending upon the response, the dose of the latter depending upon the patient's age and blood levels. These large doses will usually have to be given intravenously, with an indwelling catheter. This demands great care, and aseptic introduction, in view of the risk of inducing septicaemia with contaminating organisms. The catheter should be changed every few days. The response to treatment is judged clinically, and by observation of temperature and sedimentation rate. Failure to achieve a response in about 14 days is an indication for stopping treatment for a few days, reculturing the blood, and if an organism is not found, treating with a different antibiotic.

Valvular damage can progress very rapidly during bacterial endocarditis, and intractable cardiac failure may be a problem. Some successes have been achieved by valve replacement during the course of bacterial endocarditis, though the mortality is high. If a patent ductus arteriosus is present, it should be closed, and with other lesions, surgery may prove helpful in desperate situations.

PERICARDITIS

Pericarditis arising from myocardial infarction, acute rheumatism, renal failure, or collagen vascular disease requires management of the underlying lesion. Pericarditis arising several weeks after cardiac surgery or myocardial infarction may be improved with steroids. Anticoagulants, if being used, should be withdrawn because of the risk of pericardial bleeding and consequent tamponade. Purulent pericarditis will usually be preceded by septicaemia, but may require pericardial aspiration for diagnosis.

Tuberculous pericarditis may be diagnosed on the findings in the pericardial fluid, though this is often unhelpful, and it is sometimes difficult to distinguish this condition from non-specific pericarditis, which is probably due to viral infection in many cases. If tuberculous pericarditis is confirmed a course of streptomycin, P.A.S. and isoniazid should be given. The patient should be watched for the development of signs of constrictive pericarditis, which will require pericardiectomy.

In non-specific pericarditis, there is not uncommonly evidence of effusions elsewhere; the course is rather variable. In some patients, the condition resolves quite rapidly, leaving no sequelae. Only symptomatic treatment is required. In others, the condition may persist, with fever, pain, and in a number of cases, progression to constrictive pericarditis. Symptomatic relief is obtained using steroids, but considerable difficulty may arise if the possibility of tuberculosis cannot be ruled out. Either of two courses of action can then be adopted; to give steroids and antituberculous treatment, or to establish the diagnosis by open pericardial biopsy; the latter approach provides an opportunity for early pericardiectomy, if the pericardium is already fibrosed.

HYPERTENSION

Indications for treatment

The management of a patient whose arterial pressure is raised depends upon a number of factors, almost all of which are related to the patient, though a few are technical. The first is the level of the blood pressure. The measurement itself is liable to some technical errors, particularly in patients with fat arms. It is likely that a good deal of this kind of error may be eliminated by the use of sphygmomanometer cuffs containing a bag of sufficient length to encircle the arm completely, and it is to be hoped that manufacturers will be able routinely to supply such cuffs on all sphygmomanometers.

There is now very good evidence that blood pressure levels in any population are a continuous variable. There is also good evidence that the prognosis of patients is inversely related to the level of their pressure. This means that there is little point in attempting to provide a numerical definition of hypertension. What is important is an operational definition – the level of blood pressure at which the doctor is going to take some action. This level, of course, depends upon evidence that the treatment will be beneficial to the patient, and evidence on this point is still incomplete. There is, however, adequate evidence that treatment of patients with severe or malignant hypertension improves their outlook very considerably (Leishman 1963).

Absolute indications for rapid blood pressure control include:

(a) Malignant Hypertension, with papilloedema or 'cotton wool' exudates, is an indication for emergency treatment, since untreated malignant hypertension is very rapidly fatal.

(b) Left Ventricular Failure with pulmonary oedema, if due to hypertension.

(c) Hypertensive Encephalopathy, with impairment of consciousness and possibly fits; this will usually present with the retinopathy of malignant hypertension but occasionally this is absent. It is sometimes difficult to distinguish this condition from subarachnoid haemorrhage.

General indications for treatment

There is fairly conclusive evidence that asymptomatic middle-aged patients with diastolic blood pressures in excess of 120 mm Hg, will have a better prognosis for life if their arterial pressure is reduced. This does not necessarily mean, however, that every patient whose diastolic pressure is above this level should be treated, and common sense must be employed. The decision that a patient with hypertension requires treatment, implies either long-term administration of drugs, or fairly extensive, uncomfortable, and sometimes hazardous investigation of an underlying cause. Thus, for example, there can be little argument for treatment of an asymptomatic female aged over 70, with a pressure of 180/120 mm Hg. Treatment is not contra-indicated by any of the following:

(a) Angina pectoris, or a myocardial infarct more than two months before.

(b) Cerebrovascular disease (unless the patient has such intellectual impairment that treatment might be difficult).

(c) Cardiac failure.
(d) Renal failure.
} These conditions are positive indications for treatment.

In asymptomatic patients with diastolic blood pressure levels below 120 mm Hg there is no unequivocal evidence that treatment is beneficial. The presence of cardiac failure, however, in patients with mild hypertension is an indication for treatment. Except in emergencies, a number of blood pressure measurements should be taken before a decision is reached.

General aspects of treatment

As far as possible, the patient's activities should not be restricted. Weight reduction should be instituted in overweight patients, but in the absence of renal failure no other dietary restrictions are needed. Since patients with hypertension have a greater risk of developing myocardial infarcts than the population at large, and since there is evidence that a reduced incidence of myocardial infarcts follows the cessation of smoking, it is sensible to encourage this course.

If treatment with drugs is going to be undertaken, it will almost always have to be life-long, and continued supervision will be necessary. Certain patients will be able to manage their own drug regimes, on the basis of blood pressure measurements at home, but this does not eliminate the need for supervision.

Treatment of secondary hypertension

Hypertension may be due to a number of underlying causes. In general, extensive investigations should not be carried out, unless the physician considers that treatment is indicated, whether or not an underlying cause is found. Treatment should consist of elimination of the preliminary cause if possible, in the following ways:

Coarctation – surgical.

Phaeochromocytoma – surgical, preceeded by premedication with phenoxybenzamine and possibly propranolol and/or *α* methyl paratyrosine.

Cushing's syndrome – surgical.

Aldosteronoma – surgical.

Renal Disease. If involving both kidneys – as for essential hypertension. If unilateral, the damaged kidney is non-functional, and the other intact – nephrectomy. If the damaged kidney is functional, the decision is a difficult one, and if the patient's blood pressure is readily controlled by drugs, it is often best to leave the damaged kidney alone. Urinary infection should be treated. Oral contraceptives can cause hypertension and may have to be withdrawn.

Treatment of essential hypertension and secondary hypertension in which the primary cause is not eradicable

The object is to reduce the level of arterial pressure to as normal a level as possible, without side-effects which distress the patient. A diastolic pressure below 100 mm Hg is usually the aim.

Adrenalectomy is not now performed; sympathectomy may very occasionally be of help in a patient who is unable or unwilling to continue treatment with drugs. The drugs used fall into two general categories: those which do not require meticulous attention to dosage, and those that do. The former can be used as the sole treatment for patients with mild or moderate hypertension, or in combination with the latter type in more severe hypertension. No single drug provides the ideal treatment, and individual patients' responses may make it necessary to change from one drug to another.

(a) *Non-emergency treatment of hypertension.* Patients with diastolic pressures below 120 mm Hg can often be treated with fixed dose drugs alone, and, if there is no urgency, it is worth trying this approach, since it is relatively unlikely to give rise to side effects.

Thiazide diuretics are usually the best agents with which to begin treatment, unless the patient has gout or diabetes. There are many drugs of this type, and none has any particular advantage. Adequate doses are:

Chlorothiazide	250 mg twice daily or 500 mg once daily
Hydrochlorothiazide	25 mg twice daily or 50 mg once daily
Hydroflumethiazide	25 mg twice daily or 50 mg once daily
Bendrofluazide	5 mg twice daily or 10 mg once daily
Cyclopenthiazide	0·25 mg twice daily or 0·5 mg once daily
Polythiazide	1–2 mg once daily
Chlorthalidone (not strictly a thiazide)	50–100 mg daily.

Frusemide and ethacrynic acid are shorter acting diuretics, which do reduce arterial pressure, but they have no demonstrated advantage over the thiazides, and are more expensive than the others.

Apart from the risk of precipitating gout and diabetes the main hazard is potassium depletion, and potassium supplements should generally be given: the dose depends on the patient's response, but 13 m.Eq of potassium chloride 2 or 3 times daily, as slow-release (*not* enteric-coated) or effervescent tablets are usually adequate. If hypokalaemia is a serious problem (and this is mainly the case when digitalis is used), triamterene 50 mg daily or spironalactone 50 mg daily may be added but is seldom required. The normal diet usually contains up to 60 m.Eq of potassium daily; if a patient stops eating for any reason, he will lose this additional supply of potassium, and depletion may become more likely.

The diuretics will usually give a reduction of arterial pressure in about a week, and if this is of adequate extent, no other treatment is needed.

Should a further small reduction of arterial pressure be required, it is worth while adding a small fixed dose of a rauwolfia alkaloid to the diuretic. Reserpine in a dose not exceeding 0·1 mg thrice daily may be used, or an equivalent dose of one of the other alkaloids such as:

rescinnamine	0·2 mg twice daily
deserpidine	0·25 mg three times daily
syrosingopine	0·25 mg twice daily
methoserpidine	10 mg three times daily.

Alternatively, a number of preparations of whole rauwolfia root extracts are available. There is no convincing evidence of the superiority of any single preparation. All the rauwolfia compounds take two to three weeks to have their effect, and there is a danger of depression, with a risk of suicide with doses larger than those indicated.

With more severe hypertension, or if the above measures give inadequate control, one must employ one of the drugs, whose dose require careful regulation (Table 1); with the exception of hydralazine all these drugs interfere with sympathetic transmission and in consequence cause a greater fall in blood pressure in the standing position, with usually a further fall on exercise, often accompanied by dizziness or faintness. Pargyline is not a very satisfactory agent, as it is a monoamine oxidase inhibitor, and as such, may cause considerable side effects when certain foods or other drugs are taken. Guanoxan and Guanoclor have proved rather more toxic than the other agents. Hydralazine is used quite extensively in the United States, but little elsewhere, because of its side effects and the danger, at high doses, of inducing a state like systemic lupus erythematosis. So far as the others are concerned, there is little difference in effectiveness or incidence of side effects, though methyl-dopa causes slightly less postural hypotension than the others. (Prichard *et al* 1968). Dosage may need to be reduced in warm weather or infections. The drugs may be used in association with diuretics. If diuretics are given after a stable dose of sympathetic blocking agent has been attained, this dose will need to be roughly halved, or hypotension

Table 1

Drug	dose range per day	approximate duration of action (hrs.)	Frequency of dose modifications
Bethanidine	15–400 mg	8–12	Every 2–3 days
Methyl Dopa	750–4000 mg	18–24	Every 3–5 days
Guanethidine	10–300 mg	36–48	Every 5–7 days
Debrisoquine	10–300 mg	8–12	Every 2–3 days
Hydralazine	25–400 mg	8–12	Every 2–3 days
Pargyline	25–200 mg	Slow onset	Every 1–2 weeks
Guanoxan	20–300 mg	8–15	3–4 days
Guanoclor	20–300 mg	3–12	2–3 days

may follow. Tricyclic antidepressants should not be given to patients receiving guanethidine, bethanidine or debrisoquine, as they inhibit the hypotensive effects of these drugs.

It is better to become familiar with the use of one of these drugs, and to change, only if the patient is inadequately controlled on the first one. The general plan is to start with a small dose, and increase this at intervals shown in Table 1 until adequate control is achieved, or until side effects limit further increase. Hypotension in the morning is quite common with most of these drugs. This can sometimes be alleviated, if one of the shorter acting drugs is used, by reducing the morning dose, if symptoms appear after it is taken, or the evening dose, if symptoms occur before the morning dose is taken. In patients with renal failure the dose increments should be made at greater intervals, as these drugs are excreted in the urine, and cumulative effects are more likely in the presence of renal failure.

Ganglion-blocking agents, such as pempidine or mecamylamine are now seldom used.

The place of propranolol in the treatment of hypertension is still uncertain. Some authors have reported very good blood pressure control with this drug given in large doses of up to 1g. daily, but most physicians have found that it has relatively little hypotensive action. It can be dangerous in the presence of heart failure.

(b) *Acute blood pressure reduction.* Several methods are available:

(1) Hexamethonium tartrate I.V. 2·5 mg followed by increments of 2·5–5 mg at 2–3 minute intervals, dose determined by B.P. readings.

(2) Intramuscular guanethidine 20 mg.
(3) Intramuscular pentolinium 1–3 mg.
(4) Intravenous diazoxide 200–300 mg, injected rapidly.

Once initial control is achieved, treatment is as in the previous section.

Antihypertensive treatment and surgery

Thiazides alone do not require modification of the dose, but careful control of potassium levels is important. If possible, rauwolfia alkaloids should be discontinued 2–3 weeks before operation.

Sympathetic blocking agents should be discontinued 1–4 days before operation, if good control has been maintained for some time; guanethidine should be withdrawn 7–10 days before. In the case of emergency operations the main hazard is that of marked hypotension from slight blood loss, and volume expansion may be needed. These patients will be very sensitive to infused noradrenaline.

Hypertension and pregnancy

Patients with pre-existing hypertension may become pregnant; in these patients, the risk to the foetus is greater than in normal pregnancies, mainly because of placental insufficiency, and early induction of labour is often necessary. Apart from this, arterial pressure should be kept under strict control, by the methods previously described. No evidence has been produced to indicate that any of the drugs listed has teratogenic properties.

Women whose blood pressures were previously normal may become hypertensive during toxaemia of pregnancy. Here, control of blood pressure, together with sodium restriction, will reduce the maternal risk; there is little convincing evidence that diuretics significantly improve the prognosis of the foetus, though they may decrease the amount of time that the patient has to remain in bed.

Diet

Diet may have to be modified in obese patients, in order to lose weight. In this connection there is evidence that fenfluramine does not interfere with the hypotensive action of any of the drugs mentioned in this section. Protein restriction may also have to be introduced in the presence of renal failure. Very occasionally, in extremely difficult cases, rigid sodium restriction may be necessary. With these exceptions, there is no indication for any dietary measures in the management of patients with hypertension.

PERIPHERAL VASCULAR DISEASE

Dissecting aneurysm

There is growing though inconclusive evidence that surviving patients in whom a diagnosis of aortic dissection has been made, fare better if treated conservatively for 2–3 weeks before surgical intervention is attempted. This course is only practicable if essential arteries are spared. During this period the patient is kept strictly at rest. Hypertension, if present, should be treated and there is a theoretical argument for the use of intramuscular reserpine, 2·5 mg daily, in order to reduce the ejection rate of blood from the left ventricle. The nature of the surgical intervention depends upon the distribution and extent of the dissection.

Aortic aneurysm

The definitive and only effective treatment for aortic aneurysms is surgical. The prognosis of untreated aortic aneurysm is poor, so that surgical treatment should always be considered, unless the patient's general condition or vascular disease elsewhere precludes it.

Obstructive arterial disease

This is common, and generally affects the aorta, and its lower branches. The commonest clinical problem arises in the lower limbs. As with myocardial ischaemia, there are two main problems; influencing the course of the atheroma, and management of the symptoms produced by arterial obstruction. The first problem has not been solved. The methods employed and the evidence of benefit from these approaches, are similar to the situation in myocardial ischaemia, and will not be reiterated.

General measures include weight reduction, treatment of anaemia and the avoidance of vasoconstrictor agents such as ergot alkaloids.

The progressive occlusion of lower limb arteries causes intermittent claudication, followed by distal necrosis. The obstruction is usually in large arteries, except in diabetes, where small vessels may also be obstructed. The ideal treatment is to restore the patency of the obstructed arteries, and with obstructive lesions above the level of the knee, this is often possible by surgical means. The site of the obstructive lesion must be defined by clinical and arteriographic investigation, provided that the patient does not have serious vascular disease elsewhere.

If surgical treatment is not to be carried out, the patient will have to live within his exercise tolerance. Weight reduction may improve his walking distance. Peripheral vasodilator drugs are of no value in the management of intermittent claudication, because the limitation of flow is due to a structural narrowing of large vessels, which is not affected by vasodilators.

In these patients, the care of the feet must be exceptionally conscientious. Small superficial lesions of the skin may become severely infected, and may lead to loss of tissue. This is a particularly serious problem in diabetic patients, because of their increased susceptibility to infection and because peripheral neuropathy may cause sensory loss, so that minor trauma, as from an ill-fitting shoe, goes unnoticed.

As the disease progresses, the likelihood of tissue loss increases, and rest-pain, with impending gangrene may be present. This may require powerful analgesics. The involved limb should be kept cool to reduce tissue metabolic demands, while the rest of the patient is warmed in an attempt to reduce sympathetic tone. Sympathectomy has little part to play in the treatment of intermittent claudication, but may be of use in some patients with rest pain, but without actual gangrene. Peripheral vasodilator drugs are not generally very useful, but may be given a trial. Once gangrene is apparent, small peripheral areas may, if uninfected, be allowed to separate spontaneously, while reflex heating is continued. Gangrene of any area larger than a toe is an indication for proximal amputation and rehabilitation.

References

Gifford, R. H., and Feinstein, A. R., *New Eng. J. Med.* (1969), **280**, 351.

Leishman, A. W. D., *Lancet* (1963), **i**, 1284.

Prichard, B. N. C., Johnson, A. W., Hill, I. D., and Rosenheim, M., *Brit. med. J.* (1968), **1**, 135.

This chapter was written by Professor W. I. Cranston.

Category II

Cardio-respiratory Emergencies

Clarity of thought is indispensable, and becomes more so as the urgency of the situation increases. The patients under consideration will usually present with arterial hypotension and/or dyspnoea. Diagnosis before treatment is of the essence in the management of such patients, and unless in imminent danger of death, it is vital to obtain a history and to examine the patient thoroughly. Premature treatment undertaken blindly is only likely to conceal the diagnosis for ever.

There is an inherent difficulty in keeping to this logical path of action, posed by the fact that as patients come close to death, from whatever cause, they tend to look the same and to lose those distinguishing features by which they may be separated one from another. In a small proportion of cases, it is necessary to restore the patient in order to make an accurate assessment, but rational treatment is impossible without a diagnosis. The resolution of this dilemma can only be achieved by making a first order diagnosis, applying appropriate restorative measures, and then, with the patient partially restored, seeking the final diagnosis and definitive treatment.

The proposition that haemorrhage and heart failure should be treated in the same way is clearly ridiculous, yet both may produce a state in which the salient features are hypotension and low cardiac output. To pronounce that all patients with major derangements of the circulation are in a "state of shock", and to look for some common mode of therapy for this state, is profitless. Even when it is possible to make an accurate physiological assessment of patients suffering from acute circulatory disorders of the same aetiology, it emerges that the disease patterns differ, and the treatment requires to be tailored to the needs of each. Thus, in patients suffering from septicaemia, the emphasis may be upon hypovolaemia, myocardial failure, or the breakdown of the normal pattern of perfusion in the peripheral circulation.

INITIAL MANAGEMENT

The possible courses of action are shown in figure 1. The first action must always be to ensure that the patient has a clear airway. Subsequent management will be dictated by the state of the patient.

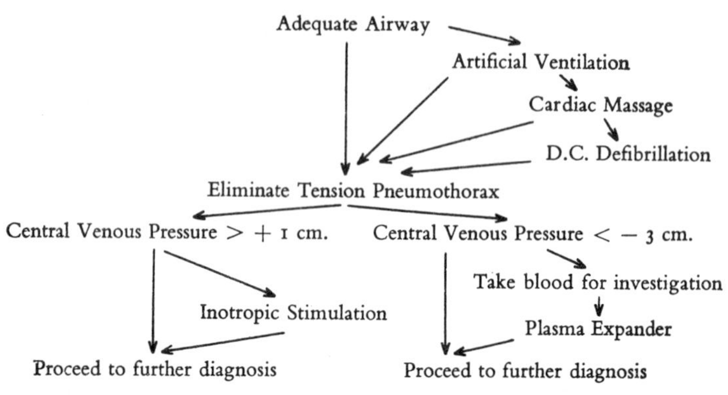

Figure 1.

If the patient's ventilation is grossly inadequate, he should be artificially ventilated with whatever apparatus is available (Brook airway, 'Ambu' bag or endotracheal tube and anaesthetic bag), preferably with oxygen. If unconscious and pulseless, the circulation should be supported with external cardiac massage. If the patient remains in a state of cardiac arrest, the degree of metabolic acidosis should be determined and corrected (0·1 m.Eq sodium bicarbonate/kg body weight/m.Eq base deficit – where the base deficit is measured in m.Eq/1); arbitrary correction with 100 m.Eq sodium bicarbonate if the arrest has been brief, or 200 m.Eq for longer periods, is a suggested approximation if measurement is impossible. An E.C.G. should be recorded. Ventricular fibrillation should be dealt with by D.C. defibrillation, starting with 100 Joules. If the ventricular fibrillation persists or returns, intravenous lignocaine 1 mg/kg body weight followed by defibrillation will increase the probability of a stable rhythm. Asystole or fine ventricular fibrillation may be converted to coarse ventricular fibrillation, or some more favourable rhythm, by the intravenous use of 5 to 10 ml of adrenaline diluted 1/10,000 (100 μg/ml), 5 to 10 ml of 2 per cent calcium chloride will increase myocardial tone, and therefore increase the effectiveness of cardiac massage in a grossly atonic heart.

Normally it is possible to proceed directly from ensuring that the patient has an adequate airway, to eliminating the possibility of a tension pneumothorax. There are two reasons for doing so at this early stage – the logical one, that the condition does not belong in either of the main groupings in the system of diagnosis to be described, and the practical one, that this is a treatable condition in which the patient's state is likely to deteriorate rapidly. In the absence of other pulmonary pathology, the physical signs are unmistakable – absent or grossly diminished breath sounds and resonance to percussion on one side of the chest, and mediastinal shift toward the opposite side.

CENTRAL VENOUS PRESSURE

Reference to Figs 1 and 2 will show the cardinal position of the central venous pressure in terms of diagnosis. Should the venous pressure be assessed incorrectly, the diagnosis must inevitably be wrong. Every possible manoeuvre must be used to establish whether the level is raised or lowered, and if there remains any uncertainty, it must be measured with a catheter in some part of the venous system within the chest. The catheter can be advanced to this point from a basilic vein in the arm, or from the subclavian, femoral or internal jugular vein. As will be seen later, a centrally placed venous line is of enormous value for many of the measures which may subsequently become necessary.

Pressures in the venous system must be measured relative to some fixed point. The sternal angle is the most convenient reference point in clinical practice, and it is to this point that the figures quoted are related.

The possible range of normal mean venous pressures is of the order plus 3 cm of water to minus 5 cm. If the venous pressure is to be used as an arbiter in patients presenting with acute cardio-respiratory disorders, the centre of the watershed can be more closely confined. All those with pressures greater than plus 1 cm are placed in the high-filling pressure group, and those lower than minus 3 cm in the low-filling pressure group.

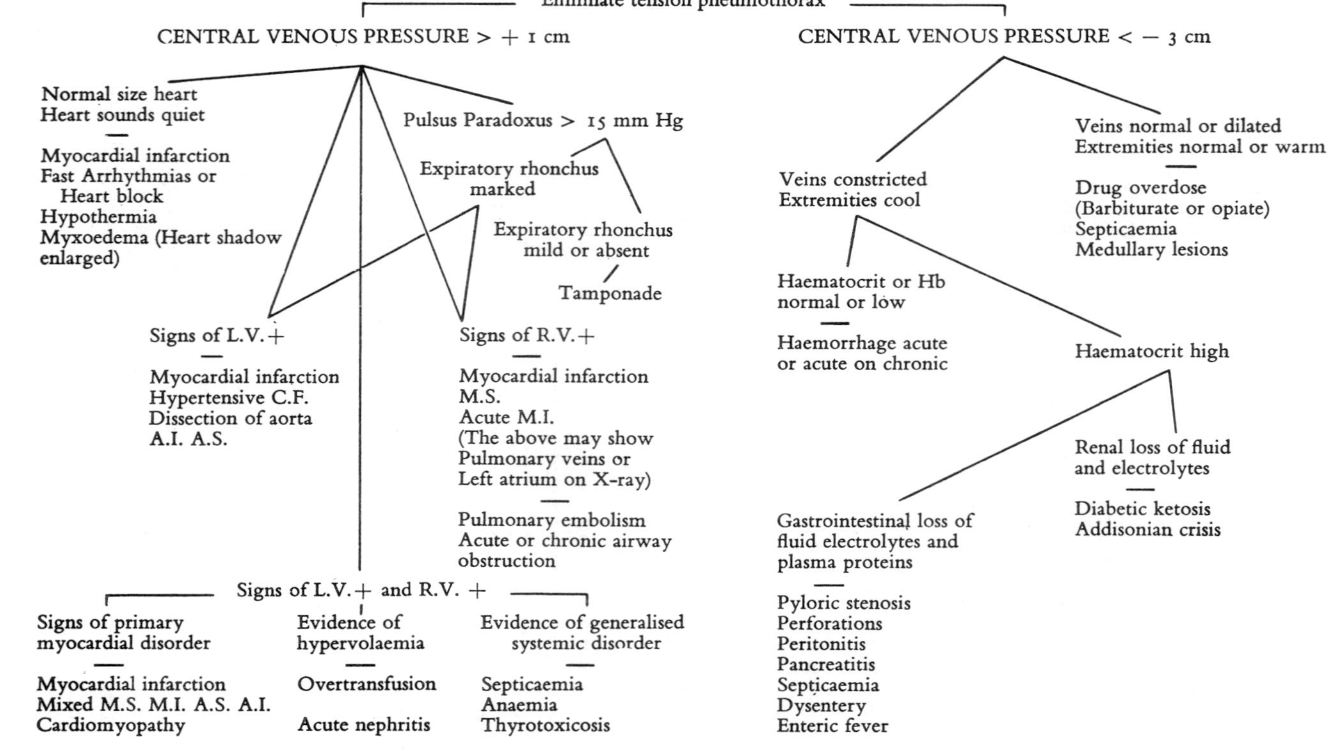
Eliminate tension pneumothorax
CENTRAL VENOUS PRESSURE > + 1 cm
CENTRAL VENOUS PRESSURE < − 3 cm
Normal size heart
Heart sounds quiet
Myocardial infarction
Fast Arrhythmias or
Heart block
Hypothermia
Myxoedema (Heart shadow
enlarged)
Pulsus Paradoxus > 15 mm Hg
Expiratory rhonchus
marked
Expiratory rhonchus
mild or absent
Tamponade
Signs of L.V.+
Myocardial infarction
Hypertensive C.F.
Dissection of aorta
A.I. A.S.
Signs of R.V.+
Myocardial infarction
M.S.
Acute M.I.
(The above may show
Pulmonary veins or
Left atrium on X-ray)
Pulmonary embolism
Acute or chronic airway
obstruction
Signs of L.V.+ and R.V. +
Signs of primary
myocardial disorder
Myocardial infarction
Mixed M.S. M.I. A.S. A.I.
Cardiomyopathy
Evidence of
hypervolaemia
Overtransfusion
Acute nephritis
Evidence of generalised
systemic disorder
Septicaemia
Anaemia
Thyrotoxicosis
Veins constricted
Extremities cool
Veins normal or dilated
Extremities normal or warm
Drug overdose
(Barbiturate or opiate)
Septicaemia
Medullary lesions
Haematocrit or Hb
normal or low
Haemorrhage acute
or acute on chronic
Haematocrit high
Renal loss of fluid
and electrolytes
Diabetic ketosis
Addisonian crisis
Gastrointestinal loss of
fluid electrolytes and
plasma proteins
Pyloric stenosis
Perforations
Peritonitis
Pancreatitis
Septicaemia
Dysentery
Enteric fever

Figure 2.

There will be a small number with mixed disease, and should a patient present with profound circulatory disturbance, whose filling pressure lies between the limits suggested above, it is well to consider the possibility of dual pathology.

Once the height of the venous pressure is known, a decision has to be made in the light of the patient's condition, for if this is deteriorating seriously, there is now information upon which to base logical supportive therapy without risk of concealing the diagnosis. There is a second consideration which may suggest such action – the patient may be in such a poor state that the physical signs upon which the diagnosis depends, will not be apparent until something has been done to improve his condition. Thus abdominal physical signs may be absent in a patient with a perforated peptic ulcer, until the circulation has been at least partially restored. The principle of diagnosis before treatment is not in fact being broken, for a first stage diagnosis has been made, which allows limited treatment.

If the patient is in the high-filling pressure group, and the circulation is inadequate, then, in general, the output of the heart can only be improved by the use of an inotropic agent. If some supportive therapy is urgently necessary, isoprenaline 1 to 2 μg/min may be given intravenously as an infusion. An acidosis will reduce the effectiveness of the drug and should be corrected. Isoprenaline may cause serious arrhythmias, making E.C.G. monitoring necessary, and if given in the presence of anoxia, it can cause myocardial damage.

Should intervention be indicated at this juncture in the low-filling pressure group, blood must be taken for haematology (Hb or haematocrit, W.B.C., platelets, grouping and serum for possible cross-matching), and chemistry (electrolytes, urea, sugar and plasma proteins), and only then the filling pressure may be restored toward normal with a synthetic plasma expander, until more is known of the nature of the fluid that has been lost. If more than one litre has to be given urgently, plasma should be used subsequently. There is nothing to be gained by raising the filling pressure above normal. If a normal filling pressure fails to produce a normal cardiac output, then there is something amiss with the heart, and the further administration of fluid may well do harm.

LOW VENOUS PRESSURE GROUP (-3 CM OR LOWER)

The further logical separation of patients with disorders in this group is not usually a matter of great difficulty.

Low venous tone group

If the cause of the fall in venous pressure is a drop in venous tone, as may occur in cases of barbiturate and opiate intoxication, certain medullary lesions and in some patients with septicaemias, then the limb veins will appear to be of normal calibre, or even dilated, the limbs will be of normal temperature, or warmer than normal, and the skin usually dry, unless the patient has become hypothermic.

These patients characteristically retain good flows, with arterial pressures as low as 50 to 60 mm of mercury, provided that they remain lying flat, and will produce urine at normal rates when the arterial pressure is above 60 mm of mercury. If the cardiac output remains low despite an adequate filling pressure, an inotropic agent should be used.

The general circulatory treatment, as opposed to specific treatment aimed at the cause, should be directed to raising the filling pressure toward normal.

In the case of intoxications, it is safer to use a synthetic plasma expander, but in patients with septicaemia who may well go on to oligaemia and require larger volumes, and who may also have thrombocytopenia and/or undergo defibrinogenation, plasma is probably the fluid of choice.

In septicaemia there is also a high incidence of pulmonary oedema, and considerable care should be taken not to overload the circulation. The most appropriate management is probably the lowest filling pressure commensurate with good systemic blood flow, and a urine output of at least 30 ml/hr. The level of the plasma proteins should be maintained in order to retain the oncotic properties of the plasma. Patients thus treated will have a normal filling pressure and a normal or raised cardiac output, depending upon heart rate, but a low arterial pressure because the systemic vascular resistance is low. Providing that the urine flow is at least 30 ml/hr, this normal flow, low pressure state, is to be preferred to the use of vasoconstrictors, since these upset the pattern of systemic perfusion more seriously.

High venous tone group

If oligaemia is the cause of a low-filling pressure, the normal vascular reflexes will produce venoconstriction and cold extremities, and the skin may or may not be sweaty. If the haematocrit or haemoglobin is normal, the probable cause is acute haemorrhage; if the haematocrit is low, acute on chronic haemorrhage. Should the haematocrit be high, renal or gastrointestinal losses of fluid, electrolytes and plasma protiens should be sought.

Common causes of gastrointestinal loss of this nature are pyloric stenosis, gastrointestinal perforations, peritonitis, pancreatitis, dysentery, enteric fever, and septicaemia. The loss may be into the lumen of the gut, or the peritoneal cavity, or both.

Renal losses on this scale occur in diabetic ketosis and Addisonian crisis.

The diagnostic scheme just described will, of course, break down, should a chronically severely anaemic patient in becoming oligaemic by loss of salt and water, raise his low haematocrit to normal. Although the diagnosis of acute haemorrhage will be incorrect, the conclusion that the oligaemia should be treated with whole blood remains true.

Ideally, oligaemia should be treated by replacement of whatever fluid has been lost. This has to be modified in practice by considerations such as the local availability of blood and blood products, their safety, and the limit set upon the use of synthetic plasma expanders by their effect upon the normal haemostatic systems, and the kidneys.

It might be thought also that the volume of the replacement should equal the volume which has been lost, and although this is probably ultimately true, it is not a particularly helpful concept. The volume which has been lost is not generally known, and although the remaining circulating volume can be estimated with isotopic techniques, replacement based upon measurements of volume in this way may cause the death of the patient. The reason for this apparent anomaly is the variability in the capacity of the vascular bed. There are few more powerfully constrictive influences upon the systemic venous capacity vessels than oligaemia.

The relation of venous tone and venous blood volume to central venous pressure can be shown diagrammatically. In Fig. 3(a), the central venous pressure is plotted on the ordinate, and the change of volume of blood in the systemic venous capacity vessels on the abscissa.

A normal man would lie at or about the origin, with a volume of 3·5 litres in the systemic venous capacity vessels, a venous pressure of approximately 0 cm water, and a normal venous tone. The line AB represents the way in which the venous pressure would rise and fall as blood is either added to or removed from the system, if the venous tone is kept constant. This line might be called an isophleb, a line of constant venous tone. There is a series of these isophlebs, each one representing the relationship between venous pressure and venous volume at a

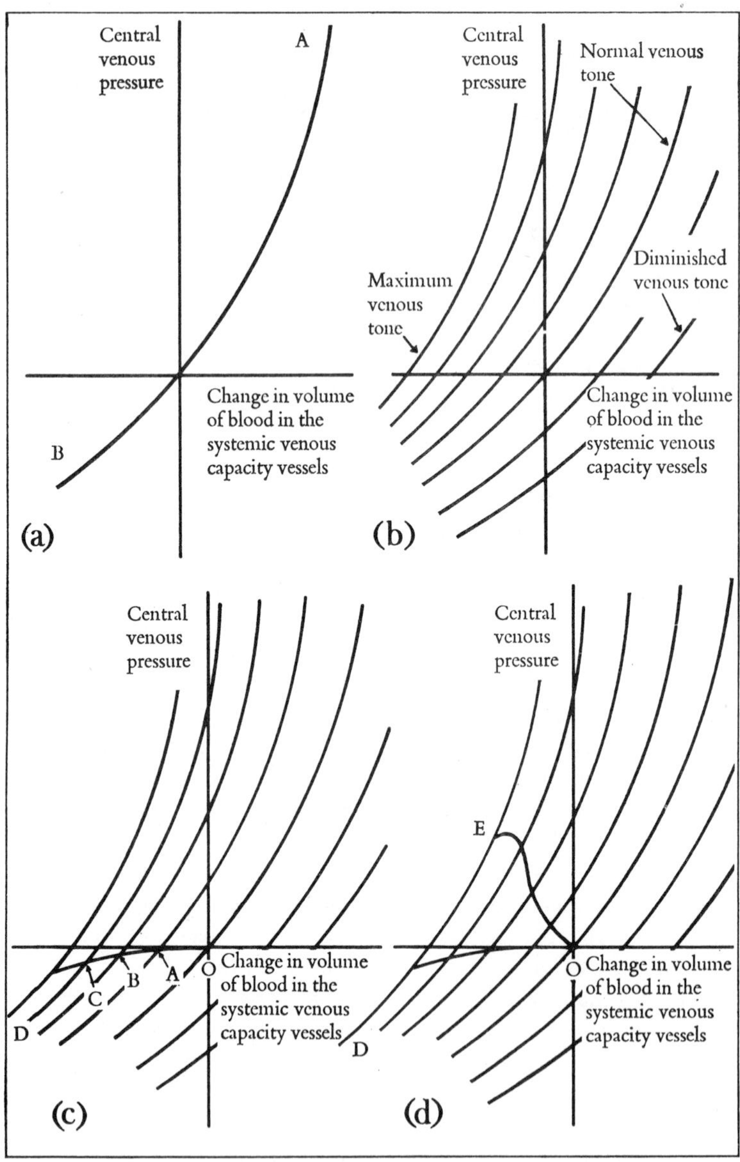
Central
venous
pressure
A
B
Change in volume
of blood in the
systemic venous
capacity vessels
(a)
Central
venous
pressure
Normal venous
tone
Maximum
venous
tone
Diminished
venous tone
Change in volume
of blood in the
systemic venous
capacity vessels
(b)
Central
venous
pressure
D
C
B
A
O
Change in volume
of blood in the
systemic venous
capacity vessels
D
(c)
Central
venous
pressure
E
O
Change in volume
of blood in the
systemic venous
capacity vessels
(d)

Figure 3.

different level of venous tone. Fig 3(b) shows a number of such lines.

During haemorrhage, volume is lost from the venous bed but initially the drop in venous pressure is very small as the veins tighten down upon the shrinking volume.

The progress of events may be followed in Fig. 3(c). As haemorrhage proceeds, the patient moves down the line OABCD. First the patient's foot veins will constrict, then the arm veins, and ultimately the venules in the skin of the face, giving the patient a characteristic pallor. With further haemorrhage, the venous pressure will fall quite sharply, and with it the cardiac output and systemic arterial pressure.

In ideal circumstances during transfusion the opposite path is retraced, and as the venous pressure approaches normal, the patient's venous system is observed to dilate; the re-appearance of the foot veins signalling a return to normality. Events may not follow such a simple course. There are a number of factors which may cause the venous system to remain tightly constricted, in spite of volume replacement. The most important appear to be anoxia, hypothermia, pain, and myocardial damage which may occur during the period of coronary malperfusion associated with a low cardiac output.

Fig 3(d) illustrates how it may come about that the venous pressure may rise to dangerous levels (E), before the volume of blood which was lost from the system has been replaced. This may be lethal if the heart is abnormal.

If the cause of the high venous tone is dealt with, or resolves spontaneously because of the increase in cardiac output associated with restoration of the filling pressure, the patient will return to normal along the hysteresis loop DEO. It is possible to avoid the danger involved in raising the filling pressure in this way, by observing the venous pressure and state of the peripheral veins, and not by measuring the blood volume. If, as the venous pressure rises toward normal, the peripheral veins do not dilate, a cause for the sustained high venous tone must be sought and corrected. It will then be possible to charge the systemic venous system to its normal capacity, the end point being signalled by dilatation of the foot veins.

(The model of the venous system which has been presented, in which the filling pressure of the right heart is the product of venous tone and volume of blood contained in the venous reservoir, is an over-simplification derived only from static considerations. The addition of dynamic considerations such as the 'sucking' effect of the right ventricle, modify the system but do not alter the conclusions.)

HIGH VENOUS PRESSURE GROUP (+ 1 CM OR ABOVE)

It is beyond the scope of this account to enter into the detailed diagnosis of all the conditions grouped under this heading in Fig 2. Some general principles are outlined in the figure; it will be seen that the breakdown into smaller groups of possibilities depends upon the assessment of the relative activity and size of the two sides of the heart. This assessment depends upon the clinical, E.C.G. and X-ray findings. Because of the difficulties of making an accurate estimate of each side of the heart, diagnosis is very much less simple here than in the low filling pressure group.

High venous pressure – normal heart size

The combination of an impalpable, or nearly impalpable right and left ventricle of normal size, a raised venous pressure and notably quiet heart sounds in a patient presenting acutely with hypotension or dyspnoea, is most commonly due to myocardial infarction. Fast arrhythmias, heart block, hypothermia and severe myxoedema can also produce these physical signs, but none of these conditions presents any diagnostic difficulty, apart from the possibility that they may be complicated by myocardial infarction.

Difficulty does arise when the signs of ventricular overactivity, which would place the patient in a different diagnostic group, are absent because of extreme reduction in cardiac output.

High venous pressure with right ventricular overactivity

The signs of right ventricular overactivity which characterise this group are a palpable right ventricular and pulmonary arterial heave, audible third and fourth sounds over the right ventricle, widened splitting of the second sound, and an intensification of the second element of the second sound. Not all may be present, and some, such as a third sound signifying dilatation of the ventricle, are of greater significance than others, for example, a fourth sound which only implies atrial overactivity and may be heard in any condition in which there is an increase in sympathetic activity, even though the atrial pressure may be abnormally low.

Within this group, myocardial infarction, acute mitral incompetence and mitral stenosis will be associated with a considerably raised left atrial pressure, whereas in pulmonary embolism, and acute or chronic airway obstruction, the left atrial pressure may be low, or at most, mildly raised. It is unfortunate therefore, that there is no physical sign related to this pressure which can reliably be used as an arbiter in all these conditions, although a straight chest X-ray in which there are prominent pulmonary veins, or a visible left atrium, is good evidence of a raised left atrial pressure.

Myocardial infarction of sufficient extent to produce signs of right ventricular overactivity will always be associated with E.C.G. changes. It is only when these changes are compatible also with acute pulmonary embolism, that diagnostic difficulty arises, and special investigations may be required.

Chronic airway obstruction and acute asthma presenting as cardio-respiratory emergencies usually declare themselves from the briefest of histories. Glottic or tracheal obstruction will usually be discovered if its existence is considered.

Acute mitral incompetence is almost always associated with a loud apical pansystolic murmur, and sometimes a thrill. The cause may be papillary muscle dysfunction or a ruptured cusp – the former associated with infarction, and the latter usually with bacterial endocarditis. Chronic mitral incompetence is, of course, associated with a dilated left ventricle. Previously undiagnosed mitral stenosis may present as an emergency, especially in pregnancy, but it is recognised by the characteristic mitral diastolic murmur, if present, or from a typical mitral configuration of the heart on chest X-ray.

High venous pressure with left ventricular overactivity

The signs of left ventricular disturbance suggestive of this group of disorders, are a left ventricular heave, apical third and fourth sounds, reversed splitting of the second sound, and the presence of pulsus alternans. Again, the fourth sound is of less account that any of the other signs as it may be heard in any state associated with sympathetic overactivity. Relatively small degrees of pulsus alternans may be detected with a sphygomomanometer; this is often precipitated by an ectopic beat, and, unless the heart rate is of the order of 200 per minute, is a reliable sign of left ventricular dysfunction.

When acute left ventricular failure occurs against a background of systemic hypertension, it is often associated with a further rise in the arterial pressure. Myocardial infarction in this setting of enlargement of the left ventricle, may present diagnostic difficulty, unless the E.C.G. changes are unequivocal, or there are enzyme changes, because the enlargement may well be due to previous infarction. Dissection of the aorta is usually suggested by the severity and sudden onset of substernal pain radiating to the back or legs, but asynchrony or absence of pulses and broadening of the mediastinum should be sought. Both aortic stenosis and aortic incompetence may present as emergencies, and are indicated by the appropriate murmurs and changes in pulse pressure.

High venous pressure with left and right ventricular overactivity

Patients in this category may be subdivided into those with primary myocardial or valvular disorders, those with hypervolaemia, and those with some general systemic disorder which occasions an abnormally high cardiac output.

Hypervòlaemia and high output states are commonly accompanied by biventricular overactivity to palpation, and audible fourth sounds at the apex and left sternal edge. Primary myocardial disorder is suggested by third sounds heard over the ventricles, and by pulsus alternans.

Those with primary myocardial disorder or valvular disease include patients with myocardial infarction, cardiomyopathies, and varying combinations of mitral and aortic stenosis and incompetence.

Hypervolaemia will be diagnosed, provided that the conditions which may give rise to this are considered – that is, overtransfusion, acute nephritis, and drug induced water-salt retention. Generalised systemic disorders, such as severe anaemias, thyrotoxicosis, and septicaemia, which may be associated with a high venous pressure and high cardiac output, do not usually present diagnostic difficulty.

Tamponade

A raised venous pressure and pulsus paradoxus in the absence of airway obstruction, are indicative of cardiac tamponade. The pressure swings in the arterial pulse due to respiration, can be measured with a sphygmomanometer. The pressure at which the pulse is just palpable at the end of each expiration is recorded, and the pressure in the cuff lowered until the pulse can just be felt continuously throughout the respiratory cycle. The second pressure recorded at this point is then subtracted from the first. In normal subjects this pressure swing is less than 5 mm Hg, but will rise to 15 to 30 mm Hg in tamponade, and may be as high as 45 mm Hg in severe asthma where it reflects the intrathoracic pressure swing.

If the heart shadow on chest X-ray is large, and there is a systolic descent in the venous pressure, the tamponade is due to a pericardial effusion. If the heart shadow is normal, or only slightly enlarged, and the descent in the venous pressure is post-systolic, or both post-systolic and systolic, the tamponade is due to pericardial constriction.

GENERAL PRINCIPLES OF ACUTE MANAGEMENT OF HIGH FILLING PRESSURE DISORDERS

The acute life-threatening problems which occur in this group of disorders are low cardiac output, pulmonary oedema, arrhythmias, cardiac tamponade, pulmonary embolism, and airway obstruction.

Low cardiac output

In those situations within the high-filling pressure group of disorders in which the cardiac output is seriously impaired, the stroke output of the heart is low, and in contrast to the normal heart does not change significantly with alterations in filling pressure. Transfusion will not. therefore, improve the cardiac output, and since it may precipitate pulmonary oedema, must be avoided.

Useful increases in cardiac output are only likely to be obtained with inotropic agents such as digitalis and isoprenaline. The agent of choice will depend upon the heart rate and rhythm; if the rate is fast, or if there is flutter or atrial fibrillation, digitalis should be used. In the presence of a slow rate, or if there is any evidence of heart block, isoprenaline should be given.

Isoprenaline sulphate as an intravenous infusion in a dose of 0·5 to 5μg/min has the great advantage that it is rapid in action, and the dosage can be modified very quickly should it cause arrhythmias. Although this drug raises myocardial oxygen consumption by increasing the heart rate, this is much modified by the reduction in the afterload upon the left ventricle which it produces by diminishing the systemic vascular resistance.

Acetyl strophanthidin has certain advantages over digoxin in acute situations; its effects appearing and passing off very much more rapidly. Digitalisation may be achieved with four intravenous doses of 0·1 mg given at twenty minute intervals.

Pulmonary oedema

Pulmonary oedema appears whenever the left atrial pressure or pulmonary venous pressure is raised above a critical value of approximately 24 mm Hg. This critical value drops to the region of 12 mm Hg if the concentration of the plasma proteins is halved. Pulmonary oedema will also occur if the basement membrane of the pulmonary capillaries loses its normal properties, as it does locally in areas of pneumonia or pulmonary infarction, and in the generalised pulmonary capillary damage which may be sustained in septicaemia. Administration of high concentrations of oxygen in the inspired air will tend to correct the fall in arterial oxygen tension produced by pulmonary oedema, but will not contribute to the dispersal of the oedema.

If the oedema has been generated by a high left atrial pressure, relief must be obtained by reducing this; the rate of disappearance of the fluid will increase according to the degree of reduction. In the case of left ventricular failure, the relation of the two sides of the heart is such that a small fall in right atrial pressure of 2 or 3 mm Hg, such as may be obtained rapidly with intravenous morphia, will produce a fall in left atrial pressure as large as 10 or 15 mm Hg.

If the heart is normal and the high left atrial pressure is due to overtransfusion, suitably large falls in left atrial pressure can only be obtained by dropping the right atrial pressure from 15 or 20 mm Hg to the region of 5 mm Hg. Pulmonary oedema due to hypervolaemia cannot, therefore, be treated with morphia, but fast acting diuretics such as frusemide or ethacrynic acid should be administered intravenously, or if the patient is anuric or likely to die before the diuretics can operate, venesection must be undertaken. It will usually be necessary to remove about 1500 ml of blood to reduce the atrial pressures to reasonable levels, and, provided the blood is taken into suitable containers, the patient's own packed cells can be retransfused, when the circulating volume has been further reduced with diuretics.

Attention is seldom paid to the level of the plasma proteins in the treatment of pulmonary oedema, but this is of particular importance in the context of septicaemia, in which the plasma proteins may be lost into the peritoneum and the gut, and there may be coexistent myocardial failure. When pulmonary oedema occurs in septicaemia due to breakdown of the pulmonary capillary membrane, there is some evidence that massive doses of steroids may help, but this complication is often fatal. Intermittent positive pressure ventilation delivered through an endotracheal tube is a most valuable supportive measure in any patient with very severe acute pulmonary oedema, from whatever cause. It may be necessary to curarise such patients, as they have a very considerable ventilatory drive and should not be allowed to breathe against the respirator as this will tend to make the oedema worse.

Arrhythmias

This brief account of the treatment of acute arrhythmias refers essentially to those occurring in association with acute myocardial infarction, but is applicable in a wider range of heart disease.

In dealing with any arrhythmia, it is essential to correct arterial hypoxaemia, to measure and correct hypo- or hyper-kalaemia, and to consider digitalis intoxication as a cause. There is some evidence also that an acidaemia should be corrected.

Supraventricular and Junctional Arrhythmias – Sinus bradycardia and nodal bradycardia only require to be treated if the slow rate is producing ectopic beats or an inadequate cardiac output, indicated clinically by poor peripheral perfusion, urine flows of less than 30 ml/hr, and drowsiness, or in the worst cases loss of consciousness.

Intravenous atropine 0·5 to 1·0 mg is probably the least dangerous method of increasing the rate. An intravenous infusion of isoprenaline 0·5 to 5 μg/min will usually produce an adequate response, but if this fails pacing may be required.

Sinus tachycardia in excess of 110 beats/min is associated with a poor prognosis if the cardiac output is low, and digitalisation should be considered.

Atrial ectopic beats may presage other supraventricular arrhythmias, but do not require treatment.

Paroxysmal atrial tachycardia, flutter, and atrial fibrillation in the presence of myocardial infarction imply either left ventricular failure or direct involvement of the atria or sinus node in the ischaemic process. In either case, digoxin is the treatment of choice, rather than D.C. shock, as all these arrhythmias tend to be recurrent. A synchronised D.C. shock may be used if there is no response to digitalisation, and this should be done under lignocaine cover within the first twenty-four or thirty-six hours of digitalisation, before the possibility of intoxication arises. The use of β-adrenergic blockers may also be considered, but D.C. shock must never be used in the presence of these agents. Paroxysmal atrial tachycardia with block and nodal tachycardia may be treated in the same way provided that there is no possibility that they are manifestations of digitalis toxicity. If this possibility exists, the digitalis must be stopped, and adequate potassium supplements given. Phenytoin is probably the drug of choice, if anything more active is felt to be necessary, in a dose of 125 mg given slowly intravenously (up to 500 mg/hr in two hours).

Ventricular arrhythmias. Ventricular ectopic beats should be treated if they occur at a greater frequency than five per minute, if they occur within the T wave of the preceding beat, if they are multifocal in origin, or if they occur in runs of two or more. Ventricular tachycardia requires treatment as a matter of moderate urgency, and ventricular fibrillation as a matter of extreme urgency.

Ventricular ectopic beats and ventricular tachycardia should be treated initially with intravenous lignocaine 1 mg/kg body weight as a bolus followed by an infusion of 1 to 2 mg/min. In the case of ventricular tachycardia this should be followed by a D.C. shock. Ventricular fibrillation has already been dealt with in the section headed 'Initial Management'.

If lignocaine fails to control ventricular ectopic beats, or the return of ventricular tachycardia, or fibrillation, there are a number of other agents which should be tried. The least depressing in terms of ventricular function is phenytoin 125 mg intravenously over five minutes which may be repeated up to a total of 500 mg in two hours. Total dose should not exceed 1 g/24 hr.

Procaine amide may be given intravenously in a dose of up to 50 mg/min for up to one hour, or from 2 to 6g. orally per twenty-four hours. Quinidine bisulphate 100 mg intravenously over five minutes followed by an infusion at 1 to 2 mg/min, although possibly the most depressing in its action on myocardial function, is also the most effective in the control of ventricular arrhythmias, and may also be given by mouth in a dose of 1·5 to 3 g/24 hr. Propranolol, bretylium tosylate and antihistamines have all been used, but appear to be less effective.

By virtue of being myocardial depressants all these drugs are relatively contraindicated in the presence of a low cardiac output, or atrio-ventricular conduction defects, or evidence of latent block such as bundle branch block, loss of septal Q waves, or widening of the QRS complex. If ventricular arrhythmias occur with severe conduction disturbances, pacemaking should be instituted first.

Heart block. Second degree and complete heart block associated with clinical evidence of poor cardiac output, Stokes-Adams attacks, or ventricular arrhythmias require treatment.

A few cases may respond to intravenous atropine 0·5 to 1 mg. The majority will respond to an isoprenaline infusion 0·5 to 5μg/min; if this fails or provokes ventricular arrhythmias, transvenous cardiac pacing is indicated.

Cardiac tamponade

Where this is sufficient to cause dyspnoea, and arterial paradox with a fall in arterial pressure such that the systolic pressure is varying between 90 and 60 mm Hg, or lower with respiration, the pericardial sac should be aspirated immediately. It is convenient to introduce a soft catheter over a Seldinger guide wire. The catheter can subsequently be left to drain attached to an underwater seal. If the tamponade is not rapidly relieved surgical intervention is required.

This chapter was written by Dr R. D. Bradley (Consultant in Clinical Physiology, St Thomas's Hospital) and edited by Professor W. I. Cranston.

Category 12

Diseases of the Lung

The greater part of this chapter is devoted to the commonest therapeutic problems in lung disease, namely infection, airways obstruction, and respiratory failure, with particular reference to diseases characterised by airways obstruction (chronic bronchitis, asthma, emphysema). Some other forms of lung disease are more briefly considered. The treatment of pulmonary tuberculosis is described in the following chapter.

TREATMENT OF ACUTE PULMONARY INFECTION

Infection may involve the airways (acute bronchitis) or the pulmonary parenchyma (pneumonia) or both. Pneumonia may be a primary lesion caused by a specific organism ('the specific pneumonias'), namely Strep. pneumoniae, Staph. pyogenes, or Klebsiella pneumoniae. More commonly, the pneumonia may follow an upper respiratory tract infection, or an acute bronchitis (aspiration pneumonia or bronchopneumonia). Such infection is particularly common in elderly or debilitated patients confined to bed, and in the post-operative state.

Acute viral infections of the respiratory tract

It is not possible to treat the virus infection directly, but the secondary bacterial infection which often follows may be treated as outlined below.

Mortality statistics show a rise in deaths from all causes during influenza epidemics, particularly from hypertension, rheumatic heart disease, chronic nephritis and diabetes. Immunisation against influenza is therefore recommended in the following conditions:

(a) Chronic lung disease (chronic bronchitis, emphysema, asthma, bronchiectasis, pulmonary tuberculosis, and fibrosis).

(b) Chronic heart disease.

(c) Chronic renal disease.

(d) Diabetes.

Acute bronchitis

There are only three therapeutic measures to be taken seriously in the treatment of uncomplicated acute bronchitis; these are the administration of antibiotics, the suppression of cough, and relief of pain.

Antibiotics should always be used in those specially at risk from bronchitis and also in those patients bringing up copious quantities of purulent sputum. It is difficult to give any clear-cut indications for, or against, the use of antibiotics apart from these. In general the authors feel that antibiotics should be given to all patients with bronchitis who are coughing up purulent sputum on the grounds that the administration of antibiotics may reduce morbidity, shorten the period off work, and prevent permanent damage to the airways. While a sputum culture before the start of treatment is desirable, it is probably not practical or necessary to do this in the majority of instances. Tetracycline (500 mg) or ampicillin (1 g.) given four times a day for three to five days is all that is required to treat the majority of patients.

Cough suppressants should never be given to patients in respiratory failure due to an exacerbation of chronic airways obstruction, for the survival of the patient may depend on the effectiveness of the cough. Moreover, most cough suppressants depress respiration. They should in theory not be given to patients with productive cough, especially during the day, for the airways are cleared of pus predominantly by coughing. However, suppression of cough and relief of pain will be necessary for some such patients at night to enable them to sleep, and are particularly indicated for those with a painful dry cough. The most useful suppressant for routine use is codeine phosphate which can be given in tablet form in a dose of 10 to 60 mg., or as linctus codeine (B.N.F.), 4–8 ml. The main side effect is constipation. When cough is particularly persistent and troublesome then morphine or diamorphine may be used but probably only in the elderly or incurable patient because of the danger of addiction.

Water will only reach the respiratory passages if droplets of water of the right size and in sufficient quantities are inhaled. If the droplets are too large they will quickly settle out and not reach the lower airways; if they are too few in number they will quickly evaporate. In theory it is possible that the deposition of water in the airways might make the sputum easier to expectorate. There is no evidence that this is true nor can one be sure with the techniques used that nebulisers or steam tents produce water droplets of the right size and in sufficient quantity in the inspired air to be of value. The recently developed 'plate' humidifiers may prove more efficient. They are not yet sufficiently developed for general use, but may be suitable for intensive care units (see Status Asthmaticus). We do not therefore feel that the provision of an aerosol or steam tent is of value in the treatment of acute bronchitis, apart from bringing symptomatic relief in a patient whose mouth and pharynx has become dry and uncomfortable due to persistent mouth breathing.

Pneumonia

The Pneumonias are often classified on anatomical grounds as localised (lobar or segmental pneumonia) or generalised (bronchopneumonia). This classification has no therapeutic value, for the treatment depends on the infecting organism.

Occasionally, the clinical picture may point to a particular organism (the specific pneumonias). The recommended initial treatment is then as follows.

Pneumonia	Organism	Recommended initial treatment
Pneumococcal	Strep. Pneumoniae	Penicillin G, 1 megaunit 6 hourly IM
Staphylococcal	Staph. aureus	Cloxacillin 500 mg 6 hourly and sodium fusidate 500 mg 8 hourly
Friedlander's	Klebsiella pneumoniae	Cephaloridine 500 mg 6 hourly IM

In practice it is rare to be able to identify the infecting organism on clinicial criteria. Usually identification rests on the results of sputum and blood culture, and until these results are available an empirical approach must be taken (see below). Initial treatment will then be modified by subsequent tests of bacterial sensitivity, especially important in staphylococcal infection. If the isolated organism is insensitive to the antibiotic initially given, and there has been no clinical response, the bacteriologist will advise on the best antibiotic or combination of antibiotics to be given.

General principles of treatment of pneumonia

(1) *Prophylaxis.* Elderly patients, smokers, patients with chronic cough and sputum with, or without airways obstruction, and patients who are to have abdominal surgery, are particularly likely to get post-operative pneumonia. The incidence of the complication will be

decreased by stopping smoking at least a week before surgery and by routine pre-operative and post-operative physiotherapy. Physiotherapy will also help to prevent hypostatic pneumonia in the elderly or debilitated who are confined to bed.

(2) *Antibiotic therapy.* In general, if the patient is less than 50, has no associated chronic respiratory disease, and has become infected outside hospital, the initial drug should be penicillin, for the causative organism will very frequently be a pneumococcus or a penicillin-sensitive staphylococcus. If the patient is over 50, has associated respiratory disease such as airways obstruction or bronchiectasis, or has become infected while in hospital, broad-spectrum therapy is required. If the illness is not serious (low-grade fever, little systemic upset, minor X-ray changes), tetracycline or ampicillin is the initial drug of choice. Many surgeons prefer to treat post-operative pneumonia by physiotherapy alone in the first instance, reserving antibiotic therapy for cases where the fever does not resolve in three or four days. If the illness is severe, a more potent bactericidal combination should be used, and culture of the blood as well as the sputum is mandatory, for the patient may be too weak to clear secretions by coughing, and the blood may be the only source from which the pathogen may be grown. Penicillin and streptomycin have been frequently used in the past, but a hospital staphylococcus is often resistant to both drugs. Ampicillin 1 g 6 hourly and cloxacillin 500 mg 6 hourly are an effective and relatively non-toxic combination, but will not control a klebsiella infection. Cephaloridine and cloxacillin together have a wider spectrum, but are a considerably more expensive combination. They will cover most important bacterial infections but not those due to pseudomonas Pyocyanea and Streptococcus faecalis, which exceedingly rarely cause pneumonia. Ampicillin and gentamycin together cover the widest spectrum, but experience with this combination is limited, and the ototoxicity of gentamycin is a serious disadvantage, especially if renal function is impaired. In general ampicillin and cloxacillin are probably the best combination for the seriously ill patient.

(3) *General measures.* A productive cough should not in general be suppressed, nor should a cough suppressant ever be given to a patient with respiratory failure. Unproductive coughs may be treated with codeine or pholcodine linctus B.P.C., 4–8 ml Pleuritic pain may be treated with local heat and simple analgesics (aspirin, paracetamol), but more powerful analgesics such as pethidine and morphine

are also respiratory (and cough) depressants. It is safest never to use them. Confusion and delirium may occur in young patients with severe pneumonia, but in elderly patients even with apparently mild infection. If this is associated with carbon dioxide retention and hypoxia, the problem is that of respiratory failure, discussed below, and oxygen therapy should be given, but with great caution. Pneumonia rarely causes carbon dioxide retention unless there is associated chronic respiratory disease. If respiratory failure is not present, chlorpromazine 50 mg is the best sedative.

THE TREATMENT OF DISEASES CHARACTERISED BY AIRWAYS OBSTRUCTION

These diseases are:

(1) *Chronic bronchitis.* Definition: a disease characterised by chronic cough and sputum (in the absence of any other cause for these symptoms such as bronchiectasis, tuberculosis, or chronic heart failure).

(2) *Asthma.* Definition: a disease characterised by attacks of airways obstruction which are reversible, i.e. between attacks the lungs are clinically normal. Sophisticated tests of lung mechanics may show abnormalities between attacks even when simple spirometric tests give normal results.

(3) *Emphysema.* Definition: a disease characterised by abnormal accumulation of air beyond the terminal bronchiole, with destruction of pulmonary parenchyma, including alveolar walls.

These definitions can hardly be regarded as satisfactory; the first is made purely on symptoms; the second on clinical and functional characteristics; and the third is a pathological diagnosis for which the best evidence in life is the chest X-ray. Nevertheless they remain the best definitions presently available.

Causes of airways obstruction. An increased resistance to the flow of gas through the airways may have several causes:

(a) The airways may be blocked by oedema fluid, mucus, or pus.

(b) The airways may be obstructed by inflamed oedematous bronchial mucosa.

(c) The airways may collapse during expiration, especially if the bronchial walls are weakened and supporting parenchyma destroyed by disease.

(d) The bronchial muscle may be inappropriately contracted.

The functional diagnosis. The effect of a bronchodilator in a classical acute asthmatic attack is obvious and requires no objective confirmation. However in patients with chronic airways obstruction, before embarking on a course of treatment which may last years, using expensive drugs which may have unpleasant side-effects, is is necessary to make sure that increased airways resistance is (a) present, and (b) responsive to the particular bronchodilator employed. Airways obstruction of clinical significance will be detected by the simple spirometric measurement of forced expiratory volume in one second (FEV_1) and forced vital capacity (FVC). If the ratio FEV_1/FVC is less than 60 per cent, there is airways obstruction. These measurements can be made as easily in general practice as in hospital practice. They can be repeated after giving a bronchodilator, when an increase in FEV_1 will give objective confirmation that the airways obstruction will be relieved by the drug. More sophisticated measurements of lung mechanics are rarely required.

Asthma

It is customary to classify asthma as extrinsic or intrinsic.

EXTRINSIC ASTHMA

This is characterised by onset of the disease in childhood and by a family history of atopy (asthma, hay fever, eczema). The lungs are usually clinically normal between attacks. An asthmatic attack may be precipitated by exposure to some substance to which the patient is sensitive (e.g. cat fur, horse hair, or house dust containing mites); by an upper respiratory infection; by exposure to cold air; or by some psychological upset.

The general principles of the treatment of asthma are to prevent attacks when possible and to abort them quickly when they occur.

Psychological factors. Although there is no doubt that some patients with asthma are neurotic, there is no clear evidence that neurosis is more common in this than in any other disease. Sometimes an attack will be triggered by an emotional upset such as a barely-avoided traffic accident, or an outburst of anger. The treatment is then that of the asthmatic attack, which will always include the psychotherapeutic effect of a firm, confident, sympathetic approach. The question is whether the number of attacks can be decreased by long-term treatment of the psychological factors. Again the psychotherapeutic effect of firm, sympathetic handling is the primary aim. One may hope, over a period of months or years, to bring the patient nearer to understanding the factors which underly the attacks, and to help him to avoid those situations which exacerbate the disease. However an attempt to do this abruptly will carry, to the patient, the implication that his condition is 'all in the mind'; this is invariably a serious, and sometimes irretrievable mistake. Some patients, particularly during periods of stress at home or at work, are helped by a mild sedative such as amylobarbitone 45 mg t.d.s., chlordiazepoxide 5–10 mg t.d.s., or diazepam 2–5 mg t.d.s. Sedation is never indicated during an acute attack. The patient is then anxious and agitated because he cannot breathe and because he fears he may die, a suspicion which occasionally proves correct. Relief of the airways obstruction will then relieve the anxiety.

Allergic factors. It may be possible to show, by skin or inhalation testing, that the patient is sensitive to a certain substance. These are usually inhaled dusts (e..g horse dander, house dust) or ingested proteins (e.g. shellfish). There are two possible approaches: first, to remove the offending substance from the environment as far as possible; second, to try to desensitise the patient. Unfortunately, neither approach has proved spectacularly profitable to the majority of asthmatic patients. Many atopic subjects will prove to be sensitive to a number of allergens; moreover, skin testing on different occasions may give different results. If in the clinical history there is a strong suggestion that one particular allergen is responsible for provoking the asthmatic attacks, and this is confirmed by testing, that allergen should obviously be avoided. This may be easy if, for example, it is an ingested substance such as shell-fish, but impossible if it is an omnipresent hazard such as house dust. Measures such as replacing feather pillows, mattresses and stuffed furniture by foam rubber materials may be beneficial, but may also involve a family in considerable expense. Again, if the clinical picture and the sensitivity tests strongly point to one particular allergen, an attempt may be made to desensitise the patient by a course of injections. Such a course may be time consuming, painful and expensive; occasional anaphylactic deaths have been recorded. Clinical benefit is far from guaranteed. In the case of pollen sensitivity however, a preseasonal desensitisation course has been shown to benefit most patients in a controlled clinical trial. In our opinion, this situation is the only one where such treatment has much likelihood of success.

Disodium Cromoglycate. This drug offers the first direct attack on the immunological reaction responsible for asthma. It has been shown by inhalation tests to inhibit both the clinical reaction due to reaginic antibodies (Type I) and that associated with serum precipitins (Type III). Most clinical trials have shown a statistically significant benefit to patients with extrinsic asthma. This has been most obvious in children and young adults, and the benefit has been measured in terms of symptoms, reduced steroid and bronchodilator dosage and, less convincingly, simple lung function tests. The drug has to be given by inhalation in powder form, and since the powder itself may cause bronchospasm in some subjects, isoprenaline sulphate is included. This cannot be regarded as a satisfactory method of administration, and it is hoped that a more convenient preparation will be developed. The drug is initially given six-hourly, or three-hourly in severe cases. However, the optimum dosage, particularly for maintenance therapy, has yet to be determined by proper clinical trial.

This drug has not yet been completely assessed; and the effectiveness of long-term therapy is not yet known. Nevertheless it is certainly worth a trial in cases of extrinsic asthma, particularly in children and young adults.

Treatment of infection. Attacks of asthma may be precipitated by upper respiratory infections or acute bronchitis. If there is fever, cough or purulent sputum a wide spectrum antibiotic (tetracycline or ampicillin) should be prescribed.

Bronchodilator therapy. In an acute asthmatic attack, a sympathomimetic drug should be given by inhalation. In general we prefer the newer drugs, orciprenaline or salbutamol, which have minimal cardiovascular side-effects. These drugs also have a more prolonged effect than isoprenaline alone. The dosage recommended by the manufacturers should never be exceeded. If there is no improvement within two hours, medical advice should be urgently sought, further treatment being discussed in the section on Status Asthmaticus.

In some cases of severe asthma, the lungs may not return to normal between attacks: some degree of bronchospasm may be present almost continuously. Oral bronchodilator therapy is then appropriate. Again we prefer orciprenaline (20 mg four times daily) to ephedrine, which may cause difficulty of micturition and insomnia especially in the elderly, but theophylline derivatives such as choline theophyllinate (0·4 to 1·6 g. daily in divided doses) are also satisfactory. There is little evidence that combinations of bronchodilators and barbiturates are more effective than a bronchodilator alone.

Rarely, extrinsic asthma may be so intractable that continuous corticosteroid therapy is needed. The danger of side-effects should then be weighed against the severity of the patient's respiratory disability. It may be possible to alleviate symptoms sufficiently by giving prednisone 5 mg four times daily on only three consecutive days in each week; corticosteroid side effects are unlikely with this regime. However, regular therapy with prednisone 5–15 mg/day may be required; a dose greater than 10 mg/day will probably cause side effects.

INSTRINSIC ASTHMA

This is characterised by onset in middle age or later, by the absence of a history of atopy, by blood and sputum eosinophilia, and by a bad prognosis. The principles of psychotherapeutic management are identical to those in extrinsic asthma. A search for allergic factors is usually unsuccessful, and the position of disodium cromoglycate in this form of asthma has not yet been fully determined, for although patients without apparent allergic factors have shown a response to the drug, the search for allergens has not usually been rigorous.

Treatment with bronchodilators may be needed continuously, since the course of the disease is often progressive rather than episodic. This should be attempted with oral therapy, reserving inhalations for the treatment of the acute attack if possible.

In the progressive form of the disease, steroid therapy will almost certainly be needed. If the patient presents with status asthmaticus, the aim should be to control airways obstruction by initial large doses (40–60 mg prednisone/day), for 4–5 days, gradually reducing the dose over about two weeks to acceptable levels if possible. If, however, the course is one of gradually increasing airways obstruction, it is probably better to start with small doses of prednisone (2·5 mg daily) and gradually work up to that dose at which life becomes tolerable for the patient. Unfortunately, in this form of asthma it is frequently impossible to make life bearable for the patient without producing the side-effects of corticosteroids. Some physicians believe that in intrinsic asthma no attempt should be made to stop steroid therapy altogether, but rather that it should be continued at the lowest possible maintenance dose for the remainder of the patient's life. This is because an attempt to withdraw steroids, however gradual, may be followed by a relapse which is resistant to steroid treatment. Although there is no firm objective evidence for this view, in terms of controlled trials, it is compatible with the authors' experience.

STATUS ASTHMATICUS

We define this as an acute attack of asthma which is unimproved by sympathomimetic drugs given sublingually or by inhalation. This is a medical emergency. The view, once widely held, that patients never die in an acute asthmatic attack, is fallacious. The recent increase in deaths from asthma is discussed below.

The traditional drug of first choice is adrenaline, 1:1000 strength, 0·5 ml being given subcutaneously over 8 minutes and repeated if necessary in 30 minutes. This treatment may now deserve reconsideration. It was undoubtedly often effective when previous treatment consisted of an inhaled bronchodilator delivered from a hand nebuliser. Such devices may not create droplets in sufficient numbers, or of correct size to reach the relevant airways. The modern 'metered-dose' aerosol canisters are certainly more efficient. In the authors' experience in hospital practice, the patient has usually already received large doses of isoprenaline or another sympathomimetic, and may have a heart rate of 150/min. In this situation, there seems little to be gained by giving another catecholamine, with risk of arrhythmias, and indeed adrenaline has rarely been effective. We therefore think that aminophylline is here the drug of first choice. However, in general practice, in milder cases where large doses of catecholamine have not been given, adrenaline should be used first. If adrenaline has no effect within 30 minutes, aminophylline, 0·25–0·5 g. in 10–20 ml sterile water, should be given intravenously. Very rarely, sudden death has been reported after the drug has been given intravenously, and this is thought to be associated with rapid injection. It should therefore be given slowly, over 5–10 minutes. If there is no effect in 20 minutes, 100 mg of hydrocortisone should be given intravenously, and the patient transferred to hospital, for even if the patient rapidly improves, close observation will be needed for at least 24 hours. It may be necessary to repeat the dose of intravenous hydrocortisone 2–4 hourly. If only one or two doses are required there is no need to follow it with oral prednisone. If more than two doses are given, oral prednisone 60 mg daily should be prescribed for 2–3 days, and the dose then gradually reduced and stopped over 10–14 days. If the attack has been precipitated by a respiratory tract infection, this should be treated; usually a wide spectrum antibiotic such as tetracycline or ampicillin is suitable.

Hypoxia and acidosis predispose to lethal arrhythmias, especially in the presence of isoprenaline. Oxygen should be given if the arterial oxygen tension (PaO_2) is less than 70 mm Hg. Bronchodilatation is frequently followed by a fall in PaO_2; oxygen should therefore be continued after the wheeze has disappeared. The hypoxic drive to breathe will thereby be removed, but in classical acute asthma this contributes only a little to the overall respiratory drive. Nevertheless the arterial CO_2 tension ($PaCO_2$) should be measured during oxygen breathing to make sure that alveolar ventilation does not decrease. A rising $PaCO_2$ may then be an indication for artificial ventilation, discussed below. Apart from the liability to arrhythmias, there is evidence that bronchodilators are less effective in the presence of acidosis; measurement of pH and $PaCO_2$ will allow this to be assessed and corrected.

Many patients with status asthmaticus are dehydrated, probably because of increased water loss through the skin and in the expired air. Blood volume may be diminished. This should be treated by intravenous fluids, the rate and amount being controlled by observation of the central venous pressure. The jugular venous pulse may be a very difficult guide, for it may be obscured by the movements of accessory muscles of respiration, and it will certainly show wide pressure swings with respiration. It is therefore highly preferable to measure the right heart filling-pressure with a right atrial catheter which may be introduced by the 'float' catheter technique.

Finally there remains the rare case which is intransigent to these measures, including intravenous steroids. The blood gases must then be measured frequently, for the main indication of impending death is a rising $PaCO_2$, and this is a late sign. If the attack is prolonged, the patient will eventually become exhausted, alveolar ventilation will decrease, and the final outcome is death in respiratory failure, perhaps with a terminal arrhythmia. A $PaCO_2$ which gradually rises to an abnormally high level (>45 mmHg) is therefore a sinister sign; at this stage preparation should be made for artificial respiration (intubation and intermittent positive-pressure respiration).

Although the precise indications for artificial respiration are not yet agreed, they basically consist of:

(a) a $PaCO_2$ of more than 60 mm Hg on admission;

(b) a $PaCO_2$ of 50 to 60 mm Hg on admission which does not fall after about 8 hours treatment;

(c) a $PaCO_2$ which rises, despite treatment, to approach 50 mm Hg; and

(d) evidence of increasing exhaustion of the patient.

One useful piece of evidence of the latter is a decrease in the pulsus paradoxus which characteristically accompanies acute asthma. The magnitude of the paradoxical pressure swing in systolic pressure is dependent on the magnitude of the intrapleural pressure swings, and hence on the amount of respiratory effort which the patient can achieve. In a deteriorating patient, a fall in the amplitude of the paradoxical systolic pressure swings may then be a useful objective index of increasing exhaustion. It should be emphasised that the presence of exhaustion and of a rising, abnormally high, $PaCO_2$ are late signs; if present, artificial respiration is urgently needed.

Post-mortem studies of lungs from patients who have died of acute asthma usually show small airways blocked by inspissated mucus. Any techniques for making these inspissated plugs less tenacious and therefore easy to expectorate would be welcome. Mucolytic drugs have been tried, but without convincing success. Bronchial lavage has been successful in some people's hands but is not without danger and should only be carried out in intensive care units by those experienced in the technique. The new 'plate humidifiers' may well be most useful in severe attacks of asthma. By adjusting the speed of vibration of the plate it is possible to produce droplets of the right size (100μ) and in sufficient quantity. At present these humidifiers are too cumbersome and experimental to be used outside hospitals or special units.

Deaths from acute asthma. There has been a recent increase in deaths from asthma. In many cases, there has been circumstantial evidence of an over-dose of a sympathomimetic drug from a 'metered-dose' aerosol canister. This suspicion has been partly confirmed by demonstration of a correlation between deaths due to asthma and prescription of such preparations. One cause of the increased death rate therefore appears to be misuse of drugs in this form. Possibly the too frequent use of a sympathomimetic drug, in circumstances where airways obstruction is unrelieved, and in the presence of anoxia, has caused lethal arrhythmias. It is therefore of the greatest importance that on prescription of a metered-dose canister, the patient should be first told never, under any circumstances, to exceed the recommended dose, and secondly instructed to seek medical help urgently should the attack not respond to the drug. For the same reason, we have suggested that these preparations should not invariably be prescribed to patients with chronic bronchospasm where a satisfactory effect can be achieved with oral therapy.

Chronic Bronchitis

The main aims of treatment in chronic bronchitis are:

(a) to remove factors which cause bronchial irritation;
(b) to treat infection;
(c) to alleviate airways obstruction.

Factors which cause bronchial irritation. It is of primary importance for the patient to give up smoking. Occupations which involve exposure to dust should be avoided.

Treatment of Infection. There is no satisfactory method for assessing the pathogenic significance of bacteria in the sputum of chronic bronchitics. An organism which can be shown to be present significantly more often in patients with purulent sputum can be assumed to be related to the infection though not necessarily causative. An organism found as frequently in patients with mucoid sputum as in those with purulent sputum can be concluded to be a non-pathogen. The pathogenic significance of organisms can be assessed by determining the clinical response to chemotherapy, e.g. the disappearance or reduction of purulent sputum, or by measuring the plasma antibody levels against the bacteria, but this is again circumstantial rather than direct evidence.

Haemophilus influenzae can be cultured from about 80 per cent of patients in remission but with purulent sputum. There is a close correlation between the presence of this organism and of sputum purulence, and specific serum antibodies are found more frequently in patients with purulent sputum (69 per cent) than those with mucoid sputum (25 per cent) and are only found in 6 per cent of normal controls. H. influenzae is probably pathogenic in about half of the acute exacerbations in chronic bronchitics but is rarely a cause of pneumonia.

Strep. pneumoniae is commonly a cause of exacerbations of bronchitis and may lead to pneumonia.

Bacteria which are rarely pathogenic. Coliform bacilli, Haemophilus parainfluenzae, Klebsiella pneumoniae, Pasteurella septica, Proteus, Staph. aureus, Pseudomonas pyocyanea and Strep. pyogenes. These organisms are more likely to be pathogenic in patients who are receiving steroids or suffering from debilitating diseases such as carcinomatosis or leukaemia.

Non-pathogenic bacteria. Diphtheroid bacilli, N. catarrhalis, Staph. albus, Strep. non-haemolyticus and Strep. viridans.

Bacterial sensitivity. The pattern of sensitivity of H. influenzae and of the pneumococcus is sufficiently constant to justify 'blind' chemotherapy.

The sensitivity of other organisms, especially Staph. aureus, is variable, and should always be determined if considered pathogenic.

The ideal goal in chemotherapy would be to attain a bactericidal concentration of antibiotic in the bronchial mucous membrane, in the micro-abscesses in the walls of the bronchioles, in the macrophages within the lung and in the sputum. The concentration of an oral antibiotic is higher in the blood than the sputum, and probably at an intermediate level in the tissues. Thus the attainment of a bactericidal concentration of antibiotic in the plasma does not imply that a bactericidal level has been reached in tissues or sputum. It is generally true that a higher antibiotic concentration can be achieved in purulent than in mucoid sputum. This is certainly true for ampicillin, and almost certainly for streptomycin and the tetracyclines.

We may now outline some broad principles for the chemotherapy of chronic bronchitis.

(a) The bacterial pathogens most likely to be encountered in chronic bronchitics are: in remission, H. influenzae; in acute exacerbations, Strep. pneumoniae and H. influenzae; in pneumonia, Strep. pneumoniae or Staph. aureus.

(b) In the majority of patients chemotherapy may be undertaken 'blind' without a sputum culture. If there is pneumonia, or a failure to respond to treatment, or the patient is very ill, the sputum should be cultured; if there is time and there is no danger to the patient, three separate cultures should be taken before chemotherapy begins.

(c) In general chemotherapy is unlikely to benefit a patient whose sputum is mucoid (non-purulent), especially if no pathogens are isolated on sputum culture.

(d) Acute exacerbations should always be treated with antibiotics or chemotherapeutic agents.

Treatment of acute exacerbations. These are usually recognised by an increase in purulence and/or volume of sputum, usually with fever and a deterioration in the patient's general clinical condition. In some patients however, sudden deterioration may occur without any immediate change in the sputum. In patients who are not severely ill ampicillin (1 g. 6 hourly) or tetracycline (500 mg 6 hourly) may be given immediately without sputum culture. A combination of trimethoprim and a sulphonamide has recently been shown to be an effective alternative. In patients who are severely ill both sputum and blood should be taken for culture before beginning treatment, and a more potent bactericidal combination should be used. The approach is exactly that of the treatment of a severe pneumonia; a combination of ampicillin (1 g. 6 hourly) and cloxacillin (500 mg 6 hourly) is probably the best initial choice, while awaiting the results of sputum and blood culture.

Treatment of chronic bronchitis in remission, but with purulent sputum. Prophylaxis. Although histological examination of the lungs in patients with chronic bronchitis suggests that bacterial infection is responsible for much of the damage, there is no direct evidence that it can be prevented by efficient bacterial suppression. However many clinical trials have shown that there is a clinical improvement in patients treated with ampicillin or tetracycline.

If the patient is in remission and has purulent sputum then the infecting pathogen is almost always H. influenzae. It is then reasonable to try bactericidal therapy, to eliminate the organism from the infected sites in the lungs and from reservoirs of infection in the upper respiratory tract. Ampicillin should be given (1 g. 6 hourly) for 4 days. There is no point in continuing this high dosage beyond four days for either the sputum will become non-purulent and bactericidal concentrations will no longer be obtained, or if purulent sputum continues it means that bactericidal concentrations have not been obtained in any case in the sputum or in the infected sites which form the reservoirs of organisms.

If bactericidal therapy is successful it can be repeated as necessary. If it fails or is followed by a rapid relapse then bacteristatic therapy should be considered; here the aim is to suppress organisms sufficiently to allow inflammation to subside. A one or two week course of ampicillin (500 mg 6 hourly) or tetracycline (250 mg 6 hourly) should be given. If the patient improves, a decision has then to be made whether antibiotics should be given continuously, or intermittently as required. This problem will now be considered.

Prophylaxis against acute exacerbations. It is likely that viral infections are responsible for starting most exacerbations and that H. influenzae and/or Strep. pneumoniae are responsible for subsequent bacterial damage. Immunological prophylaxis against viruses or the above bacteria is either impracticable or ineffective, except before an influenza epidemic, when active immunisation may diminish the severity of the illness or prevent it.

Prophylaxis against bacterial infection following viral infection can be intermittent or continuous. By intermittent prophylaxis we mean that the patient is given a supply of antibiotics to start taking immediately an upper respiratory infection starts or the sputum becomes purulent. This has been shown to decrease the severity and length of the acute exacerbation.

Continuous antibiotic prophylaxis has been shown in most trials to decrease the severity of acute exacerbations but not their number. One recent trial has shown that treatment from October to April also decreases the number of exacerbations, but that this decrease was only significant in those patients who had several exacerbations every winter. The argument is therefore not settled. In view of the disadvantages of continuous antibiotic therapy, particularly the acquisition of drug resistant organisms, it is probably best to give continuous prophylaxis only to those patients who have three or more exacerbations per winter, and intermittent prophylaxis to the rest.

The choice of drugs lies between tetracycline and ampicillin. The combination of trimethoprim and sulphonamide has not been fully assessed in this context. The tetracyclines, particularly oxytetracycline, are cheaper than ampicillin, and therefore to be preferred in long-term treatment. For continuous or intermittent prophylaxis bacteriostatic doses (tetracycline 250 mg four times daily) should normally be used. In intermittent prophylaxis each course should last 10–14 days.

Other drugs. Cough suppressants should be avoided if possible but may occasionally be needed to allow a patient to sleep. They should never be given in respiratory failure.

There are several 'mucolytic' drugs available (e.g. methylcysteine, bromhexine), which certainly alter the viscidity, quantity and microscopic structure of sputum. It is theoretically attractive to decrease the tenacity of sputum in chronic bronchitis and indeed in status asthmaticus, but there is little objective evidence of benefit from such drugs. However, one controlled trial has recently shown a significant improvement in symptoms and lung function in a group of patients with chronic airways obstruction given bromhexine.

Breathing exercises are a traditional part of the treatment of chronic airways obstruction of any cause. The aim of the treatment is to educate the subject to breathe in such a way that adequate ventilation is achieved at less energy cost, i.e. more efficiently. This is normally attempted by teaching the patient to breathe with a different rhythm from that which he would naturally maintain, and to try, at first consciously, to relax certain respiratory muscles which he would normally use. It is not clear how far these habits persist in the absence of the teacher. Moreover, electromyographic recordings have shown that the relevant muscles are not relaxed; a study of the work of breathing showed no increase in efficiency; and a controlled trial has shown no systematic change either in symptoms or lung function. We do not dispute that there may be a powerful psychotherapeutic effect.

Emphysema

The aetiology of emphysema is unknown, and there is no specific treatment. However, many patients also have chronic bronchitis, and some have airways obstruction which is partially reversed by bronchodilators. The treatment outline in the last section again applies.

RESPIRATORY FAILURE

We define this as failure of the respiratory system to maintain the arterial PaO_2 above 60 mm Hg and/or the $PaCO_2$ below 48 mm Hg in a patient breathing air and at rest.

There are two sorts of respiratory failure. In the first type, alveolar ventilation is diminished because total ventilation is insufficient, as in some cases of poliomyelitis, acute infective polyneuritis, or drug overdose. Some form of artificial respiration may be required to increase both total and alveolar ventilation. The lungs are basically normal.

In the second type, gas exchange is impaired although total ventilation may be normal or increased. The lungs are usually abnormal. The impairment of gas exchange may be characterised by an increase in venous admixture within the lung (e.g. following myocardial infarction). Arterial hypoxia will then occur without significant CO_2 retention: the treatment is to correct the hypoxia with as high a concentration of oxygen as is needed; for the removal of the hypoxic drive to breathe will rarely cause any serious rise in $PaCO_2$, and this may be checked by direct measurement. The precipitating cause, such as infarction or pneumonia, should be treated on its merits. In severe chronic airways obstruction, an increase in venous admixture initially leads to a fall in PaO_2 without a rise in $PaCO_2$. In some patients, as the disease progresses, alveolar hypoventilation occurs with a rise in $PaCO_2$. These patients are relatively insensitive to CO_2 and their chemical drive to breathe is in part due to hypoxia. It is not possible to tell by clinical examination which patients are likely to develop alveolar hypoventilation. The cause of the CO_2 insensitivity is not known.

The principles of treatment of this common form of respiratory failure are as follows:

(a) To relieve hypoxia without causing severe respiratory depression.
(b) To treat any precipitating infection and clear respiratory secretions.
(c) To relieve airways obstruction.
(d) To treat fluid retention (cor pulmonale).
(e) To avoid drugs which decrease the drive to breathe.
(f) To avoid artificial respiration if possible.

Treatment of hypoxia. The main question centres around the degree of hypoxaemia that is acceptable in these patients. All would agree that a PaO_2 of 30 mm Hg or less is unacceptable. A level of 50 mm Hg (saturation 70–75 per cent) will almost certainly avoid any serious tissue hypoxia. The aim then should be to maintain the arterial PaO_2 at 50 mm Hg, or higher if alveolar hypoventilation is not severely aggravated.

Usually an inspired oxygen concentration of 28 per cent will maintain the PaO_2 at the required level, but occasionally it may be necessary to start with 24 per cent O_2 to avoid severe alveolar hypoventilation. Oxygen at these concentrations may be given by a 'Ventimask' or by an 'Edinburgh mask'. If oxygen therapy is to lead to CO_2 narcosis it usually does so within the first few hours of treatment. The warning signs are: first, onset of mental confusion or unconsciousness; second, failure of the patient to cough and cooperate with the physiotherapist; and third, a rising arterial $PaCO_2$. It is a changing $PaCO_2$ rather than its absolute level which is the best indication that the patient is improving or deteriorating. A $PaCO_2$ of more than 70 mm Hg may be acceptable if the patient is alert, able to cough effectively, and can cooperate with the medical staff.

Once oxygen therapy has been started it should not be discontinued abruptly until the patient's condition has improved. The danger of stopping oxygen arises because of the different capacity of the stores for O_2 and CO_2; the capacity for O_2 is small, but that for CO_2 immense. When oxygen is given to a severely ill patient there is normally some alveolar hypoventilation and CO_2 retention. When oxygen is discontinued the increased store of oxygen is rapidly washed away and alveolar PO_2 falls. The CO_2 elimination is slower so that alveolar PCO_2 remains high. Since the PCO_2 is higher, the PO_2 must be lower than it was before oxygen was given. The abrupt termination of oxygen therapy, in a patient with severe respiratory failure, may lead to a level of hypoxia at which damage occurs to the central nervous system.

Treatment of infection and clearance of secretions. Bronchitis or pneumonia should be treated with antibiotics according to the principles outlined above. Prompt treatment of acute exacerbations of pneumonia may stop the patient going into respiratory failure. When respiratory failure is present, it is essential for the patient to be encouraged to cough up secretions, for accumulation at the lung bases may lead to atelectasis, abscess formation and further pulmonary damage. Postural drainage and heavy chest percussion by a skilled physiotherapist is an important part of the treatment. If the patient is too drowsy and confused to cooperate with the physiotherapist, an intravenous injection of 2 ml of nikethamide may wake the patient up sufficiently to obtain this co-operation.

Bronchospasm. Bronchospasm, if present, should be treated by bronchodilators.

Oedema. If there is congestive heart failure (cor pulmonale), diuretics should be given. There is some evidence that the use of diuretics alone produces an improvement in gas tensions. Digitalis is frequently used; there is little evidence that it is beneficial in 'pure' cor pulmonale, but these patients often have coexisting ischaemic heart disease. If there is any suggestion of a double aetiology for the congestive failure, it is certainly reasonable to digitalise the patient.

Other drugs. Cough suppressants or sedatives should never be given, as they all interfere with the clearance of secretions, and produce some degree of respiratory depression. We do not consider respiratory stimulants (analeptics) to be of sufficient benefit to justify their use, for the following reasons:

(a) they produce no useful change in $PaCO_2$ or PaO_2 in patients with chronic airways obstruction;

(b) the difference between the toxic and therapeutic dose is small (the toxic symptoms of the analeptics are apprehension, extreme fear, sweating, skin irritation, fits, nausea and vomiting);

(c) to produce any respiratory effect it is necessary to give the drug intravenously under continuous observation, with usually frequent changes in infusion rate.

The use of nikethamide when the patient is too drowsy to cooperate with the physiotherapist has been already mentioned.

Artificial ventilation. The need for tracheostomy and Intermittent Positive Pressure Respiration (I.P.P.R.) is decreased by precise control of oxygen therapy. If despite all previous measures severe alveolar hypoventilation and CO_2 narcosis develops, artificial respiration may be unavoidable. The decision to employ it rests on the following factors.

Indications: (a) failure to attain a satisfactory relief of hypoxaemia ($PaO_2 > 50$ mm Hg) without severe hypoventilation leading to CO_2 narcosis.

(b) Severe alveolar hypoventilation on admission to hospital. Occasionally through neglect, delay in treating an acute exacerbation, or the injudicious use of oxygen, immediate resuscitation is necessary. It may be possible to improve matters by temporary ventilation through an endotracheal tube, so that tracheostomy is avoided.

Contraindications: (a) severe panacinar emphysema; the most important practical diagnostic aid is a good quality chest X-ray film. By the time a patient with severe panacinar emphysema develops respiratory failure during a chest infection, lung destruction is so far advanced that a successful outcome of treatment by tracheostomy and I.P.P.R. is unlikely. Usually it is difficult or impossible to wean the patient from the respirator; even if this can be done such a patient is likely to be a respiratory cripple and succumb shortly to further infection.

(b) severe limitation of the patient's activities before the acute exacerbation. A patient who was working before the exacerbation is likely to have an adequate respiratory reserve to justify tracheostomy, while a bed-ridden respiratory cripple is unlikely to benefit.

BRONCHIECTASIS

Respiratory infections in childhood, especially whooping cough and measles, may lead to blockage of small airways by secretions with subsequent atelectasis and infection. Bronchiectasis may follow. Active immunisation has already markedly decreased the incidence of pertussis, and will probably do the same for measles in the near future.

Whether in childhood or in adult life, atelectasis with or without suppurative pneumonia should be treated with physiotherapy and antibiotics, as previously outlined.

The treatment of the established disease involves:

(a) postural drainage of the affected lobes, and

(b) antibiotic therapy, the aims being exactly as in chronic bronchitis.

Occasionally if the disease is localised to one lobe, surgical excision is indicated. Emphysema is always a contraindication to surgery.

SPONTANEOUS PNEUMOTHORAX

A tension pneumothorax should be drained immediately via a catheter in the second anterior intercostal space with an underwater seal.

If the pneumothorax is not under tension, the exact management is debatable, ranging from the conservative to the aggressive. The following regime lies somewhere between the two extremes.

(a) If the patient is less than 40, and has no coexisting respiratory disease, he may rest at home. If an X-ray film at one week shows no re-expansion at all, he should be admitted for the lung to be expanded by suction. If an X-ray at one week shows some expansion but a repeat film at 3 weeks shows the lung not fully expanded, again he should be admitted.

(b) If the patient is over 40, or has coexisting respiratory disease, he should be admitted to hospital. If there is no expansion at three days, or the lung is not fully expanded in two weeks, the lung should be expanded by suction.

(c) Once committed to mechanical expansion, the patient should have a daily chest X-ray. If the lung fails to expand because of a bronchopleural fistula, surgery will be needed. If it expands completely, suction should be mantained for 48 hours thereafter; if expansion is still complete, the tube should be clamped for 24 hours; if all is still well, it may then be removed. The maintenance of full expansion should be checked by subsequent X-rays.

(d) Recurrent pneumothorax. The occurrence of two pneumothoraces on the same side is usually an indication for surgical measures, such as pleurodesis by the installation of talc, or oversewing of bullae. A full discussion of the various surgical measures which have been employed is beyond the scope of this chapter.

SARCOIDOSIS

Lung disease is rarely an indication for treatment in sarcoidosis. The common hilar lymphadenopathy usually regresses spontaneously. The only indication for steroid therapy is progressive pulmonary fibrosis. This may be recognised by one or more of the following features: increasing dyspnoea; progression (or failure to regress) of chest X-ray changes; falling vital capacity; and decreasing transfer factor. Steroid therapy is then indicated to try to prevent further progression of fibrosis. It is reasonable to give predisone in high doses (40–60 mg/day) for three weeks followed by a gradual reduction to about 7·5 mg/day for 6 to 12 months.

CARCINOMA OF THE BRONCHUS

Radical treatment may be attempted by surgical excision or by radiotherapy. Recent evidence has suggested that for oat-cell carinoma radiotherapy is preferable to surgery. Operability was assessed without recourse to the more recently developed techniques of mediastinoscopy and mediastinotomy, and therefore surgery was attempted in cases where mediastinal spread had already occurred. Our view is that if a tumour is thought to be operable, surgery should be attempted, provided that a thorough search is made for mediastinal and other metastatic spread. Radiotherapy should be used for the inoperable case, may be used post-operatively, and is particularly indicated in palliative treatment of pain, cough, haemoptysis, or superior vena-caval obstruction.

PULMONARY EMBOLISM

The treatment of pulmonary embolism is unsatisfactory and will probably continue to be so. It is far more logical to direct therapeutic effort at the prevention, detection and treatment of peripheral venous thrombosis, especially in the legs. Certain surgical operations (particularly on the legs and in the pelvis) are known to carry a particular risk of deep venous thrombosis (DVT), and here it has been shown that prophylactic anticoagulants decrease the incidence of DVT and emboli. Elderly and immobile patients who are confined to bed are likely to get DVT, especially post-operatively. Although prophylactic anticoagulants are not indicated, regular physiotherapy and firm bandaging of the calves are reasonable precautions.

Clinical detection of DVT is notoriously unreliable, and this has made previous studies of treatment difficult to assess. Recent techniques such as phlebography, the fibrogen ^{131}I scan, and the use of the Doppler velocity probe to detect patent venous channels, should provide more exact diagnosis.

Once diagnosed, DVT is treated by promoting venous flow and by anticoagulation to prevent spread of thrombosis. The foot of the bed is raised and the calf firmly bandaged. It is customary to start anticoagulation with intravenous heparin and to continue with an oral anticoagulant such as warfarin. It is not known how long heparin should be continued, nor whether a higher dose would be preferable to those normally employed. Surgical removal of thrombi may be indicated if large unattached clots are seen on phlebography.

If a pulmonary embolus occurs, treatment depends on the clinical state of the patient. A large embolus may completely or nearly occlude the pulmonary artery and cause asystole or ventricular fibrillation. Theoretically resuscitation by cardiac massage might preserve the patient long enough for surgical removal of the clot, though such cases are rare. At the other end of the scale is the small embolus with no embarrassment to the circulation. Here anticoagulants should be started if not already given. In all cases, if a pulmonary embolus has occurred when the patient is already anticoagulated an attempt to prevent further embolism by surgery should be considered. Guided by phlebography, which will demonstrate the extent of the thrombi, the relevant veins may be tied above the level of the clot, or the inferior vena cava plicated.

Between these two extremes lie a range of cases where there is evidence of circulatory embarassment, namely raised central venous pressure, low blood pressure, tachycardia, a right sided fourth heart sound, a loud or widely split pulmonary second sound, or a cardiogram showing right heart strain. The management of such cases is extremely debatable, the main reason being the extreme difficulty in setting up proper trials.

The patient should be heparinised in an attempt at least to prevent further spread of thrombosis in the lung. Several series have shown apparently impressive results from the use of heparin in high dosage, but the observations were not fully controlled. Fibrinolytic therapy with streptokinase is theoretically attractive; impressive, though again uncontrolled, results have been published. The exact indications for its use cannot yet be defined. Surgical removal should probably be reserved for cases which show definite signs of deterioration (e.g. falling blood pressure, rising pulse rate and central venous pressure).

This chapter was written by Dr K. B. Saunders (Senior Medical Registrar, St Thomas's Hospital) and Professor S. J. G. Semple (Department of Medicine and Honorary Consultant Physician, St Thomas's Hospital) and edited by Professor W. I. Cranston.

Category 13
Infectious Diseases

MALARIA

The treatment of malaria can be described under four headings: standard therapy; therapy of complications; the problem of resistance; prophylaxis.

Standard therapy

Malignant tertian (P. falciparum) malaria responds to the prompt administration of a 4-aminoquinoline, e.g. chloroquine or amodiaquine. Delay increases the risk of serious complications. Chloroquine (as base) orally: 600 mg, 300 mg six hours later, 300 mg daily for the next two or three days. Total 1·5–1·8 g. Amodiaquine (as base) orally: 600 mg on first day, 400 mg daily for the next two or three days. Though no longer preferred drugs mepacrine and quinine are also effective though more toxic. Mepacrine hydrochloride orally 900 mg in divided doses on the first day, 300 mg in divided doses for seven days. Quinine (bisulphate or dihydrochloride) orally 600 mg thrice daily for seven days.

This treatment will also eradicate P. falciparum since there is no persistent exo-erythrocytic phase of this parasite. Benign tertian (P. vivax, P. ovale) and quartan (P. malariae) malarias in overt form also respond to the above therapy, but relapse can only be avoided by continued suppressive therapy (vide infra) or the concurrent administration of an 8-aminoquinoline, e.g. primaquine, to eradicate the extra-erythrocytic phase of these species. Primaquine (base) 15 mg is given daily for fourteen days during which the patient should remain in hospital under observation in case toxic effects should appear. These effects include cyanosis due to the formation of methaemoglobin, and intravascular haemolysis which results in serious anaemia and calls for cessation of the drug. Eradication therapy should be reserved for those who are leaving an endemic area. The alternative, suppressive therapy, except when it includes an 8-aminoquinoline, will not prevent the establishment of the exo-erythrocytic phase of plasmodia other than P. falciparum.

Therapy of complications

The most serious complications of malaria are seen in the non-immune subject with P. falciparum infection and these constitute a real medical emergency since, failing treatment, death is likely within twenty-four hours. Indications for strenuous therapy include jaundice, a falling haematocrit, prostration, hypotension, oliguria and signs of cerebral involvement such as coma or mental abnormality. In this situation chloroquine sulphate 200 mg (base) or quinine hydrochloride 600 mg can be diluted to 20 ml and given IV very slowly (10 mins) or injected equally slowly into the tubing of a continuous IV infusion. Alternatively the dose can be added to the fluid reservoir and given over one hour. The parenteral dose is repeated in eight hours if necessary, but the drug should be continued orally as soon as the patient's condition allows. Quinine should be used in patients with chloroquine resistance, and in children, as parenteral chloroquine should not be given under the age of five years.

In addition to specific treatment concurrent measures must be taken to deal with such complications as shock, haemolysis and oliguria. Blood transfusion is essential when the haematocrit is falling and steroids may help to halt haemolysis. Haemodialysis and peritoneal dialysis have much to offer in malaria with oliguria and the patient should be moved to such facilities as soon as possible. Peritoneal dialysis should be employed if the patient cannot be moved. When coma supervenes lumbar puncture allows pyogenic meningitis to be excluded and may have some therapeutic efficacy. Steroid therapy is thought to be of benefit in cerebral malaria.

The problem of resistance

The treatment of acute malaria due to resistant plasmodia is satisfactory using quinine, but is accompanied by a greater degree of toxicity than standard chloroquine therapy. The dosage is as described except in the presence of oliguria when a reduced dose of 600 mg per day has been recommended, even when the patient is undergoing dialysis. Alternatively, and where the case is less urgent, a single oral dose of sulphormethoxine 1 g. and pyrimethamine 50 mg or of sulphametopyrazine 0·75 g. and trimethoprim 0·5 g. may be given. Although the speed of action of these combinations compares favourably with that of chloroquine the severely ill patient should be given a triple drug regimen including IV quinine.

Prophylaxis

Two drugs are active not only against the erythrocytic phase of all species of plasmodia (suppression) but also against the pre-erythrocytic phase of P. falciparum (causal prophylaxis). These are proguanil (Paludrin) usually 100 mg daily and pyrimethamine (Daraprim) usually 25 mg once weekly. These drugs are ineffective against the pre-erythrocytic phase of plasmodia other than P. falciparum and should be continued for four weeks after leaving endemic areas.

Suppression of all types of malaria in the erythrocytic asexual phase is possible with any antimalarial. As an alternative to proguanil and pyrimethamine, chloroquine 300 mg once weekly can be used. Mepacrine and quinine are rarely employed in this way. Relapse can occur on cessation of the suppressive regimen unless eradication of species other than P. falciparum is carried out with an 8-aminoquinoline, e.g. primaquine, as described above.

In areas where plasmodia are resistant to pyrimethamine and proguanil either double doses of proguanil, i.e. 200 mg daily, can be used or chloroquine prophylaxis can be tried. When chloroquine resistance and multiple resistance are rife as in S.E. Asia the proguanil 200 mg regimen has been as successful as more complicated choices such as chloroquine 300 mg (base), pyrimethamine 45 mg and dapsone 25 mg weekly.

AMOEBIASIS

There are a number of effective drugs available for the therapy of amoebiasis and they have been combined in various ways which have not been exhaustively compared. Two important principles are that intestinal parasites must be eliminated and that signs of systemic invasion indicate the need for a systemic amoebicide.

Acute amoebic dysentery normally responds to the administration of a tetracycline, an indirect amoebicide which acts through its effect on the bowel flora, and diiodohydroxyquinoline, a direct amoebicide active in the lumen of the bowel. The addition of chloroquine, a systemic amoebicide, is necessary to protect the liver from invasion. These three drugs are given, simultaneously, in the following dosage:

Chlortetracycline	1 g daily for 5 days
Diiodohydroxyquinoline	600 mg t.d.s. for 20 days
Chloroquine (base)	600 mg loading dose, 300 mg 6 hours later, 150 mg 12-hourly for 14 days.

More severely ill patients require emetine hydrochloride 60 mg daily I.M. until symptoms subside or for not longer than 5 days. An alternative compound is dehydroemetine given in a dose of 80 mg daily I.M. for up to 10 days. The emetine compounds are given either along with or preceding the basic regimen for intestinal amoebiasis presented above.

Some practitioners in this field prefer to use emetine bismuth iodide (E.B.I.) to obtain the intestinal amoebicidal effect, substituting it for tetracycline, diiodohydroxyquinoline and chloroquine following the administration of emetine hydrochloride or dehydroemetine in the severely ill patient. The dose of E.B.I. is 200 mg daily for 10 days. In the moderately ill patient E.B.I. in this dosage may be combined with chlortetracycline 1 g. daily for 7 days as sole treatment.

Niridazole (Ambilhar) is a recent introduction which can replace diiodohydroxyquinoline and chloroquine and, given with chlortetracycline, is effective in acute amoebic dysentery. This drug is an orally administered effective intestinal and systemic amoebicide which should be given in a dose of 25 mg/kg daily for ten days. It is, however, toxic especially to the nervous system causing hallucinations and occasional convulsions, particularly when there is liver disease and its use in amoebiasis is diminishing.

A more successful introduction to the therapy of amoebiasis is metronidazole. It is both a systemic and an intestinal amoebicide and chloroquine need not be given in addition. As treatment for the more severe case it can replace emetine. Toxicity is very low and the dose is 800 mg thrice daily for ten days.

Alternative drugs with a luminal amoebicidal action only are diloxanide furamate 500 mg thrice daily for ten days or paromomycin, an antibiotic, in a dose of 500 mg 6-hourly for seven days. The former is suitable for the symptomless case.

Amoebic liver abscess requires an amoebicide which is active systemically. Emetine compounds and chloroquine are in this class and in practice both are usually given. Emetine hydrochloride 60 mgs per day for four days or dehydroemetine 80 mg a day for ten days should be given alone with chloroquine and diiodohydroxyquinoline in the above dosages. Niridiazole has been found effective in amoebic liver abscess and should be combined with chloroquine and, if there is dysentery, a tetracycline. Its toxicity in liver disease renders its use undesirable and the best alternative to emetine is metronidazole administered alone in a dosage of 800 mg thrice daily for ten days.

Medical treatment alone will not suffice for large liver abscesses (> 100 ml of pus) and diagnosis and localization have been aided by the development of radioisotope scanning, at least in the more advanced centres. Therapeutic aspiration is then performed as an adjunct to the administration of amoebicidal drugs.

Certain amoebicidal drugs have toxic effects. Emetine compounds have cardiovascular actions such as bradycardia, hypotension, arrhythmias, and E.C.G. abnormalities. E.B.I. orally causes nausea and vomiting to such a degree as to require antiemetics and sedatives to be administered. Niridazole also causes E.C.G. T-wave changes, but without cardiovascular symptoms. However, it should not be combined with emetine compounds.

TUBERCULOSIS

In countries where the attack on tuberculosis has been continued for many years, it is increasingly a problem of the old who are more susceptible to the toxic effects of drugs. The pool of patients, often uncooperative, with drug-resistant disease remains a problem, but with the growing appreciation of correct methods of treatment of newly diagnosed cases, it is hoped not to add to it. There is new interest in the management of primary tuberculous disease in order to prevent reactivation in later life, a step towards eventual eradication. The situation in less fortunate countries is much less satisfactory but its alleviation is proving a source of new ideas in this field.

It is wise for the inexperienced not to depart too precipitately from the accepted standard methods of therapy which have two objectives (a) to render and maintain the patient's sputum negative and (b) to avoid creating drug resistance.

The degree of infection in a case of pulmonary tuberculosis can be assessed in great detail but for simplicity a 'severe' case would be extensively cavitated and the sputum smear strongly positive for bacilli, a 'mild' case would be minimally or not cavitated and the smear either scanty or negative.

It might be desirable but it is not essential for any case of pulmonary tuberculosis to be in hospital or confined to bed. In general the newly diagnosed case should be started on triple therapy: streptomycin, P.A.S. and isoniazid. The regimen in a severe case should be:

Streptomycin	1 g. I.M. once daily
Isoniazid	100 mg twice or thrice daily
P.A.S.	5 g. thrice daily

If the patient is over 40 years the streptomycin may have to be reduced to 0·75 g. daily or be given 1 g. thrice weekly. Later, when the organism is known to be sensitive to all three standard drugs and provided progress has been satisfactory in hospital, the regimen can be continued without P.A.S. except in those patients over 40 years on reduced streptomycin. The mild case treated perhaps as an out-patient should have:

Streptomycin	1 g. thrice weekly
Isoniazid	100 mg twice daily
P.A.S.	5 g. twice daily

After the sputum is known to be negative, or the bacilli sensitive, or after discharge of a hospital patient with sensitive organisms, treatment may be continued with isoniazid 200 mg daily, P.A.S. 10 g. daily, administered together. An alternative out-patient regimen which has recently been developed to follow triple therapy is the supervised administration on two occasions weekly of:

Streptomycin	1 g.
Isoniazid	14 mg/kg body weight
Pyridoxine	10 mg

The last named is necessary to prevent the development of peripheral neuritis on this high dosage of isoniazid.

The duration of therapy need not be limited by rule and if necessary should be extended, but it will usually lie between eighteen months and two years, according to severity and progress. It is best to be generous with therapy and on its completion supervision should continue at three monthly, then six monthly intervals for at least five years.

When the above regimens are adhered to, resistance should rarely be acquired though primary resistance to at least one drug may have been present in 5 per cent of patients.

The management of resistant infection does not begin with the receipt of the first sensitivity report but with the all important interrogation of the patient. This is directed towards assessing whether or not resistant bacilli are likely to be present. Pointers to resistance are a history of irregular or inadequate therapy. At least two effective drugs should have been included in any combination.

In cases of doubt 'holding' treatment with viomycin, 2g. twice weekly and tetracycline 2 g. twice daily was formerly recommended. This is relatively ineffective, and the combination of cycloserine, pyrazinamide and ethionamide is potentially toxic. At present it is likely that patients will do best on a regime of isoniazid (300 mg daily), prothionamide (0·75 g. daily), ethambutol (25 mg/kg/day), and rifampicin (450–600 mg daily); this combination may be continued until bacterial sensitivity is known.

Once the sensitivities are known, therapy should continue as follows, reserving the latest drugs for those patients resistant to all three standard drugs.

When the organisms are resistant to streptomycin, treatment with P.A.S. 20 g./day and isoniazid 200 mg/day should suffice except for severe cases when ethionamide or pyrazinamide may be added. When resistant to P.A.S. good results can be obtained with:

Streptomycin	1 g. daily, and
Isoniazid	200 mg daily

If resistance to isoniazid is detected, streptomycin 1 g. daily and P.A.S. 20 g. daily are employed, but it is better to add ethionamide or pyrazinamide and ioniazid itself may be continued.

In cases resistant to two of the standard drugs, the third is employed along with ethionamide and pyrazinamide. In severe cases especially those resistant to both streptomycin and isoniazid, capreomycin should be added. It is probable that as experience in their use grows, the newer drugs ethambutol and rifampicin will be used at an earlier stage of resistance, in preference to ethionamide, pyrazinamide and others which are either rather toxic or provoke lack of co-operation in patients.

Sometimes all three standard drugs and one or more of ethionamide, pyrazinamide, viomycin and cycloserine are rendered ineffective by resistance. In these circumstances, with every effort to ensure patient co-operation, isoniazid should be given with ethambutol, rifampicin and prothionamide. Pyrazinamide is used when there is resistance or intolerance to ethionamide and capreomycin when neither ethionamide or pyrazinamide is effective. When rifampicin is not available pyrazinamide may be substituted or capreomycin if pyrazinamide is already in the regimen due to ethionamide resistance. When there is resistance to ethionamide and pyrazinamide and rifampicin is not available, the following should be used: isoniazid, ethambutol, capreomycin, cycloserine and thiacetazone.

Therapy with limited resources

In countries with a scarcity of resources for the treatment of tuberculosis, that which is desirable in the practice of chemotherapy has to be modified to that which is possible economically.

If the use of streptomycin is limited by expense, P.A.S. (10 g. daily) and isoniazid (200 mg daily) is a cheaper combination, but still relatively expensive; then thiacetazone may be used in place of P.A.S. in an effective regimen of isoniazid 300 mg and thiacetazone 150 mg daily in one dose. If streptomycin in a dose of 1 g. or 750 mg daily or thrice weekly can be added for two months to either two-drug regimen, the results will be better. Alternatively intermittent supervised therapy with:

Streptomycin	1 g.	given twice weekly
Isoniazid	14 mg/kg	
Pyridoxine	10 mg	

is effective and can be enhanced by the addition of P.A.S. 10 g. twice weekly until the sputum smear is negative.

On completion of a year's treatment maintenance may be with isoniazid 200 mg/day alone, except in cavitated cases when it is better to continue one of the two-drug regimens. In some circumstances, only isoniazid will be available for initial treatment when a single daily dose of 400 mg is best but may cause some peripheral neuritis unless accompanied by pyridoxine 10 mg daily or some form of vitamin B complex.

Children

As in adult disease, a severe case should have triple therapy in the following dosage:

Streptomycin	30 mg/kg/day in one dose
Isoniazid	3–5 mg/kg/day in two doses
P.A.S.	300 mg/kg/day in three doses

As soon as the organism is known to be sensitive to all three drugs in a mild case in hospital, or after three months' satisfactory progress in a severe case, streptomycin may be discontinued.

Children with mild primary tuberculosis treated as out-patients, the source of whose organisms is known to be fully sensitive or is unknown, may have:

Isoniazid 3–5 mg/kg daily
P.A.S. 300 mg/kg daily

If the sensitivity is in doubt or the case at all severe, it would be better to give streptomycin in addition, until sensitivity tests are available.

Steroids

Provided adequate anti-tuberculous cover is simultaneously administered, corticosteroids are of value in severe tuberculous meningitis, tuberculous pleural effusion and in advanced pulmonary tuberculosis. An adult dose of 30 mg of prednisolone daily may be reduced by 5 mg weekly.

Dosage of reserve drugs

Ethionamide	0·5–0·75 g. daily in divided doses
Prothionamide	0·5–1·0 g. daily in one or two doses
Pyrazinamide	40 mg/kg/day in two doses, up to 1·5 g. twice daily
Capreomycin	1·0 g. daily I.M.
Ethambutol	25 mg/kg/day for 60 days followed by 15 mg/kg/day
Rifampicin	450–600 mg daily

GASTRO-ENTERITIS OF INFANTS

At present this condition, with one recent exception (E. coli type 0:114), is generally mild in socially developed societies but is responsible for much mortality and morbidity in less hygienic surroundings. It is a syndrome in which infection with known enteropathogenic types of E. coli contributes to only one third of the cases.

Treatment should begin in the home when the infant's condition permits a period of observation. Milk feeds are withdrawn and in their place is offered half-strength saline solution (4·5 g. NaCl/litre) in a volume of 75 ml per pound (150 ml/kg) per 24 hours. This can be made up at home by adding half a teaspoonful of salt to one pint of water. Advice which should not be given and requires to be countermanded, includes total starvation and the administration of boiled water or sugar solutions of any type, particularly proprietary glucose solutions of strengths approaching 25 per cent which are dangerous. If a mother is not competent to notice further deterioration of her child, by its lethargy or refusal to accept saline solution, then the infant is better admitted to hospital at once but it is not necessary to admit every case of infantile gastro-enteritis to hospital.

If domiciliary support fails and dehydration is developing, measurement of the serum electrolytes and acid/base status is highly desirable as a guide to management in hospital. Whenever possible fluid should be offered orally in the first instance. Suitable fluid is half-strength Darrow's Solution for Acidosis. For I.V. use a mixture of equal volumes of Darrow's solution and 5% dextrose is isotonic. The daily quantity required at five days to one year old is 75 ml per pound (150 ml/kg) for the basic needs plus from 25 to 75 ml per pound to replace losses in diarrhoea. If the serum sodium is 140 mEq/L or less the replacement fluid should be added to the basic for the first 24 hours; if the serum sodium exceeds 140 mEq/L (the hypertonic case) it is better to give only the basic volume in that period. There is controversy concerning the composition of fluid for hypertonic cases. It is agreed that it should not be electrolyte-free and it should probably contain about 40 mEq/L of sodium. For I.V. use this can usually be constituted by the addition to 5 per cent glucose solution of the amount of sodium bicarbonate required to correct the acidosis (vide infra). Alternatively, one volume of Darrow's solution diluted with two volumes of 5 per cent dextrose is isotonic (one-third strength Darrow's solution). For oral therapy dilutions of Darrow's solution in water between a quarter and a half-strength are appropriate. When the fluid is given I.V. it is even more important to restrict the volume in the first 24 hours and not to infuse rapidly in the early hours of therapy of hypertonic cases. Phenobarbitone may help to prevent convulsions which tend to occur at this stage. It is vital to correct acidosis early even if this involves giving excessive sodium. 8·7 per cent sodium bicarbonate solution containing 1 mEq/ml is a useful product and the required volume can be calculated from the Base Excess (B.E.) as follows:

0·3 (weight in kg) × B.E. = mEq of bicarbonate required, or from a measure of the serum bicarbonate, or alkali reserve:

*Full-strength Darrow's Solution for Acidosis:

K Cl	2.70 g	Na	120 mEq/l
Na lactate	5.80 g	K	36 mEq/l
Na Cl	4.00 g	Cl	140 mEq/l
Aqua dest.	to 1,000 ml	HCO_3 equiv.	51 mEq/l (Lactate)

Osmolarity 313m mol/l.

$$\text{E.C.F. (litres)} \times (\text{normal } HCO_3 - \text{actual } HCO_3) \times 2 = \text{mEq bicarbonate required}$$

Further corrections of acid/base status may be required as treatment progresses.

Intravenous fluids are required for the severely hypertonic infant and for those in or near peripheral circulatory failure. In the face of continuous diarrhoea and failure to suck, attempts at oral intake should not be prolonged. If the infant shows signs of shock or impending death the best treatment is an infusion of plasma, correction of acidosis and administration of oxygen. 20 ml per kg bodyweight of plasma is given along with 15 mEq of sodium bicarbonate and 100 mg of hydrocortisone.

As soon as the infant is able to drink, replacement should begin by mouth using small volumes at first. The infusion may be discontinued when the basic requirement can be taken orally and there is no longer profuse diarrhoea.

As recovery continues and the infant can take reasonable volumes (60 ml) at intervals of two hours, milk feeds are introduced beginning with half or even quarter strength, half-cream feeds. The volume and the intervals are gradually increased until normal feeding with full strength, full-cream milk is resumed. If diarrhoea recurs clear fluids should be resumed and the process repeated in another 24–48 hours.

The place of antibiotics is controversial. They do not appear to be required in the sporadic mild forms currently prevalent and in occasional severe cases their effect is hard to judge. In an institutional outbreak of serious disease it is claimed that appropriate antibiotics not only prevent further spread but save those infants who receive them. If this is true it is likely to be a brief respite owing to the rapid acquisition by E. coli of transferable drug resistance and the routine use of antibiotics in the enteritis ward is neither necessary or desirable.

BACILLARY DYSENTERY

Dysentery has not presented in a uniform manner throughout the world and its aetiology and epidemiology have not remained constant with the passage of time. In some circumstances it is a mild illness with little more than a nuisance value to the patient, in others a severe febrile illness; it is not surprising that therapeutic trials, few of them adequate, have failed to resolve the differences of opinion which exist. Where the disease is mild the symptoms abort in forty-eight hours and spontaneous bacteriological cure follows in 50–70 per cent of patients within seven days. There is no unequivocal evidence that antimicrobial treatment alters the clinical course nor that withholding it brings an hygienic disadvantage to the community. Consequently the approach to the mild case should be expectant and the patient may remain at home if the sanitary arrangements are suitable. Simple health education should not be neglected at this stage.

When the disease presents in a severe form and rapid symptomatic relief is desired an absorbable antimicrobial such as ampicillin 50–100 mg/kg/day for 5 days should be used. In the most severe cases the parenteral route should be employed. Alteration in bowel flora occurs when this drug is administered orally, towards colonisation by Candida and the Klebsiella-Aerobacter group but no undesirable consequences have been attributed to this when the course has been restricted to 5 days.

Sulphonamides have been rendered ineffective by the development of widespread resistance and should not be used. Resistance to the tetracyclines has restricted their use which had been attended in several instances by the development of staphylococcal enterocolitis. Some British workers have claimed that non-absorbable streptomycin and kanamycin assist bacteriological clearance though neomycin does not. Others doubt the value of streptomycin.

The Shigellae in common with other members of the enterobacteriaciae can acquire and transmit both transfer factor and resistance determinants and this in the present state of our knowledge should lead to caution in their exposure to antimicrobials.

Even in the brief period of illness when Shigellosis is mild, symptomatic relief is desired and many substances such as starch, chalk, kaolin and pectin have been incorporated in antidiarrhoeal remedies. There seems to be no evidence that these have any effect.

SALMONELLOSIS

Salmonella food poisoning without evidence of invasiveness is a self-limiting condition and likely to be cured before the results of bacteriological investigation become available. The exhibition of antibiotics in this condition does not improve on the spontaneous cure rate; indeed there is mounting evidence that the (convalescent) carrier state is thereby prolonged. Except in the very ill, febrile, septicaemic patient, antibiotics should be withheld and an expectant policy followed; this implies treatment of dehydration and electrolyte imbalance. When an antibiotic is thought to be indicated the choice should be made with the help of the bacteriology laboratory but either ampicillin or chloramphenicol in a dose of 500 mg 6-hourly may be started while waiting for sensitivity reports. If a patient has been given one course of appropriate antibiotic treatment and his faeces remain positive he should not be subjected to further courses of treatment.

TYPHOID AND PARATYPHOID FEVERS

These diseases generally present as severe systemic illnesses and require a more positive approach than salmonella enteritis which is self-limiting.

In the acute phase specific therapy should be with chloramphenicol orally or parenterally. The dose for adults should be not less than 2 g. daily and should be continued for at least ten days but extended according to response. In children the dose is 100 mg/kg with a maximum dose of 2 g. daily. Longer courses or higher doses than the above will not influence the incidence of relapse or complications.

Fluid and electrolyte balance must be measured and I.V. fluids may be required if oral intake fails or is not being absorbed. If hypotension develops, plasma is the best treatment but if there has been significant haemorrhage, blood will be required. When intestinal dilatation is observed oral intake should not be trusted even if there is not a complete paralytic ileus. I.V. fluids and gastric suction may be required for many days and should not be suspended until there is good evidence of returning intestinal function. Perforation in a toxic patient is difficult to diagnose and surgery carries a high mortality. A surgeon should be consulted but operation is best avoided and the complication treated conservatively. If obstruction follows perforation, surgery will be unavoidable.

The patient who relapses usually responds to a second course of 2 g. of chloramphenicol daily for seven days.

MEASLES

No specific treatment is available for the primary effects of this virus infection. In the average case prophylactic antibiotics should have no place. Observation is all that is required during the first few days and defervescence can confidently be expected. A darkened room is not necessary and the child should be allowed up when, as his temperature falls, he requests it. In these early days generalised adventitious sounds in the chest and cough are attributable to the effects of the virus. If later complications due to bacteria are suspected they should be treated as described in the section on pneumonia. Encephalitis is a rare complication requiring specialised therapy. In an uncomplicated case the child will be up and about seven days from the onset of the rash and since he is by then non-infectios no restrictions are necessary.

MUMPS

The manifestations of this disease are due exclusively to the mumps virus and there are no complications which could be avoided by the use of prophylactic antibiotics. A child or adult with salivary involvement needs only careful oral hygiene and sufficient fluid intake. Analgesics may be required, rarely morphine, especially in mumps orchitis. Rest in bed with support for the scrotum will be desired by the patient with acute orchitis. In severe cases of orchitis a short course of steroids may lead to more rapid resolution of pain.

UPPER RESPIRATORY TRACT INFECTIONS

These infections are complex in their aetiology but in all cases except for a minority with pharyngitis or tonsillitis they are due to viruses. Clinical examination alone does not allow separation of the few due to Streptococcus pyogenes. If the throat is inflamed a throat swab is required to exclude streptococcal infection and, if the appearance is suspicious of pyogenic infection, penicillin can be administered while awaiting the result of the swab. In most cases however antibiotics should be withheld because there is no evidence of their efficacy against viruses nor as prophylaxis against bacterial superinfection. This is true whether the signs and symptoms are classified as a cold, a febrile cold, influenza, pharyngitis, tonsillitis or laryngitis or croup. If a report is received of the presence of Streptococcus pyogenes a course of penicillin should be given which should continue for ten days. Oral penicillin 250–500 mg 6-hourly is adequate for adults, 125–250 mg for children and in severe cases penicillin should be given I.M. for the first 24–48 hours. Infants with coryza may feed better after being given nasal drops of 1 per cent saline solution of ephedrine 15 minutes before feeds. Secondary infection of sinuses or middle ear may occur and penicillin should be tried first in these cases. If I.M. penicillin does not control the temperature or the local signs in 24–48 hours the possibility of infection by Haemophilus influenzae or a penicillinase producing Staph. pyogenes should be considered and ampicillin 500 mg 6-hourly and cloxacillin in the same dosage should be added. Adequate courses i.e. 10 to 14 days should be given in otitis media and the ear carefully examined for healing if the tympanic membrane had ruptured.

Most cases of croup of viral origin recover rapidly with humidification and without antibiotics but the dangerous condition of acute epiglottitis has to be remembered especially in the older child or adult. The onset is acute with fever, leucocytosis and there is rapidly increasing respiratory difficulty. The patient is prostrated, has a painful throat and the epiglottis is inflamed and swollen. There is usually a septicaemia. When this diagnosis is made tracheotomy should be performed and chloramphenicol given at once. Severe cases of croup where the epiglottis cannot be seen and those with lower respiratory tract signs may be given ampicillin 125–250 mg 6-hourly.

WHOOPING COUGH

This distressing illness is unaffected by antibiotics, active against B. pertussis, unless they are given as early as possible in the catarrhal stage. If there is a history of contact tetracycline or ampicillin or erythromycin should be given at the first sign of catarrhal symptoms. After the disease has been recognised by its characteristics it does not respond to drug therapy but it is customary to give a short five-day course to eliminate persistent organisms. A mild case is best nursed at home and only severe or complicated cases admitted to hospital. A new-born infant should not be introduced into a home where his siblings are suffering from whooping cough.

Diet and fluid intake are often a problem and require a great deal of patience to manage. Secretions sometimes require to be aspirated from the oral pharynx and humidified oxygen may be required during spasms. If clinical or radiological examination reveal collapsed lung of segmental or lobar distribution physiotherapy may help the older child. However, re-expansion of the collapsed area can be expected in up to one year and surgery should not be contemplated earlier. When secondary infection of collapsed areas is recognised antibiotics should be given and continued if necessary until the lung re-expands.

Convulsions and othere cerebral manifestations require more intensive care as a consequence of depressed reflexes, sedation, anticonvulsants and tube or parenteral feeding.

All cases, including those mild cases who have not previously had one, should have a chest radiograph just prior to dismissal or on complete recovery if they have been at home.

This chapter was written by Dr. J. C. Taylor (Senior Lecturer in Medicine and Honorary Consultant Physician, St Thomas's Hospital) and edited by Professor W. I. Cranston.

Category 14
Ophthalmology

INFECTIONS

BACTERIAL

Hordeolum is a staphylococcal infection of the lid glands with a localised red, swollen and tender area. The more superficial glands are involved in the common stye, and the deeper Meibomian glands in the internal hordeolum. Treatment is by warm compresses and antibiotic ointment four times daily.

Chalazion is a chronic granulomatous inflammation of a Meibomian gland which often, but not necessarily, follows an internal hordeolum. Usually incision and curettage are necessary for their removal. Beware of multiple recurrences at the same site which may mean a rare adenocarcinoma of the Meibomian gland.

Blepharitis is a chronic, persistent bilateral inflammation of both upper and lower eye lids with associated low grade conjunctivitis. Although staphylococcal (ulcerative) and seborrhoeic forms are described both types are usually present. The eyes are itching and burning with red margins. Scales are seen along the eye lash roots. Ulcerated areas may be present. Often seborrhoea of the scalp, eye brows and ears is associated. Treatment is by meticulous cleaning of lid margins daily with a moistened cotton applicator before applying antibiotic ointment e.g. chloramphenicol or neomycin to the lid margin. Selenium sulphide shampoo to the scalp helps in the seborrhoeic form. Although cure is rare, a mixture of antibiotic and corticosteroid ointment to the lid margins will usually keep it under control. Beware of overtreating and making an allergic blepharitis to one of the medicaments used.

Lacrimal sac infection is a common acute or chronic unilateral disease occurring in infants or in adults over 40, and is secondary to obstruction of the nasolacrimal duct. Usually it is a staphylococcal infection with pain, tenderness and swelling just below the inner canthus. In infants the dacryocystitis is secondary to delayed canalization of the nasolacrimal ducts. Treatment is by massage over the tear sac followed by antibiotic drops four times daily. If there is no improvement by 6 months of age, then probing of the nasolacrimal duct may be done under general anaesthesia.

In adults acute dacryocystitis responds to warm compresses and systemic broad spectrum antibiotics e.g. tetracyclines or the newer penicillins. The chronic form in adults rarely responds to syringing of the lacrimal passages and dacryo-cysto-rhinostomy is required.

Conjunctivitis is the commonest eye disease, usually caused by pyogenic bacteria or by viruses. In general, organisms pathogenic for the genito-urinary tract are also pathogenic for the conjunctiva.

Bacterial conjunctivitis is usually acute, with a red eye, copious tears and sticky discharge, soon becoming bilateral. It is generally self limiting, lasting 10–14 days without treatment, but only 2–3 days in the pyogenic forms with treatment.

A stained conjunctival smear usually allows bacterial identification, but cultures are necessary for study of antibiotic sensitivities. Treatment is by chloramphenicol drops 2 hourly with ointment at night to both eyes. Extra care must be taken with personal hygiene to prevent the spread of 'pink eye' through the family.

VIRAL

Viral conjunctivitis

Trachoma affects approximately 20 per cent of the world population mainly the Middle and Far East and is the commonest cause of blindness when complicated by secondary bacterial conjunctivitis. It affects mainly the upper tarsal conjunctiva and superior cornea, beginning with follicular and then papillary hypertrophy, being followed by scarring and eventually an inactive vascular pannus. Treatment is by tetracycline 250 mg tablets 4 times a day for 7 days combined with either tetracycline ointment or 10 per cent sulphacetamide drops to the eyes 5 times daily for 4 weeks.

Corneal grafting may be needed later.

Adenovirus infections tend to cause unilateral follicular conjunctivitis, with varying degrees of corneal infiltration, and tenderness of the preauricular lymph node on the affected side. The symptoms go in 2 to 4 weeks, regardless of treatment, but often sulphonamide drops are given to prevent secondary bacterial infection.

Herpes simplex keratitis

Following initial infection with the herpes simplex virus, which may be on the lips or in the eye, the virus remains latent in the affected tissue. Various resistance lowering factors such as fevers, exposure to cold or emotional upsets may start a recurrence and liberation of active virus. An initial mild herpetic conjunctivitis may be followed by a dendritic ulcer of the cornea. If suspected a dendritic ulcer can readily be seen by staining with fluorescein which shows the typical branching pattern. Treatment is by idoxuridine ointment 5 times a day for 5 days which prevents the viral replication within the corneal epithelium. Other methods of treatment include carbolization of the virus-laden epithelium, or its freezing with the cryoprobe. Steroid drops must NEVER be used in treating dendritic ulcers as they encourage deep stromal keratitis (disciform keratitis) which is followed by scarring and vascularization and a corneal graft may be needed to restore vision.

Herpes zoster ophthalmicus is an acute neurotropic viral infection of the first division of the fifth cranial nerve. Severe unilateral facial and forehead pain may precede the vesicular eruption by several days. If the tip of the nose is also involved then usually, but not always, the eye will be involved too since the naso-ciliary nerve has been affected. Keratitis, iridocyclitis and secondary glaucoma may follow. Optic neuritis and partial third nerve palsies can occur. Treatment is by ointment containing corticosteroids and neomycin to the skin lesion, local steroid drops to the eye and a cycloplegic for iritis, and acetazolamide tablets 250 mg up to 4 times daily for the secondary glaucoma.

Pain can be very troublesome, particularly in the elderly, and adequate analgesics must be used. Even so, some patients are left with a severe post-herpetic neuralgia.

TRAUMA

Ocular injuries are still common, particularly in children and in industry. Many are preventable by proper observation of safety precautions and the wearing of appropriate protective goggles. When injuries do occur their initial treatment may determine whether useful vision, or even the eye itself, can be saved.

If the patient, child or adult, is suspected of having a perforating injury it is safer to defer examination of the eye until the patient is under a general anaesthetic. A potentially salvageable eye may have its contents extruded by muscle spasm following attempts by the examiner to separate the lids.

Visual acuity should be recorded if possible in any injury as it may be important medico-legally.

NON-PERFORATING INJURIES OF THE EYE BALL

Abrasions of conjunctiva or cornea

If the patient complains of a foreign body sensation in the eye but none can be seen by bright, oblique illumination then instill a drop of sterile fluorescein 2 per cent solution, ideally from a Minims individual disposable unit. Abrasions will show up as greenish-yellow areas. Local anaesthetic such as 0·5 per cent amethocaine may be needed to permit full examination of the eye. Antibiotic ointment such as chloramphenicol, with an eye pad and bandage for corneal abrasions, hasten healing. Inspect corneal abrasions next day for infection or ulcer formation.

Contusions

Blunt trauma may cause mild to severe injuries and detailed examination and follow-up are required.

Haemorrhage and swelling of the eye lids ('black eye') mean orbital fractures must be looked for. See below. Subconjunctival haemorrhage and conjunctival oedema will clear spontaneously in 2 to 3 weeks.

Haemorrhage into the anterior chamber (hyphaema) requires strict bed rest, preferably in hospital, and patching of one or both eyes. Usually the blood is absorbed uneventfully but secondary haemorrhage may follow 3 to 6 days after the injury causing secondary glaucoma and blood-staining of the cornea. Treatment by irrigation of the anterior chamber with fibrinolysin to remove the blood clot is the best so far available.

Traumatic iridocyclitis, particularly in heavily pigmented eyes, needs cycloplegia with atropine 1 per cent drops and corticosteroids e.g. guttae prednisolone three times a day.

Ocular contusion may paralyse the pupil, rupture the root of the iris, or detach the ciliary body with a later risk of glaucoma. The lens may be dislocated, or a traumatic cataract form. Vitreous or retinal haemorrhages can occur, there may be retinal oedema especially at the macula. Traumatic retinal detachment and choroidal rupture may follow severe injuries. Treatment is mainly expectant but surgery is required for some traumatic cataracts, and the retinal detachments.

Conjunctival and corneal bodies

Foreign bodies within the conjunctival sac are among the commonest injuries. A bright light and a × 10 magnifying glass are essential to find small particles. The eye lids must be everted as a foreign body often lodges beneath the upper tarsal plate. A moistened cotton applicator may be used to wipe it away, or gentle irrigation of the conjunctival sac with sterile saline solution.

Corneal foreign bodies may respond to similar treatment after instilling 0·5 per cent amethocaine drops but if the particle is firmly embedded in the cornea then the patient must go to the ophthalmologist for careful removal under the microscope. Hyoscine 0·25 per cent drops and chloramphenicol ointment and a firm pad are applied and the patient must be checked next day to see that healing is occurring.

Burns

1. *Chemical burns.* Any chemical splashed into the eye must be washed out *at once* as the damage depends on the nature of the chemical and the time it is in contact with the cornea and conjunctiva. Immediate and copious lavage with plain tap water for 5 to 10 minutes is essential.

The lids must be held apart to ensure adequate washing out of the eye. After the initial lavage then isotonic sterile saline or buffered solutions or chelating agents can be used later. Local antibiotics and corticosteroids are applied and atropine drops.

Corneal ulceration and opacities, and adhesions between the lids and globe may still follow, particularly after alkaline burns as from cement or lime, and surgery may be required later but the results are often disappointing.

2. *Ultra-violet irradiation* from exposure to electric arc welding causes extreme pain, watering and photophobia some 6 to 12 hours later. Widespread minute fluorescein-staining spots of the cornea are seen with magnification. Treatment is by local anaesthetic drops such as amethocaine 0·5 per cent, a cycloplegic such as homatropine 2 per cent and a firm pad and bandage for 24 hours.

3. *Eclipse burns* of the macula from viewing the sun directly may cause permanent impairment of visual acuity. No treatment of any avail. Prevention is paramount.

4. *Thermal burns* of the eye lids are treated as are skin burns elsewhere.

PERFORATING INJURIES OF THE EYE BALL

In *any* perforating ocular injury always suspect, look for and X ray for an intra-ocular foreign body.

Lacerations or ruptures without prolapse of tissue

Rupture of the eye ball from direct blunt trauma may occur around the limbus with intact conjunctiva overlying the rupture. Posterior ruptures may also occur around the optic nerve.

Lacerations of the globe may follow glass or knife injuries. Direct suturing by the eye surgeon of such wounds under general anaesthesia is required. Local and systemic antibiotics are given, plus appropriate protection against tetanus infection.

Lacerations with prolapse of ocular contents

A small puncture wound of the cornea may be plugged by iris prolapse and simulate a corneal foreign body. If iris or ciliary body prolapse is small this may be abscissed and the wound sutured as described above. Any wound involving uveal tissue means that the patient must be followed closely to detect sympathetic ophthalmitis which may develop in the *un*injured eye. Sympathetic ophthalmitis can be prevented by enucleation of a severely injured eye within 10 days of the injury. This means that it is not an emergency measure to enucleate a badly damaged eye but it should first be repaired and observed for up to 10 days before making this decision.

Intra-ocular foreign bodies

If an intra-ocular foreign body is suspected, and in particular if there is a history of striking a hammar upon a cold chisel followed by pain and blurred vision in one eye, X rays must be taken.

Specialised X rays are essential to confirm and also localise any radio-opaque foreign body. Slit-lamp microscopy, or ophthalmoscopy may reveal the site of penetration and sometimes the particle itself. Iron or copper particles must be removed from the eye because of later disorganisation of the eye by electro-chemical changes. Detailed surgical management is highly specialised.

LACERATIONS OF EYE LIDS

Eye lid lacerations should be repaired early but only after lacerations of the globe have been excluded. Small superficial lid lacerations parallel to the lid margin may be sutured directly.

Lacerations involving the lid margins may form a notch if incorrectly sutured. Lacerations of the medial ends of the lid margins may sever the canaliculi and these must be repaired to avoid constant watering. Lacerations of the upper lid must be examined carefully for associated damage to the levator muscle of the upper lid with resultant ptosis. These three types of injury need specialist repair. Finally penetration of the thin orbital roof with frontal lobe damage may be found.

ORBITAL INJURIES

Bony injury

Direct trauma can fracture the orbital rim e.g. inferior orbital rim fracture with a sprung fronto-zygomatic suture from injury over the zygoma. Emphysema of orbital tissues may follow blowing the nose if the fracture extends into a sinus.

Blunt trauma to the globe by a fist or similar sized convex object can cause a blow-out fracture of the thin orbital floor and leave the rim intact. These patients may present with just a 'black eye' but have paraesthesiae in the upper lip on that side from infra-orbital nerve involvement, and diplopia, particularly on trying to look up or down. This is due to trapping of the inferior rectus muscle within the fracture or haemoutoma of the muscle. As oedema of the lids settles then enophthalmos and depression of the globe may be found. X rays will confirm the herniation of orbital contents into the antrum. Surgical intervention is not always required for a radiological floor fracture and may be deferred for up to 10 days if there is no enophthalmos and the diplopia is resolving spontaneously. If operation is necessary a direct approach can be made along the orbital floor, or a Caldwell-Luc approach to the antral roof and the prolapse and fracture reduced. Various materials can be used to reinforce the orbital floor, such as silicone rubber.

Penetrating injuries

Any penetrating injury of the orbit may involve the sinuses or anterior cranial fossa too. Foreign bodies must be localised carefully to distinguish them from intra-ocular ones. Many intra-orbital foreign bodies are best left alone.

Pulsating exophthalmos may result from a fracture involving the cavernous sinus and causing a direct arterio-venus shunt which transmits the pulse to the orbital contents.

Differential Diagnosis of the Red Eye

	Acute Conjunctivitis	Corneal trauma or keratitis	Acute Iritis	Acute Glaucoma	Spontaneous Sub-conjunctival Haemorrhage
Symptoms	slightly gritty, sore eye	irritation and pain	aching eye	severe pain, nausea and vomiting	none
Vision	normal	slightly blurred	slightly blurred	marked blurring	normal
Discharge	sticky	watery	none	none	none
Conjunctival Injection	generalised	mainly around the cornea	mainly around the cornea	generalised	localised patch of blood
Cornea	clear	abrasion patch, or dull, opaque area of ulceration	clear, with keratic precipitates	steamy	clear
Pupil, size	normal	small	normal or small, irregular	dilated, irregular	normal
Pupil, light reaction	normal	normal	sluggish	minimal	normal
Tension to palpation	normal	normal	normal	rock hard	normal
Management	smear for microscopy and culture, local antibiotics	investigation antibotics mydriatics	full medical investigation mydriatics cortiscosteroids	emergency treatment, miotics, acetazolamide, surgery	check blood pressure, blood film and for bleeding tendency

NEVER USE CORTICOSTEROID EYE DROPS UNTIL THE DIAGNOSIS HAS BEEN MADE

GLAUCOMA

Glaucoma is a disease in which the intra-ocular pressure is elevated to levels that cause loss of vision by pressure damage on the optic nerve. More than 2 per cent of the population over 40 years have glaucoma and it is a common cause of blindness.

Open-angle glaucoma is the major problem.
The normal intra-ocular pressure of 14 to 18 mms of mercury is necessary to keep the eye ball a constant shape so that its optical focusing properties remain stable. This pressure is maintained by the production of aqueous humour by the ciliary body which flows forwards through the pupil into the anterior chamber and drains through the angle between iris and cornea into the canal of Schlemm and eventually into the venous system. If the outflow resistance is increased then the intra-ocular pressure will rise and if this pressure stays high then vision will be insidiously lost.

Early diagnosis is difficult. All patients over the age of 40 years should have the intra-ocular pressure measured and this can be done by the general practitioner with a Schiotz tonometer. If the pressure is 25 mms of mercury or higher the patient should be referred to the ophthalmologist. The optic disc appears cupped, with a grey rim and nasal displacement of the retinal vessels. Careful measurement of visual fields is essential in making the diagnosis and in evaluating the effect of treatment. Medical treatment comprises pilocarpine 1 to 4 per cent drops four times daily. In addition, eserine 0·25 per cent or neutral adrenaline 1 per cent may be used. These drops increase aqueous outflow. Acetazolamide tablets 250 mg up to four times daily may also be required to control the pressure by reducing aqueous production. Only if control cannot be adequately maintained by these means will surgical methods of increasing aqueous drainage be used.

Angle closure (acute) glaucoma

This is an ophthalmic emergency. The patient has blurring of vision in one eye with severe ocular pain, headache and even nausea and vomiting. This is due to the iris being pushed forwards peripherally so that the drainage angle is completely blocked and intra-ocular pressure rises rapidly. Many of these patients give a history of slight blurring of vision in the dark and of seeing coloured haloes around lights due to mild corneal oedema. These mild attacks usually subside during sleep.

Contributing factors to the development of angle closure are a shallow anterior chamber, high hypermetropia, a large lens within the eye and pupillary dilatation. For routine fundoscopy a short-acting mydriatic such as cyclopentolate 0·5 per cent or phenylephrine 2·5 per cent should be used, and a miotic instilled after the examination.

In the acute attack of glaucoma the eye is red, the cornea hazy, the pupil irregularly dilated and the eye feels rock hard to palpation.

Treatment is by intensive miotics, usually pilocarpine 4 per cent every 15 minutes, intravenous acetazolamide 500 mg followed by oral acetazolamide. Orally 3 ml/kg bodyweight of 50 per cent glycerol may be used as a dehydrating agent, provided the patient is not a diabetic. Morphine 15 to 20 mg for pain also helps with miosis.

Intravenous mannitol, 1·8 g./kg bodyweight, may also be used to bring down the pressure as an immediate pre-operative step. Once the intra-ocular pressure has been lowered a peripheral iridectomy should be done to prevent further attacks. The second eye usually will be found to have a similar predisposition to angle closure glaucoma and many surgeons advocate later prophylactic peripheral iridectomy to this eye.

Infantile glaucoma is raised intra-ocular pressure occurring within the first three years of life. In this age group, the raised pressure causes haziness and enlargement of the cornea, with lacrimation and photophobia as prominent signs. The raised pressure is due to abnormal development of the anterior chamber angle, but once diagnosed early surgery can help up to 80 per cent of these infants.

Secondary glaucoma may follow iritis, trauma to the eye, lens dislocation etc. Treatment is aimed at the causative condition.

SUDDEN LOSS OF VISION

ACCIDENTALLY DISCOVERED POOR VISION

Poor vision in one eye may be accidentally discovered when the patient chances to cover one eye, or at a routine eye sight test such as school children have.

Refractive error in one eye may be responsible e.g. marked myopia, hypermetropia or astigmatism. Measure the patient's visual acuity looking through a pinhole. If this improves vision to nearly normal it means that spectacles can do the same.

Strabismic amblyopia due to a squint is preventable provided it is detected early enough. All children should have their visual acuity in each eye tested by 5 years of age, and preferably by their 4th birthday. If acuity is low on one side refraction under a cycloplegic should be done and the ocular media and fundi checked for any obvious cause of poor vision. If none is found then spectacles will be worn if indicated and the fixing eye patched to make the vision develop properly in the 'lazy eye'.

Once equal visual acuity has been obtained in the two eyes then the eyes must be made straight. Sometimes glasses alone suffice, or with the addition of miotic drops. In other patients surgery is needed to reposition the extra-ocular muscles.

Visual field loss affecting one eye severely may be due to glaucoma which has destroyed the sight on one side and already affected the other eye before being discovered. Lesions affecting the visual pathways may do the same, e.g. pituitary tumours. Confrontation testing of visual fields will indicate the degree of field loss in the remaining eye. Refer to the ophthalmologist or neurologist.

TRANSIENT LOSS OF VISION

Papilloedema due to raised intracranial pressure may cause blackouts lasting 5 to 15 seconds only, or a patchy blurring of vision. Headaches, nausea and vomiting may be present and general examination is required since the prime causes are cerebral tumours and hypertension. Appropriate treatment is then instituted .

Carotid artery insufficiency causes unilateral blindness 'like a curtain coming down over the eye' and returning to normal in 4 or 5 minutes. It occurs as a warning symptom in 50 per cent of cases of carotid occlusion. Transient contralateral limb pareses may occur. Listen along the course of the carotids for bruits. Examine the fundi for bright cholesterol embolic plaques in the arterioles. Refer the patient for assessment for possible surgical endarterectomy, or long-term anticoagulants.

Basilar artery insufficiency produces varied symptoms, including dysphagia, dysarthria, dysphonia and numbness of the lips. 80 per cent of patients with basilar insufficiency have ocular signs including diplopia, usually from VIth nerve involvement. Scintillating scotomas and various field defects may be present. Horizontal or vertical gaze palsies can occur, as may vestibular nystagmus. Visual hallucinations and diplopia are never found in carotid insufficiency.

Migraine typically presents a zig-zag flashing before the headache develops. The visual loss may progress to a hemianopia lasting 15 to 30 minutes. Often migraine will be aborted by ergotamine tartrate taken at the first warning of an impending attack. Prolonged and even permanent hemianopia following migrainous symptoms means that arteriovenous anomalies must be suspected.

LONGER LASTING OR PERMANENT LOSS OF VISION

Central retinal artery occlusion causes sudden and often permanent loss of vision. A pale oedematous area of the posterior pole is seen with a red patch at the macula. With branch occlusions of the retinal arterioles the embolus may be visible. Most emboli are atheromatous in older patients, but in young adults heart disease, particularly the rheumatic type, may be responsible. Treatment if it is to have any hope of success must be prompt. Methods of attempted vasodilation to allow the embolus to pass peripherally into the retina include intermittent globe massage with the fingers, breathing a 95–5 per cent mixture of oxygen and carbon dioxide, intravenous acetazolamide 500 mg to soften the eye, and paracentesis of the anterior chamber. Retrobulbar injections of acetylcholine may also be tried.

Central retinal vein thrombosis may be complete or partial. A dramatic fundus picture of dilated and tortuous veins is seen. Causes of both primary and secondary polycythaemia must be searched for and treated. No treatment for the eye is effective but surprisingly good visual acuity sometimes returns after several weeks. Other cases progress to thrombotic glaucoma.

Ischaemic optic atrophy causes sudden visual loss, usually of the lower field with a pale and swollen optic disc, sometimes accompanied by splinter haemorrhages. Later neovascularization of the optic nerve head develops. Systemic corticosteroids may be tried.

Cranial (temporal) arteritis is followed by blindness in half the patients within a period of weeks. General malaise, weight loss and insomnia with severe headache and localised tenderness over the superficial cranial arteries may be found. Ophthalmoplegias occur in 15 per cent of cases. Rarely is sudden blindness the first symptom. The erythrocytic sedimentation rate (ESR) is usually well over 40 mm in one hour and a temporal artery biopsy confirms the diagnosis. Emergency medical treatment with 60 mg of prednisolone a day is started but must be reduced and continued at least 6 months, the dosage being adjusted according to the ESR.

Optic neuritis may be due to a wide range of causes of which the commonest are multiple sclerosis and the toxic amblyopias. The latter include tobacco, methyl alcohol, quinine and salicylates.

The optic disc has blurred margins, filling of the physiological cup, distended veins and surrounding retinal oedema. It must be differentiated from papilloedema on the associated findings.

Retrobulbar neuritis means that the optic nerve is affected posteriorly so that no changes are visible ophthalmoscopically.

In retrobulbar neuritis, the patients present with sudden loss of vision, rarely total, and a central scotoma can be shown. There is pain on eye movement and the pupil shows a poorly sustained constriction to light. Visual improvement occurs in the ensuing 2 to 3 weeks and there is no conclusive evidence that treatment with systemic corticosteroids helps. Only 50 per cent of patients with retrobulbar neuritis will develop later evidence of multiple sclerosis.

The toxic amblyopias all require drug withdrawal. In addition the tobacco amblyopia responds to vitamin B supplements and the use of intramuscular hydroxocobalamin. For methanol poisoning the acidosis must be controlled by alkali therapy with monitoring of the blood CO_2 combining power. Ethyl alcohol helps by inhibiting the toxic degradation of methanol to formaldehyde.

Vitreous haemorrhages cause sudden visual loss and may take weeks or months to clear. Often diabetic retinopathy or hypertensive retinopathy will be seen in the other eye. Treatment is for the systemic condition.

Retinal detachments may be preceded by sudden floating spots or flashes of light with later loss of visual field and then of visual acuity as the detachment spreads to include the macula.

References

1. *General Ophthalmology* by D. Vaughan, R. Cook and T. Asbury, 5th edition, 1968, published by Lange, U.S.A.
2. *Neurology of the Visual System* by D. G. Cogan, 1st edition, 1966, published by Charles C. Thomas, U.S.A.

This chapter was written by Mr P. Fells (Institute of Ophthalmology, Honorary Consultant Surgeon Moorfields Eye Hospital) and edited by Professor W. I. Cranston.

Dr. Fry considers the treatment and diagnostic problems that common disease presents to the doctor of first contact. The analysis of incidence and the assessment of the most effective forms of treatment that appear in this section are based on many years of practical experience as a family doctor.

Common Emergencies

by

John Fry

General Practioner, Beckenham, England

Introduction

It is a truism that 'common diseases commonly occur and rare diseases rarely happen'.

In approaching the management of the so-called 'common emergencies' it is appropriate first to consider the meaning and significance of all these terms, – common, emergency and management.

This part is designed to assist the physician to deal with emergency situations that he may expect to encounter on a number of occasions in any one year. The management is considered from the viewpoint of the young physician in hospital or in general medical practice.

Each section sets out to present a profile of the condition, its presentation and diagnostic procedures and its management in an emergency situation.

ACUTE BACK

The 'acute back' is a frequent cause of sudden disability seen in general medical practice.

The annual prevalence is 25 per 1,000, so that the general practitioner or primary physician who cares for a population of 2,500 may expect to treat at least one such case each week.

More frequent in males than in females, the age-prevalence shows that it is a condition of active adult life with a peak in the sixth decade (50–59). This type of age-prevalence curve suggests a mixture of degeneration and physical overactivity. Below middle-age the lumbosacral region is still supple enough to tolerate the stresses to which it is subject and after the age of 60 there occurs a natural rigidity and less activity. It is important, nevertheless, to appreciate the natural tendency to spontaneous decline in prevalence, since it will influence our management of a condition that is likely to improve naturally with age.

The causes of the 'acute back' syndrome are many and various. Most frequently it results from sudden damage to either intervertebral joints, discs or ligaments in the region of the lumber 4th and 5th and 1st sacral vertebrae. Rarely is it secondary to some more serious conditions such as secondary malignant neoplastic deposits from a primary in the breast, bronchus, prostate, thyroid or kidney, or myelomatosis; to osteoporosis which may be idiopathic or associated with hyperparathyroidism; to ankylosing spondylitis; to spondylolisthesis or following a missed vertebral fracture; or from osteomyelitis caused by tubercle, staphylococci or other organisms.

Presentation and Diagnosis

The common history is that of a sudden incapacitating pain in the lower lumbar and sacral region following a trivial movement such as stooping to tie a shoelace, making a bed or on lifting heavy weights. The pain is disabling and all movements tend to be restricted. The back is held in an erect position with considerable spasm of the sacrospinalis muscles.

Examination may help to localise the site of the causal lesion. Pain may occur on stretching the sacro-iliac joints and there may be limitation of the straight-leg-raise indicating a probable lesion at the level of the 5th lumber and 1st sacral vertebrae. Referred pain down the legs (sciatica) occurs in approximately 20 per cent of acute backs but signs of nerve root pressure, such as loss of ankle jerk, weakness of calf or thigh muscles or anaesthesia over the appropriate nerve segments of the skin, are found in less than 5 per cent of episodes.

No examination is really complete without a palpation of the rectum to exclude a possible carcinoma of the prostate or other pelvic lesions.

Special investigations are not indicated initially in most cases but where there is no improvement within one or two weeks then a radiograph of the lumbo-sacral region, haemoglobin level, white blood cell count and erythrocyte sedimentation rate and serum phosphatase (alkaline and acid) are indicated.

The course in most cases is a rapid improvement. Two-thirds will recover within three weeks irrespective of the treatment given and only 5 per cent will still be disabled after two months.

Management

The simplest therapy is the most successful. Rest, heat and analgesics should be tried first and persevered with for at least 2–3 weeks. Rest should be in the most comfortable position. This most often is lying flat and supine in bed with a board, to avoid sagging, between the mattress and bedstead.

Heat may be with hot water bottles, electric blankets or hot baths at home, or with infra-red lamps.

Analgesics such as aspirin or paracetamol are usually adequate, but rarely opiates such as morphine injection or its derivatives, such as pethidine, may be necessary to control severe pain.

If no improvement has begun to occur within 2–3 weeks, then various physical therapies may be considered such as support to the lumbar spine through a spinal corset or plaster of paris cast; traction to distract lumbar vertebrae and in theory allow replacement of a prolapsed intervertebral disc; or manipulation by those who believe in intervertebral joint displacements and who are experienced in the techniques. Alternatively, injections of local anaesthetics, such as ½ to 1 per cent lignocaine, can be given either into areas of local tenderness or into muscle 'nodules' if they can be demonstrated or into the epidural space by those experienced in the technique.

Surgery such as removal of prolapsed intervertebral discs or bone grafts to stiffen the lumbo-sacral region are required in very few cases. The indications for surgery are persistent nerve root pressure and particularly if there is pressure on the cauda equina with interference of micturition, or, repeated severe attacks, when a bone graft may occasionally be considered.

In my own experience some 90 per cent of 'acute backs' will settle with simple measures, 10 per cent will require physical therapy and less than 0·1 per cent will be operated upon.

THE ACUTE NECK

The syndrome of acute pain in the neck with radiation down the arms and up the neck and head has a similar age prevalence to that of the acute back but in contrast the acute neck syndrome affects more women than men.

The cause is that of a degenerative spondylosis affecting intervertebral joints and a narrowing and collapse of the intervertebral discs. These changes lead to nerve root pressure and referred pain.

Presentation and Diagnosis

Pain and stiffness of the neck may occur suddenly and spontaneously, often on awakening or following an incident such as a jolt or 'whiplash' injury in a motor car accident.

Radiation of pain depends on the nerve roots affected and there is often wasting of the muscles supplied by the affected nerves.

The diagnosis is confirmed by radiographic signs of cervical spondylosis with narrowing of disc spaces and osteophyte formation around the intervertebral joints.

Management

Rest and analgesics are the sheet anchors of management.

Rest with restrictions of movements is supplemented by local immobilisation with a felt or plastic collar, which should be worn until pain ceases, which may be a month or longer.

Analgesics are as for management of the acute back.

Physical measures involving cervical traction and manipulation have never been proved conclusively to be more effective than less active therapy.

Surgery, involving the removal of prolapsed intervertebral discs and bone grafting to fix segments of the cervical spine, should never be undertaken without a great deal of consideration, because of the general tendency for the acute conditions to settle with less drastic measures.

ACUTE ABDOMEN

A section on the 'acute abdomen' in a medical textbook is not misplaced. The diagnosis and management of this condition faces all physicians who practise in the medical front line.

Although not required to undertake definitive technical surgical procedures the primary physician, whether in hospital or in the community, has the responsibility of early diagnosis and making the vital decision on when to refer the patient for surgery.

In making the diagnosis the physician should not be too concerned to fit the exact aetiological and pathological label but rather to answer the question, is there an acute intra-abdominal crisis present that requires urgent surgical care or is it a condition that can continue to be managed by the physician?

There are numerous non-surgical conditions with similar clinical manifestations which have to be excluded.

Aetiological Types

The annual prevalence of the acute abdomen is approximately 3–4 per 1,000. This means that the primary physician with 2,500–3,000 patients to care for will encounter some 7–12 cases each year or less than one each month, and the large district general hospital may expect to admit around 250–300 'acute abdomens' each year, or one a day.

There are many possible types of 'acute abdomen' and some of these may be non-surgical. Table 1 gives a list of these in the order of frequency as seen by the primary physician.

Clinical Presentation and Diagnosis

The prominent symptoms of an acute abdomen are abdominal pain and vomiting. Any abdominal pain that persists for more than six hours is increasingly likely to be due to a surgical cause.

Abnormal signs may consist of abdominal tenderness, rigidity and distension. General features of collapse and shock may be present.

A systematic diagnostic approach is essential for correct management.

The history, possibly, is of greater importance than the examination or even the investigations and as much time should be allowed for talking with the patient and relatives as for examination and investigation.

Since pain is the most striking symptom, attention must be paid to its analysis.

The exact time and mode of onset are helpful. The most sudden and dramatic onset is with perforation of a gastric or a duodenal ulcer or with conditions such as a rupture of the abdominal aorta with dissection and tracking of the blood. Equally dramatic is the collapse and faint that may accompany an acute pancreatitis or rupture of a pregnant uterine tube.

A more gradual build up of pain occurs in appendicitis, the colics and intestinal obstruction, but where there is strangulation of bowel or torsion of a cyst then the onset usually is quite sudden. With medical conditions the onset tends to be gradual except in rupture of the abdominal aorta; and in some cases of myocardial infarction and pneumonia and porphyria.

Table 1 Surgical and non-surgical causes of the acute abdomen syndromes. (In order of frequency.)

Surgical	'Medical' (non-surgical)
1. Acute appendicitis	1. Acute tonsillitis (in young children)
2. The colics – renal and biliary	2. 'Spastic colon', 'The periodic syndrome' and other psychosomatic conditions
3. Acute intestinal obstruction	3. Pneumonia
4. Diverticulitis of colon	4. Cardiac and vascular – myocardial infarction, pericarditis, dissecting aneurysm and mesenteric thrombosis
5. Perforation of peptic ulcer	5. Herpes Zoster (T.8–12)
6. Haemorrhage (intra abdominal)	6. Bornholm disease (epidemic myalgia)
	7. Intestinal worms
	8. Acute haemolytic crises in malaria, sickle cell trait and other haemolytic anaemias
	9. Diabetic pre-coma
	10. Acute porphyria
	11. Tabes dorsalis

Information on the nature of the pain depends on the ability of an acutely sick person to tell his story. In intestinal obstruction and the colics the pain is intermittent and in women is likened to labour pains, in appendicitis it is constant, dull and aching, in a perforated gastric or duodenal ulcer it is diffuse, burning and immobilising, in dissecting abdominal aneurysm it is tearing and in acute pancreatitis it is agonising and unremitting.

The site may be fixed or the pain may shift or radiate. In a perforation it is usually 'all over the abdomen' from the start. Small intestine and appendicular pain is felt first in the epigastric and umbilical regions. Pain from the large bowel is generally in the lower abdomen. Biliary colic is referred to the epigastric or to the right subcostal region and renal colic to the loins and groins.

Pains referred to the abdomen from non-surgical conditions are generally mid-abdominal. Thus pain from a myocardial infarction, diabetic pre-coma or hiatus hernia tend to be epigastric, whereas in the 'periodic syndrome' of children and in tonsillitis, porphyria and haemolytic crises the pain is central or lower abdominal.

Vomiting may occur as a result of obstruction of the bowels, ureters or biliary ducts or from reflex nervous irritation. Pain tends to precede vomiting in most acute abdominal conditions and it occurs earlier with reflex causes as in the colics and appendicitis that with obstructions of the small and large bowel.

Any significant change in bowel habits is important. Constipation with no flatus may be indicative of a large bowel obstruction but this may occur over a few days. Diarrhoea is a confusing symptom. It is dangerous to assume that it is suggestive of a common enteritis; in association with lower abdominal pain and tenderness it may well be a feature of a much more serious pelvic peritonitis. The presence of blood is always highly significant and may occur in intussusception or with a neoplasm of the large bowel or rectum.

Special attention should be paid to the menstrual pattern and any changes or characteristics suggestive of ovulatory pain and irregular losses together with a late onset of a period may occur in a tubal pregnancy or in an abortion.

The examination of a patient with an acute abdomen must always include a rectal and vaginal examination, as well as a routine examination of the chest, cardiovascular and central nervous systems.

Investigations are by no means always necessary to establish the diagnosis but should always be carried out in assessing a patient for possible surgery.

Radiographs of the chest and abdomen may be required. The former to exclude an intra-thoracic lesion or to assess the state of the lungs and the size of the heart in surgical cases and the latter in possible cases of intestinal obstruction to observe distension of coils of intestines and fluid levels, in cases of an intussusception following a barium enema and in biliary or renal colic to detect calculi.

Blood examination should check the level of haemoglobin and the various indices, a blood smear should be examined for leucocytosis, abnormal red blood cells (sickling and spherocytosis), white blood cells (leukaemia) and malarial parasites. Serum electrolytes should be measured in order that any correction by intravenous therapy may be made.

The urine must always be examined not only for albumin and sugar but also on a slide for pus and red blood cells. In difficult and uncertain situations the urine should also be tested for porphyrins.

Management

The physician has a number of decisions to make and to make them fairly quickly.

1. Is the condition an 'acute abdomen' or is it secondary to some other disorder?
2. Is it surgical and therefore referred to a surgeon?
3. If uncertain can one wait and observe and investigate or proceed to more active measures?

These decisions must be taken alone or in consultation on the clinical diagnostic bases enumerated. It is best always, and it should be possible, to seek the advice of a surgeon when in doubt over diagnosis or management.

In general terms the management comprises the following components. During the first 24–48 hours it is advisable to withold solid food but to allow fluids if there is no vomiting.

Vomiting, if it is repeated, will require tube-suction in association with intravenous fluids.

Control of pain will generally require potent analgesics such as morphine or pethidine, but it is dangerous and unsafe to rely on these before a diagnosis has been made and a plan of management decided upon. Specific therapy must depend on the causal condition.

ACUTE VOMITING AND/OR DIARRHOEA

There are two main portals of entry into the human body – through the respiratory and the alimentary tracts. It is not surprising therefore that both tracts are liable to suffer from infections and irritants that are inhaled and ingested, and that respiratory and gastrointestinal infections are the two most common disorders in the community.

Not only is the alimentary tract affected directly by infection or irritation but it can be affected also indirectly through metabolic disturbances as in diabetes, pregnancy, thyroid and renal disorders and through the central nervous system by involvement of the vomiting centre in the brain.

The most frequent cause of vomiting and diarrhoea are acute infections. It is possible that most of these are viral when no pathogenic bacteria can be found on investigation. The condition is more or less endemic in all places with bouts of extra cases that may add up to local epidemics on occasions. Local inhabitants appear to become resistant to these local organisms but visitors, especially to the tropics, soon succumb but even here often no specific bacterial organisms can be isolated from the stools.

Of course there are specific bacterial infections such as dysentery, typhoid fever and cholera but these are much more rare, particularly typhoid and cholera, than the non-specific and possibly viral gastro-enteritis.

In infants certain strains of E. Coli are pathogenic and may in institutions assume epidemic proportions, whilst in certain situations such as after prolonged antibiotic therapy in debilitated patients the staphylococcus pyogenes may cause severe and dangerous entero-colitis.

Food Poisoning

Food poisoning may occur from bacterial toxins, bacterial infection, chemical contaminants or allergy.

Staphylococcal food poisoning is caused by the ingestion of preformed toxins which have accumulated in foods such as artificial cream, custards, trifles and cream cakes. The foods are contaminated by handlers with staphylococcal lesions and the organisms and their toxins are not destroyed by cooking.

The onset with vomiting occurs a short while after ingestion (1–3 hours) and is followed by diarrhoea and a variable degree of malaise and collapse.

Cl. Welchii is another organism that causes a toxin type of food poisoning. It is transmitted by stored or recooked meat products such as meat pies.

Bacterial food infections are caused by the salmonellae, especially salmonella typhimurium, dysentery, staphylococci or occasionally streptococci.

The onset usually is delayed until the ingested bacteria have grown sufficient in numbers to cause symptoms that is 24–36 hours after infection. Profuse diarrhoea is the main symptom and in a salmonella infection is likely to persist for many days unless treated with antibiotics.

Chemical, plant or allergic food poisoning from cooking vessels, cooking ingredients, fungi and berries or shellfish results in vomiting followed by diarrhoea within two hours of ingestion.

Vomiting

Apart from accompanying the common acute gastro-enteritis this vomiting may occur without diarrhoea. Epidemics of vomiting do occur and are probably also caused by a variety of undefined viruses. The so-called 'epidemic winter vomiting' disease is one such syndrome.

Repeated and sudden vomiting may occur in cases of duodenal ulcer when obstruction as a result of spasm, oedema or scar stenosis develops.

As part of the 'acute abdomen syndrome' vomiting usually follows pain.

Acute vomiting may occur in myocardial infarction in association with chest pain and collapse, in renal conditions such as renal colic, acute nephritis and anaemia, in diabetic precoma and glaucoma.

Vomiting may be the first feature of pregnancy and when a young woman previously fit, comes with recent nausea and vomiting as symptoms the first question that should be asked is the date of her last menstrual period.

In migraine, vomiting follows headache and in other central nervous system conditions such as meningitis and space occupying lesions the vomiting is but one feature, the others being headache and disturbance of consciousness.

Acute Diarrhoea

Infections, already referred to, are the most frequent causes of acute diarrhoea but on rare occasions ulcerative colitis with slime, pus and blood in the faeces, and cancer of the colon and rectum may present acutely.

Clinical Presentation and Diagnosis

Nine out of ten cases of acute vomiting and diarrhoea are caused by an infection.

Vomiting followed a few hours later by watery diarrhoea and accompanied by abdominal pain, fever and various degrees of malaise and collapse are the clinical features of a gastro-intestinal infection.

The course in most instances is towards a natural and spontaneous resolution within 2–3 days.

In the majority of cases special investigations are unnecessary and unhelpful. It is only when some unusual cause or epidemic is suspected such as food poisoning, a metabolic disease, an intracranial lesion or an acute abdomen, or if the condition is not beginning to settle within 48 hours, that special investigations are indicated.

If food poisoning is suspected then specimens of or the whole remnant of the possible causal food should be sent for bacteriological examination, and faeces should be examined for salmonella and dysentery organisms.

If the person has collapsed then blood examination for electrolyte and haematocrit levels is necessary as a preliminary to possible intravenous fluid therapy.

Management

On the assumption that most cases will resolve spontaneously within 48 hours and providing that no other serious condition is suspected and that the general condition is good then 'expectant measures' are all that is required.

These measures consist of avoiding solid food, taking fluids by mouth if they are retained, and rest. If it is felt that the patient expects some medication then a mixture of kaolin, 10 ml. two hourly, is reasonable.

It is quite wrong to give antibiotics or sulphonamides or some other chemical antiseptics blindly on the assumption that the cause is a bacterial infection. In the great majority of the common infections no pathogenic bacteria can be detected and the condition settles rapidly and well without these potent drugs.

It is also wrong to take prophylactic antibiotics (these themselves can cause diarrhoea) or chemical antiseptics on travelling to foreign lands. There is no proof that they are helpful.

Naturally specific conditions once diagnosed will require specific remedies and in severe cases dehydration will require intravenous fluids, particularly in infants and in the aged.

GASTRO-INTESTINAL HAEMORRHAGE

Bleeding from the gastro-intestinal tract may occur from any part but in practice it is the oesophagus, and stomach duodenum and the large bowel that contain the lesions which account for most of the incidents.

Bleeding from the oesophagus, stomach and duodenum is manifest by vomiting of blood (haematemesis) but if some of the blood passes through the stomach and intestines it will pass through and be excreted as black altered blood (melaena). Bleeding from the small and large intestines tends to be unaltered and bright red.

Serious gastro-duodenal haemorrhage is not all that frequent in practice. A primary physician caring for a population of 2,500–3,000 may expect no more than 1–2 cases a year, whereas a large district hospital may admit annually between 50–100 cases.

Profuse bleeding from the lower bowel is less frequent, although minor bleeds are common and present as diagnostic rather than therapeutic problems.

Causes

Haematemesis and Melaena

Acute and chronic gastric and duodenal ulcers account for 85 per cent of all cases. The acute erosive ulcers occur chiefly in the stomach and are a separate condition from the chronic penetrating varieties. In many acute ulcers there is a history of ingestion of aspirin or similar drugs immediately before the bleeding occurs and it is likely that these substances are responsible.

Bleeding from oesophageal varices which develop from cirrhosis of the liver or some other obstruction of the portal circulation accounts for between 2·5 and 5 per cent of all cases, depending on the prevalence of chronic alcoholic cirrhosis.

Hiatus hernia and gastro-oesophageal reflux (2·5 per cent) cause an oesophagitis with occasional ulceration of the lower oesophagus. This tends to cause chronic bleeding but on occasions this may be acute and profuse.

Other possible causes are gastric or oesophagael neoplasms (2·5 per cent), rupture of the lower oesophagus (Mallory–Weiss syndrome) (2·5 per cent), and a variety of conditions such as rupture of an aortic aneurysm, gastric polyps and acute gastritis.

A condition of uncertain origin causing diffuse bleeding from the stomach is gastrostaxis. This is rare but extremely difficult to treat.

When considering haematemesis it is always necessary to differentiate between a true bleeding from the gastro-duodenal region and vomiting of swallowed blood after dental or nasal haemorrhage.

Bleeding through the Rectum

Blood per rectum may originate anywhere along the intestinal tract from the duodenum downwards. Blood that has passed through the stomach by regurgitation will be altered and black (melaena) but blood from the small and large bowels may pass through quickly and be bright red in colour.

Causes of sudden and profuse bleeding per rectum are in order of frequency, melaena from bleeding gastric or duodenal ulcers; haemorrhoids, although usually the bleeding is slight and recurrent; rectal or colonic neoplasms that have eroded largish vessels; polyps of the small and large intestines; ulcerative colitis (although rarely is bleeding profuse, more often it is of small amounts and mixed with slime and pus); an ectopic gastric ulcer in a Meckel's diverticulum; lesions in the terminal ileum such as ileitis; and sometimes in spite of repeated investigations no cause for a single sudden and profuse bleed can be found.

Gastro-intestinal haemorrhage may occur in a haemorrhagic disorder such as thrombocytopenia or telangiectasia, or in someone on anticoagulants, and this possibility should be borne in mind when no clear explanation is evident.

Clinical Presentation

The case may present clearly with a history of vomiting blood or bleeding per rectum, but it is not unusual for it to present as some feature of a sudden and hidden internal haemorrhage.

Vomited blood may be either fresh, but darker than normal, or it may appear as 'coffee grounds' as a result of some retention and digestion in the stomach.

Blood per rectum may be black and tar-like if its passage has been through the stomach and intestines or bright, red from lesions in the large intestine.

Sometimes the first feature is not an obvious bleed associated with vomiting or passage of blood per rectum but an effect of the sudden and severe hidden internal haemorrhage. An unexpected faint in a previously fit man; collapse with malaise, headache, pallor, thirst, cold sweat and dyspnoea; and sudden onset of angina of effort and even myocardial infarction, all these may delay the early diagnosis unless specific questions are asked about the colour of the stools and nature of any vomit.

Diagnosis

Cause of the Bleeding

Remembering that more than four out of five gastro-duodenal bleeds are caused by acute or chronic ulcers, it is possible from the history, physicial examination, endoscopy and radiography to establish an accurate diagnosis in the majority.

A history of intermittent dyspepsia supported by a positive finding after a barium meal makes a chronic ulcer likely.

Acute gastric ulcers or erosions have no previous history of dyspepsia but often are associated with taking aspirin, alcohol, phenylbutazone and similar drugs, or corticosteroids.

Oesophageal varices should be considered where there is a palpable spleen, spider naevi, 'liver palms' and of course a history of alcoholism.

Alteration of bowel habits, symptoms of intermittent intestinal obstruction, colicky abdominal pain and distension, are suggestive of neoplasms of lower bowel and all cases must have a rectal examination performed.

The extent and detail of investigations must depend on the state of the patient, on the available facilities and expertise and on the confidence in the clinical assessment. In most specialist units oesophagoscopy and gastroscopy and sigmoidoscopy with the less traumatic fibrescopes and radiology with barium or gastrografin contrast media are possible within a few hours after resuscitation.

Assessment of Blood Loss

It is dangerous and inaccurate to rely solely on the history and the general state of the patient to assess the amount of blood loss. A persistent pulse rate of over 100 per minute and a systolic blood pressure below 100 mm. Hg. make blood transfusion urgently necessary. An initial level of haemoglobin may be fallacious as it may be falsely high before haemodilution has taken place.

Haematocrit levels and indices such as M.C.V. and M.C.H.C. are more useful.

General Investigations are designed to determine the presence of any coincident diseases and a chest radiograph, electrocardiograph, urinalysis and estimation of blood urea, serum electrolytes and blood cells may be indicated.

Management

Although the bleeding ceases spontaneously in many instances it is safer to transfer to hospital all cases with anything more than apparently small bleeds. However, no cases should be transported if in a state of severe shock. It should be possible to resuscitate the patient, at home or wherever the incident has occurred, with intravenous fluids and other measures before the ambulance ride which may itself be traumatic and disturbing.

In general the following steps should be taken in hospital after the preliminary case history has been taken and examination carried out.

Arrangements for possible Blood Transfusion

A blood sample should be taken for haemoglobin and other blood examination and for blood grouping and cross matching with at least 2–3 litres of blood, which must then be kept available constantly. Blood transfusion is indicated in patients who appear clinically shocked with a pulse rate of over 100 and systolic blood pressure below 100 mm hg. It is indicated particularly in the elderly but here the dangers of circulatory overloading are very real.

Constant Observation and Assessment

Pulse rate and blood pressure levels should be recorded every half-hour and close attention paid to any clinical deterioration.

Rest and Sedation

Bed rest is essential until it becomes clear that bleeding has ceased and the general condition is improving.

In spite of theoretical objections, morphine in 15 mg subcutaneous injections every 4–6 hours still is, in my opinion, the best sedative in these cases.

Gastric aspiration is indicated only with repeated vomiting and where it is thought that there is residual blood in the stomach.

Diet

A light diet with adequate fluids should be allowed from the very onset. Starvation does not prevent re-bleeding and leads rapidly to dehydration.

Surgery

Gastro-intestinal bleeding is a situation for joint action by physician and surgeon. Emergency surgery is now relatively safe, even in the elderly, and it will be indicated when bleeding continues or recurs over 2–3 days, in the elderly more than in the young and middle-aged, and where there are causal lesions that may require definitive surgical treatment.

The results of management of gastro-intestinal bleeding severe enough to require hospitalisation should aim at a mortality of less than 1 per cent in those under the age of 60, and less than 10 per cent in those over 60.

ACUTE POISONING BY OVERDOSAGE OF DRUGS

In the United Kingdom there are 24,000 attempted suicides admitted to hospital each year and 6,000 suicides. This means that there will be 1–2 cases annually per general practitioner and more than one case admitted each week to a large district hospital.

More than two-thirds of these suicides and attempted suicides are the results of overdosage with drugs.

Acute poisoning by drugs comprises two other smaller groups – accidental poisoning, most often in young children who discover some attractive-looking pills and eat them, and, criminal poisoning in an attempt at murder.

The whole question is associated with emotional drama, legal and police involvement.

The following are the most usual drugs that are responsible for acute poisoning:

1. Barbiturates	60 per cent	2/3 of total cases
Tranquillizers	5 per cent	
2. Salicylates	15 per cent	
3. Coal gas	10 per cent	
4. Others	10 per cent	

The high frequency of poisoning by barbiturates and similar preparations is a result of the prevalent use of these drugs for persons suffering from depression and other emotional disorders. It is not surprising therefore that access to an accumulating quantity of sleeping pills offers ready opportunities for overdosage.

The specific effects of the common poisons depend on the individual drug but in large doses they affect the central nervous system, respiration and circulation and when death occurs it is due to the depression and ultimate failure of these systems.

Presentation and Diagnosis

The presentation is dramatic. The victim usually is discovered by friends or relatives in a drowsy or unconscious condition. The situation is full of emotion and upset.

As much information as possible should be obtained from all available sources on the recent mental state of the victim and on previous physical and mental illnesses. Suicide notes are useful guides. The approximate time of the ingestion of the drugs is important in assessing the duration of its action. Identification of the drug should be established as soon as possible. Some may remain and the name of the drug may have been written on the container.

The case may present as one of 'coma' and in the elderly and the middle-aged, overdosage of drugs must be considered in the differential diagnosis of a cerebrovascular accident.

If the victim is not found for some hours, and particularly if he decides to perform the act of suicide out of doors, there will be the added dangers of exposure and hypothermia.

General Management

The aim of treatment of acute poisoning must be to save life and restore the victim to health. Under modern conditions in a well-equipped and staffed unit it should be possible to reduce the mortality, in patients admitted alive, to below 1 per cent.

The general management comprises a mixture of supportive measures and active therapy and skill lies in arriving at the best mix of the two.

It is safer to admit to a hospital with necessary services, all patients who have taken an overdose of drugs, either intentionally or accidentally. The primary physician has the role of making the probable diagnosis of overdosage, of collecting information on the drugs ingested and in applying emergency aid and arranging for the transfer of the patient to hospital. It may be necessary to carry out resuscitation and intubation and mechanical ventilation prior to moving the patient in severe cases.

The definitive management consists of the following steps:

1. Keeping the patient alive.
2. Removing the poison.
3. Increasing the elimination of the drug.
4. Managing any underlying psychiatric condition that led to the self-poisoning and arranging for after-care of the individual.

5. Deciding on the steps, if any, to be taken to inform the police or other authorities.

6. Applying, if in difficulty, to an information service e.g. ('Poisons Bureau' – or the drug manufacturer) on the nature and content of preparations ingested and on the correct management.

Keeping the Patient Alive

During the journey to hospital it is essential that the airway be kept clear in the unconscious patient who should be transported in the semi-prone position with an airway in place.

Admission should be to a ward or unit equipped for intensive care and blood-gas analysis.

If the patient is deeply unconscious then the airway must be maintained by means of a cuffed endotracheal tube which can be left in place for up to 72 hours.

Oxygen should be given in high concentration. Bronchial and tracheal secretions should be aspirated and assisted mechanical ventilation started if the patient is cyanosed with feeble spontaneous circulation or if the blood-gases are seriously disturbed.

Shock and hypotension should be treated by elevating the foot of the bed and injecting intramuscularly metaraminol 5 mg and repeated once only after ½–1 hour if necessary. If there is no response and blood pressure remains low then blood transfusion or the infusion of plasma or dextran should be started and the amounts given controlled by frequent recording of the pulse rate and blood pressure and by monitoring the central venous pressure.

For dehydration and electrolyte balance in the patient who is unconscious for more than 24 hours, one litre of 5 per cent dextrose and half a litre of normal saline in alternation should be administered (in 24 hours).

Cardiac failure requires rapid but careful digitalisation and cardiac arrhythmias, which are likely with overdose of the tricyclic antidepressants should be controlled with lign ocaine or propranolol.

Convulsions may occur in unconscious patients in poisoning with tricylic antidepressants and phenothiazines, and curarization with controlled ventilation may be necessary.

Prophylatic antibiotics are rarely necessary and should be used only when there is evidence of respiratory infection. Bladder catheterization is not required and analeptics have no virtue.

Successful outcome will depend to a large extent on a high standard of nursing team care.

Removal of the Poison

If the poison has been swallowed then removal can be helped by vomiting and washing out the stomach.

If the poison has been inhaled then the patient should be moved into the fresh air and oxygen administered.

If the poison has been absorbed from the skin then the clothes should be removed and the skin washed.

Most poisons are ingested. It is dangerous to induce vomiting in the drowsy or unconscious patient. Ipecacuanha and apomorphine should not be used. Vomiting should not be induced in the very old and the very young, in petroleum or corrosive poisoning, in those with previous gastric operations and in alcoholics, and it is useless to wash out the stomach more than four hours after ingestion.

In the conscious patient vomiting can be induced by drinking salt water or by inserting fingers down the back of the mouth.

In the unconscious patient the stomach can be washed out through an adequately sized tube (Jacques 30 English gauge) but only with a cuffed endotracheal tube in place.

Elimination of Poison

There are no general antidotes. Most cases of poisoning through over-dosage will recover without active measures designed to increase elimination provided that supportive measures are adequate.

If increased elimination is required then forced diuresis (by frusemide or intravenous mannitol), peritoneal dialysis, haemodialysis, passage of blood over ion-exchange resins or even exchange transfusions may be considered.

Barbiturate Overdosage

Poisoning with barbiturates accounts for 60 per cent of all cases of poisoning) and most of these occur in patients already being treated for depression or other psychiatric illnesses. The risks should be appreciated whenever these drugs are prescribed and when they are all containers should be labelled with the name of the contents.

The effects of excessive barbiturates are depression of the central nervous system leading to drowsiness and coma, to depression of respiration and respiratory failure, to depression of the vasomotor centre with shock and hypotension, and to interference with temperature control and thus leave a liability to hypothermia.

Diagnosis depends on a good history, the identification of the ingested preparation and on the level of blood barbiturates.

The prognosis depends on the degree of severity which is measured by the depth of unconsciousness.

Mild cases (60 per cent of all barbiturate poisoning) are those who are drowsy but conscious.

Moderate cases (30 per cent) are stuporose but responsive to painful stimuli.

Severe cases (10 per cent) are comatose and non-responsive. Assessment of these grades is often more accurate clinically than biochemically.

The levels of serum barbiturates are useful. With moderately quick-acting barbiturates levels of more than 2–3 mg per 100 ml are indicative of a severe overdose and the rapid absorption of the drug, and with slow-acting barbiturates a level of more than 8–10 mg per 100 ml of barbiturate suggests severe overdose.

Management

The mild cases do not require any specific therapy but should be seen and assessed by a psychiatrist prior to discharge. He should arrange after-care and support.

The moderate cases who are stuporose but rousable require the application of standard methods.

The respiration must be maintained through a clear airway (intubation if necessary) with oxygen and assisted mechanical ventilation if necessary.

The stomach may be washed out (with endotracheal tube in place) up to four hours of ingestion.

Shock and hypotension may require raising foot of bed, metaraminol and transfusion.

The severe cases in order to maintain life may require increased elimination of drugs by forced diuresis with intravenous dextrose and saline, mannitol or frusemide, or by peritoneal or haemodialysis.

Salicylates

Ingestion of large numbers of aspirin tablets is the second most common form of drug overdosage (15 per cent of all poisoning).

The effects are to cause salicylism with ketosis, respiratory alkalosis and metabolic acidosis. Accompanying this there is dehydration and acid-base upsets.

Clinically there is vomiting, tinnitus, deafness, dizziness and excitability. There is sweating, overbreathing, fever and dehydration. Eventually, in severe cases, coma, collapse and death ensue.

Blood salicylate levels offer a guide to severity. In adults cases are considered to be severe when the blood salicylate level is more than 70 mg per 100 ml, and moderate when it is over 50 mg per 100 ml. In children a level of 30 mg per 100 ml and over, is dangerous.

Management

Up to twelve hours after ingestion a stomach wash out with sodium bicarbonate under suitable precautions is advisable.

Mild cases can be treated with copious oral fluids.

Moderate cases showing a blood salicylate level of over 50 mg per 100 ml should have forced diuresis encouraged with intravenous saline, dextrose and sodium lactate.

Severe cases in coma and with a salicylate level of more than 70 mg per 100 ml may require haemodialysis in a special unit.

Iron

Ingestion of brightly coloured iron tablets is a hazard in young children and causes a haemorrhagic gastritis and acidosis.

Many cases settle spontaneously under observation.

In severe cases the chelating agent desferrioxamine should be used to inactivate the iron as soon as possible. It can be used intravenously, instilling 80 mg/kg over 24 hours, or by intramuscular injection 2 g. – 12 hourly until the condition improves. It is also useful to wash out the stomach and leave a 5 g. solution in 50 ml of fluid in the stomach.

ACUTE CORONARY ARTERY DISEASE

The clinical spectrum of acute coronary artery disease is a wide one.

Sudden and unexpected deaths account for 20 per cent of all forms. There is usually a preceding history of 'indigestion' that may be worse on effort, for a few hours or even days before the victim is found dead or collapses and dies within minutes.

Angina is the first sign of acute coronary artery disease in another 20 per cent of cases. The presternal pain that radiates down the left or both arms is brought on by effort, cold or emotional upsets.

In myocardial infarction the chief clinical feature is a heavy and constant presternal pain that persists for hours.

The category of acute coronary artery insufficiency is unnecessarily confusing and represents a mild form of infarction rather than a specific category.

Clinically three grades of severity can be recognised.

The 'mild' myocardial infarction (12 per cent of all presenting types) is that type where the patient often walks into the consulting room with a history of classical coronary chest pain for variable periods during the preceding days associated with 'indigestion'. Electrocardiography confirms the diagnosis of myocardial infarction.

In the 'moderate' variety (35 per cent) the patient is often seen at home, or is brought to hospital, with a history of severe anterior chest pain for an hour or longer. The patient is distressed but there are no signs of shock or cardiac failure. The pain and general condition improve and then clear within a few hours after an injection of morphine, or similar analgesic.

In the 'severe' type (13 per cent) there is shock, hypotension, collapse and heart failure often from the very onset.

Coronary artery disease is a condition of ageing and degeneration and is not one affecting only middle-aged men, although it is this group that tends to present most suddenly and dramatically.

The place and time of the sudden deaths are of relevance. In a study on my own practice I found, for example, that sixty-five per cent of all deaths from coronary heart disease occurred on the first day.

Of these 'first-day deaths' 70 per cent occurred in the victim's own home, 13 per cent in hospital and 17 per cent elsewhere.

Fifty per cent were 'instant' within 15 minutes of onset, 30 per cent within 15–60 minutes of onset and 20 per cent between 1–24 hours.

In theory, after excluding instant deaths and those with associated conditions that would have made resuscitation impossible, it was found in 36 per cent of these sudden first-day-deaths resuscitation would have been possible and feasible – but 72 per cent of these 'possibles' died at home and 80 per cent within the first hour, so that speedy resuscitation outside hospital would have to be available.

Presentation and Diagnosis

The presenting clinical features of an acute myocardial infarction may be – pain, collapse, dyspnoea or arrythmia.

The pain is most often presternal. It is a heavy pain as 'though someone is sitting on me' or 'crushing' or 'constricting'. It may radiate down the arms (left more often than right), up to the chin or through to the back. It may occur only at the referral sites namely arm, chin or back. The severity varies and the mild types may be regarded by the patient as unimportant 'indigestion'.

Diagnosis

The electrocardiogram (E.C.G.) is the most useful investigation. Characteristically positive findings of a transmural infarction are deep Q waves, elevation of the S–T segments in leads facing the damaged area with reciprocal S–T depression in remote leads and symmetrical T wave inversion (further reference to a standard book on this subject should be made—see references).

When present these changes are confirmatory but they may take a few days to develop and in some instances may never appear even in otherwise definite cases of myocardial infarction. In my opinion more reliance should be placed on the clinical assessment than on an E.C.G., and other tests, and if it is considered clinically that the patient has sustained a myocardial infarction then, and if there is no evidence of other conditions, he should be managed as such in spite of repeated negative E.C.G. changes.

A chest radiograph should be taken when diagnosis is uncertain to exclude other conditions such as pericardial effusion and lung lesions.

An elevation of the temperature often develops and persists for several days and like an elevated erythrocyte sedimentation rate (E.S.R.) and polymorph leucocytosis, is evidence of muscle damage.

Serum enzyme levels may be helpful with equivocal E.C.G. tracings.

The serum glutamic oxaloacetic transaminase (SGOT) reaches its peak level 24–48 hours after infarction and should be tested for only at this time.

The serum lactic dehydrogenase (SLDH) is maximal later at 48–72 hours.

Management

The objectives of management are to save life during the immediate acute stage, prevent complications and rehabilitate to normal life whenever possible.

The most dangerous period is the first day and in particular the first hour after infarction. If care is to be optimal then the feasibility of special emergency ambulances staffed by physicians able to use resuscitative equipment should be considered. These ambulances are being used successfully in the large cities such as Moscow, Leningrad and Kiev in U.S.S.R., and in Belfast in Northern Ireland.

Whilst it is not possible to predict the course of any myocardial infarction and complications may occur even in 'mild' cases, in the first few days after onset, the course and outcome are related closely to the clinical severity. The primary physician therefore is in a dilemma when faced with the management of the 'mild' and 'moderate' cases. Complications may occur but the course is benign in the majority of these cases. In an ideal situation the patient with a proven (or probable) myocardial infarction should be admitted to a hospital coronary care unit, equipped to deal with all possible complications, for 2–3 days. It is of doubtful value for the patient to be admitted to a hospital without such facilities, and he might as well be nursed at home.

The steps in management are:

1. Diagnosis and resuscitation at home or wherever the victim is found.
2. Transport to hospital if admission is considered necessary.
3. Intensive care and supervision for 2–3 days.
4. Progressive care in hospital for up to 2 weeks.
5. Rehabilitation at home.

The possibility of resuscitation at home by an emergency team has been referred to and facilities for resuscitation should be available also in the ambulance taking the patient to hospital A sizeable proportion die in transit and if intensive care is to be given then it should commence as soon as skilled assistance reaches the patient.

Intensive care implies constant supervision by trained nursing staff, E.C.G. monitoring and appropriate treatment for any complications that may arise.

Since the danger period is chiefly in the first two or three days after the infarction the patient's stay in the unit need not be any longer, unless he is on active treatment for a complication.

From the intensive care unit the patient is transferred to the general hospital wards where progressive ambulation can be carried out over the following weeks. Complete bed rest is not necessary and the aim should be for the patient to be ambulant in the ward within two weeks in an uncomplicated case.

Immediate Care

Pain must be controlled and morphine is still the analgesic most widely used, 15 mg intramuscularly, or 5–10 mg intravenously for severe pain, should be given at once and repeated within an hour if there is no relief. Vomiting occurs in a proportion of patients after morphine, and diamorphine (heroin) is recommended by some as a better preparation in similar dosage. Those who do not wish to use opiates because of respiratory depression give pethidine 100 mg intramuscularly.

Oxygen is given when available at a rate of 4 litres per minute.

Anticoagulants are effective in reducing the likelihood of thrombo-embolic complications. They have no effect on the infarction. They are safe and should be given to younger patients, up to 65, and for all severe attacks unless there is a history of active peptic ulcer, presence of a pericardial friction rub, suggesting a transmural infarct, or a history of haemorrhagic disorders.

To effect immediate anticoagulation heparin in an initial intravenous dose of 10,000 units should be followed by an intravenous infusion for 48 hours. This should contain 40,000 units of heparin in one litre of 5 per cent dextrose per 24 hours and will keep the whole blood-clotting time at twice the normal. Oral phenindione should be started on admission at 100 mg daily and the dose controlled by estimation of prothrombin time.

Complications

The death rate of patients admitted to hospital with acute myocardial infarctions is still between 15 and 30 per cent.

The causes of death are:

Arrhythmias – 50 per cent
Shock and heart failure – 43 per cent
Thrombo-embolism – 5 per cent
Ruptured myocardium – 2 per cent

Arrhythmias should be detected by the continuous E.C.G. monitor. Digoxin 0·5 mg followed by 0·25 mg 6 hourly is indicated for persistent atrial tachycardia and fibrillation (providing there is no history of previous digitalisation, when the dose must be modified.

Frequent ventricular ectopic beats predispose to ventricular fibrillation and are best prevented by adding lignocaine into the intravenous drip. The dose will depend on what is needed to achieve control of the arrythmia but up to 6–8 g. can be given in 24 hours. Alternatively oral propranolol up to 40 mg 6-hourly can be used.

Ventricular fibrillation is an emergency that is best treated by immediate electrical version with a synchronous D.C. defibrillator. If this is not available up to 50 mg of lignocaine should be injected slowly.

Cardiac arrest is due either to a systole or ventricular fibrillation. Mouth to mouth respiration and external cardiac massage should be started immediately and assistance summoned. Endotracheal intubation should be carried out and mechanical ventilation with oxygen commenced.

For ventricular fibrillation correction should be attempted with the defibr illator and for asystole,pacing with an intracardiac pacemaker is indicated.

Metabolic acidosis should be anticipated and once the heart beat has been restored intravenous infusion with some bicarbonate (100 m.Eq initially) should be started.

Complete heart block is an early complication if it occurs and should be treated by pacing with an intracardiac pacemaker until rhythm is restored and the pacemaker should be left in situ for 5 days more. If not available then a long acting isoprenaline (such as 'saventrine') may restore normal rhythm and prevent recurrence. Atropine by injection may be tried also.

Hypotension in association with shock is difficult to manage and when persistent carries a bad prognosis.

Raising the foot of the bed, oxygen and intravenous therapy are all that can be done.

Cardiac failure is treated with digitalisation, and diuretics.

CARDIAC ARRHYTHMIAS

Cardiac arrhythmias are not infrequent as medical emergencies. Some are benign and may occur in normal and healthy persons and others are the results of various disorders of the heart itself or conditions affecting the heart.

There are two groups. The ectopic tachycardias, including atrial, nodal and ventricular tachycardias and various forms of heart block.

Extrasystoles

Extrasystoles may occur in young persons with no cardiovascular abnormalities. There is no reliable treatment that controls them and reassurance with, perhaps, a sedative or minor tranquillizer, are all that is required.

In the middle-aged and elderly the appearance of extrasystoles may be the result of ischaemic heart disease and when they occur after an acute myocardial infarction they often are danger signals that herald paroxysms of ventricular tachycardia or fibrillation.

Extrasystoles may result from excessive dosage with digitalis and coupled rhythm is almost always due to this cause.

Control of extrasystoles that may be associated with ischaemic heart disease may be treated with digitalis (provided that it has not been given in the past few weeks), or with quinidine.

Paroxysmal Supraventricular Tachycardia

This usually occurs in young persons who often give a history of repeated attacks which start and stop suddenly. The function of the heart is usually not disturbed and the rhythm is regular. However, some cases may be associated with various underlying conditions such as thyrotoxicosis, rheumatic fever and ischaemic heart disease. Digitalis overdosage may cause a dangerous form of paroxysmal tachycardia in persons with heart failure and potassium depletion.

The attacks may last a few seconds or up to some hours. The rate is around 170–200 and the diagnosis is confirmed by E.C.G.

The management should be non-specific unless serious functional disturbance occurs.

Reassurance and sedation are necessary. Simple manoeuvres such as holding a deep breath, massage of the carotid sinus, eyeball pressure or an ice-cold drink may all cut short an attack.

Specific measures are rapid digitalisation, provided it has not been used in the past few weeks, quinidine, propranolol or electroversion.

Atrial Flutter and Fibrillation

These conditions are almost always portents of serious underlying disorders such as ischaemic heart disease, hypertension, rheumatic heart disease and thyrotoxicosis.

Paroxysmal bouts may occur for some years before a persistent arrhythmia is established.

Functionally, atrial fibrillation and flutter interfere with the work of the heart and may lead to left or right cardiac failure, and because there is some stagnation of blood in the atria, thrombi may form, and produce emboli in the lungs or peripheral arteries.

In atrial flutter the jugular vein pulsation is often more than twice the ventricular rate. The pulse is regular. Fibrillation produces a completely irregular pulse.

Diagnosis should be confirmed by E.C.G., which in flutter shows an inverted 'saw-tooth appearance' and in fibrillation a totally irregular ventricular rhythm with normal QRS complexes and fine coarse irregular 'f' waves.

Management of the acute case is by full digitalisation. An initial dose should be given of digoxin 1·0 mg followed by 0·5 mg 6-hourly for 48 hours and then 0·25 gm two or three or four times a day until control with minimal dosage is established.

In flutter the rhythm may be converted to fibrillation and then normality; fibrillation may persist; or the rhythm returns to normal. Recurrences are not uncommon.

In fibrillation the objective is primarily to control the heart failure and not simply the irregular rhythm.

In cases with a sudden and recent onset there is a place for electroversion. This has now replaced quinidine for this purpose.

Paroxysmal Ventricular Tachycardia

This is associated with ischaemic heart disease and carries a serious prognosis and a high risk of death. There is always considerable functional disturbance with breathlessness, low blood pressure and raised venous pressure.

The E.C.G. shows wide bizarre splintered complexes.

The most satisfactory treatment is electroversion. If this is not available then intravenous lignocaine should be given.

Heart Block

Complete heart block is most frequent in old persons. It is most likely to be associated with ischaemic heart disease.

Heart block by itself causes little serious functional disturbance if it is stable. It is the Stokes-Adams attacks of syncope or near-syncope that occur with complete heart block, and when there is a change from partial to complete block, that require emergency care.

The attacks occur when the heart rate suddenly drops to an unacceptable level of 10–15 beats per minute or ceases altogether for a few seconds. There may be transient loss of consciousness with convulsions at times which may be confused with epilepsy. In other attacks consciousness is not lost but there is faintness, giddiness and a feeling of dying.

In most attacks the heart beat soon returns to its regular rhythm of around 30–40 beats per minute and consciousness returns and circulation is restored. If this does not happen then a pacemaker (external or internal) is needed but this is not often readily available. Isoprenaline should be given intravenously or even intracardially.

The most satisfactory drug for prevention is the long-acting preparation of isoprenaline, saventrine, which is given in 30 mg doses every 3–6 hours.

ACUTE DYSPNOEA

In practice there are two important groups of sudden and severe breathlessness.

There are the various conditions that lead to acute left ventricular failure and those that lead to acute pulmonary insufficiency.

A result of better care and facilities for controlling the causes of both groups, has been that the numbers that present as emergencies has fallen – and since these were the reasons for many 'night calls', so have the number of night calls.

Acute Left Ventricular Failure

The condition occurs when the left half of the heart pump suddenly fails and the function of the right half remains unimpaired. The effects fall largely on the lungs and there is a build-up of back pressure in the small alveolar and pulmonary vessels with a slowing of blood flow and an outpouring of fluid into the alveoli, to produce pulmonary oedema.

The pulmonary venous engorgement and oedema fluid in the alveoli and connective tissues of the lungs, result in a decrease of lung compliance – leading to increased efforts to breathe, and a disturbance of ventilation and perfusion relationships. These abnormalities in function, and the nerve reflexes from the distended tissues, lead to the severe dyspnoea of left ventricular failure.

The causes are:

1. Myocardial infarction. Acute myocardial infarction may present as acute left ventricular failure but more often it develops from the myocardial weakness some time after the acute episode.

2. Hypertension is found frequently in those who suffer from left ventricular failure. The reasons for its sudden appearance at night are

uncertain but presumably it is as a result of strain on the left ventricle from attempting to circulate the blood against the high arterial resistance or as a result of the recumbent posture.

3. Less frequently the condition may complicate aortic valvular disease (aortic stenosis or regurgitation or mitral regurgitation).

4. Rarely paroxysmal tachycardias, intracardiac tumours and cardiomyopathies may also cause acute left ventricular failure.

5. Iatrogenically overloading the circulation in too rapid, or too profuse,intravenous transfusions may lead to pulmonary oedema and breathlessness.

Clinical Presentation

Although the severe attacks of breathlessness occur at night, often in the early hours between 11 p.m. and 1 a.m., there is usually a history of some dyspnoea and cough on exertion for a few days before the acute episode.

The patient awakens with a 'heavy' 'tight' chest, severe breathlessness and a dry cough. Sitting up on the edge of his bed helps, but not very much. Clothes are then removed or loosened and finally the victim gets out of bed on to an open window to try and overcome the frightening suffocation. After a while the cough becomes bubbly and productive of a large amount of thin, frothy pink, blood-stained sputum.

There is extreme distress and fear. The patient is ashen grey in colour with a cold and clammy skin. Auscultation reveals fine crepitations that are most marked at the lung bases. Triple rhythm of the heart is usual and often better felt than heard.

The rapid and alternating pulse may be felt or detected on measuring the blood pressure with a sphygmomanometer.

Management

No time should be lost in carrying out any further investigations such as chest radiography and electrocardiography.

The patient should be propped up in bed, if he is not already sitting up. Oxygen, if available, should be given at a rate of 6–8 litres per minute through a face mask until the breathing improves.

Morphine is the drug of choice and 15 mg should be given intramuscularly, or 10 mg intravenously in severe cases. The danger of morphine when there is uncertainty over the differentiation of this condition from chronic airway obstruction has been exaggerated and, as it is a life-saving measure, decision and action must be taken quickly.

The response is often dramatic and within 10–15 minutes breathing is easier and the patient relaxed and comfortable. If there is no satisfactory response then aminophylline 0·25 g. should be given slowly intravenously. Intramuscular and rectal routes are unsatisfactory.

Diuretics should always be given. A useful 'cocktail' is a mixture of morphine 15 mg and mersalyl 2 ml given intramuscularly. If more rapid action is considered necessary, intramuscular mersalyl takes 15–30 minutes before diuresis commences, then intravenous frusemide, 20 mg can be given.

The subsequent (within hours) treatment of the causes may include digitalisation, control of hypertension, management of the myocardial infarction and assessment of valvular lesions and possible surgical treatment.

Venesection used to be recommended as a heroic measure for acute left ventricular failure. It is a messy and unsatisfactory measure but it may have a place when the condition is the result of circulatory overloading by transfusions.

Acute Pulmonary Insufficiency

Acute dyspnoea from pulmonary causes may be the result of the following:

1. Acute airways obstruction associated with wheezy bronchitis and bronchopneumonia or asthma. The obstructed airways may extend from the larger bronchi down to the smallest bronchioles and alveoli. The factors concerned in the obstruction may be contraction of the bronchial muscles, mucosal swelling from congestion and oedema, plugging by viscid mucus and collapse of the smallest airways due to destruction and other damage.

2. Spontaneous pneumothorax is most often a disease of young healthy adults with no serious underlying disease. The cause is rupture of a small bulla or other lesion on the surface of a lung. This spontaneous rupture leads to a communication between the vacuum of the inter-pleural space and the air containing lung. Air is rushed into the pleural cavity until the defect closes. The size of the pneumothorax depends on how much air escapes before self-closure of the defect. After closure the air is reabsorbed gradually and the lung expands. Recurrences are frequent.

Occasionally the defect may remain patent with a valve-like effect allowing air to escape into the pleural cavity but not to re-enter the lung. A gradual build up of positive intrapleural pressure results, this tension pneumothorax may compress vital mediastinal structures and lead to death. Occasionally spontaneous pneumothorax may complicate chronic airways disease and here it is always a most serious matter.

3. Massive lung collapse occurs most often after abdominal operations due to blockage of the large airways by sticky mucus and weak respiratory movements. This leads to an absorption collapse of the lung distal to the block.

Other causes of massive collapse are found in catarrhal children and chronic bronchitics whose thick, sticky and profuse sputum may cause similar blockage and distal collapse.

4. Laryngitis Stridulosa. Although not strictly a pulmonary defect, inflammation and swelling of the larynx cause a 'croupy' cough and dyspnoea.

Clinical Presentation

In acute airways obstruction there is the shortness of breath accompanied by generalised expiratory wheezing in the chest and areas of collapse and crepitations. Severe obstruction results in carbon dioxide retention and hypoxaemia with cyanosis, confusion and restlessness, hot hands, rapid bounding pulse and signs of cor pulmonale (raised jugular venous pressure, triple rhythm and accentuation of pulmonary second round).

There is almost always a history of previous attacks and 'chest troubles' with cough and sputum.

Spontaneous pneumothorax, when large enough, is detected clinically by reduced air entry, hyper-resonance, lack of movement and displacement of the mediastinum.

Diagnosis

Clinical findings are most helpful but in hospital a chest radiograph, sputum culture and measurement of arterial carbon dioxide and oxygen levels are useful.

Management

Acute airways obstruction is managed in the same way, whatever the cause.

1. Oxygen should be given with caution because with hypercapnia a vicious cycle may result with excessive oxygen, due to an unresponsive respiratory centre.

2. Bronchodilators. Aminophylline 0·25 g. intravenously is safest for quick action. Corticosteroids should not be withheld for long in severe asthma and they may be beneficial also in chronic bronchitis and emphysema. If given by mouth a loading dose of up to 80 mg prednisone on the first day followed by a reduction of 5 mg daily is appropriate. In emergencies 100 mg of hydrocortisone hemisuccinate can be injected intravenously and then followed by oral prednisone.

3. Broad-spectrum antibiotics such as oxytetracycline or ampicillin 0·25 g. 4-hourly should be started and continued until the results of sputum culture are available.

Differentiation between Acute Cardiac and Pulmonary Dyspnoea

Because management of these two types of dyspnoea is different, differentiation is important.

It is usually not difficult and the following are useful clinical points.

1. A history of previous chest illnesses is always present with pulmonary causes, but it may well be that a respiratory cripple may suffer occasionally from an acute left ventricular failure.

2. Wheezing and rhonchi are features of pulmonary dyspnoea, bubbling and crepitations are characteristic of left ventricular failure.

3. In acute cardiac dyspnoea there are generally other features of heart trouble such as triple rhythm, alternating pulse, and features of causal disease such as myocardial infarction, hypertension or valvular heart disease.

SUDDEN COMA

The list of possible causes of coma is long and includes many unusual situations. For practical purposes the most frequent types of sudden coma (prolonged unconsciousness) encountered in primary medical care are, in order of descending prevalence:

1. Cerebro-vascular accidents. (Strokes)
2. Head injuries
3. Drug overdosage (including alcoholism)
4. Epilepsy
5. Intracranial neoplasms
6. Meningitis and other intracranial infections

7. Metabolic disturbances such as uraemia, hypoglycaemia and diabetic coma.

The approach to any cause in coma must be orderly and systematic. It is necessary first to make as accurate a diagnosis as possible in order that suitable management may be carried out.

Although the initial situation is dramatic, once steps have been taken to ensure a free airway and satisfactory respiration, further diagnostic assessment need not be hurried.

Clinical Presentation

The ways in which the case presents depend on the cause of coma, and the form of onset and the circumstances in which the patient is found, will be helpful in diagnosis.

There may be a history of past disease as in diabetes, epilepsy and the immediate history may suggest possible causes such as trauma, overdose with drugs, infections which may be related to a meningoencephalitis, or a history of progression to coma, as in some cerebro-vascular occlusions and haemorrhage.

Diagnosis

The clinical examination, whilst concentrating on the central nervous system must cover all systems.

Examination must be delayed until respiration is adequate and cerebral anoxia due to respiratory distress has been corrected.

The examination should be conducted towards answering questions that will influence management.

1. Is the cause intracranial?

2. Are there any specific and urgent therapeutic measures that ought to be taken?

In the central nervous system the pupils, fundi, muscle tone and reflexes must be examined and an assessment made of the level of consciousness. This is best tested by noting the response of the patient to certain stimuli such as shouting, shaking, pin pricks and pressure of the tendo-achilles. These tests should be repeated at regular intervals and a comparative record made.

Investigations should include urinalysis, radiograph of skull, blood count, E.S.R., and Wassermann and Kahn tests.

A lumbar puncture and examination of the cerebrospinal fluid should be made unless there is thought to be a raised intracranial pressure, with papilloedema when it would be a dangerous act.

Management

The first essential is to ensure a free airway with adequate oxygenation. Routine care must include attention to posture, care of the skin, the state of hydration and control of urinary incontinence by an indwelling catheter.

Specific therapy will be necessary once a diagnosis has been made as in the management of drug overdosage, diabetes, hypoglycaemia, uraemia and meningitis.

Surgical intervention may be needed for head injuries and the possibilities of extradural or subdural haematomas should be borne in mind even after minor trauma.

ACUTE CHEST INFECTIONS

Acute Bronchitis and Pneumonia

Acute chest infections are the most frequent group of major (life-threatening) diseases in the community.

In the United Kingdom the annual prevalence rate of these conditions is 30 per 1,000 and the general practitioner with a practice of 2,500 may expect to treat 75 cases each year. Of these less than 10 per cent require admission to hospital. The others respond satisfactorily to treatment at home.

Certain groups are particularly vulnerable and liable to chest infection. Males at all ages are more vulnerable than females; the young and the old are the age groups most likely to suffer and in children the peak prevalence is between 4 and 7 years of age, and in the elderly there is a gradual rise with age from 50 onwards. Sufferers from other chest conditions such as chronic bronchitis and emphysema, asthma, pneumoconiosis and other pulmonary fibroses and bronchiectasis are particularly liable to recurring infections; tobacco smokers and those living in atmospherically polluted areas and the lower social groups all suffer from more than average amounts of chest infection.

The *classification* of acute chest infections may be on an *aetiological* basis where the condition is related to the specific causal organism or on a more practical *clinical or radiological* basis of presenting signs.

Aetiologically, chest infections may be caused by bacteria such as streptococcus pneumoniae, staphylococcus pyogenes, haemophilus influenzae, Klebsiella pneumoniae, tubercle bacillus, or mycoplasma or viruses such as adenovirus, respiratory syncytial virus, the ornithosis-psittacosis group, Q-fever, influenza and measles.

Unfortunately there is no clear and ready correlation between the causal organisms and the presenting clinical picture and often there is a mixture of organisms responsible.

Clinically, diagnostic terms such as acute bronchitis, bronchopneumonia and various forms of pneumonias such as lobar, lobular, aspiration and segmental are described. However in practice it is better to rely on a combination of a number of co-ordinates such as the general condition of the patient, the clinical and radiological picture and the results of bacteriological and virological tests.

It should be recalled always that the acute chest infection may be secondary to a lesion such as a carcinoma of bronchus or some other primary condition of the lungs.

Physio-pathological Effects

The two major effects of acute chest infections are the infection and the results of interference with aeration because of airways obstruction with infiltration and oedema of the alveoli and pulmonary parenchyma. This results in anoxaemia, retention of carbon dioxide and acidosis. Interference to, and obstruction of, the pulmonary blood flow leads to pulmonary hypertension which may in turn lead to cor pulmonale or right heart failure.

Presenting Clinical Features

Cough with sputum that is generally yellow or green in colour and which may be blood-stained, shortness of breath and pain in the chest are the local symptoms that suggest an acute chest infection. More generally, there is fever, with rigors on occasions and malaise, and there may be cyanosis.

The signs in the chest fall into four main groups.

'Acute wheezy chests' with bilateral rhonchi and rales represent the diffuse type of acute bronchitis or bronchopneumonia. It is impossible to differentiate between the two clinically except on severity of illness and on radiographic signs of patchy consolidation. The acute wheezy chest is the most frequent clinical type of acute chest infection, accounting in the United Kingdom for more than one-half of all cases.

Segmental pneumonia denotes a specific clinical syndrome with irritating cough and some mucopurulent sputum and only a minor or moderate degree of illness. Chest signs are those of a local area of inspiratory moist rales or crepitations usually at one or other base (of the lower lobes) or over the lingula or middle lobe. This type of acute chest infection is also very frequent and accounts for up to 40 per cent of all cases.

Amongst the remaining 10 per cent of cases there are lobar pneumonias with a more severe illness and clinical signs of consolidation, the empyemata and other effusions which are now rather uncommon, acute pleurisy with a pleural rub as the only abnormal sign and others which may be variants of all the types or which may yield no abnormal physical signs although there is radiological evidence of infection.

Clinical evidence of a high carbon dioxide retention (more than PCo_2 of 49–50 mm Hg) is hypercirculation with hot hands and a bounding pulse, congested retinal veins, and papilloedema on occaions, mental confusion and drowsiness and tremor of the hands.

Cor pulmonale (right heart failure) may be recognised by a raised jugular venous pressure, enlargement of the liver, oedema of the legs and sacral pad and an accentuation of the second pulmonary heart sound.

Investigations must include a chest radiograph, bacteriological and possibly virological examination of the sputum, haemoglobin, E.S.R., and white blood cell count and possibly levels of PCo_2 and $P.O_2$. An electrocardiograph may also be useful.

Management

There are four parts to the management of acute chest infections.

1. Control of infection
2. Clearing airways obstruction
3. Management of respiratory failure
4. Management of heart failure.

1. *Infection*

Treatment should be started at once in most cases without waiting for the result of the bacteriological identification of the causal organism, which is only possible in less than one-half of all cases.

The antibiotics most suitable are either intramuscular penicillin 1 mega unit 8–12 hourly, oral ampicillin 0·25–0·5 g. 6-hourly or oxytetracycline 0·25–0·5 g. 6-hourly. One of these preparations should be started and the progress reviewed. If there is no improvement within 36–48 hours, or if the report on the sputum suggests resistant organisms then other antibiotics should be considered.

2. *Airways Obstruction*

It is the 'acute wheezy chest' that presents the greatest problem with a mixture of bronchospasm, oedema and mucus obstruction. Aminophylline by intravenous injection (0·25 g.) or by suppository; corticosteroids by intravenous injection of hydrocortisone (100 mg) or by oral prednisone, up to 60–80 mg daily to start with; or various antispasmodics such as ephedrine (30 mg) or orciprenaline (20 mg) – 4-hourly – all these may be tried, but often without much success.

3. *Respiratory Failure*

In respiratory failure carbon-dioxide retention occurs and the respiratory centre becomes less sensitive to the stimulus of the circulating levels of oxygen and carbon dioxide.

Whilst oxygen is essential for respiratory failure it must not be given continuously or in too high a concentration too quickly, because this may lead to even greater hypercapnia.

When the respirations are weak and there is difficulty in expectoration then aspiration and sucking out of bronchial secretions through a bronchoscope may be necessary and in more severe cases a temporary tracheostomy or intubation and mechanical ventilation may be indicated.

4. *Cor Pulmonale*

When present treatment should be by digitalisation and diuretics.

ASTHMA

It is difficult to separate 'asthma' from the other types of 'acute wheezy chests'. It is true, as Chevalier Jackson remarked many years ago, that 'not all that wheezes is asthma'.

In looking at 'acute wheezy chests', we find that age-prevalence is a U-shaped curve with greatest involvement of the young and elderly.

The syndrome of the acute wheezy chest includes three definable and separable types – wheezy children, acute episodes in chronic bronchitis and emphysema and asthma.

Acute wheezing in the chest affects no less than one child in every four in their first decade (Fry, J. 'The Catarrhal Child', 1962, London).

The great majority (95 per cent) cease these attacks, which are a response of a sensitive and immature respiratory tract to infection, as they grow older and fewer than 5 per cent become true asthmatics.

Acute exacerbations of chronic bronchitis are characterised by wheezing in the chest and dyspnoea and have to be distinguished from asthma.

Excluding these two large groups of chest wheezers there is asthma which may be defined as 'paroxysmal attacks of acute airways obstruction unassociated with any underlying pulmonary disease'.

Asthma

The annual incidence in my own practice over 20 years has been 2 per 1,000, which means that in a country such as the United Kingdom there are 1 million asthmatics (or 2 per cent of the population).

The annual mortality from 'asthma' in the United Kingdom is 2,000 but this may include a number of non-asthmatic chronic bronchitics. Over the past five years there has been a sudden and unexpected increase in deaths of young asthmatics and it is believed that these have been iatrogenic as the result of over-treatment with the newer aerosol sprays of isoprenaline and similar antispasmodics.

It is customary to divide asthma into extrinsic (allergic) and intrinsic (non-allergic) types. The allergic type tends to start in early childhood and the non-allergic in adult life. Asthma is a genetic condition and in one-quarter of the cases there is a near relative with asthma.

The natural history of asthma shows a strong tendency to spontaneous improvement, particularly in those whose attacks begin in childhood. In a long-term follow-up of asthmatics in my own practice I found that only 15 per cent were disabled after 20 years.

Effects of Asthma

An attack of asthma is produced by an acute airways obstruction due to a combination of spasm of the bronchiolar muscles, oedema of the bronchial and bronchiolar mucosa and excessive production of sticky mucus which causes plugging of the smaller bronchioles with some alveolar collapse.

This results in difficulty in breathing with consequent anoxaemia and hypercapnia and acidosis and respiratory failure – if the condition continues in a severe form.

Clinical Presentation

There is almost always a history of previous attacks.

The patient is breathless, sitting up, with the accessory muscles of respiration being used and there is expiratory wheezing to be heard in the chest. The severity of attack varies from a minor inconvenience on effort or associated with some other trigger-factor to very severe distress, breathlessness, cyanosis, shock and even sudden death.

Signs of danger the indicate the need for urgent and intensive care are:

1. Increasing restlessness and confusion indicating cerebral anoxia.
2. Increasing breathlessness with decreasing wheeze suggesting more complete obstruction of the airways.
3. Decreasing expectoration with retention of bronchial secretions and further increase of obstruction and collapse of alveoli.
4. Increasing pulse rate and evidence of right heart failure with cyanosis, gallop rhythm, raised jugular venous pressure and E.C.G. features of cor pulmonale.
5. Exhaustion and peripheral circulatory failure.

Diagnosis

Conditions to be considered in differential diagnosis are acute left ventricular failure, acute wheezy chests associated with an exacerbation of chronic bronchitis and spontaneous pneumothorax. In relation to the latter it should be remembered that pneumothorax may sometimes complicate an acute attack of asthma and may be the reason for a sudden and serious deterioration of the patient's condition. Likewise, acute left ventricular failure may occur in patients with a previous history of asthma.

Investigations

In an acute asthmatic attack there is no need to await investigations before commencing treatment. A chest radiograph is useful to exclude any local lesions and in particular pneumothorax. Radiological features in asthma are over-inflation of the lungs, and patchy collapse.

If the attack follows an acute respiratory infection and the sputum is purulent than bacteriological examination for antibiotic sensitivity is useful, but should not delay antibiotic therapy.

In prolonged attacks knowledge of the blood levels of Po_2 and PCo_2 is necessary to control therapy.

Management

Many chronic asthmatics have become able to abort and control their acute attacks with a variety of preparations such as adrenaline and isoprenaline inhalers and antispasmodics such as ephedrine.

The physician is only called in to help these chronic asthmatics when the attack is particularly severe or when there is no response to their usual measures.

The physician on seeing the patient in an acute attack has to make an assessment of severity, based on duration of the attack, the general state of the patient, including the pulse rate, degree of dyspnoea and cyanosis and the nature of previous attacks.

On this assessment a decision has to be made whether the patient is to be treated at home or admitted to hospital. Whatever the decision, and each situation has to be managed individually, the following are the most useful measures.

1. *Reassurance and Confidence*
Although the role of emotions in an acute asthmatic attack are secondary to the physical effects, a vicious circle is created if the victim is tense, anxious, unsure and afraid. A part of successful management is the instillation of confidence and assurance by the physician.

2. *Bronchodilators*
Bronchospasm is only one reason for the acute airways obstruction and hence oral and inhalant bronchodilators are not always successful once the attack has persisted for more than an hour or so. They are helpful however in aborting some attacks and in long-term management.

A dangerous situation arises when there is no response and the patient is tempted to increase the number of ephedrine and similar tablets taken and to use more frequently his aerosol inhalers of isoprenaline. The over-use of such preparations may lead to dangerous levels in the body and cause death from acute heart failure.

If there has been no response to the patient's usual preparations after an hour then intravenous aminophylline (0·25–0·5 g.) should be given slowly, or alternatively a subcutaneous injection of adrenaline (0·5– 1·0 ml of 1 in 1,000 solution) may be used.

3. *Oxygen*
Oxygen is essential in all severe attacks and can be given in high concentration, providing there is no history of chronic airways obstruction with a raised arterial PCo_2 when a lower oxygen concentration should be given.

4. *Steroids*
Corticosteroids should be given early in a severe attack of asthma. They are safe preparations given intermittently and in large doses for short periods.

They are best used in high dosage for a few days followed by a gradual reduction over 2–3 weeks.

In a severe attack an initial injection of 100 mg of hydrocortisone hemisuccinate should be given followed by 80 mg of oral prednisone daily for 2–3 days and then reduction by 5–10 mg daily providing that satisfactory improvement occurs.

5. *Antibiotics*
Respiratory infection is a frequent precipitating cause of an attack and broad-spectrum antibiotics such as oxytetracycline (0·25–0·5 g. 6-hourly or ampicillin 0·25–0·5 g. 6-hourly) should be given whenever infection is suspected or the sputum is purulent.

6. *Sedation*
In the past asthmatics were over-sedated. Asthmatics are anxious because they cannot breathe. Once they have responded to treatment they become less anxious. Sedatives are not an important part of treatment. If one is considered necessary, then chlorpromazine 50 mg intramuscularly can be given, and repeated, or administered orally every 6–8 hours.

7. *Expectorants*
There are no reliable expectorants or mucolytics. Dehydration is one cause of increasing viscosity and intravenous therapy should not be delayed, if clinical dehydration is present.

8. *Mechanical Ventilation and Bronchial Lavage*
When the attack fails to respond to the above regime and there is danger to life because of respiratory and circulatory failure then the possibility of assisted mechanical ventilation, aspiration of the bronchi and even bronchial lavage must be considered urgently, but provided at a special centre.

9. *After Care*
Successful management of an acute attack must be followed by long-term supervision of the patient in order to try and prevent further attacks.

SPONTANEOUS PNEUMOTHORAX

Spontaneous pneumothorax is not uncommon, with an annual incidence of approximately 1 per 5,000, implying that a primary physician may see a new case every two years.

It is a condition of young adults, apparently in good health and in the great majority it is not associated with any underlying primary disease. It is often recurrent and this suggests some local structural defect of lung or pleura.

The condition is believed to be due to small sub-pleural bullae which rupture, and when this happens air is sucked into the vacuum in the pleural space causing a collapse of the lung. The pleural defect generally seals itself off and the lung re-expands within a short time, depending on the size of the pneumothorax. Occasionally the pleural opening acts as a one-way valve allowing air out of the lung but not back again. This leads to a build-up of air under pressure in the pleural cavity with displacement of vital mediastinal structures producing circulatory and respiratory embarassment and failure.

Rarely the pneumothorax may be secondary to pulmonary diseases such as tuberculosis, primary or secondary neoplasms, asthma, or chronic bronchitis.

Clinical Presentation

The presentation generally is undramatic with a vague pain in the chest followed by some breathlessness. The pain may be sharp and pleuritic at first but soon becomes an ache. The degree of breathlessness depends on the extent of the pneumothorax and on the state of respiratory function.

Examination of the chest reveals hyper-resonance, diminished air-entry and, perhaps, shift of mediastinal contents away from the side of the chest that has a sustained pneumothorax.

The course in the majority of cases is towards gradual absorption of air within 2–4 weeks, but recurrence on the same side or on the opposite side is not uncommon.

Tension pneumothorax results in considerable breathlessness, distress and shock and urgent treatment is required.

The diagnosis is confirmed by chest radiography.

Management

In most cases no special intervention is necessary and unless there is appreciable dyspnoea the patient should be managed by close supervision with radiographic control until the lung re-expands. Tension pneumothorax, when it occurs, does so from the start and is not a later complication.

There is no need to admit these patients to hospital unless there is some complication or primary disease that requires special investigation.

If there is increasing breathlessness or other evidence of tension pneumothorax then it is necessary to release air from the pleural cavity. This is carried out by inserting a wide bore needle or intra-pleural catheter through the second or third anterior intercostal spaces or the fourth intercostal space in the axilla.

Recurrent attacks may require pleurectomy or other surgical measures to seal the pleural defect and to obliterate the inter-pleural space.

ACUTE THROAT INFECTIONS

Acute throat infections are common in any community. The annual prevalence is between 30–40 per 1,000. They are chiefly conditions of children and young adults.

Aetiologically, in approximately one-half of cases a pathogenic organism will be isolated from a throat swab. Thus in 46 per cent Streptococcus pyogenes will be grown and in 3 per cent a variety of organisms such as Vincent's organisms (B. fusiformis and S. vincenti) and Candida albicans but in 50 per cent no bacteria are isolated and it is assumed that the cause is a virus. Diphtheria is now an extremely rare cause of an acute throat infection but must always be borne in mind as a possibility, particularly in patients in developing countries.

Acute throat infections may also be the presenting feature of blood disorders such as glandular fever (infectious mononucleosis), leukaemia or agranulocytosis.

Clinical Presentation

Sore throat, fever and malaise are the presenting features.

There is tonsillar swelling, if the tonsils are present, with a follicular, gelatinous or membranous exudate. It is quite impossible to make an accurate aetological diagnosis from the appearance of the fauces because the appearance is similar, irrespective of the cause. The condition is not usually confined to the tonsils and the adjacent pharynx and soft palate are generally red and swollen. A punctate erythema of the soft palate sometimes occurs in glandular fever. A solitary dirty ulcer in one tonsil with foul breath is suggestive of an infection with Vincent's organisms.

The degree of general disturbance is variable, ranging from sudden onset of high fever and prostration to a sore throat that is only an inconvenience in one's daily routine.

Cervical glands are usually tender and palpable With streptococcal infections, glandular fever and some viral infections, skin rashes may occur. These are a diffuse scarlatiniform erythema with streptococci, blotchy pink macules over the neck and trunk in glandular fever and a more generalised confluent rash in viral infections.

Diagnosis

A throat swab should be examined for causal organisms in all cases that do not resolve quickly and a differential white blood cell count and a Paul-Bunnell test to exclude glandular fever or other blood conditions.

Course

The natural course is for the condition to clear over 4–7 days. Complications are unusual and consist of peritonsillar infection (quinsy). Acute nephritis and rheumatic fever are, nowadays, rare complications of streptococcal infections. Recurrences are frequent.

Management

One-half of all acute throat infections are caused by viruses which do not respond to antibiotics. The results of a bacteriological examination take 1–2 days. Antibiotics may be prescribed for all but the mildest cases in the knowledge that in some they will be ineffective, or they can be withheld for 48 hours to see if natural resolution will occur.

Penicillin is the most effective antibiotic and in my opinion, should be given intramuscularly, 1 mega unit twice daily for 48 hours followed by oral penicillin 0·25 g. 6-hourly for a further 4–5 days. Improvement should occur within 2–3 days. If this has not occurred then bacteriological investigations and blood tests (white cell differential count and Paul-Bunnell test) should be carried out.

Glandular fever is a condition of adolescents and young adults with the main age-prevalence in the teens (13–20). It presents as a sore throat, enlarged cervical glands and fever. These persist in spite of treatment with penicillin. The acute phase lasts 1–3 weeks often followed by weakness and malaise for some months.

It is diagnosed by a mononucleosis and a positive Paul-Bunnell test.

The cause is unknown and the condition does not respond to antibiotics. In severe cases with considerable local and systemic disturbance corticosteroids (prednisone 50 mg each day for 3 days and then a daily reduction by 5 mg), may have dramatic beneficial effects.

ACUTE LARYNGEAL DYSPNOEA

The causes of acute laryngeal obstruction are:

1. Acute laryngo-tracheo-bronchitis (croup)
2. Acute epiglottitis
3. Diphtheria
4. Angioneurotic oedema
5. Foreign body or other laryngeal irritants
6. Acute retropharyngeal abscess
7. Papillomata of the larynx.

Acute laryngo-tracheo-bronchitis (Croup)

This is a frequent condition in young children (6 months–3 years). Most cases are associated with a viral upper respiratory infection but the same syndrome may be caused by such bacteria as haemophilus influenzae, streptococci and pneumococci.

The onset often is sudden and in the middle of the night. The child awakens with a dry, irritating, barking and seal-like cough with hoarseness and an inspiratory crowing and breathlessness.

The child is frightened and is usually sitting up in bed or on the parent's lap with the accessory muscles of respiration being used. In severe cases cyanosis is present and sudden death may occur.

Fortunately most cases are not severe and will settle with simple measures such as warm moist air – a steam kettle is an excellent improvisation at home – and oxygen, if available.

Severe cases with considerable respiratory distress, restlessness and cyanosis should be admitted to hospital speedily with oxygen and medical supervision during transport.

Tracheostomy may be a life-saving measure and should not be over-delayed. Alternatively endotracheal intubation may be attempted.

The question of antibiotics is a difficult one because many cases are caused by viruses. To start with, until bacteriological investigations are available, a mixture of intramuscular penicillin and streptomycin is reasonable.

Acute Epiglottitis

This is a condition of young children caused by viruses. Since the inflammation is above the larynx there is no hoarseness or stridor. The main feature is an obstructive dyspnoea.

The appearance of the fauces is characteristic – on depressing the tongue the epiglottis is seen as a red cherry-like swelling behind the tongue.

The condition is a serious one with an appreciable mortality and the child must be admitted to a hospital able to deal with the management of this form of respiratory obstruction quickly by intubation or tracheostomy, supported by antibiotics.

Laryngeal Diphtheria

This is now a rare condition but should be considered in all cases of laryngeal dyspnoea. A membrane may not be seen and the child may have a history of immunisation.

If there is any suspicion of diphtheria an immediate intramuscular injection of 24,000–48,000 units of diphtheria antitoxin should be given pending the results of throat swabs.

Angioneurotic Oedema

Laryngeal obstruction in angioneurotic oedema is accompanied usually by other features such as swelling of the face and generalised urticaria.

Treatment is with subcutaneous injections of adrenaline (0·5 ml of 1/1,000 solution) repeated in 5 minutes if no improvement has occurred.

INFLUENZA EPIDEMICS

The impact of an influenza epidemic is considerable on all local medical services and emergency actions are required to cope with the rush of patients who require treatment for the primary infection and its complications.

Influenza or the 'flu' is massive and unpredictable. The 2- or 3-yearly epidemics are unexpected and disorganising, but the pandemics that seem to occur once every 10–20 years are disastrous, not only in toll of life but in their economic effect on the community as well.

The influenza viruses belong to the myxovirus group. There are three types, A, B and C. Each type is antigenically distinct and there is no cross immunity.

Influenza A causes the most serious epidemics and pandemics.

Influenza B is responsible for milder but local epidemics.

Influenza C has been blamed for only minor epidemics in closed communities.

The extent and severity of an epidemic of influenza depend on the virulence of the organisms and the prevailing state of mass immunity.

The most severe epidemics occur when a new mutant strain of influenza virus develops and gains a foothold on an unprotected population.

The effects of the influenza viruses are on the respiratory tract causing damage to the mucosa and making a secondary bacterial infection likely. The clinical features are those of an acute respiratory infection and complications tend to be limited to the lungs.

An epidemic lasts some 6–8 weeks. Starting insidiously with a few sporadic cases. By the end of the second week, with a build-up of cases, it becomes obvious that an epidemic is on. As a rule school children tend to be the first to be affected, then their families and the elderly are affected only in the later stages or may escape altogether.

The peak of the epidemic is reached after 3–4 weeks and is followed by a gradual decline in the number of cases over the following month.

Clinical Features

The onset is sudden, often the victim is able to record it to the minute. Intense malaise with aching limbs, back, head and eyes predominates. Coughing, sore throat and nasal discharge denote involvement of the respiratory tract. Additional symptoms may be present, such as vomiting, diarrhoea and abdominal pain, but these are not necessarily evidence of viral involvement of the gastro-intestinal tract but more likely to be general non-specific reactions to an acute infection.

The course of an uncomplicated attack is for a slow improvement over 4–5 days followed by a period of weakness and depression.

Complications

The case fatality of influenza overall is less than one per 1,000. Complications are almost confined to the respiratory tract and consist of pneumonia, acute bronchitis, otitis media or sinusitis.

Over nine influenza epidemics during the past 20 years (1950–1970) the rate of chest complications in my own practice has been 11 per cent. These complications principally affected young children and old persons and the chronic bronchitic and cardiac cripples.

Management

There is no specific treatment of the acute attack. It is best treated with bed rest, fluids, analgesics and a linctus that relieves the irritating cough.

Vulnerable groups such as those with a history of chronic bronchitis or other chronic chest conditions or those with cardiac failure should be given broad-spectrum antibiotics such as ampicillin or oxytetracycline prophylactically (0·25 g. 6-hourly) during an attack.

Chest complications should be treated with these broad-spectrum antibiotics and if there is no improvement within 48 hours then the sputum should be tested for possible resistant bacteria.

Prevention: Influenza vaccines are available but it is difficult quickly to prepare the vaccine appropriate to the strain and type of influenza virus causing the epidemic. There are no influenza vaccines that will protect against all types of infection because of the changing antigenic strains of the viruses. The beneficial effects of any vaccine will last for only 2–3 years.

The best approach is to prepare as quickly as possible a vaccine suitable against the type of virus causing the epidemic, and once available, use it selectively for certain vulnerable individuals such as chronic chest and cardiac cases and for key workers such as physicians, nurses, hospital and ambulance workers and others particularly exposed to the infection.

ACUTE OTITIS MEDIA

Pain in the ear due to an acute otitis media is a common emergency in practice.

Acute otitis media is now quite a different condition from that of twenty years ago. With the availability of antibiotics and because of the lower virulence of causal organisms it has now lost the earlier terrors of mastoiditis and even death. Yet, in spite of the success of antibiotics in controlling the acute infection, many problems remain. Slow resolution and persistent and sometimes permanent deafness are dangers which have to be controlled, and avoided.

Frequency

Acute otitis media is now chiefly a condition of children although attacks do occur in adults, particularly recurrent attacks in already damaged ears. No fewer than one-third of all children in the United Kingdom suffer one or more attacks of acute otitis media during their first ten years. In any year a physician with a population of 2,500 to care for may expect to treat 50–60 children with attacks of acute otitis media.

The age distribution is characteristic of all forms of respiratory infection in childhood, namely, a rising prevalence from the age of 2, a peak between 4 and 8, and then a rapid decline which continues in adult life. This pattern is explained by the time at which children are most exposed to cross infection, that is when they start to mix with other children and begin to attend school. It seems that after 2 or 3 years the child builds up a natural resistance to infections which then become less severe and less frequent.

Clinical Pathology

Acute otitis media is part of the catarrhal child syndrome, namely, recurrent coughs, colds, sore throats, wheezy chests and ear infections.

Infection of the middle ear is secondary to an upper respiratory infection, which is often viral. The ear infection, however, is caused usually by pneumococci, streptococci, haemophilus influenzae and staphylococci bacteria. This secondary infection reaches the middle ear along the eustachian tubes which become obstructed by inflammatory swelling or pressure by enlarged adenoids. Infection with an obstructed eustachian tube leads to accumulation of muco-pus in the closed middle ear space with interference with movement of the ossicles and swelling and inflammation of the drum.

The symptoms related to these changes are pain due to inflammation, deafness from accumulation of fluid, and some discharge from a perforation of the drum.

Complications such as mastoiditis, brain abscess and chronic otitis media are rare now but deafness may occur due to the persistence of thick mucus in the middle ear (serious deafness or 'glue ear').

Clinical Presentation

The painful red drum is the most usual type. Nine out of ten cases present in this way. The child is unhappy and feverish. The older child is able to localise the trouble and complain of earache but in younger children and infants the presentation may be that of high fever and malaise. Examination of the ears, imperative in all sick children, reveals a red drum, sometimes bilaterally.

The discharging ear may on occasions be the first symptom in a disturbed child (in 10 per cent of cases), but more often any discharge, when present, follows earache.

Deafness to some degree occurs in all attacks.

Course

In the typical case the acute phase with pain and fever persists for 3–4 days and then proceeds to a natural resolution. This tendency to natural resolution should be recalled since it is likely that even without antibiotics most ears would resolve. Although the pain and fever soon settle the appearance of the drum may not return to normal for 1–4 weeks and with redness and swelling of the drum deafness is present. Discharge generally settles within 2–3 weeks, but there are a few cases in which it continues in spite of antibiotics.

Recurrent attacks are frequent and two-thirds of children with otitis media suffer more than one attack.

The final outcome is related to social factors as well as clinical severity. Thus, the outlook is worse in lower social groups, in larger families (of any class) – the more children making cross infection more likely – and where there is a family history of ear disease or deafness.

Management

1. *Antibiotics*

Although it is so easy and cheap now to prescribe oral antibiotics it is salutary that I use them in less than one-half of all attacks, with good results. My indications for antibiotics are the severity of pain and fever, presence of discharge, recurrences and where there has been no improvement within 2–3 days of onset.

Penicillin is still the most satisfactory antibiotic, either by intramuscular injection or by mouth.

2. *Myringotomy (or Aspiration)*

Myringotomy or aspiration of mucus from the middle ear is now reserved for those cases in which there is persistent deafness after some weeks and where the cause is considered to be a 'glue ear'.

3. *Adenoidectomy*

This is a useful procedure with recurrent attacks where it is considered that the enlarged adenoids obstruct the eustachian tube.

4. *Follow Up*

An essential part of management must be careful and continuing follow-up of all cases until the drum and hearing have returned to normal. Ideally all children old enough to cooperate should have a pure-tone audiogram carried out 3–6 months after the attack.

COMMON EMERGENCIES IN CHILDREN

The three most frequent emergencies in children are acute chest infections, diarrhoea and vomiting, and dehydration and convulsions.

The approach to these must be systematic and the first step is an accurate diagnosis followed by appropriate therapeutic measures. Not only has the child to be treated but the parents have to be managed and it is important to develop good rapport and communication with them and explain in understandable terms the situation and the steps being taken.

Acute Chest Infections

These have been referred to already in general terms.

Acute chest infections are frequent in early childhood with the peak prevalence between 4 and 8 years of age.

The 'acute wheezy chest' is the most common type and it is an acute diffuse bronchitis with airways obstruction. It is not the forerunner of asthma in later life.

Segmental pneumonia, presenting as cough, and variable malaise and fever with a local area of inspiratory rales at one or other base, is the next most frequent type.

A less common but important type is acute bronchiolitis of infants. Most cases are caused by the respiratory syncytial virus but other viruses and bacteria can produce the same condition. The infection affects the smaller bronchioles which become obstructed with secretions and inflammatory oedema.

Following an upper respiratory infection there is a fairly sudden onset of breathlessness with a frequent spasmodic cough. There is difficulty in both inspiration and expiration with indrawing of the lower chest wall. The child becomes restless and agitated and grey.

There are many scattered rales and rhonchi in the chest and the radiograph shows hypertranslucency and depression of the diaphragm with no consolidation and little collapse.

The management of these cases is based on antibiotics, treatment of respiratory distress and failure, and general care.

Although many of the infections are caused by viruses and are insensitive to antibiotics, it is impossible to differentiate these cases and it is safer to prescribe one of the broad-spectrum antibiotics such as ampicillin or oxytetracycline.

Humidified oxygen is necessary when there is respiratory distress and if the condition continues to deteriorate then bronchoscopic suction or even tracheostomy with mechanical respiration or bronchial aspiration must be considered as life-saving procedures.

Although less of an influence than in the past, good skilled nursing makes a great contribution to the care of the really sick child.

Gastro-enteritis and Dehydration

Diarrhoea and vomiting is second only to acute respiratory infections as the most frequent condition in children.

Caused by a variety of organisms and irritants most cases will settle quickly by withholding food, but not fluids, for 12–24 hours. It is not necessary to give antibiotics because only a small number are caused by sensitive bacteria.

In management, care has to be taken to distinguish in these children the presenting symptoms from a possible 'acute abdomen' or secondary to infection elsewhere, such as acute throat or chest infections.

Dehydration is suggested by anxiety, restlessness, throat and dry tongue, weight loss and oliguria requires hospitalisation and fluid replacement under biochemical control.

Convulsions

There are many causes of convulsions in childhood but the commonest are the 'febrile convulsion' and epilepsy.

The febrile convulsion occurs in an apparently normal child at the height of some acute infection with high fever. Rare before six months and after three years, it often recurs in the same child in subsequent fevers and there is frequently a family history of similar episodes.

The convulsions are usually generalised tonic and clonic seizures. Usually the fit is solitary and of short duration. Attacks which continue to recur or last for more than ½–1 hour raise more serious possibilities, such as meningo-encephalitis.

In most cases no special treatment is necessary because the convulsion does not last very long. More important than treating the convulsion is the establishment of an accurate causal diagnosis.

Continuing convulsions require attention to maintaining a free airway and administration of anticonvulsants such as paraldehyde (1 ml per 7 Kg of body weight) or sodium phenobarbitone (60 mg at 6–12 months and 120 mg at 2–3 years), intramuscularly.

Repeated bouts require further investigations to consider the possibilities of epilepsy, intracranial lesions or metabolic disturbances.

ANAPHYLAXIS, URTICARIA AND ANGIONEUROTIC OEDEMA

Three forms of allergic reactions are anaphylactic shock, angioneurotic oedema and urticaria.

Anaphylactic shock is a violent systemic reaction to foreign proteins and other substances to which the patient has become previously sensitised. Injections of serum, vaccines, especially those grown in chick embryos, and penicillin are the most frequent causes.

The reaction may be immediate or delayed depending on the dose of allergen and the route of administration.

The patient complains of feeling unwell with pallor, vomiting, tightness in the chest, abdominal pain and a feeling of impending doom. The blood pressure falls, the pulse becomes rapid and thready with a shock-like state. Cardiac arrest may occur or the patient may become comatose. Death may occur.

Obviously before potentially dangerous drugs which may cause anaphylactic shock are given the patient must be questioned as to any previous reactions.

Once the reaction occurs the patient should be laid down. Adrenaline 0·5 ml of 1/1,000 solution should be injected intramuscularly at once and repeated in 5–10 minutes if no response. Oxygen should be administered. If there is no response in 5–10 minutes an intravenous injection of hydrocortisone hemisuccinate 100 mg should be given. When bronchospasm is marked and persistent in spite of adrenaline and hydrocortisone administration, then aminophylline (0·25 g.) should be given intravenously.

With cardiac arrest, mouth to mouth breathing and external cardiac massage should be applied.

Angioneurotic oedema occurs in sensitive individuals as a result of ingesting a food to which the victim has been sensitised. There is swelling of the lips, tongue, eyelids and face and there may be generalised urticaria as well.

The swelling may involve the perilaryngeal tissues and cause an acute respiratory obstruction.

Adrenaline should be injected immediately (0·5 ml intramuscularly) and repeated in 5–10 minutes if no response. Hydrocortisone hemisuccinate (100 mg) may be given intravenously and if successful prednisone should be continued by mouth in reducing dose from 50 mg per day.

If there is severe laryngeal obstruction then intubation or tracheostomy may be required urgently.

Urticaria of the skin is a common condition, but its cause is often undetermined. Most frequent in children it tends to recur.

As it does not usually last for more than a few days, symptomatic measures are all that are required. Where there is considerable distress antihistamines or corticosteroids may be given. Chronic urticaria is a very troublesome condition which may persist for years and which, in the main responds poorly to most of the standard forms of treatment.

Dr. Lascelles' article is a guide to the most important laboratory tests at present available and to the significance of abnormal results. Many of these tests are now standard practice in hospitals and a knowledge of them is becoming increasingly important to the practising doctor.

Current Trends in Laboratory Investigations

by

P. T. Lascelles

Consultant Chemical Pathologist, The National Hospital, London

Introduction

The vastly increased use of the hospital laboratory particularly in the biochemical investigation of patients, has led to a radical reorganisation of the chemical pathology services. Automation of analytical techniques and of data handling have become essential to deal with the work load and to increase efficiency and accuracy in the larger laboratories [1]. Moreover, the ability to perform a large number of tests on one sample of blood collected from every patient has led to a re-evaluation of the normal range of constituents in plasma and blood and correlations have been made with variations in age and sex [2]. Race, diet, time of day as well as method by which the sample is taken and analysed must also now be considered in evaluating the normal range. Recent surveys have confirmed earlier observations on the type of distribution of commonly assayed constituents in normal subjects [3].

Newer techniques particularly Radio-immuno-assay and saturation analysis have been increasingly applied to the routine investigation of patients and more sophisticated laboratory equipment has enabled greater use to be made of the highly sensitive and specific fluorometric methods of analysis particularly in the investigation of disorders of the adrenal cortex and medulla [4].

It has been known for a long time that extracellular fluid including plasma is chemically highly unrepresentative of body fluid as a whole, and recently more attention has been focused on 'Intracellular Chemical Pathology' [5]. Most important in this respect are assays of tissue enzyme levels whether quantitatvately in red cells (e.g. glucose-6-phosphate dehydrogenase) and in white cells (e.g. alkaline phosphatase) or semiquantitavely by histochemical techniques in muscle biopsy material (e.g. enzymes of the anaerobic glycolytic cycle in suspected cases of muscle glycogen storage disease). Moreover, reports of specific enzyme deficiencies in hereditary diseases, including those in which mental retardation is part of the syndrome continue to grow. (For a comprehensive review see 'Clinical Pathology in Mental Retardation', by Eastham and Jancar.) [6]

LABORATORY TESTS OF ENDOCRINE FUNCTION

THE THYROID GLAND

The Protein Bound Iodine (PBI) remains a widely used and extremely useful test for the diagnosis of both thyrotoxicosis and hypothyroidism, representing in about 90 per cent cases an estimate of total hormone bound to protein in the peripheral blood. Automation of the assay has solved some of the problems of sample contamination in the laboratory and Butanol Extractable Iodine (BEI) differentiates the PBI from contamination by inorganic iodide. Unfortunately organic iodide which includes that used in contrast radiography of the gall bladder, kidney and bronchial tree, still causes prolonged interference, for months, and in some instances for greater than 20 years.

PBI results must be interpreted with care in patients on replacement therapy with Triiodothyronine (T3) or Thyroxine (T4) as the PBI reflects the total T4 level while metabolic activity is dependant on free thyroid hormone which is markedly influenced by T3. A change in the T3/T4 ratio can therefore lead to confusion.

A further complication is that a change in concentration of thyroid binding globulin (TBG) influences the PBI. This can be caused by many currently used drugs and hormonal preparations. ^{131}I-Triiodothyronine Resin uptake (^{131}I-T3 Resin Test) is a useful screening test for assessing thyroid function. It is probably of less value for assessing hypothyroidism than hyperthyroidism but even in the latter false negatives are not infrequent. Accurate assessment of thyroidal status depends on normal T3:T4 ratio; thus invalid results may be obtained with patients on Triiodothyronine therapy. Moreover, many conditions affecting the plasma proteins (and therefore TBG) including liver disease, and the nephrotic syndrome interfere with this test. Drugs including hormonal preparations also interfere by competing for binding sites with TBG. However, most iodine containing compounds except sodium Ipodate (ORAGRAFIN) do not interfere and the ^{131}I-T3 test may be helpful in a situation where the PBI is valueless. Better diagnostic discrimination is now thought to be given by the ^{131}I-T3 test than by the ^{131}I-T4 test.

Free Thyroxine Index, can be calculated in relative terms from the PBI and ^{131}I-T3 Resin values, by a number of equations of varying complexity [7]. This parameter of thyroid activity may be used in situations where there is no contamination with iodine but where there is a change in TBG level, and is a particularly useful thyroid function test in pregnancy, or for women on oral contraceptives.

Thyroid Stimulating Hormone Test (TSH Stimulation Test) [8]
The thyroidal uptake of ^{132}I is measured before and after a single intramuscular injection of TSH, though if there is a subnormal response repeated injections may be necessary. This test is mainly of value in diagnosing early hypothyroidism, for confirming the diagnosis of myxoedema after substitution therapy has been started and for differentiating primary hypothyroidism from that secondary to pituitary insufficiency.

Triiodothyronine Suppression Test (T3 Suppression Test) [8]
40 μgm T3 is given eight hourly for six days and the thyroid uptake of ^{132}I is measured before and afterwards. The main indications for this investigation are the diagnosis of early hyperthyroidism whether due to Grave's Disease or a toxic nodular goitre, the confirmation of thyrotoxicosis after treatment has commenced, and in the differential diagnosis of exophthalmos.

THE ADRENAL CORTEX

Urinary Unconjugated 11-Hydroxycorticosteroids
The diagnosis of early Cushing's syndrome and particularly its differentiation from simple obesity is still a difficult clinical problem. The most valuable biochemical criteria for establishing the diagnosis, namely the cortisol secretion rate and urinary cortisol excretion, are too elaborate for routine purposes, but it has been shown that the urinary 24-hour excretion of unconjugated 11-Hydroxycorticosteroids correlates well, over the required range, with cortisol secretion rate and that this assay can be adapted as a simple fluorometric assay for routine purposes. Further experience has confirmed that this test is much more satisfactory for the diagnosis of Cushing's syndrome than assay of urine 17-Hydroxycorticosteroids or 17 oxogenic steroids [9].

Single Dose Dexamethasone Suppression Test [10]

This varient of the Dexamethasone Suppression Test is a simple and reasonably reliable screening procedure for Cushing's syndrome. Dexamethazone is given orally in the late evening, and the following morning the plasma 11-Hydroxycorticosteroids are measured and compared with a base-line level taken the previous morning. Normal subjects show a fall of >70 per cent to a level of <6.5 μgm/100 ml while most patients with Cushing's syndrome fail to suppress significantly on this régime.

Connolly, however, has shown that some hospital patients not suffering from Cushing's syndrome do not suppress satisfactorily and that this test should be regarded only as a screening test particularly for outpatients [11].

Stimulation Test of the Adrenal Cortex

The standard adrenocorticotrophic hormone (ACTH) stimulation test has been used to differentiate primary atrophy of the adrenal cortex from that secondary to pituitary insufficiency and to assess adrenal cortical function after prolonged treatment with steroids. In 1965 the Synacthen test was introduced [12] and more recently reviewed [13]. Synacthen (CIBA) is a synthetic peptide and consequently there is less chance of allergic responses to its administration than with natural ACTH. The test requires only two venepunctures, the results can be obtained the same day and it may be adapted as an outpatient procedure, the rise in plasma 11-Hydroxycorticosteroids over a 30 minute period in response to a single intramuscular injection of 250 μgm Synacthen being measured.

THE PITUITARY GLAND

Anterior Pituitary

A large number of tests is now available for the assessment of pituitary function and reserve. A knowledge of the latter is essential when attempting to predict a patient's response to stressful situations such as anaesthesia, air encephalography or surgery. Radio-immuno-assay of peptide hormones particularly adrenocorticotrophic hormone and Growth hormone have helped enormously in this field, but a number of tests still rely on measuring the response of the adrenal cortex to stimuli applied to the hypothalamus and pituitary.

Plasma ACTH Assay

Homologous Radio-immuno-assay of plasma corticotrophin has been shown to be of practical value in elucidating the cause of Cushing's syndrome [14]. Patients with untreated Cushing's disease showed morning plasma levels of 40–200 $\mu\mu$gm/ml (normal range 12–60 $\mu\mu$gm/ml). Even higher levels were found in patients with adrenocortical hyperplasia associated with ectopic ACTH production. By contrast, plasma ACTH was undetectable in 5 patients with adrenal tumours (4 adenomas and 1 carcinoma). Further studies demonstrated the absence of circadian rhythm in all patients with Cushing's syndrome from any aetiology.

Plasma Growth Hormone Assay

Assays of plasma Growth hormone (and plasma cortisol) before, 20, 30, 60, 90 and 120 minutes after the intravenous injection of insulin have proved a valuable means of assessing hypothalamic and pituitary reserve function [15]. *Adequate precautions must be taken however when administering insulin to patients with suspected pituitary insufficiency.*

Abnormal responses were found in patients with hypopituitarism, anorexia nervosa, prolonged corticosteroid therapy, chromophobe adenoma and acromegaly. In the patient with acromegaly it was found that the high resting levels of Growth hormone were paradoxically decreased rather than increased in response to the production of an adequate hypoglycaemia. Moreover, the response to oral glucose load (resulting in a diabetic sugar curve) was a further increase of the high resting level rather than a fall.

Metopirone Test

The Metopirone test of pituitary reserve has now been available for a number of years during which several reports of its efficacy have appeared, one recent trial being reported by Metcalf et al [16]. Metopirone is a specific inhibitor of the adrenal 11-hydroxylating system in man and animals.

Experimental protocol has varied with different workers, but a satisfactory régime would be the administration orally of 0·75 g. Metopirone four hourly for 48 hours. Under these circumstances there is a significant decrease in plasma cortisol level resulting in stimulation of the pituitary to produce ACTH. This in turn stimulates the adrenal cortex to produce, on average in the normal, a sixfold increase of the immediate non-11-hydroxylated steroid precursors of cortisol in the urine.

These may be measured in several ways, usually as 17-oxogenic steroids or 17-Hydroxycorticosteroids. An impaired rise in urinary steroid excretion is found in patients with organic pituitary disease, with pituitary suppression secondary to steroid therapy and in association with the concurrent administration of tranquilizer drugs.

The disadvantages of this test are that it is time-consuming and unphysiological in that it necessitates the reduction in level of what may be an already low plasma cortisol. Thus it is not entirely without danger, particularly in children.

This test correlates well with the clinical status of patients but is relatively insensitive, some 80 per cent gland destruction being necessary before a definitely positive result is obtained. Quantitative evaluation of results is probably unwise.

Lysine-vasopressin Test

Following the demonstration that vasopressin stimulates the hypothalamo-pituitary-adrenal axis, synthetic Lysine-vasopressin was introduced as a test of pituitary function. It was originally thought that this compound acted at the level of the pituitary, being both a stimulator to the secretion of and releaser of ACTH [17]. Thus it was hoped to be able to differentiate by a battery of tests hypothalamic from pituitary insufficiency. Unfortunately more recent evidence is against the exact site of Lysine-vasopressin being at the level of the pituitary [18]. Moreover, there is conflicting evidence as to the value of Lysine-vasopressin in differentiating the pituitary origin of Cushing's syndrome from the other causes of adrenal hyperfunction [19, 20] and the current view is that from the practical point of view it does not add much to the information obtained from other tests [18].

The Pyrogen Test

In this test the response of plasma 11-Hydroxycorticosteroids to an intravenous dose of a bacterial pyrogen (ORGANON) is measured. A deficient response to this test is seen less often in patients with untreated pituitary tumours than with other 'stressful stimuli' including the metopirone test, hypoglycaemia and Lysine-vasopressin [18], and when present indicates a more severe impairment of corticotrophin production by the pituitary. The test is an unpleasant one for the patient but the symptoms may be amelierated by the administration of aspirin without interfering with the biochemical response and the results may be obtained quickly. Hydrocortisone must be available for intravenous administration in the rare event of circulatory collapse occurring.

Posterior Pituitary

The differentiation of Pituitary Diabetes Insipidus from psychogenic water drinking can still be a considerable problem due mainly to the variable responses which may be obtained to any particular test. Reliance may have to be placed on the response to long term vasopressin administration, patients with diabetes insipidus being improved while those with psychogenic water drinking are not, on account of the chronic manifestations of water intoxication.

Most tests now employed depend on osmolality measurements in plasma and urine and the responses to vasopressin and dehydration.

The saline infusion test however, has been re-evaluated [21] with attention directed to raising the plasma osmolality above the 'osmotic threshold for vasopressin release' and the measurement of free water clearance.

THE PARATHYROID GLANDS

In recent years a number of specialized tests for the early diagnosis of parathyroid disease have been described but none have been entirely satisfactory for routine use. They have included the infusion of calcium, phosphate, parathormone, radioactive strontium turnover studies and parathyroid scanning.

In practice reliance should still be placed on the *accurate* repeated measurement of serum and urine calcium and the assessment of renal phosphate handling [22].

With regard to the diagnosis of minimal hypoparathyroidism, particularly following thyroid surgery, reliance should still be placed on the Sodium Phytate Test [23] and not on the Trisodium Edetate Test which appears to be less satisfactory.[24].

LABORATORY TESTS OF CARBOHYDRATE METABOLISM

Glucose Tolerance Test

In recent years the concept of diabetes mellitus has been greatly widened in an attempt to elucidate the fundamental mechanisms underlying this condition in man. The Glucose Tolerance Test however, remains the essential diagnostic aid but there is now an increasing tendency to measure other parameters of carbohydrate metabolism simultaneously including Growth hormone, plasma insulin and non-esterified fatty acids.

Recently the normal limits of the standard oral glucose tolerance have been correlated with age, sex and race. Correlation was also made with response to glucose of insulin, cholesterol and glycerides [25, 26, 27].

Glycogen Storage Diseases

The number of glycogen storage diseases in which specific enzyme deficiencies have been described continues to grow. Although extremely rare, those presenting as muscle disorders in adolescence or adult life have attracted considerable attention in the literature and have recently been reviewed [28, 29].

Elaborate biochemical investigations are required to discover which enzyme of the anaerobic glycolytic cycle is deficient, but the ischaemic exercise lactate test is a useful screening procedure [30] in all these conditions, and if positive is an indication for further studies.

VITAMIN B GROUP DEFICIENCIES

The Pyruvate Metabolism Test [31]

The Pyruvate Metabolism Test is useful in the confirmation of suspected vitamin B_1 deficiency particularly in patients presenting with polyneuritis and a history of alcoholism or with Korsakow's syndrome. These show a rise in blood pyruvate after glucose which is corrected by vitamin B_1 therapy. It is essential that the test be carried out before the patient resumes a normal diet. Fallacious results may be obtained in patients with congestive cardiac failure and in diabetic patients.

Where there is no improvement following vitamin B_1 therapy, the patient may be suffering from heavy metal intoxication, pernicious anaemia or Wilson's disease. In the latter two situations, the pyruvate metabolism test reverts to normal after appropriate therapy.

Red Cell Folate Assay

Extracellular folic acid concentrations as represented by serum folate levels are now regarded as a poor index of total body folate stores. It is probable however, that there is a better correlation with red cell folate and that this will prove to be a better index of folate deficiency. Methodological problems still exist and it is difficult to compare the results in different series due to variations in technique. In one series [32] red cell folate activity correlated well with megaloblastic anaemia subsequently shown to respond to folate therapy, but was low in only 8 out of 29 other non-anaemic patients whose plasma folate was below 2·0 mμgm/ml.

In another investigation [33] whole blood folate activity (which reflects mainly red cell folate) was assessed as a screening test for coeliac disease in childhood. The results suggest that a normal whole blood folate value may be used with confidence to exclude the clinical diagnosis of coeliac disease in childhood.

Red Cell Transketolase Activity

Transketolase, which is a 'transferase' enzyme found in red and white cells but not in serum, catalyses a number of reactions in the pentose phosphate pathway. It has been shown to require thiamine pyrophosphate (TPP) as an essential co-factor.

Ribose-5-phosphate is used as substrate and incubated with a red cell haemolysate after which analysis is made for remaining pentose and formed hexose. When haemolysates from thiamine deficient subjects are employed, there is a decreased rate of conversion but more important, a marked increase of activity is obtained on adding thiamine pyrophosphate to the system (TPP effect). The TPP effect is regarded as a specific and sensitive index of thiamine deficiency.

METHYLMALONIC ACID EXCRETION

Vitamin B_{12} has been shown to be an essential co-enzyme for the conversion of methylmalonic acid to succinic acid. Methylmalonic acid is excreted in small amounts in normal urine, but is present in excess in vitamin B_{12} deficiency. A simplified method for its estimation in urine has been described and a test devised, after Valine loading, for the rapid diagnosis of vitamin B_{12} deficiency in anaemic patients [34].

Vitamin B_{12} Chromatography [35]

Methods for separation and quantitation of individual plasms cobalamins, by chromatography, bioautography, and photometric scanning, have recently been published, together with normal values. It is reported that the ratio between the two major components, methylcobalamin and deoxyadenosyl coenzyme B_{12}, shows a characteristic alteration in overt or incipient B_{12} deficiency, methylcobalamin being disproportionately reduced. Alterations in this ratio may also occur, in certain cases, in the presence of a normal total plasma B_{12} concentration. Cyanocobalamin is normally present only in traces. It is increased after oral or parenteral administration of cyanocobalamin, and in certain ophthalmological disorders, including some cases of tobacco amblyopia, Leber's optic atrophy, and dominantly inherited optic atrophy. The technique appears to have considerable diagnostic potential in the investigation of disorders of B_{12} metabolism.

Fat Absorption Test [36]

Penfold has described a test in which serum lipid levels are assayed following a standardised fatty meal as a test for steatorrhoea. Good separation was obtained between normal subjects and patients with malabsorption, by taking a rise of total serum lipids of 90 mg/100 ml as the lower limit of normal. This test avoids the inaccuracies of faecal collection and the results can be obtained in one day.

Pentagastrin Test Meal [37]

In a recent study, comparison has been made between the gastric response to pentagastrin, histamine and histalog. It was found that the short test using intramuscular Pentagastrin gave a reliable assessment of maximal acid secretory capacity. This procedure will probably be more acceptable to patients than the augmented histamine test meal and appears to be adequate, both for the diagnosis of achlorhydria and for discriminating between high and low secretions of gastric acid.

This survey of current trends in biochemical laboratory investigations is necessarily incomplete, but some attempt has been made to present the more important applications of recent research, which at the present time appear to be of genuine help in the management of patients.

The sections that follow contain, in addition to tables of normal values, practical details of the more commonly used tests of function, with short notes on their interpretation.

I am grateful to Dr. P. F. Mitchell-Heggs* for the section on Pulmonary Function Tests, and to Dr. D. M. Matthews for the section on Vitamin B_{12} Chromatography.

* Present address: The Brompton Hospital.

Table of Normal Laboratory Values of Clinical Importance—Chemistry

Range of normal values for blood

Investigation	Specimen	Normal Range	Notes
Aldolase	Serum	1·5–6·8 I.U./L.	
α Amino-nitrogen	Plasma	3·5–7.0 mg/100 ml	
Amylase	Serum	< 4,000 I.U./L.	
Base excess	Serum	−2·3 to + 2·3 mEq/L.	
Bicarbonate (alkali reserve)	Plasma	24–32 mEq/L.	Collect under paraffin
Standard bicarbonate	Plasma	22·4–25.8 mEq/L.	
Bilirubin	Serum	0·1–0·5 mg/100 ml	
Caeruloplasmin	Serum	23–44 mg/100 ml	
Calcium	Serum	4·5–5·5 mEq/L. (9–11 mg/100 ml)	
pCo_2	Whole blood	34–45 mm Hg.	Arterial blood
Chloride	Serum	97–107 mEq/L.	
Copper	Serum	85–110 μg/100 ml	
Creatine	Serum	0·2–0·6 mg/100 ml	
Creatine phosphokinase	Serum	♂ 10–66 I.U./L. ♀ 10–43 I.U./L.	
Creatinine	Serum	0·9–1·7 mg/100 ml	
Fibrinogen	Plasma	200–400 mg/100 ml	
Folic acid	Serum	6–19 mμg/ml	
	Red cells	80–470 mμg/ml	
11-Hydroxycorticosteroids	Plasma	5·0–15·0 μg/100 ml	10 a.m.–6 p.m.
Iodine (Butanol Extractable)	Serum	3·5–6·5 μg/100 ml	
Iodine (protein bound)	Serum	3·5–8·0 μg/100 ml	
Iron	Serum	♂ 80–175 μg/100 ml ♀ 60–160 μg/100 ml	
Iron combining capacity	Serum	♂ 250–385 μg/100 ml ♀ 205–430 μg/100 ml	
Saturation of combining capacity		♂ 25–56 per cent ♀ 14–51 per cent	
Lactic acid	Whole blood	6–18 mg/100 ml	Specimen pipetted at once into fresh cold TCA; patient fasting at rest
Lactic dehydrogenase	Serum	145–375 I.U./L.	
Lead	Heparinized Whole blood	< 50 μg/100 ml	
Lipids			
Total Lipids	Serum	400–800 mg/100 ml	
Total cholesterol	Serum	140–250 mg/100 ml	
Total fatty acids	Serum	9–15 mEq/L.	
Free fatty acids	Serum	0·3–0·7 mEq/L.	
Neutral fat	Serum	up to 200 mg/100 ml	
Total phospholipids	Serum	7·6–11·5 mg/100 ml expressed as lipid P. [38]	

Investigation	Specimen	Normal Range		Notes
Triglycerides	Serum	25–150 mg/100 ml		
Magnesium	Serum	1·5–1·8 mEq/L.		
Non-protein nitrogen	Serum	18–30 mg/100 ml		
5-Nucleotidase	Serum	1·6–17 I.U./L.		
Osmolality	Plasma	274–286 mOsmols/Kg		
pO_2	Whole blood	90–110 mm Hg.		Arterial Blood
O_2 Saturation	Whole blood	95–98 per cent		Arterial Blood
pH.	Whole blood	7·37–7·42		Arterial blood
Phosphatase (acid)		$<$ 5·5 I.U./L.		
Phosphatase (alkaline)		20–90 I.U./L.		
Phosphorus inorganic	Serum	2·5–4·5 mg/100 ml		Separate serum quickly from cells
Potassium	Plasma	3·6–5·4 mEq/L.		
Protein	Serum			
Total protein		6·3–7·8 g./100 ml		
		g./100 ml	*Per cent total protein*	
Albumin		3·5–5·3	50–65	
Globulin total		1·8–3·6	35–50	
α_1 Globulin			1–5	
α_2 Globulin			4·5–9·5	
β Globulin			11–16	
γ Globulin			14–20	
Immunoglobulins Ig		*mg/100 ml*	*Per cent Ig*	
IgA		50–200	15–20	
IgM		40–120	5	
IgG		800–1,500	75–80	
Pyruvic acid	Blood	0·5–1·0 mg/100 ml		Pipetted at once into fresh cold TCA; patient at rest and fasting
Sodium	Plasma	132–148 mEq/L.		
Sugar	Blood	80–120 mg/100 ml		Fasting
Glucose	Blood	60–100 mg/100 ml		Fasting
Sulphur	Serum	0·5–1·5 mEq/L.		
Abbott's Kit T3 resin test	Serum	25–35 per cent		
Transaminases				
SGOT	Serum	2–20 I.U./L.		
SGPT	Serum	2–15 I.U./L.		
Thymol turbidity	Serum	0–4 units		
Urea	Blood	20–40 mg/100 ml		
Uric acid	Serum	1·5–4·5 mg/100 ml		
Vitamin A	Serum	30–100 I.U./100 ml		
Vitamin B_{12}	Serum	190–950$\mu\mu$gm/ml		
Vitamin C	Blood	0·4–1·5 mg/100 ml		
Zinc sulphate turbidity	Serum	2–8 units		

Range of Normal Values for Urine

Investigation	Excretion/24 unless otherwise stated	Notes
α Amino nitrogen	47–293 mg	
δ Aminolaevulinic acid	0·01–0·57 mg/100 ml	
Calcium	♂ <300 mg ♀ <250 mg	
Catecholamines (free total)	<240 μg	Expressed as Adrenaline
Copper	<50 μg	
Creatine	0–50 mg	
Creatinine	♂ 1·5–2·0 g. ♀ 0·8–1·5 g.	
17-Hydroxycorticos-steroids	♂ 8·0–21·8 mg ♀ 4·6–17·0 mg	Varies with age
Lead	<80 μgm	
Oestrogens	♂ up to 25 μg ♀ up to 60 μg	
Osmolality	40–1,200 mOsmols/Kg	
17-Oxosteroids	♂ 9–24 mg ♀ 5–17 mg	Depends on method of assay and on age of patient
17-Oxogenic steroids	♂ 8–20 mg ♀ 6–18 mg	
pH	4·5–7·8	
Porphobilinogen	0·0–0·2 mg/100 ml	
Porphyrins		
Coproporphyrin	60–280 μg	
Uroporphyrin	5–30 μg	
Potassium	80–200 mEq	Depends on diet
Pregnandiol	♂ 0·4–2·4 mg ♀ 0·1–3·0 mg	
Sodium	80–200 mEq	Depends on diet
Specific gravity	1·002–1·032	
Titratable acidity	20–30 mEq	
Urea	16–35 g.	Depends on intake of protein
Uric acid	0·1–2·0 g.	
Urobilinogen	<2.0 mg	
Vanillylmandelic acid	1·8–7·1 mg	

The Cerebrospinal Fluid

Pressure	70–180 mm water
Appearance	Clear and colourless
Cells	Up to 4 lymphocytes per cmm
Sugar	50–100 mg/100 ml
Chloride	120–130 mEq/L
Protein–Total	Lumbar fluid up to 40 mg/100 ml (average) but rises with age up to 60 mg/100 ml in seventh decade γ globulin usually about 10 per cent of total protein

Ventricular fluid 5–10 mg/100 ml.

Phospholipids in CSF

Total phospholipid content 12–20 μg/ 100 ml P.

Differential phospholipid content	Per cent [39]	
Lysolecithin	14·6	Range ± 5 per cent of these values
Sphingomyelin	27·9	
Lecithin	36·0	
Serine	5·9	
Ethanolamine	10·1	
Phosphatidic acid	4·1	

Haematology – Normal Values

(from 'Practical Haematology' 4th Edition, J. V. Dacie and S. M. Lewis)

Haemoglobin	♂ 13·5–18·0 g./100 ml
	♀ 11·5–16·5 g./100 ml
Red cells	♂ 4·5–6·5 million/cmm
	♀ 3·9–5·6 million/cmm

Packed Cell Volume (Haematocrit)

♂ 40–54 per cent

♀ 36–47 per cent

Mean Corpuscular Volume (MCV) 76–96 cμ

Mean Corpuscular Haemoglobin (MCH) 27–32 μμg

Mean Corpuscular Haemoglobin Concentration (MCHC) 30–35 per cent.

Leucocytes

Total leucocyte count 4,000–11,000/cmm.

Differential leucocyte count

Neutrophils	40–75 per cent	2,500–7,500/cmm
Lymphocytes	20–45 per cent	1,500–3,500/cmm
Monocytes	2–10 per cent	200–800/cmm
Eosinophils	1–6 per cent	40–400/cmm
Basophils	1 per cent	0–100/cmm

Reticuloyctes 0·2–2·0 per cent
Platelets 150,000–400,000/cmm
Bleeding time (IVY'S method) 0–11 minutes
Coagulation time (Lee and White's method 37°C) 5–11 minutes
Prothrombin time (Brain-thromboplastin time, 1-stage (quick)
10–14 seconds

Prothrombin consumption index 0–30 per cent
Serum Haptoglobins 30–200 mg. Hb – binding per 100 ml
Erythrocyte sedimentation rate (Westergren 20°C ± 3°C)
♂ 0–5 mm/hour
♀ 0–7 mm/hour.

Blood Volume

Red cell volume	♂ 26–33 ml/kg
	♀ 22–29 ml/kg
Plasma volume	40–50 ml/kg
Total blood volume	60–80 ml/kg.

FUNCTION TESTS

Glucose Tolerance Test

The patient should be on a diet containing 300 g. carbohydrate for 3 days prior to the test.

50 g. glucose are given orally in the morning to the fasting patient. Venous blood is collected at 0, 30, 60, 90, 120 minutes and urine at 60 and 120 minutes.

Normal response:

Fasting <120 mg/100 ml sugar.

Peak value (30 min.) <180 mg/100 ml sugar.

Normal fasting level should be regained by 120 minutes.

No glucose should appear in the urine.

True glucose levels are approximately 20 mg/100 ml lower than sugar values.

Used in the diagnosis of diabetes mellitus. A prolonged Glucose

Tolerance Test (5 hours) may be helpful in the diagnosis of reactive hypoglycaemia.

Cortisone-Glucose Tolerance Test

This test is similar to the Glucose Tolerance Test above except that the patient is given 50–62·5 mg cortisone orally 8½ and 2 hours before the glucose load.

Normal response:

As above. Used in the diagnosis of 'pre-diabetes'.

Tolbutamide Tolerance Test

The patient should be on a diet containing 300 g. carbohydrate for 3 days prior to the test.

1 g. Tolbutamide is given intravenously over 2-minute period to the recumbent patient fasted overnight.

Blood is taken for *glucose*, prior to Tolbutamide administration and afterwards at 10, 20, 30, 90, 120 and 180 minutes.

Intravenous glucose and hydrocortisone should be available to terminate the test quickly if necessary.

Normal response:

Maximal fall of blood glucose is at 20–45 minutes. The level to which the blood glucose falls is less significant than the level at the end of 3 hours which should be at least 70 per cent of the fasting level. Used in the diagnosis of insulinoma.

Pyruvate Metabolism Test [31]

The patient is fasted and rested overnight. Two oral doses of 50 g. glucose are given at 0 and 30 minutes and blood is taken for pyruvate assay, prior to the first glucose load and at 60 and 90 minutes.

Normal response:

Fasting pyruvate $<$ 1·0 mg/100 ml.

60 minute sample $<$ 1·3 mg/100 ml.

90 minute sample $<$ 1·3 mg/100 ml.

A normal fasting pyruvate followed by an excessive and prolonged rise after glucose, which reverts to normal after vitamin B_1 therapy, is indicative of vitamin B_1 deficiency.

Insulin Tolerance Test

The patient should be on a diet containing 300 g. carbohydrate for 3 days prior to the test.

0·1 unit soluble insulin/Kg bodyweight is given intravenously and blood samples for *glucose* are collected prior to the injection of insulin and at 5, 10, 15, 20, 45, 60, 90 and 120 minutes.

Normal response:
Blood glucose should fall to 50 per cent fasting level within the first 20–30 minutes and return to the fasting level within 2 hours.

Provided a blood glucose of $<$35 mg/100 ml is achieved, measurements of plasma Cortisol and Growth hormone may be made as additional functional parameters of the hypothalamico-hypophyseal-adrenal axis [15].

This test may be dangerous in patients with pituitary insufficiency, in whom an initial test using 0·03 units/Kg insulin should be tried. In all cases, intravenous glucose should be available for immediate administration.

The Insulin-Glucose Test is a modification of the Insulin Tolerance Test in which 0·8 g. glucose/Kg bodyweight is given within the first 30 minutes of the standard I.V. dose of 0·1 unit/Kg bodyweight of insulin.

Normal response:
Fall of blood glucose to 50 per cent fasting level at 30 minutes, followed by a sharp rise at 60 minutes to between 100 and 200 mg/100 ml and then a gradual fall. Used as a test of pituitary 'reserve function'.

Glucagon Test

The patient should be on a diet containing 300 g. carbohydrate for 3 days prior to the test.

1 mg glucagon is given intramuscularly to the fasting patient, and blood samples are taken for *glucose* assay, prior to the injection and at 15, 30 minutes and half-hourly for 3 hours.

Normal response:
Rise of blood glucose of 40 mg/100 ml or more in first ½-hour and a peak increase over the fasting level of 30–90 mg between ½ and 1 hour. and returning to near the fasting level within 3 hours. Useful in the recognition and differential diagnosis of spontaneous hypoglycaemia and in the investigation of glycogen storage diseases.

Ischaemic Exercise Lactate Test [30]

The patient should fast overnight and should have been lying at complete physical rest in bed for at least 1 hour before commencement of the test.

Blood should be withdrawn by venepunture and placed *at once* into a heparinized tube. Immediately 2 ml (exactly) of this should be pipetted at the bedside into a universal bottle containing *exactly* 10 ml of freshly prepared cold (2°C) 10 per cent Trichloracetic Acid.

A sphygmomanometer cuff is placed around the patient's wrist and another around the upper arm.

The *lower* cuff is inflated to 200 mm Hg and after 45 seconds blood is withdrawn from the ante-cubital vein without inflating the upper cuff.

The upper cuff is then also inflated to 200 mm Hg and the patient exercises ischaemically by opening and closing the hand vigorously for 50 seconds or until fatigued.

A needle is inserted into the ante-cubital vein, the upper cuff is released and after 10 seconds blood is withdrawn.

3 further samples of blood are then withdrawn at 2 minute intervals.

The lower cuff remains inflated and the upper cuff deflated throughout.

The lower cuff is then deflated.

2 further samples of blood are taken at 10 minutes and 15 minutes also with the upper cuff deflated but the lower cuff is inflated 45 seconds before each sample is taken and released immediately after the blood is withdrawn.

Normal response:

The normal base-line blood lactic acid is 6–18 mg/100 ml. After ischaemic exercise under the above conditions there is a rapid rise of lactate in the first 2 blood samples often to 40 mg/100 ml or more, followed by a more gradual return to the base-line level within 15 minutes.

In McArdle's syndrome and other disorders of muscle glycogen storage in which there is a deficiency of enzymes in the anaerobic glycolytic cycle, there is a failure of the blood lactate to rise under these conditions.

Synacthen Test [12]

Blood is collected in the morning for estimation of plasma 11-Hydroxy-corticosteroids, after which a single intramuscular injection of 250 μgm of the synthetic polypeptide β^{1-24} corticotrophin (Synacthen) is given. A further blood sample is taken 30 minutes later.

Normal response:
Basal plasma 11-Hydroxycorticosteroids should be not less than 6 μgm/100 ml, and 30 minutes plasma 11-Hydroxycorticosteroids should be not less than 18 μgm/100 ml with a rise of not less than 7 μgm/100 ml. Used mainly in suspected Addison's disease as a test of the adrenal's ability to respond to stimulation.

Single Dose Dexamethasone Suppression Test [10]
2 mg Dexamethasone is given orally to the patient between 11.30 p.m. and midnight. The following morning blood is withdrawn for estimation of plasma 11-Hydroxycorticosteroids and the level compared with that of the previous morning.

Normal response:
The plasma 11-Hydroxycorticosteroids after Dexamethasone should be suppressed by at least 70 per cent to less than 6·5 μgm/100 ml. Patients with Cushing's syndrome show a fall in plasma 11-Hydroxycorticosteroids of less than 30 per cent in most cases with absolute levels of 13 μgm/100 ml or more.

Metopirone Test
24-hour collections are made before, during and after the administration of Metopirone 0·75 g. orally every four hours for 48 hours.

Normal response:
A four to six-fold increase in the 24-hour excretion of 17-Oxogenic Steroids or 17-Hydroxycorticosteroids represents a normal pituitary reserve [16]. Used as a test of pituitary functional reserve. No operative procedures of any kind should be carried out during or immediately after the test.

Pyrogen Test [18]
A bacterial pyrogen (ORGANON) is given intravenously in a dose of 0·005 μgm/Kg bodyweight, and blood is taken for estimation of plasma 11-Hydroxycorticosteroids immediately before and three hours after the injection.

If the patient complains of headache or muscle cramps, aspirin may be given without interfering with the test.

Intravenous hydrocortisone should be available for immediate termination of the test in the event of signs of collapse in patients with poor pituitary reserve.

Normal response:
Mean increase in plasma 11-Hydroxycorticosteroids of 22·1 μgm/100 ml with standard deviation of 10·7. Used as a test of pituitary functional reserve.

TESTS OF POSTERIOR PITUITARY FUNCTION [40]

1. Plasma Osmolality

In a patient with polyuria and on free fluid intake, a plasma osmolality of greater than 290 mOsmols/Kg favours a diagnosis of diabetes insipidus, while a value of less than 275 mOsmols/Kg favours psychogenic water drinking.

2. Vasopressin Administration while on Free Fluid Intake

Vasopressin Tannate in oil 5 units is given intramuscularly while the patient is on free fluid intake. There should be a rise in urine osmolality to at least 500 mOsmols/Kg and usually much higher, e.g. 800 mosols/Kg in normals, patients with psychogenic water drinking and patients with pituitary diabetes insipidus. Patients with nephrogenic diabetes insipidus (hereditary and acquired) do not respond. Note that this test may lead to water intoxication in patients with psychogenic water drinking.

3. Water Deprivation and Vasopressin Administration

The patient is deprived of all fluid until there has been a loss of 4 per cent bodyweight. Urine samples are collected and the osmolality measured.

Normal subjects and patients with psychogenic water drinking will show a rise in urine osmolality, and this will be greater than after vasopressin. Patients with pituitary diabetes insipidus will show no rise. If however, vasopressin is now given, there will be a rise in urine osmolality in those with pituitary diabetes insipidus and this may be more marked than their response to vasopressin on free fluid intake.

TESTS OF THYROID FUNCTION

Basal Metabolic Rate [41]

Robertson and Reid standard. Normal Range +15 to −15 per cent. Used in the diagnosis of Hyperthyroidism and Hypothyroidism.

Urine Excretion of Radioactive Iodine (^{131}I)

Normal Range

30–70 per cent of the administered dose in 24 hours.
44–88 per cent of the administered dose in 48 hours.

Hyperthyroidism <20 per cent in 24 hours.
<35 per cent in 48 hours.

Hypothyroidism 70–92 per cent in 48 hours.

Protein Bound Radioactive Iodine (^{131}I)

Normal Range: less than 0·3 per cent of the administered dose per litre of plasma at 72 hours.

Thyroid Uptake of Radioactive Iodine

Normal Range: 20–50 per cent of administered dose in 24 hours (^{131}I).
11–31 per cent of administered dose in 4 hours (^{131}I, ^{132}I).

Hyperthyroidism >40 per cent in 4 hours.
>55 per cent in 24 hours.

Hypothyroidism <10 per cent in 4 and 24 hours.

TSH Stimulation Test Using the Thyroid Four-hour ^{132}I Uptake [8]

The thyroid four-hour uptake of ^{132}I is measured before and 22 hours after an intramuscular injection of 2·5 units TSH. In the normal subject, the uptake is increased to between 35 and 56 per cent (mean 45·7 per cent) of the administered dose. In Hypothyroidism stimulation is to <35 per cent.

T3 Suppression Test Using the Thyroid Four-hour ^{132}I Uptake [8]

40 μgm Triiodothyronine is given 8 hourly for 6 days and the thyroid four-hour uptake of ^{132}I is measured before and afterwards. In the normal subject the uptake is decreased to 16 per cent or less, of the administered dose.

The ratio of the ^{132}I uptake before and after suppression lies within the range 2·0–4·8 (mean 3·1). Hyperthyroidism there is failure of suppression to <20 per cent. Ratio of uptake before and after suppression range 0.32–1·7 (mean 1·0).

PARATHYROID FUNCTION TESTS [22]

Renal Phosphate clearance (PC) 6–15 ml/minute
Tubular Reabsorption of Phosphorus (TRP) 84–97 per cent
Phosphate Excretion Index (PEI) 0·0 ± 0·09

	PC	TRP	PEI
Hyperparathyroidism	↑	↓	↑
Hypoparathyroidism	↓	↑	↓

Some of these indices overlap with the normal but if all are calculated often, a clear pattern emerges.

Sodium Phytate Test for Latent Hypoparathyroidism

The patient is placed on a low calcium diet, and sodium phytate 9 g. daily in divided doses with the main meals is given for one week. The serum calcium is assayed before and during phytate administration.

Parathormone Test for Pseudo-Hypoparathyroidism

The patient should preferably be on a low phosphate diet prior to the test and should fast and rest overnight. Water intake should be encouraged to ensure an adequate urine output. Urine is collected hourly for 3 hours before and for 5 hours after an intravenous injection of 200 units fresh Parathormone. Blood may be collected before and after the injection for phosphate clearance studies.

Normal response:

A marked phosphate diuresis (e.g. 100 mg/hour or a 2–3 fold increase of phosphate output) and an increase in phosphate clearance following parathormone differentiates hypoparathyroidism from pseudo-hypoparathyroidism.

It is advisable to carry out a control test with a normal subject to ensure the potency of the parathormone preparation.

Cortisone Test for Hypercalcaemia

Cortisone 150 mg daily by mouth in divided doses is given for 10 days as a diagnostic test to patients with hypercalcaemia. In those with sarcoidosis or vitamin D intoxication, there will be a significant decrease in the serum calcium but there will be no change in patients with hyperparathyroidism.

LIVER FUNCTION TESTS

Bromsulphthalein (BSP) Excretion

5 mg/Kg bodyweight Bromsulphthalein is injected intravenously in a 5 per cent solution. The patient should be fasting as turbidity of serum

interferes with the assay. Blood is withdrawn at 45 minutes for assay of Bromsulphthalein remaining in the serum. Blood may also be taken at 1 minute to check that the initial concentration is 10 mg/100 ml.

Normal response:
Less than 5 per cent of injected dose remains in the serum at 45 minutes. A sensitive test of hepatic function in the absence of jaundice.

Oral Galactose Tolerance Test (Dangerous in patients with Galactosaemia)
40 g. galactose is given orally to the fasting patient in the morning.

Normal response:
Less than 3 g. galactose should be excreted in the urine in 5 hours.
A test of hepatocellular function.

RENAL FUNCTION TESTS. Corrected to 1·73 sq m **surface area** [40]

Renal Plasma Flow 612 ± 68 ml/minute

Endogenous Creatinine Clearance 112 ± 15 ml/minute

Urea Clearance maximal urea clearance 75 ml/minute

Maximal Glucose Reabsorption Capacity (TMG) 323 ± 64 mg/minute

Maximal PAH Excretory Capacity, TM PAH 68 ± 11 mg/minute

Water Excretion Test
The patient is fasted overnight and the bladder emptied in the morning. 20 ml/Kg bodyweight is drunk within 30 minutes and the urine is collected hourly for 4 hours.

Normal response:
50 per cent or more of the total volume ingested should be excreted during the first 2 hours and approximately 80 per cent or more during the 4 hours. The urine specific gravity should fall to 1·002 (osmolality 40–80 mOsmols/Kg) during the test.

Abnormal result in pituitary insufficiency, Addison's disease, malabsorption syndrome, congestive heart failure, advanced liver disease and renal failure.

If the test is repeated 4 hours after oral administration of 100 mg cortisone, an improved result would point to the original diagnosis being pituitary insufficiency or primary adrenocortical failure.

Phenolsulphonephthalein (PSP) Excretion

The bladder is emptied and the patient drinks approximately 600 ml water. 6 mg PSP is given intravenously and urine samples are collected at 15, 30, 60, 120 minutes.

Normal response:

15 minutes 28–51 per cent administered dose in this sample.
30 minutes 29–31 per cent administered dose in this sample.
60 minutes 9–17 per cent administered dose in this sample.
120 minutes 3–10 per cent administered dose in this sample.
Total excretion in one hour 40–60 per cent administered dose in this sample.
Total excretion in two hours 63–84 per cent administered dose in this sample.

Water Concentration Test

All fluids are withheld from 8 a.m. and the bladder emptied at 8 p.m. Urine is collected as passed until 8 a.m. the following morning. The specific gravity and osmolality of all specimens passed during the second 12-hour period are measured.

Normal response:

In at least one specimen the specific gravity should be greater than 1·022 or the osmolality greater than 800 mOsmols/Kg.

GASTRIC AND INTESTINAL FUNCTION

Augmented Histamine Test Meal

The patient fasts for 12 hours, after which the whole of the resting gastric juice is aspirated.

100 mg Mepyramine Maleate is given intramuscularly and the gastric juice aspirated every 5 minutes for the next 30 minutes and added to the resting sample. Histamine acid phospate 0·04 mg/Kg bodyweight is injected subcutaneously and the gastric juice aspirated every 5

minutes for the next 60 minutes, being placed into 4 containers 0–15 minutes, 15–30 minutes, 30–45 minutes, 45–60 minutes.

Normal response:
Maximal secretion of acid occurs in period 15–30 minutes, up to 11·6 mEq/minute. Used for assessing gastric acid secretion in pernicious anaemia, gastric ulcer, duodenal ulcer and Zollinger-Ellison syndrome.

Pentagastrin Test Meal [37]
6 μgm/Kg bodyweight is injected intramuscularly after an overnight fast and gastric juice is collected by continuous suction for 30 minutes in three 10-minute samples.

Normal response:
Maximal secretion occurs in 10–30 minute period and results calculated on this are similar to those of the augmented histamine test meal.

Daily Fatty Acid Excretion
On an ordinary hospital diet containing 50–150 g. fat, the normal daily range of faecal fat excretion in an adult is 2–8 g. as fatty acid with *a four day average of 5 g. or less* (and 4 g. in children).

If the dietary fat intake is known, a percentage absorption of 90 per cent or more is normal in adults and children.

Fat Absorption Test [36]
The patient is fasted overnight and blood samples are taken before and 2 and 4 hours after a meal containing 100 g. fat, for assay of serum total fatty acids.

Normal response:
A rise of 90 mg/100 ml or more in serum total fatty acids in either the 2- or 4-hour sample. Used for diagnosis of malabsorption syndromes.

Xylose Absorption Test
25 g. d-xylose are given orally to the patient fasted overnight. Blood is collected between 90 and 120 minutes and urine over a period of 5 hours. It is important to maintain an adequate urine flow by giving the patient water to drink (500 ml) during the test.

Normal response:
Blood level 25–40 mg/100 ml.

5-hour urine excretion >4·2 g.

Used to confirm that malabsorption not due to pancreatic disease.

Vitamin A Absorption Test [42]
For this test the patient is *not* fasting.

Blood is taken for vitamin A assay and again 5 hours after the oral ingestion of 350,000 I.U. vitamin A in arachis oil.

Normal response:
The normal response is somewhat variable, thus low plasma levels do not necessarily confirm the presence of malabsorption. A rise of plasma vitamin A to 500 I.U./100 ml is much stronger evidence for excluding malabsorption.

Vitamin B_{12} Absorption Test [43]
In this modification of the Schilling test, serum vitamin B_{12} radioactivity is measured as well as the urine excretion. The patient is fasted overnight. An oral dose of 0·5 μgm (approximately 0·5 μc) ^{57}Co Cyanocobalamin is administered together with 1000 μgm stable vitamin B_{12} intramuscularly and the fast continued for a further two hours. A 24-hour sample of urine is collected as from the administration of vitamin B_{12} and blood for serum assay at 8 hours.

Normal response:
Urine radioactivity 10·5–25·7 per cent administered dose in 24 hours. 8-hour serum radioactivity 0·56–1·54 per cent of administered dose/litre. Used to confirm pernicious anaemia particularly after vitamin B_{12} therapy has commenced.

TESTS OF VITAMIN DEFICIENCY

Tryptophan Loading Test for Vitamin B_6 Deficiency
24-hour urine collections are made before and after an oral dose of 2 g. l-tryptophan, and preserved with 25 ml normal hydrochloric acid. The urine is analysed for xanthurenic acid.

Normal response:
Normal subjects excrete 1–3 mg xanthurenic acid/24 hours after the tryptophan load.

Patients with vitamin B_6 deficiency may excrete up to 60 mg/24 hours after tryptophan load.

Vitamin C Saturation Test
Ascorbic acid 70 mg/Kg bodyweight is given daily by mouth at 10 a.m. Urine is collected between 4 and 6 hours later, into a container with 20 ml glacial acetic acid and sent at once for analysis.

Normal response:
At least 50 mg ascorbic acid will be found in the 2-hour period urine sample on the first or second day.

PULMONARY FUNCTION TESTS

There are two aspects to be considered in the assessment of lung function; first the assessment of the ability of the individual to move volumes of gas in and out of the chest and the times required for these procedures (Tests of Ventilation); secondly, the assessment of gaseous exchange between the environment and the pulmonary capillary blood (tests of gas transfer).

TESTS OF VENTILATION

1. *Vital Capacity (VC)*
The volume of air expelled by a voluntary effort after maximal inspiration. The volume can be measured using a recording spirometer.

Normal Values:

4 litres	aged 20	men	6 litres maximum
2·5 litres	aged 70		
3 litres	aged 20	women	4·5 litres maximum
2 litres	aged 70		

2. *Forced Vital Capacity (FVC)*
The volume of air expelled by a forcibly rapid expiration after a maximal inspiration. The spirometer is again used. Normal values are the same as, or slightly less than, those obtained for vital capacity.

3. *Forced Expiratory Volume in One Second (FEV_1)*
The volume of air expelled from the lungs during the first second of a forcible expiration, after maximal inspiration. The spirometer is again used.

Normal Values Vary with Age and Height:

1·5 litres to approximately 3·2 litres men
maximum approximately 5 litres
2·5 litres to approximately 3·5 litres women
maximum approximately 4 litres

$\frac{\text{FEV}}{\text{FVC}} \times 100$ 70 per cent at any age; about 80 per cent in younger subjects. Useful indication of degree of airways obstruction.

4. *Peak Expiratory Flow Rate* (*PEFR*)
Maximum expiratory flow rate during a forced expiration.

Measured with a Wright's meter: maximal forcible expiration causes movement of a spring loaded vane proportional to the force of expiration. The vane is maintained in the maximal displacement position by a ratchet and attached to a pointer and dial for direct reading.

Normal values:

men	700 minus ($^9/_2 \times$ age) litres/minute
women	200 litres/minute lower than men

Variation with height and age:

average man aged 30	600 litres/minute
man aged 66	500 litres/minute

Other Tests of Ventilatory Function Requiring More Specialised Apparatus

5. *Functional Residual Capacity* (*FRC*)
The volume of air in the lungs after a normal expiration measured by (a) nitrogen washout, (b) helium dilution.
Average normal values:
approximately 2–4 litres
variation with height, age and sex.

6. *Total Lung Capacity*
The volume of air in the lungs after a maximal inspiration.
Average normal values:
5·5–6 litres.

TESTS OF GAS TRANSFER

1. *Estimation of arterial blood gases*
Normal values:

Pa O_2	110 mm Hg
O_2 sat^n	95–98 per cent at sea level
Pa CO_2	38–43 mm Hg

2. *Estimation of $PaCO_2$ by rebreathing method*
This estimates mixed venous PCO_2 which is 6 mm higher than $PaCO_2$; 6 mm Hg is therefore subtracted from this estimation for comparison with $PaCO_2$ estimations.

This method has the advantage of simplicity and may be used at the bedside. It may be repeated regularly without undue distress to the patient.

3. *Estimation of Transfer Factor for Carbon Monoxide* (Diffusing capacity)
Two methods are available differing in technique and results obtained.

1. 'Steady state' technique
   average normal values 10–25 ml/min/mm Hg men
   8–21 ml/min/mm Hg women
2. 'Single breath' technique
   average normal values 11–38 ml/min/mm Hg man
   6–32 ml/min/mm Hg women.

PULMONARY FUNCTION TESTS IN CERTAIN DISEASES

Two patterns of abnormality are well defined, both cause ventilatory insufficiency but affect gas transfer differently. The characteristic feature in one is airways obstruction, and in the other limitation of lung expansion due to tissue changes in the lung itself, or to abnormalities in the thoracic muscles or bones.

Interpretation of Results

1. *Obstructive*

The main deficiency is in ventilation.

FEV_1 decreased
FVC decreased
$\frac{FEV_1}{FVC} \times 100$ 70 per cent often reduced well below this figure
PEFR reduced
TLC increased (maybe).
Blood gas estimations show decrease in PaO_2 often below 70 mm Hg
Blood gas estimations show increase in $PaCO_2$ above normal levels.
Transfer factor is decreased, often to very low levels.

Changes of $\frac{FEV_1}{FVC}$ ratio, PEFR, FEV_1 and FVC with 'bronchodilator' agents indicate some element of reversibility of the airways obstruction and may be used as guidelines in the therapy of these conditions.

Examples are asthma, bronchitis, emphysema.

2. *Restrictive*

The main deficiency is in gas transfer.

FEV_1 decreased
FVC decreased
$\frac{FEV_1}{FVC} \times 100$ normal or 80 per cent
PEFR normal or decreased
TLC decreased.

Blood gas estimations show decrease in PaO_2
Blood gas estimations show normal or low $PaCO_2$ (due to hyperventilation).
Transfer factor is reduced, often markedly.
Examples are fibrosing alveolitis, asbestosis, farmer's lung.

References

1. College of Pathologists' Symposium, *J. Clin. Path.* (1968), **21**, 231.
2. Flynn, F. V., *Ann. Clin. Biochem.* (1969), **6**, 1.
3. Wootton, I. D. P., *Lancet* (1953), **i**, 470.
4. Udenfriend, S., In *Fluorescence Assay in Biology and Medicine* (1962), Academic Press.
5. Baron, D. N., *Proc. Royal Soc. Med.* (1969), **62**, No. 9, 945.
6. Eastham, R. D., and Jancar, J., In *Clinical Pathology in Mental Retardation* (1968), Pub. John Wright and Sons Ltd. (Bristol).
7. Osorio, C., *J. Clin. Path.* (1967), **20**, 351.
8. Bayliss, R. I. S., *Suppl. J. Clin. Path.* (1967), **20**, 360.
9. Mattingly, D., and Tyler, C., *Brit. med. J.* (1967), **4**, 394.
10. McHardy-Young, S., Harris, P. W. R., Lessof, M. H., and Lyne, C., *Brit. med. J.* (1967), **2**, 740.
11. Connolly, C. K., Gore, M. B. R., Stanley, N., and Wills, M. R., *Brit. med. J.* (1968), **2**, 665.
12. Wood, J. B., Frankland, A. W., James, V. H. T., and Landon, J., *Lancet* (1965), **i**, 243.
13. Greig, W. R., Boyle, J. A., Jasani, M. K., and Maxwell, J. D., *Proc. roy. soc. Med.* (1967), **60**, No. 9, 908.
14. Besser, G. M., and Landon, J., *Brit. med. J.* (1968), **4**, 552.
15. Greenwood, F. C., and Landon, J., *J. Clin. Path.* (1966), **19**, 284.
16. Metcalf, Mary G., Beaven, D. W., *Amer. J. Med.* (1968), **45**, No. 2, 176.
17. Wied, D. de, Bohus, B., Ernst, A. M., Jong, W. de, Nieuwehuizen, W., Pieper, E. E. M., and Yasumara, S., *Proc. roy. soc. Med.* (1967), **60**, No. 9, 907.
18. Jenkins, J. S., Else, W., *Lancet* (1968), **ii**, 940.
19. Webb-Peploe, M. M., Spathis, G. S., and Reed, P. I., *Lancet* (1967), **i**, 195.
20. Mackay, J. S., Montgomery, D. A. D., and Kennedy, T. L., *Lancet* (1967), **ii**, 211.
21. Moses, A. M., and Streeten, D. H. P., *Amer. J. Med.* (1967), **42**, No. 3, 368.
22. Hodgkinson, A., *Clinical Science* (1961), **21**, 125.
23. Smith, J. W. G., Harrard Davis, R., and Fourman, P., *Lancet* (1960), **ii**, 510.
24. Stowers, J. M., Michie, W., and Frazer, S. C., *ibid.* (1967), **i**, 124.
25. Boyns, D. R., Crossley, J. N., Abrams, M. E., Jarrett, A. J., and Keen, J., *Brit. med. J.* (1969), **1**, 595.

26. Abrams, M. E., Jarrett, R. J., Keen, H., Boyns, D. R., and Crossley, J. N., *ibid.* 599.
27. Rubenstein, A. H., Seftel, H. C., Miller, M., Bersohn, I., and Wright, A. D., *ibid.* 748.
28. Selter, R. H., *Lancet* (1968), **i**, 1301.
29. Mahler, R., *Suppl. J. Clin. Path.* (1969), **22**, 32.
30. McArdle, B., *Clinical Science* (1951), **10**, 13.
31. Joiner, C. L., McArdle, B., and Thompson, R. H. S., *Brain* (1950), **73**, 431.
32. Spray, G. H., *J. Clin. Path.* (1969), **22**, 212.
33. McNeish, A. S., and Willoughby, M. L. N., *Lancet* (1969), **i**, 442.
34. Green, A. E., and Pegrum, G. D., *Brit. med. J.* (1968), **3**, 591.
35. Linnell, J. C., Wilson, J., and Matthews D. M., *Clin. Sci.* – In Press.
36. Penfold, W. A. F., *Proc. Ass. Clin. Biochem.* (1967), **4**, No. 7, 205.
37. Forrest, A. P. M., *et al.*, *Lancet* (1969), **i**, 341.
38. Cumings, J. N., Shortman, R. C., and Skribic, T., *J. Clin. Path.* (1965), **18**, 641.
39. Cumings, J. N., Personal Commun.
40. Wardener, H. E. de, In *The Kidney* (1967), 3rd Ed. pub. A. Churchill Ltd.
41. Douglas Robertson, J., and Reid, D. D., *Lancet* (1952), **i**, 940.
42. Patterson, J. C. S., and Wiggins, H. S., *J. Clin. Path.* (1954), **7**, 56.
43. Donaldson, D., Personal Commun.

The general principles in the treatment of alcohol and drug dependence, both physical and psychological, are presented in this section. Various types of dependence are discussed and methods of help and treatment, both medical and social, are examined in depth.

A Guide to the Treatment of Alcoholism and Drug Dependence

by

M. M. Glatt

Consultant Psychiatrist, St. Bernards Hospital, Middlesex, and a member of WHO Expert Advisory Panel on Drug Dependence

As the discussion of these subjects is bedevilled by a great deal of semantic confusion, we should like to quote the definitions in which the relevant terms are used in the present article.

Alcoholism (following the recommendation of the World Health Organisation (1952): 'Alcoholics are those excessive drinkers whose dependence upon alcohol has attained such a degree that it shows a noticeable mental disturbance or an interference with their bodily and mental health, their interpersonal relations, and their smooth social and economic functioning; or who showed the prodromal signs of such developments. They therefore require treatment' [1].

Following recent WHO recommendations the embracing term **'drug dependence'** is here used in place of the formerly popular terms 'drug addiction' (which in the strict pharmacological meaning would be roughly 'physical plus psychological dependence') and 'drug habituation' (psychological dependence). The term 'dependence' is now defined as 'a state arising from repeated administration of a drug on a periodic or continuous basis' [2] and in each individual case it is essential to specify the type of drug involved, e.g. dependence of the Morphine type, Cannabis type etc.

Drugs affecting the CNS may produce a 'psychological dependence', i.e. '. . . a state of mind . . . a psychic drive which requires periodic or chronic administration of the drug for pleasure or to avoid discomfort' [3]. Some such drugs also provoke 'physical dependence, an adaptive state characterised by intense physical disturbances when administration of the drug is suspended or its action is counteracted by a specific antagonist' (e.g. in the case of the Morphine type of dependence by nalorphine).

GENERAL PRINCIPLES IN THE TREATMENT OF ALCOHOL AND DRUG DEPENDENCE

Before describing the therapy in some detail, a few general principles should be briefly discussed. This, it is hoped, will despite certain overlapping greatly simplify later discussion and general understanding.

The division of dependence-producing drugs into those producing psychological dependence only and those also capable of producing physical dependence is of considerable therapeutic significance. Drugs which stimulate the CNS, such as cocaine, the amphetamines and Khat [66], as a rule produce psychological dependence only and, at least clinically, no evidence of physical dependence (although workers in Edinburgh have described sleep pattern alterations, indicated by EEG and eye movement changes, on sudden withdrawal of amphetamines). Likewise LSD and Cannabis apparently produce psychological dependence only. In view of the lack of the risk of a physical abstinence syndrome, cessation of drug intake in people dependent on such drugs can be sudden and complete (although an eye should be kept on such mental withdrawal symptoms as depression etc.).

Drugs which depress the CNS often produce, apart from **psychological dependence,** also a state of **physical dependence.** In these cases, because of the danger of a physical abstinence syndrome on sudden withdrawal, the drug should either be tapered off gradually (e.g. in the case of barbiturate dependence) or temporarily replaced by an adequate substitute (e.g. by methadone in the case of heroin addicts). Physical (as well as psychologically) dependence producing drugs include opiates, the hypnotic-sedatives (in particular barbiturates, but also most non-barbiturate hypnotics) the tranquilliser meprobamate (the benzodiazepines Chlordiazepoxide and diazepam only in exceptionally high doses and when administered for a long period) [35, 41] alcohol and possibly also nicotine. In alcoholics and addicts to hypnotic drugs, the physical abstinence syndrome includes withdrawal convulsions and delirium tremens, and therefore requires the prophylactic administration of anticonvulsants and powerful tranquillisers. Provided this precaution is taken, alcoholics as a rule can be – at least in hospital – suddenly and completely taken off alcohol.

It is popularly assumed that physical dependence is more dangerous than psychological dependence. However, whilst it is true that as regards risk to life the physical abstinence syndrome is more important than the psychological withdrawal symptoms supervening on sudden cessation of dependence provoking drugs, from the aspects of relapse and rehabilitation psychic dependence is more important, once the period of drug withdrawal has been completed. Thus alcoholics, barbiturate and opiate addicts relapse as a rule not because of physical but mainly because of psychological dependence or as a consequence of factors such as 'the original psychological conflicts or a simple social situation which invokes drinking – or also 'social dependence', i.e. their involvement with their 'sub-culture', which exerts a strong attraction on them, induces them often to return to their former drug taking habits [9].

Therefore sobering-up the drunk and detoxifying the drinker and the drug taker are by themselves no more than first aid measures, curtain raisers which have always to be followed up by **long-term and rehabilitation measures.** Otherwise all that will have been achieved is to render the alcoholic and the drug addict fit to resume drinking and drug taking in a better physical state, with renewed vigour and fervour. Or to put it another way: initial therapy of the state of physical dependence and intoxication – by means such as tranquillisers, vitamines, fluids etc. – is vital but must always be followed up by the therapy aimed at neutralising and removing the effects of psychological and social dependence [4]. For example, if drug takers after treatment in hospital are sent out without provision being made for their living in a drug-free environment, without having been put in touch with new friends, without attempts at vocational guidance and assistance, they will drift back to their old haunts, their former drug-taking friends and subculture – and to certain return to their drug taking habits [9].

The relationship between psychological and physical dependence is as yet obscure. Three characteristics of any state of drug dependence include craving or pathological desire for the drug effects, a state of tolerance (requiring increasing dosage to get the same effect) and the supervening of psychological and/or physical abstinence symptoms on sudden cessation (or even too rapid reduction of the dosage) of the drug. The length of time that has to elapse between onset of drug taking and of psychological and/or physical dependence varies with several factors, e.g. with the 'agent', i.e. the pharmacological nature of the drug (dependence in general arising more rapidly with the opiates than with the barbiturates, and with these more rapidly than with alcohol), with the dosage employed and the 'predisposition' or emotional vulnerabilty of the 'host'. However, recent work carried out at the Addiction Research Foundation in Ontario – one of the leading centres in the world – suggest that 'the physical dependence aspect of alcoholism is not, as previously though, the cumulative result of years of abuse; instead, it can be brought on by repetitive drinking over a few weeks and can be reversed when drinking stops' [5]. Thus, as Archibald remarks in his paper, 'one does not have to become a socially or psychologically deteriorated alcoholic in order to experience physical dependence; one simply has to drink large enough quantities during a short period of time' [5].

This conclusion fits in with the present author's experience of heavy drinkers sometimes experiencing physical abstinence symptoms at the sudden ending of a severe bout without having been long-standing alcoholics. There is, also the well-known finding that drinkers may develop the definite physical or mental complications of so-called 'chronic alcoholism' (Jellinek's 'Beta alcoholism') [6] without having been necessarily dependent on alcohol, but just as a consequence of habitual heavy drinking (e.g. 9 ounces of whisky or 21 ounces of wine or 5½ bottles of beer per day, every day in the year) [5]. Naturally other factors, such as nutritional status and a balanced food intake, may here also be closely involved.

To what extent these findings hold good also for drugs other than alcohol, is not yet clear. However, in view of many other similarities it would seem not unlikely that similar factors may also be at work in the case of these 'other drugs'. This is only one of many examples showing the need for much further research in the field of alcohol and other drug dependence.

Whilst there are many similarities between alcohol and other drugs, there are also many dissimilarities. In view of the similarities, e.g. in causation and treatment [7, 13], the WHO Committee on 'Services for the Prevention and Treatment of Dependence on Alcohol and Other Drugs' (1967) [8] recommended a 'combined approach' (possibly 'coordinated' would be a more suitable description) to problems of alcoholism and drug dependence. Such a **'combined approach'** – in the Committee's view – would apply most usefully to research, least to control measures, with treatment and education taking an intermediate position. One important reason for recommending a 'combined approach' was the feeling that in recent years the approach to alcoholism as an illness and to the alcoholic as a sick man had become increasingly accepted – e.g. both in England and North America; whereas in many parts of the world (including North America) drug addicts were still mainly regarded as criminals. It was hoped that such a 'combined approach' would in time also make drug dependence more widely acceptable as an illness. In the UK drug 'addicts' have in principle for many years been considered to be sick people in need of help, whereas in the USA 'dope fiends' have been widely approached as criminals, with medical men until recently taking very little active part in their management. In very recent years, however, whilst in the UK addicts to the opiates are still treated as sick men, their treatment has become less 'permissive' in the sense that only specially licensed doctors can prescribe such drugs [9], whereas in the USA quite a few centres have recently begun to treat heroin addicts by such means as 'Methadone Maintenance' [60, 61] or blockade with opium antagonists, such as Cyclazocine [64]. Again, differences in national and local situations, in public image and in legal provisions offer an opportunity for research, comparing and contrasting the methods and results obtained under varying conditions in these two countries.

Whilst the **aetiology** of alcohol and drug dependence is still rather obscure, clearly three different sets of factors are involved in dynamic interaction with each other in the individual patient [10], i.e. the mental make-up (the role of a predisposing physical make-up, though often hypothesized [6, 65], is as yet not definitely proven, though it may quite possibly turn out to be important in certain types of alcoholism and dependence on other drugs), factors connected with the environment (e.g. cultural or religious factors, availability at times of stress) and, finally, the pharmacological nature of the drug concerned. To draw a rough analogy with conditions pertaining in infective diseases (and the spread from person to person in certain types of drug dependence in recent years has often been likened to the contagiousness of the infective diseases) [11] factors connected with the 'host', the 'environment' and the causative 'agent' play a role. Therefore in the prophylaxis and the management of the health problems involved, it is obviously not enough to limit oneself to measures directed at the legal control of the drug ('agent') but attention has also to be directed to the personalities involved ('host') and environmental conditions [10, 12].

Moreover, in view of the multifactorial causation, it is clear that one and the same treatment cannot be the best for every individual involved. Different types of personalities take drugs of widely varying composition and effect for varying reasons under widely different conditions for varying lengths of time in greatly varying amounts. Therefore treatment, too, should be as far as possible individualised and tailored to the requirements of the individual patient. Treatment should always be preceded by an investigation and an assessment of the causative factors involved in the individual patient. The question is therefore not – as sometimes debated – 'Pavlov or Freud' – implying that such a choice may be rather independent of the exigencies of the case concerned. Whether to employ methods based predominantly on Freud or on Pavlov, should be decided only after an assessment of the individual patient's needs, and very often there may be a need for combining various techniques based on different therapeutic philosophies.

Though often expected by patients or their relatives, there is in fact no hope for a miraculous 'cure' by 'chemotherapy' at the present state of knowledge. In general, most observers would regard treatment by drugs as adjuncts to the more fundamental tasks of an emotional reorientation of the patient's attitudes and 'life style' by relatively brief psychotherapy – individual or in groups – and of social therapies, giving assistance to his social problems such as domestic, housing and occupational difficulties. In most cases a comprehensive approach – combining psychological, social and pharmacological techniques – is nowadays regarded as the best form of treatment in alcoholism and dependence on other drugs.

Clearly such multidimensional comprehensive therapy cannot be carried out by members of one therapeutic discipline, but is the responsibility of a well-integrated **multidisciplinary team,** whose members have to work in close cooperation with each other. Medical men, social workers, sociologists, nurses, priests, probation officers, the alcoholic's family, recovered alcoholics (AA) and addicts, personnel managers, employees of local authorities and voluntary welfare agencies, at times also magistrates, lawyers, police etc. are all members of the therapeutic team [10]. Sometimes the team member first approached by the patient or his family may not be the best one to help in this individual case – and he must then be prepared to refer him to a member of the team who may be better qualified or in a better position to assist him, such referral serving the purpose not of shifting responsibility but of sharing it. There is no place here for interdisciplinary rivalry, jealousy or warfare, but a need for the closest interdisciplinary collaboration and pooling of experiences and forces. In fact, representatives of one discipline must have a fair notion of the functions of the other team members: e.g. the psychiatrist must have some idea of the work and the role of the sociologist and vice versa, and he must not exclusively consider psychological but also social causative factors involved.

Alcoholism and drug dependence are both diseases of the whole family. Treatment cannot be regarded as complete without also including other members of the **family** in the treatment situation [10]. Often the family constellation may have greatly contributed to setting the patient initially on the road to his excessive drinking or drug taking. In the case of the alcoholic, sometimes the wife (who may frequently be older or the more dominating partner compared to the emotionally often much more immature alcoholic husband) may have married him primarily because of unconscious personality needs of her own. In the case of the young drug addict he often, rightly or wrongly, blames the misunderstanding by his parents for his 'opting out' of the family circle, his tuning in to the gang subculture and turning to drugs. At any rate, secondarily the alcoholic's or drug addict's behaviour must exercise considerable influence and have wide repercussions on the attitudes, feelings and behaviour of the whole family, e.g. the alcoholic's wife and children. Thus the family needs help often as much as the patient himself. Moreover, among environmental factors – which are so important in deciding on the patient's success or failure in the tasks of resocialisation and rehabilitation – none is more important than his family's attitude. His relatives – like the patient himself – have to become acquainted with and learn to accept emotionally the illness concept of these conditions, so that they are in a better frame of mind to understand his otherwise unpredictable and incomprehensible behaviour, and ease his way back to family and the community as a whole. Faulty patient's and family attitudes can otherwise lead to a persistence of mutual misunderstanding and recriminations.

Is dependence on alcohol or other drugs a **'symptom'** of underlying psychological or social problems or a **'disease'** in its own right? In the past, psychiatrists usually regarded alcoholism solely as a symptom of underlying psychopathology; they therefore tended to neglect the 'symptom' – excessive drinking – as being of relative minor interest, hoping that by diagnosing and remedying the underlying psychological cause the need for excessive drinking would disappear. However, it is only fair to say that approaches based on such reasoning as a rule failed to get anywhere, and there is little evidence that orthodox psychoanalysis had any success with alcoholism [46]. In practice, AA, who look at alcoholism as a 'disease' without (in theory) caring much about the underlying psychopathology, had much more success in the 'treatment' and rehabilitation of alcoholics.

There seems, at any rate, no reason why these two approaches could not be successfully combined, in the sense that alcoholism and drug dependence can both be looked at as conditions which in many (certainly not all) cases may have started as symptomatic of underlying psychological problems (Jellinek's 'alpha alcoholism') [6] but which in the course of time may have outrun their original purely symptomatic function and have assumed the extent and the importance of a 'disease' in their own right, for example causing, in turn, physical and mental complications. In group sessions with alcoholics and drug dependent individuals at the Alcoholism and Drug Dependence Unit at St. Bernard's Hospital, discussions deal both with psychological (and social) problems which may originally have caused excessive drinking or drug-taking, as well as with difficulties in inter-personal relationships (quickly becoming manifest whilst living in close proximity in the therapeutic community) and with events arising during, and as a consequence of, their drinking or drug-taking career [10]. Thus psychiatrists, GPs, etc. can well work together with AA, their work often being a good and frequently necessary complement to each other.

Whether these conditions are in fact 'diseases' in the strict pharmacological meaning of the term has often been hotly debated. Regarding alcoholism, the most widely accepted view is the one proposed by E. M. Jellinek in his important book 'The Disease Concept of Alcoholism' (1960) [6]. He rightly stresses that, in view of the great multiplicity of types of alcoholism, one should speak of the 'alcoholisms' rather than of alcoholism, and he delineates a minimum of five varieties of alcoholism; 'Alpha' (or symptomatic) alcoholism, 'Beta' alcoholism (already mentioned above, where – even in the absence of dependence on alcohol, and possibly as a consequence of such factors as impaired nutritional status and poor habits – definite mental or physical complications may arise, such as liver cirrhosis, peripheral neuropathy or alcoholic dementia); 'Gamma' or 'loss of control' alcoholism (in predominantly spirit-drinking countries); 'Delta' or 'inability to abstain' alcoholism in predominantly wine (or beer drinking) countries; and 'Epsilon' alcoholism (periodic alcoholism). He regards as 'addictions' or as 'diseases' in the strict pharmacological connotation of the term only the gamma and delta varieties, because in these the organism has temporarily become reliant on the presence of alcohol, so that sudden discontinuation of the supply leads to a physical abstinence syndrome. Just as there is no such person as 'the' alcoholic, so there is, of course, no such man as 'the' drug addict, and possibly similar considerations might to a certain extent apply to other forms of drug dependence [7, 13].

Whether one regards alcoholism and drug dependence as essentially a 'symptom' or as an 'illness' or 'disease', there is no doubt that they are (though not exclusively) the responsibility and province of the healing professions, and that **doctors** are – or should be – vitally interested. Naturally, these conditions constitute also a social problem, an economic, a financial, a theological, a criminological problem, but this does not exclude that they are not also an important medical problem. This, of course, does not mean that doctors should make a 'takeover' bid – a fear that was expressed to the writer at a recent conference by the well-known Finnish sociologist Kettel Bruun regarding conditions pertaining to alcoholism in his country. But a fear of a 'takeover' bid by doctors in problems of alcoholism and drug dependence can certainly be discounted, as far as the UK and probably also as far as the USA is concerned. Unfortunately the danger here is that as in the past – though fortunately to a gradually decreasing extent – doctors have all too often opted out from taking an active and leading interest in these conditions. This may have been to a large extent the consequence of inadequate teaching of these subjects in the medical curriculum [10]. For instance, alcoholism, if mentioned at all to undergraduates, meant no more than its rare complications, such as liver cirrhosis, so that doctors, further on in their professional life, thought of a possible diagnosis of alcoholism only when a patient exhibited such late (and fortunately relatively rare) complications – so that a great majority of cases of alcoholism (in England perhaps 13–14 out of 15 alcoholics on the average GP's list) are never known to their GPs. Regarding other types of drug dependence, until recent years, the term 'opium addiction' probably often conjured up notions of some exotic, oriental affliction hardly ever seen in Western countries – until the UK doctors and the general public in the 1960s had a rude awakening for which they were totally unprepared. Then again, the fact that 'respectable' drugs, such as barbiturates and amphetamines, could produce dangerous states of drug dependence was until recently hardly known to the great majority of doctors, one of the consequences being that quite a few GPs by their liberal and generous prescribing habits contributed greatly to the spread of 'epidemics' [9].

There is therefore a great need for adequate **teaching** at undergraduate level in the subjects of alcoholism and drug dependence (and equally, of course, of students of other professions concerned with alcohol and drug dependent individuals). This would not only lead to earlier diagnosis and detection of cases of alcohol and drug misuse, thus allowing earlier treatment with prevention of further complications – ('secondary' prevention) – but would gradually also alter the attitude of doctors; they would no longer look at these people as time wasters who could do better if they only tried, but rather as sick human beings in need of help. This would also have the effect that alcoholics and addicts (and their families) would no longer keep away from the GP as long as they could (or present themselves under the guise of sufferers from headache, backache, stomach-ache, injuries etc.) because they fear moralising lectures, but come forward at an earlier phase where often the chance of successful help and rehabilitation would be much greater than later on when easily irreversible complications might have set in. As a consequence of a positive attitude of the medical profession towards these sufferers, in time also the attitude of the community at large would follow suit – so that the stigma attached to these conditions would gradually fall by the wayside. Again this would lead to an earlier coming forward of these patients for help [10].

In as far as the patient's own attitude to himself – e.g. his guilt feelings and the need to 'project' them on to his family and the community at large – is to a large extent a reaction to family and community attitudes, altered, positive medical attitudes by changing family and public attitudes would also constructively influence the alcoholic's and addict's own attitude to himself. He might then no longer regard himself as a hopeless misfit, as having to live up (or rather 'down') to Society's prophecy about himself, and finally to die outside the 'fold', but instead come to look at himself in a more hopeful light and be encouraged to cooperate actively in his own rehabilitation.

From the point of view not only of treatment but also of prevention (education of the general public, changing public attitudes, research) it is vital that the medical profession takes a leading, active part in the management of problems of alcoholism and drug dependence [10].

How poor the education of medical practitioners is, in regard to these conditions, can be seen from the relatively high proportions of doctors who become alcoholics and drug addicts. As regards 'other drugs', professionally, doctors are easily exposed to constant temptation and opportunity (as are nurses, pharmacists, etc.) but their knowledge should prevent them from taking unnecessary risk. Anyway this consideration does not explain the relatively high incidence of alcoholism in doctors (which is not really reflected in the standard mortality rate – in England, two and a half times that of the average population, and probably kept low artificially by the unwillingness of doctors to certify liver cirrhosis as the cause of death in a colleague).

Neither alcoholism nor dependence on other drugs is a respecter of social class, occupation, race or religion. A **comprehensive programme** must therefore cater for everybody, in particular for all social classes. For some reason or other in England it is in the main Social Classes I and II alcoholics who turn up at the treatment facilities. This does not necessarily mean that there are proportionately more alcoholics among them but that the illness concept of alcoholism and the knowledge that alcoholics can be greatly helped has as yet not become known widely among other social classes.

Conversely, formerly in the USA it was mainly the slum area youngsters who became drug abusers and dependents. In England, on the other hand, youngsters from all social classes were always represented among those becoming dependent on drugs in the 1960s. In recent years the situation in this aspect has begun to alter also in the US.

At any rate, any (comprehensive) treatment programme for alcoholics and addicts has therefore to make provision for the care and management of alcoholics and drug dependents of all classes and all types, by in-patient, out-patient facilities, halfway houses, community treatment, connections with other treatment and after-care agencies etc.

In 1962 the Ministry of Health recommended for the hospital treatment of alcoholics the establishment of regional alcoholic units [10]. There are now in the UK about fifteen such regional units, one in Scotland and one in Wales, apart from a number of smaller units. The Ministry memorandum rightly stressed the need for such in-patient units to work closely together with GPs, social services, local authorities and voluntary organisations such as AA. In our own view, the whole complex of in- and out-patient facilities, halfway houses, domiciliary visits etc. should be regarded as the 'unit' and not merely its in-patient facility [10, 14]. In such a way, the unit should be able to cater for all types of alcoholics in all phases of the condition, even if such patients may not fit into a therapeutic community geared to group discussions. It is obvious that it must not limit itself to the treatment of patients who seem to have a fair prognosis.

The question is often raised whether **in-patient or out-patient therapy** is preferable for alcoholics and drug addicts. This seems, however, to be more than an academic problem [10], as there will always be patients who, at least to start with, will require hospitalisation. The lesser the stigma, the more likely will be the number of those who will present themselves at such an early stage of development that the whole treatment can be carried out without hospital admission – e.g. by the GP, possibly with the help of health visitors, AA, etc. The question should rather be for what type of patient is in-patient, for which type is out-patient treatment indicated, and to this purpose much further research will be necessary. The answer to this question may be determined not wholly by the type of patient and the stage of the development of the condition, but also by the number and type of specially trained staff or suitable facilities available. Where, for example, special hostels are available, many patients who otherwise would have to stay in hospital for longer periods could leave hospital earlier; and quite a few homeless and friendless patients might avoid hospitalisation altogether. Such hostels should probably cater exclusively for alcoholics and drug addicts respectively as it often has been found that they do not fit in well into therapeutic communities consisting in the main of other types of patients. The same principle holds good, very probably, also for the treatment of alcoholics in hospital. However the question of forming communities exclusively consisting of drug addicts probably requires much further research.

The length of hospitalisation may also depend largely on the type of aftercare available, including assistance from voluntary organisations and local authorities. For example, in areas where there is a strong and good AA group, patients can often be discharged earlier from hospital.

Not all alcoholics, and perhaps not all addicts, require medical care and attention, though probably in all such cases the **GP** could be of the greatest help. The GP is in a key position, in as far as he knows the family background and often the history of such a patient from childhood onwards. He is in a position to explain the illness concept of dependence to the patient and to his family, and thereby remove obstacles which stand in the path of their applying for help. He could carry out a certain part of the treatment himself, or refer the patient to the facility best suited to his condition, and he could collaborate with bodies such as AA; he could supervise the aftercare (e.g. disulfiram administration in the case of alcoholics) after discharge from hospital. He has the chance, based on his intimate knowledge of the home situation and the family background, to spot early behavioural changes and thus to make an early diagnosis, to win the patient's confidence and cooperation and to impress on him and his family the need for treatment and the chance – provided there is cooperation – of recovery or at least marked improvement. In helping the families of alcoholics and drug addicts to regard the conditions as illnesses rather than as a vice, crime, character weakness etc., the GP can do a great deal to alter a negative home atmosphere into one that is constructive and helpful [10].

The **treatment goals** should be realistic and aim at the optimum attainable in each given patient. The ideal goal is, of course, total abstinence from alcohol or from addictive drugs respectively, combined with effective and satisfying social-occupational functioning. The goal of total abstinence from alcohol in the case of alcoholics should in general be strictly adhered to, notwithstanding occasional reports of erstwhile alcoholics having become moderate drinkers. It is certainly true that quite a few alcoholics can for very brief periods using special 'techniques' get away with drinking (or 'nibbling') a few drinks [10], but the great majority of alcoholics trying moderate drinking very soon fall by the wayside; and many alcoholics must have gone to their graves, attempting up to the bitter end to prove to themselves that they could become moderate drinkers. Helping alcoholics to achieve total abstinence is usually the first step in therapy, because as a rule only after he has stayed sober for some time, is the alcoholic in a fit state to understand and to grapple with underlying psychological and social problems. On the other hand, in drug addicts as in alcoholics, personality defects may prevent such people from being helped beyond a certain potential, and in such people one has often to be satisfied with a more modest goal, falling far short of life-long abstinence and full, independent socio-occupational functioning. Chronic drunkenness, offenders, for example who never in their life had been 'socialised', may sometimes require lifelong emotional and social support.

The task of a realistic attainable goal becomes even more complex in the case of drug dependent individuals. Ideally addicts should be weaned off their drugs and be helped to learn to live fully and happily without them. But so many young drug addicts are emotionally so unstable, immature and 'dependent' that sometimes one wonders whether they will ever be in a position to function without drugs. Similarly in the case of certain amphetamine or barbiturate users who have functioned fairly well over years as long as they were given a moderate 'maintenance' dose of their drugs, but go to pieces after this is discontinued, it might be difficult to decide whether insistence on total 'abstinence' from their drug in such exceptional cases is essential [74]. In the case of narcotic addicts the question of 'stabilised addicts' is sometimes brought up. They must be rare and far between, as tolerance usually forces the addict to push his dose upwards – and so many narcotic addicts do not function well anyway whilst taking these drugs. Rarely one comes across addicts who seem to function reasonably well on small doses of Heroin (and even Cocaine, the latter, for example, in the case of a few jazz musicians who have managed to restrict their habit to sniffing it – though of course this too should be strongly discouraged), or – in the USA – on high doses of methadone. On the other hand, it is clear that before agreeing to such maintenance therapy in the case of young newcomers who claim that they could not live without their drugs, stringent precautionary clinical and laboratory investigations should be carried out. In the UK, for example, the present drug epidemic amongst youngsters was directly helped on its way by the ease with which a few London GPs agreed to prescribe largish amounts of amphetamines, Heroin, Cocaine and more recently barbiturates to youngsters appearing on their doorsteps and clamouring for such drugs [9, 6].

Thus whilst as a rule ideal goals should be aimed at, one has sometimes to be satisfied with less complete, intermediate goals, with the patient's improvement rather than full recovery, with reduction of drug amount as far as possible, and with his functioning at a level of socio-occupational and emotional stability, that is not too unsatisfactory for him and that frees him from the need to indulge in subsocial activities.

The treatment procedure and the **phases of treatment** in cases of alcoholism and other forms of drug dependence follow in general a similar order. Treatment starts in general with the gradual or abrupt withdrawal of the drug and detoxification. This is followed by the long-term treatment and finally the rehabilitation phase, though clearly no strict demarcation line exists between them. In fact, the rehabilitation task begins in most cases with the first time such a patient is seen. Aftercare is the most important phase. In many patients it will be necessary also to treat complications, such as malnutrition, overdoses, injuries, etc. so that any treatment facility specifically dealing with these conditions should have immediate and rapid access to medical and surgical establishments. Very often – i.e. as a rule in drug 'addicts' and commonly in alcoholics – the withdrawal and detoxification treatment will require hospitalisation, whereas the long-term and rehabilitation treatment will take place in the community. Whether the immediate post-withdrawal and the initial steps of the long-term therapy will be carried out on a residential or non-residential or non-residential basis, will depend on a number of factors, such as type of drug dependence, severity of individual case, treatment philosophy (e.g. therapeutic community facilities aim at much more than mere drug withdrawal, e.g. at emotional re-orientation etc.), availability in the community of adequate after-care facilities or self-help organisations, etc.

The question of **compulsory treatment** in patients suffering from alcoholism or drug dependence is complex and controversial. It is often said that it is no use to treat such patients unless they are 'ready', although on the other hand the former view that, for example, alcoholics cannot recover until they have reached their 'rock bottom' has now been abandoned. 'Rock bottom' is not a static point and does not mean that a sufferer must have lost family, home and health, but is an individual experience at a juncture at which the sufferer realises that he cannot any longer continue with his drinking or drug-taking in his old way. Everyone agrees, of course, that it would be preferable that such patients would come voluntarily for treatment, but what is one to do if one sees such people going downhill rapidly, adamantly refusing treatment despite their obvious urgent need for it. Anyhow probably the great majority of so-called voluntary (in the UK 'informal') patients are voluntary in name only: very often they come pushed along by the threat of divorce or loss of job. In such cases the 'rock bottom' experience has been hastened by external agents and one wonders whether this principle could not with advantage – and sometimes possibly with health – and life-saving effect – be employed more often. Use is made of it for example in the case of many American firms whose constructive policy in regard to their alcoholic employees consists in helping them to have treatment whilst keeping their jobs open, but in threatening dismissal if they fail to undergo and to cooperate with treatment [15].

It is often maintained that treatment is useless unless patients are 'motivated', but many experiences have shown that even patients who at the beginning were totally unmotivated, sooner or later acquired 'insight' into their illness and their need for treatment [10]. Likewise the argument that treatment results with compulsorily treated patients were poor, does not dispense with the need occasionally to consider the possibility of compulsory therapy. Many alcoholic patients have in fact recovered although their treatment was initiated without their consent [10]. As regards people dependent on other drugs, at the present juncture results unfortunately are often equally unsatisfactory whether they are treated 'voluntarily' or 'compulsorily' [4].

Finally, there is the often used argument of the 'liberty of the subject'. Yet it is difficult to see how one could speak of the freedom of an habitually intoxicated alcoholic or a continually 'stoned' drug addict to make a rational choice: such people are more or less continually prevented by their intoxicated state from making any free decisions. Only if treatment has helped them, for several weeks at least, to abstain from alcohol or drugs would they be rendered rational enough to take such a decision whilst in a mentally fit state to do so.

It is sometimes argued by sociologists [16] that psychiatrists calling for compulsory treatment measures may hide their essentially 'punitive' attitudes and 'authoritarian techniques of social control' behind a mantle of humanitarianism. However, those not directly involved in active therapeutic measures might easily overlook the need for active steps which may seem necessary in the interests of the individual's own health as well as (often) that of his family. After all, the alcoholic and drug dependent destroy not only their own health but also that of those nearest and closest to them, and desperate appeals for help coming from the family are only too well known to those charged with looking after such patients.

Clearly, care will have to be taken that compulsory treatment does not degenerate into mere 'custodial care', that as far as possible the therapy within the hospital is carried out exactly as for voluntary patients, e.g. within the framework of a 'therapeutic community', and that the compulsory label is discontinued as soon as possible. Such compulsory treatment should be followed by an adequate period of aftercare and supervision after discharge, and hospital treatment could possibly often be cut short by a system of parole, e.g. to a hostel. As in all such schemes, built-in research evaluation programmes should be part and parcel of such programmes.

However, in general, arguments and discussions about the need or otherwise for compulsory treatment measures are usually shelved on the grounds that there is no adequate proof that it would work, and that 'voluntary' measures would be better. While everyone would agree that voluntary treatment would be preferable – if patients would agree to have it, the present laissez-faire policy, in this writer's view, means that quite a few sufferers from alcoholism and drug dependence whose health could at least be temporarily restored or at least greatly improved, will die prematurely or unnecessarily.

One difficult point in this connection must still be remembered. Just like 'voluntary' treatment, compulsory therapy could be expected to work best in the case of those people for whom one would be most reluctant to employ it, e.g. the middle-aged, fairly stable alcoholic who in the past has achieved a fair degree of socio-economic stability and has since fallen on bad times. On the other hand, little success could be expected in the case of the young anti-social alcohol or drug user suffering from an underlying character disorder, who usually can expect little help from voluntary treatment either.

In the UK under the Mental Health Act 1959, Sections 29, 25, 26 and 60 provide in certain cases grounds for the hospital admission of alcoholic or drug dependent patients – though not primarily because of alcoholism or drug dependence but because of their disturbed mental state in general [17]. Similarly Section 4 of the Criminal Justice Act makes it possible, with the consent of the sufferer, to impose a Condition of Residence in hospital of up to one year.

Although alcoholics and drug addicts are sick people, for some reason or other there will always be those among them who, because of offences related to their compulsive drinking or drug taking, will find themselves in **prison.** A recent Home Office Working Party Report on Habitual Drunken Offenders [17] recommended a whole series of changes, including sobering-up stations and varying types of hostels for such people, which should replace the present useless cycle of repeated fines or short term imprisonment. However, it is clear that some time will elapse until these suggested changes can be implemented. Until then such people – of whom a considerable proportion are genuine alcohol 'addicts' with evidence of chemical dependence [18] – will often be sent to prison, as may be other alcoholics and drug dependent individuals who run foul of the law. It should be possible to establish in a few selected prisons proper 'units' for their treatment, to be run on the lines of therapeutic communities, with a well-trained and sympathetic, understanding staff, possibly with the provision that a certain period, in the case of cooperative offenders, could be spent in hostels whilst working outside prison; any misdemeanours would automatically lead to loss of privileges. In this way a more constructive regime could be established which might help in the rehabilitation of a certain proportion of these people [4, 10].

In the 'host', predisposition or 'vulnerability' often plays an important role in the causation of alcohol and drug dependence; care has to be taken whilst treating such patients not to **substitute** one type of drug abuse and dependence for another. For example, the 'psychogenic' alcoholic (whose alcoholism is psychological in origin) – in contrast to the 'sociogenic' alcoholic (whose alcoholism is mainly social in origin) – may often act as if he feels two tablets might do him double as much good as one. Thus a practitioner who prescribes barbiturates in an attempt to wean him from his alcoholism, might possibly succeed, but only at the high price of substituting a state of barbiturate dependence in place of alcoholism. In fact, barbiturates and alcohol in some ways resemble each other so much that World Health Organisation experts placed these two drugs into one and the same bracket [19]. But alcoholics have also been found to readily abuse non-barbiturate hypnotics, such as glutethimide, methyprylone paraldehyde, methaqualone (in the form of the proprietary preparation 'mandrax'), etc., the tranquilliser meprobamate, and the stimulating amphetamines. Thus great care must be taken in the treatment of alcoholics to minimise or to avoid the prescribing of these dependence-producing agents, and as far as possible non-dependence-producing drugs should be prescribed instead. Naturally the same principle holds good for addicts to 'other drugs'. It is interesting to note that many of the drugs more recently favoured by young drug 'addicts' are the same which years ago were formerly (and still are today) abused by alcoholics. Thus in recent years on the English drug scene many youngsters abused amphetamines, including drinaryl methylamphetamine, and more recently barbiturates and 'mandrax' – often refusing the alternatives offered to them by the doctor, such as the benzdiazepines (chlordiazepoxide, diazepam) or the hypnotic nitrazepam; and Glutethimide at one time was very popular among American drug addicts [20]. Likewise in our experience among alcoholics the abuse of amphetamines, barbiturates, mandrax, and glutetimide ('Doriden') in the past was common, of the benzdiazepines very rare [10]. Changing over from alcohol to the opiates among recovered alcoholics and vice versa, from opiates dependence to alcoholism, seems much rarer in England than in the USA. But quite clearly the possibility that emotionally unstable and 'vulnerable' personalities with a psychological readiness [6] to escape into drug abuse, may easily switch from one addictive agent to another must always be kept in mind in the treatment of these people.

Naturally the therapeutic use of tranquillisers, hypnotics and anti-depressants cannot always be avoided in these patients who so often suffer from anxiety, tension, depression, insomnia etc., especially in the early post-withdrawal as well as during the withdrawal period. Probably no CNS-affecting drug is quite free from the risk of leading to dependence, particularly in unstable personalities, and in particular in those individuals who have already proven themselves 'prone' or predisposed towards the development of dependence in the past. But care should be taken to choose those drugs which seem, so far, to have shown relatively less abuse liability; among the tranquillisers the phenothiazines and the benzdiazepines; among hypnotics non-barbiturates, in particular (at the present state of knowledge) nitrazepam; and the modern non-stimulating anti-depressant drugs in place of the CNS stimulating amphetamines. Care should also be taken to discontinue all such drugs used as soon as possible, as for example even chlordiazepoxide and diazepam have been found occasionally, after much heavier and prolonged administration, to lead to dependence [35, 41].

Another question to be considered is the use of these drugs in later phases, during the after-care and rehabilitation period (as different from the withdrawal and immediate post-withdrawal period), as for, example, in the alcoholic who from time to time may be assailed by what AA members call 'dry drunk' episodes of tension or depression, and these can of course be quite common in drug addicts who try to keep away from their drugs of dependence. In principle, it would of course be better to keep away from CNS-affecting agents altogether in the long-term therapy of such people. But although 'hope is better than dope' [21], sometimes judicious, temporary, moderate employment of mild tranquillisers and antidepressants may help these patients to get over periods of tension and depression which might otherwise carry a great risk of provoking a relapse into drinking. From his knowledge of the patient's personality and vulnerability, the doctor has the very difficult task to assess whether the patient may be capable of tolerating this particular episode of tension and overcoming the hurdle without the help of drugs – and thereby use it as a challenge, an opportunity to grow up emotionally and to develop his own adaptive potentialities – or whether he will be more likely to fall by the wayside, so that for a period tranquillisers or antidepressants may be indicated [22]. However, in the long run, clearly the alcoholic's and drug addict's hope of a happy future rests on the foundations of re-education and emotional reorientation, rather than on chemical tranquillisation, sedation or stimulation [22].

In the hands of various observers, quite different therapeutic techniques have achieved success in the case of some alcoholics and drug addicts, only to fail abysmally in the hands of others. It has therefore been argued that possibly all these different techniques may work on the basis of a **common denominator,** i.e. the *breakdown* of old-established, long cherished *attitudes* to such an extent that the way is free for the development of diametrically opposite attitudes, and a totally changed outlook [23, 24]. Such personality disruption might, for example, possibly result from the chemical aversion therapies for alcoholism (by apomorphine or emetine, rarely used in the past also for other forms of drug dependence), the frightening, fear of death provoking experience of the disulfiram-alcohol reaction, Wesley's technique of frightening his listeners with 'hell and brimstone' before offering them a way out, the 'conversion' experience of some AA members, and also the 'rock bottom' concept of AA. Similarly, there is the uncovering process of analytic psychotherapy, and the frequently very aggressive, possibly often traumatic techniques employed by the newer self-help organisation of drug 'addicts' such as 'Synanon' and the 'encounter' groups of 'Phoenix' and 'Marathon'. Possibly all these techniques may be so traumatic to the patient's ego that his old attitudes become shattered and he becomes ready and 'motivated' to search for alternative, more constructive ways of trying to cope with his inner (emotional) and external problems and obstacles.

However, a common denominator might also lie, perhaps, not so much in the type of therapeutic techniques used but in the attitude of the therapist, i.e. his ability to 'get through' to the patient and to build up a *helping relationship* to him [10]. After all, the same techniques which proved so valuable in the hands of some therapists, failed with others; and many wonder-drugs and techniques over the years have come (found extremely helpful by their initiators, who had extreme faith in them) and gone, because others lacking belief in their value failed to reproduce the successful results of the originator of the new technique. Nobody is likely to have much success in treating alcoholics (or drug addicts) who approaches them with a censoring, moralistic, or even ridiculing attitude, and in a 'holier-than-thou' spirit. On the other hand, an approach based on understanding and genuine emotional acceptance (which implies much more than just paying lip-service to the disease concept of alcoholism or drug dependence) will often get a long way. Understanding and accepting such patients does, of course, not mean that all their activities are approved of, but, on the contrary, the therapist who has been able to build up such a genuine, helping relationship to the patient, will often be in a good position to convey to him that certain behaviours are in fact not in his best interest – and the patient will be willing to accept such strictures from this therapist whilst rejecting them scornfully, and as evidence of rejection, when coming from another therapist.

Obviously, success or failure in the treatment of alcoholic and drug dependent patients rests on many factors, among the most important ones probably being the degree of emotional stability of the underlying personality, and – to some extent correlated with it – record of his past social (domestic, occupational, residential) stability. The greater this stability, the better – provided other factors are equal – his **prognosis.** Thus it is impossible to compare the treatment results obtained by different authors with each other, without having an idea of the composition of the 'material'. Most therapists will do well if the great majority of their patients are basically well adjusted, relatively stable personalities who became dependent on alcohol or other drugs either at a time of abnormally severe emotional stress (e.g. death of a close relative) or perhaps as a consequence of social pressure – such as the need to conform to the customs of their immediate social environment, their 'subculture' (so important in the case of the modern young drug addict) [9] – or as a result of continual occupational exposure and temptation, which may explain the prevalence of alcoholism in such occupations as publicans and their wives, waiters, journalists, merchant seamen, etc., or of drug dependence in doctors, nurses, etc. Even in such groups, clearly not all people exposed to the same experiences and influences become dependent, so that the 'host' factor must play a certain role even then. But provided environmental manipulation, removal of precipitating traumatic factors etc., to a certain degree is possible, the outlook for such patients is not too bad. On the other hand, all therapists will have a high proportion of therapeutic failures if among their patients there happen to be a high proportion of 'psychopathic' patients whose basic trouble is the underlying character disorder, with alcoholism or drug dependence no more than one – and possibly not the most important – facet of their emotional disturbances.

Whether social or psychological therapy [25] is relatively more important, may to some extent depend on the circumstances in which a person became dependent. In countries [6] (or occupational groups) [10] in which drinking or drug taking is widespread and socially accepted, even emotionally relatively stable personalities may take to heavy drinking or to drug taking: thereby under such conditions even the fairly stable may become heavy drinkers (and some among them alcoholics) or become dependent on drugs – and without necessarily feeling very guilty or secretive about it. Such personalities may require less psychotherapy, though supportive advice or 'counselling' may be necessary, and attention will have to be directed to their social or occupational environment, as, for example, removal from the influence of their 'subculture'. On the other hand, in countries, or socio-occupational groups where heavy drinking is taboo (and similar considerations may apply to heavy drinking in women), in the main psychologically 'vulnerable' personalities will expose themselves to the risk of social censorship and become excessive drinkers or drug takers. In such cases, psychotherapy will play a more important role – e.g. such people may also be more beset by guilt feelings, depression, and their prognosis as a group will be less favourable than that of the first group. Jellinek developed this **acceptance-vulnerability theory** [6] with regard to the national differences between the more sociogenic French alcoholic and the more 'psychogenic' Anglo-Saxon alcoholic.

The **prognosis** is in general better for alcoholics than for people dependent on other drugs – perhaps partly for the reasons discussed in the preceding paragraph. As in Western culture alcohol has become a 'domesticated drug' [6] and its consumption sanctioned by tradition and culture and encouraged by society, even relatively stable people can become excessive drinkers and thereby run the risk of alcoholism. Because of this, their personality and social stability will be on the average better than that of the hypothetical average drug addict who, in Western culture, had to break social taboos and the law in order to get hold of drugs (e.g. opiates, cocaine) e.g. by manipulating doctors into prescribing excessive amounts for him, or by forging prescriptions etc. Thus often the future addict's personality may have been from the beginning more unstable than that of the future alcoholic. For similar reasons, women alcoholics may be on the average more unstable personalities than male alcoholics, and in general young alcoholics and drug addicts more unstable than the middle-aged: after all, it often took the middle-aged alcoholic many years before his personality resistance was so broken down that he became an overt alcoholic, whereas the resilience of the younger alcoholics was probably slight from the beginning. Again, prognosis on the whole would be better in such persons who have become alcoholics or drug addicts mainly (or at least partly) because of occupational temptation and exposure, or because of social pressure exerted by a 'subculture' e.g. publicans who drifted into alcoholism, doctors and nurses who become dependent on barbiturates or opiates, or students who started on cannabis and later LSD use mainly because it was the 'done' thing in their circles), should, on the whole, have a fair prognosis. But clearly this may again depend largely on the possibility to change the 'noxious' environment, as otherwise the temptation and exposure will continue. As such a change is as a rule not possible in the case of people whose livelihood is involved, treatment in these, too, may mainly consist in helping them to adjust, and learn to adopt better 'coping' mechanisms than in the past.

In general, prognosis for alcoholics is much better than generally believed by the lay and professional public alike; roughly two alcoholics in three – in an unselected sample – can be expected to improve greatly under an adequate therapeutic regime [10]. This knowledge, if imparted by doctors to alcoholics and their families, should give them hope and encouragement. Many female alcoholics too – though their outlook may be on the whole less good – can recover or improve greatly. Unemployed, single, homeless alcoholics etc. naturally require a more comprehensive regime of support and after-care than employed, skilled alcoholics with family support [17]. The length and strength of support and after-care required in alcoholics and addicts is inversely proportional to the stability of personality, and the availability of stabilising factors in terms of family, employment, residence, etc.

The prognosis of addicts to other drugs, as a whole, is by no means as hopeless as often assumed. Some years ago a WHO Study Group [26] pointed out that the majority of addicts the world over belong to the category of 'easy amenability to treatment', i.e. those whose drug dependence was 'not due to a primary personality disorder': e.g. those whose drug dependence originated from incidental stress, especially in countries where the drugs used were freely available and inexpensive; or mainly from social, environmental or cultural factors; or during the course of serious illness. Fortunately the group of those drug dependent individuals who were 'less amenable to treatment' and whose drug dependence was superimposed on 'a basically pathological character structure' was held to be numerically smaller, consisting of immature, narcistic personalities with low frustration tolerance and 'poorly developed ego and superego'.

However, even in the young, immature, narcotic addicts – with possibly the worst prognosis of all forms of drug dependence – one has to remember that only recently have definite attempts been made to learn more about them and to carry out proper research into adequate methods of treatment and rehabilitation. Various, newer techniques have helped in the recovery of a minority among them. Possibly, as suggested by Winnick [27] some narcotic addicts may in their thirties 'mature out' of their addiction – and methods which help them to stay alive up to then, may therefore assist greatly in their ultimate recovery. Here again, better training and greater interest of doctors should in the future play an important role.

Doctors, like all other healing professions, should keep in mind that all forms of drug dependence are essentially **relapsing disorders,** and that many patients only recover after a number of unsuccessful attempts. Early failures should therefore not be regarded by the doctor as a failure of all therapeutic attempts but as a challenge to try again – and again; and such failures should not be taken by the doctor as a personal affront. Again, as already stressed before, in many patients with a very limited personality potentiality, even partial successes and realistic goals are important.

As so many alcoholics and drug addicts will fail to recover, clearly the task of **prevention** is all-important. We have already seen how doctors by instituting research, by setting an example to the general public in accepting and propagating the illness concept of alcoholism, and thereby reducing the stigma, and by early detection and diagnosis ('secondary prevention') can greatly contribute in this task [10].

However, complete preoccupation and reliance on the task of prevention to the exclusion of therapy – with the implication that interest in treatment may detract from taking prophylactic measures – is surely unrealistic. Drug addicts often claim that all their troubles stem from malaise of society, and similarly some sociologists [16] state that the only sensible approach would be to eradicate these ills of society which give rise to drug dependence. That social factors are of the utmost importance to the health of the community and thereby also to the prevention of drug dependence and alcoholism is beyond doubt, and they therefore require urgent attention. It is therefore right and proper to be concerned with the 'macroproblem of the society which nurtures' alcoholics and drug addicts; but 'as the hope of total prevention of drug dependence (and alcoholism) seems Utopian, the community will have to go on working steadily towards perfecting its methods of rehabilitation' [4] and like the arguments 'out-patients versus in-patients' or 'physiological v. physical v. social therapies,' so also the question 'is prevention or rehabilitation the main priority?' seems mainly academic: there is an urgent need for both, and doctors must be vitally interested in both.

Likewise the argument put forward by some sociologists [28] that society pays so much attention to problems of drug use and abuse, because it needs a scapegoat to deflect attention from its own inadequacies, is surely more than doubtful: any doctor who has been called upon to treat youngsters who have become victims of the drug abuse habit can think of quite a number of other reasons why society and the medical profession must be interested in the plight of the young drug abuser.

In general it may perhaps be said that in the withdrawal and post-withdrawal phases, drug therapies are relatively more important (although the rehabilitation process and the attempt to establish a helping relationship to the patient should already have started then), and that psychological and social methods of therapy become relatively more important in subsequent phases. However, certain **specific pharmacological therapies** are employed in the long-term treatment, i.e. the alcohol-sensitising treatment in the case of alcoholism – i.e. disulfiram or CCC (citrated calcium carbimide) and narcotic blocking agents (methadone) and narcotic antagonists (e.g. cyclazocine) in narcotic dependence. Although the modes of action in these therapeutic approaches to alcoholism and drug dependence are quite different from each other, there is that similarity between them that in either case the specific drug therapy aims at dissuading the alcohol and narcotic addict respectively from continuing with his drug of dependence by pharmacological interference with the effect of his addictive drug on him: 1. in the case of the alcoholic by (the fear of) producing a very unpleasant and dangerous reaction through stopping the further metabolic break-down of alcohol (at the acetaldehyde stage), 2. in the case of the narcotic addict by (a) either producing cross-tolerance between methadone and the opiate (such as heroin) on which the addict had become dependent, and by reducing the craving for the opiate, or (b), by preventing through the use of narcotic antagonists, the opiate addict from finding 'relief' when taking his narcotic, through the precipitation of abstinence symptoms, and by helping to forestall the development of dependence in those 'dabbling' and experimenting with opiates.

It is not too much to say that the approach to alcoholism has been revolutionised since the advent in 1935 of the fellowship of Alcoholics Anonymous [10] which in many extents has been also a forerunner of and (with several modifications) the model for several **self-help organizations** for addicts formed over the past few years. Whatever other methods may be used in the treatment of alcoholics, the therapist will find an invaluable ally in AA, the fellowship of recovered, and recovering alcoholics. Here the alcoholic – feeling misunderstood, rejected and ostracized by society – finds a body of people who have undergone similar experiences to his own, and where he feels understood, accepted, and can get a feeling of belonging; and by helping other alcoholics he gains self-confidence, self-respect and satisfaction. Meeting in AA other alcoholics who have in the past used overtime the same defence mechanisms as he has done, he soon finds he can no longer get away with these rationalisations, projections, repressions and denials. He is thus encouraged to allow his façade to disappear and learn to face up to reality.

In principle the same basic approach is employed by the addicts' newer self-help organisations [29] – Synanon, Daytop, Phoenix, Marathon, Odyssey; indeed, the first, Synanon, was started by a recovered alcoholic. Compared with AA, they are more 'aggressive' in the sense that the attitude change – which takes place more gradually in those alcoholics who stick to the AA 'programme of recovery' '12 steps' – is 'helped along' more actively by such means as the 'encounter groups' of Phoenix and Marathon, during which accusations pour forth, there is a controlled release of anger and verbal aggression, with the purpose of encouraging members to become honest and to express emotions, and so to acquire new modes of behaviour, attitudes and values. Another difference between AA and these addicts' self-help groups is the fact that AA is non-residential (although there are now all over the world also many AA groups in hospitals and prisons), AA meetings being attended, as a rule, by alcoholics who live in their own homes, who often follow their occupations etc., and who meet usually at 'closed meetings' (for alcoholics only) or at open and 'public' meetings, which are open to family, friends and the general public. Probably because of the (usually) greater disturbance of personality in narcotic addicts and of the mode of living brought about by narcotic dependence, their greater degree of immaturity and social deviance, to some extent connected with their usually much younger age than alcoholics, their greater social disruption (estrangement from parental home, lack of residence, etc.) the addict's self-help communities are residential, being run (like units and hostels for alcoholics and addicts) on the lines of a 'therapeutic community'. Apart from Synanon, the aim is usually – after dependency of the drug has been altered temporarily to a dependence on the therapeutic community – to assist their members towards a 're-entry' into the community at large.

Both AA and the addicts' self-help groups are also of great value as means of education and enlightenment of the general public. AA, for example, has shown to the professional and lay public (as of course also to alcoholic newcomers) that alcoholics in their thousands can recover, and has thus helped to change the former picture of doom and gloom into one of hopefulness. In time, one may hope, these addicts' self-help organisations, may assist, too, in the gradual change of the public image of the drug addict.

The principle of the **'therapeutic community'** – employed by the addicts' self-help organisations – is also the basis of the approach in alcoholism and addiction 'units' and hostels [4, 10]. For example, in the UK two Government Memoranda have recommended — for those alcoholics who require hospitalisation-treatment in regional alcoholism units (of which there are now about 15) which are to work in association with GPs, local authorities, voluntary organisations, AA, etc. The 'therapeutic community' approach – introduced into psychiatry by Maxwell Jones [30] – in such units is combined with another basic principle, discovered by AA, i.e. the ability of alcoholics easily to identify with each other and thereby to learn from and to help each other by mutual understanding. In a therapeutic community the old hospital hierarchical system has been abandoned, and all grades of staff and patients work together towards a common goal, aiming at on as much active patients' participation, initiative, responsibility and self-government as possible. Everything occurring during the 24-hour day in close living, working, playing together can be observed and discussed, and thus used to therapeutic purpose. The aim of treatment in such a therapeutic community goes thus far beyond mere withdrawal and detoxification – which is largely a chemical process – and deals also with post-withdrawal and the early rehabilitation phases, though it is impressed on the patient that it still constitutes only the first step in a much longer drawn-out, long-term rehabilitation process [4].

Obviously such 'units' – which should have out-patient and hostel facilities, etc. – should also provide help with social and occupational problems, they should have access to facilities for vocational guidance and possibly occupational training, facilities for education, etc. They also provide excellent opportunities for professional and lay education and for research [10, 14].

Similarly alcoholic hostels, such as those for discharged hospital patients, for ex-prisoners or for habitual drunkenness offenders (for example Rathcoole House in London [18]) are largely based on similar considerations. As already discussed – these various types of alcoholics require a tailoring of the exact therapeutic and management regime to their varying socio-occupational-educational backgrounds and potentialities, etc.

Most alcoholism and drug dependence units and group-therapy sessions nowadays probably mix male and female patients, but should treatment facilities, for example residential units, cater both for alcoholics as well as for addicts to 'other drugs', or should they be treated separately? Should those dependent on 'soft drugs' (amphetamines, barbiturates, hallucinogens) be treated alongside opiate addicts, or not? Should those injecting the drugs – skinpoppers (i.mu.) and 'mainliners' (i.v.) – be mised with those taking them orally?

Clearly these are all questions which, for their definite answer, require much more planned research. At present opinions vary greatly. Most therapists separate alcoholics and addicts, but in our units where they have been mixed [31], despite initial difficulties – arising for example from the great differences in age between the middle-aged alcoholics and the younger addicts – in the course of time certain advantages were observed, in as far as some more mature alcoholics were able to relate well to and to help the much more immature addicts. Tensions between the more 'conforming' alcoholics and the non-conforming addicts, created by different values and life styles, abound with therapeutic opportunities which can be utilised [33] – including the possibility of 'bridging the generation gap'. Obviously the risk of bringing in drugs into open establishments (and nowadays the units for alcoholics are usually 'open') create additional surveillance problems, which in at least one instance led to the abandoning of one such experimental programme in the USA [33]. However, in our experience **mixing** in the same unit of middle-aged, 'therapeutic' (i.e. with the drug originally prescribed by a doctor) amphetamine and barbiturate **addicts and alcoholics** – with often similar psychopathology – never produced any real difficulties. We now have in our set-up alcoholics and all types of addicts living in the same wards, i.e. in the same therapeutic community, but we include the middle-aged amphetamine and barbiturate addicts in the group-therapy sessions of the alcoholics, and have separate group sessions for the younger addicts.

Likewise there are different views held about the advisability or otherwise of mixing soft and hard drug users [34]. Some observers feel that amphetamine users of the 'adaptive' type (i.e. essentially middle-aged abusers bolstering up their otherwise conventional social functioning) should not be treated in proximity with 'escapists' (i.e. usually younger amphetamine abusers escaping from conventional social functioning), or with most narcotic addicts, but in proximity with other 'medicine abusers' (of tranquillisers, antidepressants and 'some analgesic addicts who had medical or accidental onsets' [35]. Dependence on these latter types of drugs seems rare in our experience, though analgesic abuse and dependence is quite common in such European countries as Switzerland [38]. It has also been claimed that because of the risk of 'seduction', amphetamine abusers should not be treated alongside narcotic addicts, and 'fixers' – who inject their drugs (for example methylamphetamine) – not alongside oral amphetamine abusers. In our experience – administrative reasons forced us in the early 1960s to mix soft and hard drug addicts – cases of such 'seduction' were extremely rare, and did not really produce any great problems – but certainly, as already said, much further research is necessary in this field.

Care must be taken in each case not to overlook **complications** which may have arisen as direct or indirect consequences of drug abuse. These may include, for example, overdosage (common in the case of hypnotics and narcotics), possibly leading to respiratory depressions (necessitating resuscitation, narcotic antagonists, etc.) neglect of personal hygiene and food intake, to the mimicking of many neurological diseases by habitual barbiturate overdosage, infections (often – in the case of injections – a consequence of unsterile 'gear') with local and general sepsis or viral hepatitis; injuries; and mental complications such as paranoid psychosis (amphetamines), anxiety, tension, aggressive behaviour (stimulating drugs) or depression (LSD and 'come down' from stimulating drugs) with risk of suicidal attempts or gestures; states of confusion, disorientation (e.g. hypnotics, LSD), anxiety, paranoid states, panics (cannabis, LSD), 'flashbacks' into a hallucinatory state days or weeks after LSD has been taken, etc.

In all types of drug dependence withdrawal treatment must be followed by measures aimed at long-term therapy and rehabilitation. Here measures will often have to be quite different in the case of the modern type of unstable, immature, **young** multi-drug abuser, the more stable, **middle-aged** 'therapeutic' or 'professional' addict and those individuals whose drug abuse was precipitated by episodes of extreme stress, or by social pressure, such as 'subcultures' encouraging drug use. Factors depending on 'host', environment and 'agent' have all to be taken into consideration, when mapping out rehabilitation programmes in individual cases. The task is often much less difficult in the middle-aged, educated, skilled individual who has the support of family and the sheet anchor of a steady, interesting job, who often may require no more than an understanding family doctor and possibly temporarily a regime of tranquillisers and antidepressants, perhaps combined with counselling of the family; and similar conditions may prove helpful in the case of the middle-aged, barbiturate (or amphetamine)-dependent housewife. Much wider rehabilitative efforts – involving psychotherapeutic measures, education, vocational guidance, occupational training, finding of congenial homes and friends – may be needed in the case of the younger, non-therapeutic drug abuser who has in recent years become so much more common at the cost of the therapeutic, middle-aged drug abuser [9].

Measures of **prevention** will naturally cover a wide field and will have to be directed at the 'host' (for example by measures of mental hygiene in childhood by helping youngsters to find an identity somewhere else than by drug taking and antisocial activities etc.) and environment (for example influencing social attitudes, improving socio-economic conditions – although it must not be forgotten that despite modern situations of affluence drug abuse has greatly intensified) – as well as at the 'agent' (by legislative measures, as, for example, those incorporated in the new Misuse of Drugs Act 1971).

In the field of prevention of drug abuse and dependence the GP has a very important, direct role to play. To a large extent – for example in the great majority of cases of drug abuse by the middle-aged – the condition has been 'iatrogenic', the drug concerned first prescribed by a GP, and then often prescribed again and again, often in increasing doses, though usually at the insistent demand of the patient. If a patient comes again and again, insisting that only a special type of drug is of any use to him, if he keeps asking for increasing amounts etc., the greatest care is obviously necessary – but in spite of this one comes across many patients who have obtained increasing, large doses of dependence producing drugs from their own GP for longish periods, and also from doctors who did not know them whom they attended as 'temporary patients'. Even greater has been the responsibility of those few doctors who through gross over-prescribing – whatever their motives – were largely responsible for the development of the Heroin-Cocaine [9, 38] and later the methylamphetamine epidemics in England in the 1960s. Obviously better instruction in medical school [9] on the problems of drug dependence is vitally necessary. A voluntary ban on the prescribing of amphetamines has been recommended by the British Medical Association, as – narcolepsy and possibly hyperkinetic children apart – they have hardly an indication that cannot be equally well or better fulfilled by other, less harmful drugs; in particular there is no indication for their formerly so prevalent use in obesity (which caused many cases of dependence on amphetamines and phenmetrazine [Preludin]) and in depression. The tricyclic antidepressants (e.g. imipramine and related drugs such as amitriptyline and protriptyline) have so far not shown evidence of leading to dependence, whereas there have been a few cases with the MAO Inhibitors such as 'Parnate' (tranqylpromine), in particular when given in the form of 'Parstelin' (tranqylpromine plus trifluoperazine). The MAO drugs are therefore, perhaps best avoided in the treatment of alcoholics and drug abusers — the more so as they potentiate or prolong the action of opiates.

Equally there seems to be no indication for prescribing of barbiturates to young patients (except during withdrawal, and in special circumstances such as the need for phenobarbitone in epilectics etc.) or to 'temporary' patients of any age group not on the particular GP's list, without prior reference to the doctor on whose list they are. And although methadone as yet can still be prescribed to addicts by a GP, it would surely be better that newcomers, not previously notified to the Home Office, should be referred immediately for investigation to a Treatment Centre, rather than being first supplied by a GP for a few weeks with methadone, before being referred to a Treatment Centre as otherwise they can then claim that meanwhile they surely had become dependent and that they quite legitimately required further supplies.

There is another, indirect way in which medical practitioners – in particular GPs but also hospital doctors – can help in the task of prophylaxis. By becoming less generous in their prescribing of CNS affecting drugs – even considering the pressure presented by the insistent demands of too many patients clamouring for such drugs, and the insufficient time at their disposal to discuss the pros and cons with such patients in greater detail – doctors could in time begin to counteract the ever-increasing 'legitimate' drug abuse in this 'drug age'. Young drug abusers often are indignant because only their drug taking is under criticism, not that of their elders who not only drink and smoke cigarettes a great deal but who also swallow all types of pills to tranquillise or pep themselves up at daytime and to put themselves to sleep at night. Some youngsters started their drug using career by taking some of the tranquillising or stimulating tablets prescribed to their mothers by their GPs. In 1968 psychotropic drug prescriptions in Great Britain under the NHS made up one sixth of all NHS prescriptions [39]. Out of a total of 58·4 million prescriptions (which did not include hospital and private prescriptions) approximately 25 millions were for barbiturates, 12½ million for benzodiazepines, 6 million for phenothiazines, 5·5 million for non-barbiturate hypnotics, 5 million for tricyclic antidepressants, 4 million for amphetamines, nearly ½ million for MAO Inhibitors. To these prescriptions came another 20 million prescriptions for various analgesics. The journal '*Drugs in Society*' [40] comments that the 6·1 million prescriptions for phenothiazine tranquillisers represent approximately enough tablets for a month's treatment to every tenth person in the UK; there was double this number of prescriptions for the minor tranquillisers (the benzodiazepines) and the total of (barbiturate and non-barbiturate) hypnotic tablets prescribed amounts to enough pills 'to make every tenth night's sleep in the UK hypnotically induced'. Many of these prescriptions are for drugs which may more or less readily lead to dependence such as the barbiturates, the non-barbiturate hypnotics and the amphetamines. Sir Derek Dunlop [39], reporting the above figures, commented that it looked as if 'the overworked medical profession in this country may be unduly concerned with satisfying the public's "wants" rather than what we think it "needs" ', and that the extent of drug seeking by patients and the accession to such demands by doctors are disturbing features of modern medicine.

Apart from producing dependence, there are other hazards associated with the widespread use of psychotopric drugs, such as accidental and intentional self-poisoning or impairment of driving. For all these reasons it is vital that doctors should exercise great restraint in prescribing such drugs: they are not placebos and should not be the immediate, automatic answer to each and every one of the frustrations, disappointments, despondencies and anxieties' of everyday life. [39]. In this way the medical profession may contribute towards stemming the ever rising tide of consumption of such psychotropic drugs. It may thereby forestall not only many possible occurrences of deliberate and accidental overdosage and habitual drug abuse and drug dependence among their patients, but also reduce the risk of a further progression of our times into a 'drug age', where youngsters may be only too inclined not only to follow but to outdo their elders in the dangerous habit of swallowing more and more pills for less than adequate reasons.

TREATMENT OF THE VARIOUS FORMS OF ALCOHOL AND DRUG DEPENDENCE

World Health Organisation Expert Committees have listed the following main types of drug dependence [19, 37].

Alcohol type (which because of many close similarities, and of marked cross-tolerance, is often coupled with the barbiturates into a barbiturate-alcohol type)
Barbiturate type
Morphine type
Amphetamine type
Khat type
Cocaine type
Cannabis type
Hallucinogen type.

However, it must be kept in mind that in contrast to former years, among young drug addicts nowadays – in particular those in the younger age groups – the most common form of drug abuse and dependence is probably that of **misusing several types of drugs** at the same time. It is not unusual to meet young drug abusers who take any drug they can get hold of, often without bothering to ask what type of drug it is, whether it has sedative or stimulating effects, of what strength the tablets they buy on the illicit market are, etc. In England at present among youngsters attending the 'Treatment Centres' where they receive Heroin and/or Methadone, they may also at the same time buy on the illicit market the so-called 'Chinese Heroin' (containing, apart from Heroin, also caffeine and sometimes also quinine or barbiturates), amphetamines, the non-barbiturate 'Mandrax', cannabis (usually in the form of the resin Hashish) and LSD; they may also obtain some proprietary cough mixture preparations, and they often manage, by attending various GPs as 'temporary' patients, to obtain barbiturate tablets which they dissolve and inject intravenously, often together with Heroin or methadone. The result therefore is a mixed type of dependence. As far as the treatment of the acute state is concerned, as a rule, in such cases any sedative-hypnotic or narcotic drug should be tapered off gradually – for fear of the development of a physical abstinence syndrome, whereas the stimulating drugs (amphetamines and Cocaine – the abuse of the latter has over the past three years become very rare) are cut off suddenly (watching for evidence of development of depression) as are Cannabis and LSD. The doctor nowadays being called upon to treat a young drug 'addict' must therefore take great care to elicit by careful history taking, not only from the patient but also, if possible, from family and friends which combination of drugs he has been taking, for how long and in what amounts – although unfortunately this may often have to remain a counsel of perfection. This should be followed by physical examination and laboratory tests (chemical analyses of blood or urine), and by close observation after the treatment has started.

ALCOHOLISM

Acute Stage

Although sudden withdrawal of alcohol – a CNS depressing drug – occasionally leads to a severe physical abstinence syndrome – including epileptiform convulsions on the first 12–36 hours, and subsequent delirium tremens – abrupt, sudden cessation of alcohol, rather than gradual tapering off is now the method favoured by most therapists. In heavy drinkers, where the possibility of such complications is feared, it is wise to give prophylactically such medication as phenytoin (epanutin) 100 mg t.d.s., and tranquillisers (phenothiazines, benzodiazepines, or possibly chlormethiazole [10, 43, 44] (see below).

Dehydration,, salt depletion, malnutrition and restlessness require methods such as liberal administration of fluids and salt orally or parenterally, vitamins (especially the B complex) at first parenterally ('parentovite' is a favourite preparation) i.v. or i.mu. – and later orally, and tranquillisers to calm the tense, anxious, agitated and restless patient. Among tranquillising drugs all major and minor tranquillisers have been used, such as the phenothiazines: chlorpromazine (Largactie, Thorazine) 50–100 mg t.d.s. (despite the theoretical risk of liver toxicity which in practice does not seem to have provided a great problem), promazine (Sparine) 50–100 mg t.d.s., trifluoperazine (Stelazine) 5–10 mg t.d.s. and thioridazine (Melleril) 50–100 mg t.d.s. (in higher doses an anti-Parkinsonian drug should be given with the phenothiazines, e.g. Benzhexol ('Artane'). Of the 'minor' tranquillisers the benzodiazepines chlordiazepoxide (Librium) 10–30 mg t.d.s. or diazepam (Valium) 5–10 mg t.d.s. have been widely used, apparently in the USA all of them in somewhat higher dosage than in the UK. Unlike the barbiturates and meprobamate, these drugs – phenothiazines and benzodiazepines in ordinary usage carry hardly any risk of dependence (though after daily prolonged dosage of 100–150 mg Diazepam or 300–600 mg Chlordiazepoxide withdrawal convulsions have been noted [35, 41]. A recently recommended drug is Doxepin (25 mg t.d.s.) [43]. All these tranquillisers can in an average case be gradually withdrawn within about one week.

Insomnia may require the administration of hypnotics at least for the first few nights, and as barbiturates and other non-barbiturates (the latter to a somewhat lesser extent) have proved 'addictive', nitrazepam (Mogadon, 0·5–1·5 g nocte) seems at present the safest drug for that purpose.

DT

In prevention and treatment of DT the same drugs can be used, though in somewhat higher dosage or parenterally. On the European continent, especially Sweden and Germany, and also in our own experience, both for prevention and treatment of DT chlormethiazole (Heminevrin) has proved an excellent sedativehypnotic [43, 47]. It is derived from the thiazole part of the Vitamin B_1 molecule, and is available as 0·8 per cent solution for i.v. injection or infusion, and as 500 mg tablets. In severe cases of DT, treatment starts by i.v. injection of 40–60 ml of the 0·8 per cent solution over a period of 3–5 minutes, and continues (or more usually immediately starts) by an oral regime of 2–4 tablets, to be repeated within 1–2 hours, the aim being to produce profound sedation or sleep; ordinarily a maximum dosage of 9–10 g a day should not be exceeded. We have used this drug also as our routine in ordinary cases of alcohol withdrawal in alcoholics [44]. The drug should be discontinued after 6 days, as, like other CNS depressing drugs, it carries a risk of psychological and also, more rarely, physical dependence. For this reason it should not be employed as a routine hypnotic or daytime sedative in alcoholics or drug addicts. Because of some evidence that alcoholics prone to develop DT are less likely to develop dependence on 'other drugs' [45], the drug could be employed for somewhat longer periods in DT patients, if required.

A point probably not sufficiently stressed and as yet not widely appreciated even in medical circles concerns the risk of dangerous physical withdrawal symptoms supervening in heavy drinkers – such alcohol abstinence syndrome, like the barbiturate abstinence syndrome, is possibly more dangerous than the much more widely known opiate abstinence syndrome. In fact, one often hears of alcoholics who have suddenly made up their minds to give up drinking and to 'sweat it out' at home. Unless skilled medical help and nursing supervision is available at home, in the case of heavy drinkers it seems much safer under such circumstances to 'taper off' – by gradually reducing the amount of drink over the next few days – than to cut alcohol out suddenly. Much more preferable, of course, would be the admission of such a patient to detoxification centres [17] (pioneered in Czechoslovakia and Poland and proved of value in the USA – e.g. in St. Louis – and which, one hopes, will be established in the UK in the near future) or to a general hospital for a few days.

Another point concerns the frequent tendency of many (particularly the mainly psychogenic) alcoholics to take also other drugs habitually to excess, especially barbiturates. All alcoholics should therefore be questioned about their drug taking habits. Should they also habitually have taken barbiturates to excess, these should be tapered off gradually. Where they deny taking barbiturates but where there is some suspicion or doubt, phenobarbitone 100 mg t.d.s. (rather than phenytoin) should be given for the first 3–4 days and then gradually reduced and stopped. The fact that like alcohol, so also barbiturate withdrawal can lead to DT must be kept in mind.

LONG-TERM TREATMENT AND REHABILITATION [10]

Following withdrawal and detoxification, the earlier phase of the long-term treatment and rehabilitation programme could be carried out with the alcoholic remaining an in-patient – for example in a therapeutic community set-up. On the other hand, after initial withdrawal and detoxification the alcoholic could leave hospital and continue treatment as out-patient whilst living in the community. The principles were all discussed in the general section. Treatment involves a combination of psychological and social approaches with physical therapies as adjuncts.

Psychotherapy and supportive counselling

There is in general no need for a deep form of psychotherapy and psychoanalysis has not proved successful in the treatment of alcoholism [46]. Brief eclectic psychotherapeutic techniques (often based on psychoanalytic principles) have found widespread employment. The large number of alcoholics in need of treatment practically precludes individual psychotherapy for the great majority anyway, but, anyhow, partly because of the urgent need of alcoholics for resocialization, group psychotherapy is being increasingly employed as a valuable, acceptable (to patients) and effective method. The aim is for the alcoholic to gain some insight into his problems and personality difficulties – which he has tried to solve by taking recourse to drink (or drugs), and to learn to cope with tensions, anxieties etc. in a more mature and less self-destructive manner than searching oblivion in drink or drugs. That social class is often a factor in alcoholism treatment, has recently been stressed by Canadian research workers [47] who found that current clinical treatment of alcoholics favours patients from higher social classes, perhaps partly because of verbal skills involved in psychotherapy and the middleclass background of most therapists. Clearly care should be taken to make allowances for that, possibly by forming a greater variety, socially more homogeneous groups presenting fewer social barriers to interaction.

Social methods

Social support is necessary in a great many alcoholics, its extent depending on the lack of social adjustment, home and occupational circumstances etc. The need to include the patient's family in the treatment situation, to assist the patient in finding suitable accommodation (including hostels), a congenial job, etc. has already been stressed.

Physical treatments

Two different types of approaches have found more or less widespread use:

(*a*) Drugs which sensitise the body to alcohol, such as disulfiram ('antabuse') and citrated calcium carbimide ('abstem', 'temposil'). They act as conscious deterrents against drinking, provided the alcoholic has become fully convinced that if he were foolish enough to risk drinking within 3–4 days, or 36 hours, on top of disulfiram and CCC respectively, he would be likely to suffer extremely distressing (and dangerous) symptoms: e.g. flushing, feeling faint and sick, breathless, feeling like dying etc. Most observers no longer regard a preliminary alcohol-disulfiram test as necessary. The procedure is for the alcoholic regularly to take a maintenance dose – for example ½ tablet of 'antabuse' (i.e. 200 mg) in the evening, or a tablet of 'abstem' (1 g) in the morning. CCC is slightly less effective than disulfiram, its 'protective' effect starts more rapidly and also wanes earlier than that of disulfiram. Given such minimum maintenance dosage, serious side effects from taking these drugs, for example peripheral neuropathy, are very rare. Obviously it is easy for the alcoholic to stop taking these tablets – and, as in the case of any other method, its success depends on the therapist's ability to arouse a motivation in the alcoholic to try to abstain from drinking. Thus these drugs – like other physical treatments are no more than adjuncts to the more fundamental socio-psychological techniques. Yet in the hands of the GP who is able to establish a positive relationship to his alcoholic patient, his use of such drugs, perhaps combined with referral to AA, may in many early-stage alcoholics provide a very efficient and successful approach.

A more recently introduced drug – metronidazole ('Flagyl') – claimed to have some disulfiram-like properties, and to diminish alcohol withdrawal symptoms and craving [48], has not yet been sufficiently evaluated to allow more definite conclusions.

(b) Aversion techniques: pharmacological methods (apomorphine [49] or emetine [23] and, more recently reintroduced, electric shock techniques have been employed to induce in the alcoholic a conditioned aversion towards the sight, smell and taste of alcohol. The principle consists in associating the taking of alcohol with an unpleasant experience. These methods have, of course, to be carried out in hospital. Although at one time very popular, especially in private practice, nowadays consensus of opinion is probably that at best such conditioning techniques are no more than adjuvants to psychosocial methods.

Clearly, before carrying out any of these physical techniques, a thorough physical and laboratory investigation is required, including urinalysis, liver function tests and ECG and probably blood analysis; and in the case of the aversion techniques, nursing staff well versed in these particular methods must be available.

(c) Other drugs sometimes employed: LSD for some time enjoyed a certain vogue in the treatment of alcoholics, but again it is probably fair to say that few therapists would now feel that there is a real indication for it in the treatment of alcoholics – although further research is indicated [50].

The occasional use of tranquillisers and antidepressives [51] (but not barbiturates or amphetamines and related drugs) to tide alcoholics over occasional emotional crises and periods of difficulties has already been referred to.

Alcoholics Anonymous

AA and its 'sister' organisation – Al Anon (and also Alateen, for the adolescent relatives of alcoholics) are the most valuable allies of the doctor in the rehabilitation of alcoholics. On its own AA – without any professional help – has assisted more alcoholics to a contented state of sobriety than all professional disciplines taken together. AA regards alcoholism as a sickness of body, mind and spirit, social (group), psychological and spiritual factors all entering into the AA programme of recovery. Some of its principles have been discussed above. AA is only too happy to cooperate with doctors and other professionals. There are now groups all over the British Isles (and even more so in the USA, where it was founded 37 years ago). Two additional points: as the image of 'the' alcoholic is based on the 'loss of control' alcoholic – the person who having had one drink, cannot be certain of being able to call a halt on that occasion – the GP when recommending other types of alcoholics to 'join' AA, should explain the difference to his patient so as to forestall misunderstandings. The GP, too, who has recommended disulfiram or CCC to his patient, should stress to him not to be put off taking these tablets by occasional ill-informed adverse comment from a few over-enthusiastic AA members who feel that because they have done well with AA alone, any drug treatment is superfluous. Just as doctors have no monopoly in treating alcoholics and should cooperate with AA as far as possible, it is likewise clear that by itself no single agency – not even AA – can successfully treat all alcoholics. By itself, AA is probably the most successful single agency, but as there are so many different types of alcoholics, there is an absolute need for close, integrated collaboration of all interested agencies.

The GP will also find the greatest help from close cooperation with Al Anon, the organisation of families of alcoholics. Referring the desperate wife of an alcoholic to that organisation where she finds kindred souls with similar experiences, frustrations etc., such a wife (or husband of an alcoholic woman) will find great help from finding others in a similar position. She may thus develop a different attitude, find new hope, and in this altered frame of mind may be able to approach her alcoholic husband in quite a different way from before – which in turn may have positive consequences on his behaviour in the future.

Complications

Prior to establishing a treatment programme, a full physical examination and certain laboratory tests should be carried out. Alcoholism, like all other forms of dependence, apart from the socio-psychological consequences arising out of the state of dependence, can lead to physical complications. Some of these are reversible, such as polyneuropathy (treated by Vitamin B complex in high doses, to start with parenterally, later orally, physiotherapy etc.) sometimes associated with memory defects and confabulations (Korsakoff's Syndrome – which may improve to a major or lesser extent), Wernicke's Syndrome (high Vitamin B complex parenterally), reversible fatty infiltration of the liver; or irreversible liver cirrhosis – which, however, under a regime of total abstinence and balanced diet, may be stationary for many years. These physical as well as the mental complications (alcoholic paranoia, dementia etc.) require separate treatment – quite apart from the overriding need for lifelong abstinence.

Can alcoholics learn to drink in moderation?

In spite of the publication of occasional case reports of a few 'cured' alcoholics apparently having managed for years to drink in moderation, at the present state of knowledge the rule must still remain that alcoholics have to learn to accept, without resentment or bitterness, the fact that drink is definitely out for them. Quite a few alcoholics manage in fact to drink moderately for short periods, by clinging to certain rules: such as beer or wine only, drinking with meals and in company only, drinking very small amounts only, or only when in a cheerful, relaxed frame of mind etc. [10]. But sooner or later in almost all cases these attempts are doomed to failure. It is true that the future for an alcoholic who for so long had considered alcohol as practically his only ally and standby, initially may sound bleak and miserable indeed without alcohol; but the GP can make use of a technique used by AA, i.e. for the alcoholic to live a day at a time: he may find the task of living without alcohol for one day easily manageable, and tomorrow is another day which will be tackled when it comes along. In this way, the sober days will mount to weeks, then to months – and the doctor will be able to assure the alcoholic that once he has managed six and more months without a drink, the going will become easier [52] – though every alcoholic must for ever beware of neglectful overconfidence. The doctor can also reassure his alcoholic patient that many thousands of male and female alcoholics have found life without alcohol not only tolerable but also happy and full. Naturally, when joining AA he will meet numerous examples of recovered alcoholics, a visual demonstration which will give him hope. By helping other alcoholics, once he himself has been off alcohol for a certain period, he will also do a great deal to help himself (AA's '12-Step' Work, 'Sponsorship').

In the overall approach to alcoholism the family doctor has a key role to play: not only as a very important member of the therapeutic team but also by setting an example to the general public in, and in educating it towards, accepting the alcoholic as a sick man who can be helped and who is well worth helping.

DEPENDENCE OF THE BARBITURATE TYPE

Whilst the protagonists of this type are the barbiturates, very similar features occur also in the case of dependence on non-barbiturate hypnotics and sedatives, and the tranquilliser meprobamate [41]. Though not yet included in the WHO descriptions, chlormethiazole dependence seems to belong to the same type (as does paraldehyde). There is development of psychological dependence and – after consumption of slightly more than the usual therapeutic dose for some time (e.g. 0·6–0·8 g/day for 35–57 days [53] – also physical dependence, with the supervening of a dangerous physical abstinence syndrome when dosage is suddenly reduced below a critical level. Because tolerance is irregular and incomplete, there is disturbance of behaviour and a state of chronic intoxication which often resembles that seen in long-standing alcoholism. Treatment in all these forms of dependence resembles that described for alcohol dependence.

Acute stage

These drugs must never be suddenly withdrawn but 'tapered off' gradually, in the case of barbiturates for example by about 0·1 g every second day. Reduction should be stopped temporarily for a few days when signs such as tremor, anxiety, insomnia etc. appear. In cases of persistent anxiety and depression following withdrawal, smallish doses of benzodiazepines and antidepressants (not amphetamines) could be given. Vitamin medication is indicated where there is evidence of undernutrition, as for example in the modern type of youngish 'mainliners' of barbiturates. In cases of insomnia, Nitrazepam seems the most suitable drug at the moment. During barbiturate withdrawal watch should be kept for evidence of serious depression and possible suicidal attempts.

In the modern cases of multiple drug dependence, withdrawal of the various drugs can be carried out simultaneously. In the case of dependence on the popular barbiturate-amphetamine preparations (e.g. 'drinamyl') the drug should be tapered off as described above.

Withdrawal DT

The best method is probably to reintroduce smaller doses of the drug concerned, and withdraw it slowly after a few days. Alternatively, high doses of a phenothiazine (e.g. chlorpromazine 100–150 mg t.d.s.), or paraldehyde 10 mil i.mu. or, perhaps best, chlormethiazole (as described in the alcoholism section) can be given.

Post-withdrawal phase, long-term treatment and rehabilitation

The principles have been outlined in previous sections. There is, of course, a great difference here between the rehabilitation needs of the modern young initially and of the **middle-aged addicts** – who usually have been introduced to the drugs by their GP ('therapeutic addict'). The latter may often still have the stabilising influence of home, husband and family, and although in their case, too, the condition may tend to relapse, their chances are not too bad. It is interesting to note that under similar conditions of stress where men may tend to fall back on alcohol, women may often prefer to rely on barbiturates. This probably reflects an environmental factor, i.e. the different social attitude towards public heavy drinking by females as compared to heavy male drinking.

The state of **chronic intoxication** – with features such as ataxia, confusion, disorientation, slurred speech etc. – usually responds fairly rapidly to the regimen of rest, gradual reduction of barbiturates, vitamin medication (if there is evidence of neglect of nutrition), non-barbiturate hypnotics when an hypnotic is needed, possibly followed later on in states of continuing tension or depression, by minor tranquillisers and/or antidepressants. In as far as, to a certain extent, the psychopathology of middle-aged barbiturate abusers resembles that of alcoholics, we have for many years included such patients in groups formed predominantly by alcoholics. There seemed little difficulty in mutual identification, in particular as the alcoholics' groups always included a certain proportion of drinkers who also had habitually misused barbiturates.

Individual psychological support, counselling, or brief psychotherapy may occasionally be required to help these patients to cope with inner stresses and outer problems (domestic, marital, business etc.) from which they initially had sought refuge in excessive drug taking. In general, as with alcoholics, the outlook for middle-aged barbiturate addicts is not too bad – though probably less good than in the case of alcoholics, depending again mainly on the ego strength and stability of the underlying personality, his or her history of residential, domestic and – in male addicts – occupational stability, and the support available from family, friends and occupation. No drug therapy comparable to disulfiram is available in the case of dependence on barbiturates (or on other 'soft' drugs).

Quite different is the case of the **young barbiturate abuser.** Whereas in the USA barbiturates have always been abused also by young drug misusers, youngsters in the UK until a few years ago always maintained that hypnotic drugs (and alcohol) were not for them: they – the youth – wanted stimulation (by amphetamines) or consciousness – expansion by cannabis and hallucinogens, not 'sleepers'. However, over the past few years, English drug addicts have also taken to the misuse of barbiturates – mainly 'Nembutal' and 'Tuinal' – which they dissolved and mainlined. Another great favourite is the non-barbiturate hypnotic 'Mandrax' (the hypnotic methqualone combined with the antihistamine diphenhydramine) which is taken orally. All these drugs are often taken in greatly excessive doses, producing a state of subacute or chronic intoxication, with the danger of acute overdosage – not infrequently fatal; local abscesses at the site of injection, septicaemia etc., viral hepatitis etc. (Mandrax, incidentally, is claimed by these youngsters to give them rapidly a feeling of 'high' or of being intoxicated, especially if combined with a few drinks). The complications arising from intravenous self-injections are worse in the case of barbiturates than with methylamphetamine, opiate and cocaine injections – but at any rate in the UK practically all youngsters taking barbiturates to excess are multi-drug abusers, as a rule also taking cannabis and amphetamines, and often Heroin, methadone and LSD. After the gradual withdrawal of the barbiturates and attention to the physical state and complications, the treatment and rehabilitation problems are therefore the same as discussed in the case of other young drug abusers in the following chapters. In fact, as a rule, young British barbiturate abusers claim that they have been 'driven' to the use of 'sleepers' as a consequence of the policy of the specialised Treatment Centres which did not provide them with as much 'stuff' (Heroin, or more recently methadone) as they 'need'. The problem of barbiturate abuse by British youngsters is therefore intimately bound up with the approach to the problem of the young heroin addict.

DEPENDENCE OF THE MORPHINE TYPE

This type, with strong psychological dependence, rapid development of physical dependence and tolerance, is seen in habitual misusers of opium, morphine, heroin etc., as well as of synthetic products, such as methadone, pethidine, dextromoramide etc. As in the case of the barbiturates, there is in many ways a fundamental difference between young non-therapeutic addicts on the one hand and the relatively more stable middle-aged addicts on the other. The latter may have started their drug abusing career as a consequence of being prescribed opiates during the course of a severe, painful illness ('therapeutic addicts'). These few may later have managed to keep on a relatively stable dosage and to function fairly well ('stabilised addicts'), although such occurrence by and large seems to be relatively rare. There is also the group of usually middle-aged 'professional addicts' (doctors, nurses etc.) in whom easy access and availability may have been important factors once such people at a time of strain and stress had started on the drug. Similarly the largely middle-aged opium smokers in the Far East seem a very different group [53] from the young, modern type of narcotic addicts in the UK and in the USA, their opium smoking in the 'dens' to a large extent being related to long-standing customs and poor material living conditions (in this respect resembling the Heroin abuse among New Yorks's slum dwellers) rather than to marked personality problems. Given the possibility of changing environmental conditions to a certain extent – in cases where such dependence was mainly a consequence of environmental, social, cultural factors (e.g. acceptance of drug taking among a certain group) – many such addicts would come under the heading of 'easy amenability to treatment'. The problem is much greater in the group of youngish Heroin addicts in whom personality instability may have been a marked contributory factor in the escalation from 'soft drugs' (cannabis, amphetamines) – used widely among their peers – to the 'hard drugs' (from which the majority of their peers had shied away). 'Subcultural' factors often also play a role in these young drug abusers; and in treatment both sets of factors – personality and environment – require urgent and often long-continuing attention, by such means as psychotherapeutic support, counselling, help with social problems etc. It must be remenbered that addicts – in particular narcotic addicts – do not revert to ordinary 'normal' functioning for some time after withdrawal, and that psychological after-effects may linger on for a long period.

Withdrawal

After full assessment of the personality and environmental factors in the given individual, after physical examination (complications) and laboratory investigations, it may occasionally be decided to delay withdrawal in view of certain physical complications (infections, severe malnutrition, etc.) or because for some reason or other a 'maintenance' or a very gradual method of withdrawal is adopted. Where it is decided to proceed with withdrawal immediately, the addict's fear of the 'cold turkey' – i.e. withdrawal without any adequate substition drugs – should be allayed: narcotic withdrawal symptoms (diarrhoea, severe abdominal cramps, aches all over etc.) can often be indeed very severe, and it would seem inhumane to subject addicts to such a regime when today adequate, humane and effective methods of withdrawal are available. It is necessary to state this clearly, as very often addicts use their fear of the 'cold turkey' as an alibi not to come for withdrawal treatment at all, and to continue their drug taking. It is remarkable, however, that the narcotic drug self-help organisations manage to tide their newcomer addicts over these very distressing withdrawal phases without the help of drugs, mainly by support from the groups – which of course reflects the very high motivation of addicts who have decided to join these organisations. But in hospital or in prison there is no place for such severe regimes.

Methods of withdrawal

Of the regimes formerly described in textbooks and, for example, in a report of a Study Group of the WHO in 1957 [26] most have been abandoned by now, such as the withdrawal of narcotics under cover of such substances as barbiturates or meprobamate (a treatment regime which itself carried the hazard of additional forms of dependence), scopolamine, or with the help of ECT or insulin. In certain circumstances gradual withdrawal under cover of phenothiazines – as mentioned in that report – may possibly still be tried. Certain supportive therapy, such as intravenous fluids, cardiovascular stimulants etc., will be required occasionally and should be readily available. However, the method usually employed nowadays for rapid withdrawal, very effective and carrying little risk, is the substitution method with methadone.

Methadone (known in the UK under its proprietary name 'Physeptone') is a synthetic opiate analgesic with similar actions to morphine, but longer lasting. It produces psychic and physical dependence; withdrawal symptoms are less severe (though more prolonged) than those of morphine or heroin dependence. In the withdrawal treatment of heroin and morphine addicts methadone is temporarily substituted for H or Mo and then itself gradually withdrawn over a period of roughly 7–10 days, the amount and the duration of the medication depending on objective abstinence signs and not on the history as given by the patient. Methadone is usually given orally (parenteral medication only rarely being necessary) – for example as Syrup of Methadone in a dose of 10 or 20 mg, to be repeated when abstinence signs persist. According to Blachly [55], American addicts only rarely require more than 40 mg during a 24 hour period; English addicts who, at least in part, have often taken a higher Heroin dosage may sometimes need a greater amount of methadone. When withdrawal symptoms subside, methadone is gradually withdrawn, the dose being reduced by 5 mg every 12 or 24 hours. 1 mgm methadone is said to equal 1 mg Heroin, 3 mg morphine (and 30 mg Codeine) [55].

Methadone, of course, is itself an addictive drug; at present the number of 'known' English addicts using methadone is higher than that of Heroin addicts. A drug found to carry only a slight addictive risk and, because of its unsuitability for parenteral injection, having a much smaller hazard of misuse, is the anti-diarrhoeal agent, diphenoxylate, a congener of Pethidine [56]. Preliminary trials of diphenoxylate (in form of 'Lomotil') – combined with the hypnotic-sedative drug chlormethiazole – have shown it to be a possible alternative to methadone in the withdrawal treatment of opiate addicts. The dosage employed was 1 to 2 'Lomotil' tablets (Diphenoxylate hydrachloride 2·5 mg plus atropine sulphate 0·025 mg), and 2–4 Chlormethiazole tablets (0·5 mg) [not exceeding 16 Chlormeth. tablets per day] every four hours, for a period of 4 to 7 days [57]. This combination of Lomotil with a tranquilliser has proved effective in the treatment of the heroin abstinence phase, but requires – and deserves – further trials [57, 58].

Frequently, the heroin addict suffers from complications – such as intercurrent infections, local or general sepsis, hepatitis, under-nutrition – which require urgent attention; in such cases, withdrawal will usually have to be carried out more slowly.

At any rate, the withdrawal treatment will always have to be followed up by the much more important **long-term and rehabilitation** treatment, which should enable him, as far as possible, to cope with life without recourse to dependence-producing drugs. He will as a rule require long-continued support from professional workers, local authorities, voluntary agencies, family, friends, the Church, etc. Often a gradual process of weaning from reliance on the security and shelter of the hospital – such a transfer from closed wards (which will not always be necessary) to open wards, then to half-way houses and later to a controlled and supported home environment before complete independence at home – may be advisable and necessary. The final phase of adjustment will have to take place in the community, and long-term support and assistance from many community agencies (which for example, could help in vocational rehabilitation and finding suitable employment) may often be required. Individual and group counselling of addicts and their families may often be very helpful, apart from educational and vocational training. Long-continued out-patient supervision by parole officers has proved helpful in civil commitment programmes for narcotic addicts. A 'rational authority' (as contrasted with the 'punitive approach') approach has been described by L. Brill) and Jaffe [59]: here a court agency and a Rehabilitation Centre work in close cooperation, sharing information casework planning and decision making: coercive measures and controls being employed (or kept in the background as possible deterrents) in order to anchor the addict firmly in the treatment situation. Some units in England have used Section 4 of the Criminal Justice Act – Probation Order with a condition of Residence or Attendance at an out-patient clinic – with a similar purpose in mind [4].

Comprehensive programmes aiming at rehabilitation of narcotic addicts all include a variety of psychological, pharmacological and social approaches. The two most widely employed approaches nowadays are the chemical methods (maintenance or, more rarely, antagonists) on the one hand, and the self-help organisations on the other.

Chemotherapy

Maintenance

(*a*) Methadone Maintenance [59, 60]—This method was introduced in 1964 by Dole and Nyswander [61]. High maintenance doses of say, 80 – 120 mg of Methadone prevent the addict from getting any kick from heroin, cross tolerance leading to a 'blockade' of the Heroin effects; somewhat smaller doses, moreover, eliminate narcotic 'drug hunger'. Thus the way is paved for effective rehabilitation. In a Methadone maintenance programme addicts report once daily to receive their dosage of 100 – 180 mg in orange juice; this large dosage is effective for about 24 hours. The Heroin addict is thereby helped to keep off Heroin, to take up employment, and to readjust his life. Many former Heroin addicts have thus been helped to function within the community and to adjust socially and occupationally without further criminal involvement. Not much research seems to have been done as yet to decide whether after a period of Methadone maintenance it might be possible to get the addict also off the Methadone to live free from addictive drugs – and to what extent it may be advisable or otherwise to try to achieve this goal.

It has been stressed that Methadone maintenance should be employed only under the auspices of clinics or hospitals which have the required wide range of services needed at their disposal, and is thus unsuitable for use by the individual medical practitioner. Much further research is required in regard to Methadone maintenance. For example, under present circumstances this approach is probably more suitable under American than under British conditions, as in Britain it might often be difficult to establish that the newcomer – when first appearing at the Out-patient Treatment Centre – has in fact been dependent on a narcotic for any length of time [4].

(*b*) The so-called 'British Approach'—Until 1968 any British medical practitioner was allowed to prescribe Heroin to addicts. To a large extent, because of the over-prescribing of Heroin (and Cocaine) by a small number of London GPs under this now abandoned over-permissive 'British System', a Heroin-Cocaine epidemic arose in

England in the early 1960s [96, 62]. Since 1968, only doctors at the newly established Treatment Centres (of which there are about 15 in the London area and a few in the provinces) are permitted to prescribe Heroin and Cocaine to addicts. In general the policy adopted by the Treatment Centre doctors is (apart from virtually eliminating the prescribing of Cocaine) as far as possible to cut out the prescribing of narcotics altogether, or at least to substitute Methadone in place of Heroin. As a consequence of such a policy the number of Methadone addicts 'notified' to the authorities is now greater than that of Heroin addicts. Methadone is used in these British clinics by and large in much smaller doses than in the American maintenance programmes [63], and probably not so much with the aim of a prolonged maintenance programme, but in the hope that at some time in the future at least some addicts may become 'motivated' to stop all addictive drugs. Moreover, probably more addicts receive Methadone in form of ampoules than in form of the oral tincture – largely perhaps, because addicts resist giving up 'fixing' and the therapist may fear that if he insisted on oral medication the addict may stop coming to the Centre, with the loss of any hope of establishing a therapeutic relationship.

As it is, although the number of 'known' narcotic addicts in the UK – which kept on rising until 1968 – has now begun to drop, addicts are buying and selling drugs on the Black Market; among them Methadone; the risk of 'addiction' is of course much greater when Methadone is injected (as is often the case in England) than when taken in oral form (as in the American maintenance programme) [61]. It seems that in the UK very few addicts are by a deliberate prescribing policy stabilised on Heroin, so that it is quite wrong to compare and contrast American Methadone Maintenance programmes with a policy of 'Heroin Maintenance' in the UK. At any rate, because of differences between conditions in America and the UK (for example, sociocultural and legal differences, differences in personalities of drug abusers and in doctors' prescribing habits), methods proving successful in one country may not necessarily be so in another. Careful assessment, close supervision (including urinary monitoring) and controls are necessary in the British Treatment Centres as in the American maintenance programmes to minimise the danger of abuse, for example in avoiding the 'spilling over' of prescribed drugs to the 'Black Market'.

Whilst recently the number of officially known Heroin addicts has gone down and Cocaine abusers have become few and far between, Black Market abusers of cannabis, LSD, 'Chinese Heroin' (see p 699), Methadone, amphetamines and barbiturates have risen in numbers although obviously not even approximate estimates are available. However, there seems to be no organised illicit trade and no marked increase of crime as a result of reduction of the prescribing of Heroin. Clearly as in the USA the situation is very fluid and requires constant vigilance, as the British Drug Scene seems to be changing continually and multidrug abuse is nowadays common, as are septic complications arising from the use of unsterile syringes and needles.

Narcotic antagonists

Cyclazocine is an orally effective narcotic antagonist, whose regular administration (on an Out-patient basis) to volunteer Heroin addicts of good motivation has been found helpful (in the USA) in preventing return to narcotic drug use, as it reduces the mental and physical effects of Heroin and other opiates [59, 64]. A single oral dose of 4 mg Cyclazocine was found in the USA to prevent the effects of Heroin administration for a period of 20–28 hours, with its peak effects after 6–8 hours. As long as the addict continues to take cyclazocine, Heroin – unless taken in large amounts – will have little effect on him. Thus, it is hoped in time to bring about extinction of conditioned physical dependence and of drug-seeking behaviour. Before starting the antagonist, the narcotic must first be withdrawn.

Cyclazocine has a number of unpleasant side-effects. These are not present with another opiate antagonist, Naloxone, which, however, is too expensive, and is even shorter-acting than cyclazocine, its antagonism to opiates lasting 3–4 hours [64]. Research is being carried out to develop new drugs which lack cyclazocine's side-effects and are longer-acting. The final place of the antagonists in the treatment of narcotic drug dependence cannot yet be assessed.

When considering the value of all these chemotherapeutic approaches, it should be kept in mind that nowadays many addicts are multi-drug abusers, and that 'cured' Heroin addicts may continue or start abusing 'soft' drugs, such as amphetamines or barbiturates or also alcohol. Such drug therapies should be regarded as part and parcel of an overall comprehensive rehabilitation programme (for which, indeed, they may sometimes pave the way) and which – as already said – should include vocational guidance, educational training or retraining, resocialisation, assistance by welfare and social workers or probation officers, etc. As drug dependence, as a rule, is symptomatic of underlying psychological or social problems, psychosocial therapies will have to accompany or follow Methadone or cyclazocine treatment.

Self-help organisations

In contrast to the chemotherapeutic approaches, the 'therapeutic community' approach treats alcoholics and drug addicts essentially as people suffering from underlying psychological problems, such as emotional instability or immaturity. However, drug abuse, having started as a symptom, in time has led to secondary changes, so that later on addicts have many common features – even if originally their personalities varied a great deal. Because of such later changes brought about in the course of their drug taking career, drug addicts find that they have a lot in common which enables rapid, easy identification. This principle, as already discussed, is made use of in special units, halfway houses etc. by professional workers, but also in self-help organisations, run by addicts themselves, often with the help of recovered addicts.

The principles have already been discussed above; as a rule they form residential groups, members helping each other; no drugs are given, even during drug withdrawal; and the addicts participate in often very outspoken group discussions in which members severely criticise each other. However, it is hoped that group support will enable the criticised member to 'survive' such critical remarks and in time benefit from them, leading to a change in his immature outlook and behaviour and to emotional growth. New members start at the 'bottom', being called upon to perform the most onerous and menial duties, but are gradually able to work their way up towards positions of trust and responsibility. There are now quite a number of such organisations, varying slightly in their approaches and in their co-operation with professional bodies. Visitors are certainly impressed by the way in which formerly antisocial and irresponsible individuals cooperate with the group code, but again it is probably much too early to try to assess the long-term fate of those who have left the residential communities and returned to ordinary living, where they are no longer able to depend on the support of the group.

DEPENDENCE ON STIMULANTS, HALLUCINOGENS AND CANNABIS

As these drugs produce no physical abstinence syndrome there is no need for any special withdrawal regime. As regards long-term therapy of the state of psychological dependence, no specific chemotherapy is available, that could be compared with the maintenance Methadone programme or the antagonists in the case of the opiates, or with the sensitising drugs in the case of alcohol. The general principles applicable to the withdrawal phase and the long-term approach have been outlined above. As in other forms of drug dependence, after the withdrawal and detoxification phase is over, attempts must be made to establish a long-term after-care and rehabilitation regime by a combination of physical, psychological and social approaches.

Certain features sometimes observed among these types of drug abusers deserve brief mentioning. The **amphetamine** 'high' [9, 65, 66] is often followed by a psychologically painful 'come down' experience, so that a watch should be kept for depressive symptoms possibly accompanied by suicide attempts in this phase. Antidepressant (but not the CNS stimulating) drugs may have to be used at the time in spite of the delay of action and although in general they are not greatly appreciated by such patients. Impulsive, irresponsible, aggressive, and violent behaviour sometimes noticed in habitual amphetamine abusers may require the administration of tranquillisers. Paranoid psychosis – a not uncommon complication of habitual amphetamine abuse – necessitates treatment by major tranquillisers, such as phenothiazines; fortunately the prognosis is good, the psychosis as a rule clearing up rapidly when the consumption of amphetamines comes to an end.

Whilst – as already discussed – there are very few indications for starting amphetamine medication in new patients, the question may sometimes arise as to whether middle-aged people who have for years functioned satisfactorily on slightly excessive doses of a drug such as 'Drinamyl' (dextroamphetamine combined with amylobarbitone) should be given further 'maintenance doses' or not. One might feel that in such cases – with the number of tablets perhaps no greater than 4 to 5 per day, with no evidence of a desire for increase of dosage etc., and where attempts at reducing and withdrawing these tablets lead to persistent complaints of lethargy, depression, inability to work etc. – it might perhaps be better to leave things well alone.

The acute and prolonged reactions which may occur in **LSD** users

[29, 65] may necessitate – apart from such general measures as attempts at reassurance ('talk down') and psychological support – medicinal treatment in the form of tranquillisers, for example phenothiazines (chlorpromazine i.mu) during the acute panic reactions, during the 'flashback' phenomenon following some time after the drug has been taken, during an acute or prolonged LSD psychosis etc. Prolonged psychological support will be necessary in such patients for some time after the acute manifestations have passed off. Phenothiazines are said to be contraindicated in cases where STP (and not LSD) has been consumed because of the danger of potentiation [65]. Untoward reactions following cannabis use (as a rule much milder and much less common than in the case of LSD) require similar symptomatic treatment as the LSD reactions.

Where individuals in states of psychological dependence on amphetamines, LSD and Cannabis ask for help, they are initially probably best treated in hospital, to be followed by prolonged medical and social supervision after discharge. In as far as habitual Cannabis users as a rule see nothing wrong with this drug and (rightly or wrongly) claim that they could give it up any time they want to [9], they usually lack any motivation to cooperate with any treatment suggested to them.

CONCLUSION

Much progress has been made during the past decades in the understanding and the treatment of alcoholism and drug dependence, but a great deal more remains badly understood and requires much further research. Much remains to be done, for example, in the fields of treatment, education and prophylaxis. Alcoholism and drug dependence are problems of multifactorial causation requiring an integrated multi- and inter-disciplinary approach: for example in treatment by the employment of psychological, social and pharmacological techniques. (Incidentally, the features of some of the drugs referred to in this section are discussed in greater detail in Section C: Drugs in Current Use (e.g. phenobarbitone, phenytoin sodium, artane, barbiturates, non-barbiturate hypnotics, [including glutethimide, paraldehyde, nitrazepam, methaqualone], narcotic analgesics [including morphine, diamorphine or heroin, codeine, nalorphine, methadone, dextromoramide, pethidine], 'minor analgesics' such as phenacetin, antidepressants, such as imipramine, amitriptyline, nortriptyline, protriptyline, iprindole, tranylcypromine; 'major tranquillisers', such as chlorpromazine, promazine, fluphenazine, thioridazine; 'minor tranquillisers', such as chlordiazepoxide, diazepam, oxazepam, meprobamate, chlormethiazole; psychomimetic drugs, such as lysergide; sympathomimetic drugs, such as amphetamine, dexamphetamine, methylphenidate, methylamphetamine; vitamins, such as thiamine, riboflavine nitotinic acid). As important members of the therapeutic team, 'doctors should be in the forefront in the task of preventing and fighting alcoholism and drug dependence, but they need to be better equipped by adequate education in this field during their student days. This important task can no longer be left to the postgraduate private enterprise of a few individuals' [67].

References

1. World Health Organisation Alcoholism Subcommittee. *Wld Hlth Org. techn. Rep. Ser.* (1952), **48,** 16, 33.
2. World Health Organisation, *Wld Hlth. Org. techn. Rep. Ser.* (1964), **273,** 9.
3. World Health Organisation, *ibid.* (1964), **287,** 4–6.
4. Glatt, M. M., *Brit. J. Addict.* (1969), **64,** 165.
5. Archibald, D., Third Leonard Ball Oration (1970), Melbourne. p. 9.
6. Jellinek, E. M., *The Disease Concept of Alcoholism* (1960), Hillhouse Press, New Haven, Conn. pp. 36/39, 92, 146, 155.
7. Glatt, M. M., *WHO Chronicle* (1967), **21,** 293.
8. World Health Organisation (1967), *Wld Hlth Org. techn. Rep. Ser.,* **363,** 8.
9. Glatt, M. M., Pittman, D. J., Gillespie, D. G., and Hills, D. R., *The Drug Scene in Great Britain* (1969), E. Arnold Ltd., London. (Revised reprint). pp. 19, 43, 80, 101, 106, 115.
10. Glatt, M. M., *The Alcoholic, and the Help he needs* (1970), Priory Press, Royston, Herts. pp. 41, 72, 102 (Part 1); pp. 1, 3, 7, 12, 22, 29, 45, 60, 78 (Part 2).
11. Bejerot, N., *Addiction and Society* (1970), Ch. C. Thomas, Springfield, Illin. p. 91.
12. Halbach, H., *Brit. J. Addict.* (1959), **56,** 27.
13. Glatt, M. M., in *World Dialogue on Alcohol and Drug Dependence* (1970), ed. E. D. Whitney. Beacon Press, Boston. p. 311.
14. Glatt, M. M., in *New Aspects of the Mental Health Services* (1967), ed. H. Freeman and J. Farndale. Pergamon Press, Oxford, N.Y. p. 115.
15. C. D. Smithers Foundation, *Understanding Alcoholism* (1968), C. Scribner's Sons, New York p. 138.
16. Cohen, S. (ed.), *Images of Deviance* (1971), Penguin Books. p. 11.
17. Home Office. Report of the Working Party, *Habitual Drunken Offenders* (1971), H.M.S.O., London.

18. *The Drunkenness Offence* (1969). Eds. T. Cook, D. Gath, and C. Hensman. Pergamon Press, Oxford, N.Y. pp. 9, 51, 99, 109.
19. Eddy, N. B., Halbach, H., Isbell, H., and Seevers, M.A., *Bull. Wld Hlth Org.* (1965), **32,** 721.
20. Nyswander, M., in *Drug Addiction in Youth* (1965). (Ed. E. Harms), Pergamon Press, Oxford, N.Y. p. 126.
21. Asher, R., *Lancet* (1958), **i,** 954.
22. Glatt, M. M., *Brit. J. Addict.* (1959), **55,** 111.
23. Williams, L., *Alcoholism* (1956), Livingstone, Edinburgh, London. p. 39.
24. Sargant, W., *Proc. R. Soc. Med.* (1949), **42,** 3.
25. Glatt, M. M., in *Colloque International sur la sujetion aux drogues.* Quebeck (Sept. 1960). Optat, Quebeck. p. E1. (also: *Brit. J. Addict.* 1970, **65,** 51.
26. World Health Organisation Study Group, *Bull. Narcot.* (*U.N.*) (1957), **9,** 36.
27. Winnick, C., *Bull. Narcot.* (*U.N.*) (1962), **14,** 1.
28. Wiener, R. S. P., *Drugs and Schoolchildren* (1970), Longman, London. p. 165.
29. Louria, D. B., *The Drug Scene* (1968). McGraw-Hill Book Cy., N.Y., Toronto. p. 182.
30. Jones, Maxwell, *Social Psychiatry in Practice* (1968), Penguin Books.
31. George, H. R., and Glatt, M. M., *Brit. J. Addict.* (1967), **62,** 147.
32. Ottenberg, D. J., and Rosen, A., *Quart. J. Stud. Alc.* (1971), **32,** 94.
33. Neumann, C. P., and Tamerin, J. S., *ibid.* (1971). **32,** 82.
34. Connell, P. H., In *Drugs and Youth* (1969), Eds. Wittenborn, J. R., Brill, H., Smith, J. P., Wittenborn, S. A. Ch. C. Thomas, Springfield.
35. Chambers, C. D., and Brill, L., *NACC Reprints* (1971), **4,** No. 1. Narcotic Addiction Control Commission, New York State.
36. Kielholz, P., *Schweiz. med. Wschr.* (1957), **87,** 1131.
37. World Health Organisation, *Wld Hlth Org. techn. Rep. Ser.* (1965), **312,** 8.
38. *Drug Addiction*, Report of an Interdepartmental Committee (1961). H.M.S.O., London.
39. Dunlop, Sir Derrick, *Proc. Roy. Soc. Med.* (1970), **63,** 1279.
40. Annot, *Drugs in Society*, June 1971, p. 12.
41. Essig, C. F., In *The Addictive States* (1968), ed. A. Wikler, William and Wilkins Cy., Baltimore, p. 188.
42. Butterworth, A. T., *Quart. J. Stud. Alc.* (1971), **32,** 78.
43. *Chlormethiazole* (1966), ed. E. P. Frisch. Munksgaard, Copenhagen.
44. Glatt, M. M., George, H. R., and Frisch, E. P., *Brit. med. J.* (1965), **2,** 401.
45. Lundquist, G., In *Chlormethiazole* (1966) (*cf.* ref. 43), p. 203.
46. Alexander, F., *Fundamentals of Psychoanalysis* (1949), London, p. 24.
47. Smart, R. G., Schmidt, W., and Moss, M. K., *Int. J. Addict.* (1969), **4,** 543.
48. Taylor, J. A., *Bull. Los Angeles Neurol. Soc.* (1964), **29,** 158.

49. Dent, J. Y., *Anxiety and its Treatment* (1947), 2nd ed. Mullan, Belfast.
50. Smart, R. G., Storm, T., Baker, E. F. W., and Solursh, L., *LSD in the Treatment of Alcoholism* (1968), University of Toronto Press, Toronto.
51. Dally, P., *Chemotherapy of Psychiatric Disorders* (1967), Logos Press, London.
52. Glatt, M. M., *Acta psychiat. Scand.* (1961), **37**, 143.
53. Wikler, A., In *Drug Abuse* (1970) (ed. P. H. Blachly). Ch. C. Thomas, Illin. p. 283.
54. Glatt, M. M., and Leong Hon Koon, *Psychiat. Quart.* (1961), **35**, 1.
55. Blachly, P. H., *Amer. J. Psychiat.* (1966), **122**, 742.
56. Fraser, H. F., Isbell, H., *Bull. Narcot.* (*U.N.*) (1961), **13**, 29.
57. Glatt, M. M., Lewis, D. M., and Wilson, D. T., *Brit. J. Addict.* (1970), **65**, 237.
58. Goodman, A., *Southern med. J.* (1968), **61**, 313.
59. Brill, L., and Jaffe, J. H., *Brit. J. Addict.* (1967), **62**, 375.
60. Second National Methadone Maintenance Confer. (1969), *Internat. J. Addict.* (1970), **5**, 341–591.
61. Dole, V. P., *ibid.* (1970), **5**, 359.
62. Interdepartmental Committee on Drug Addiction, Second Report (1965) H.M.S.O., London.
63. Glatt, M. M., *Internat. J. Addict.* (1972), **7** (in the press).
64. Brill, L., and Laskowitz, D., *Cyclazocine*. Eastern Psychiatric Rsrch. Assoc (1970), 15th Ann. Meet. (Nov. 8). New York City.
65. Cohen, S., *The Drug Dilemma* (1969), McGraw-Hill Book Cy., New York, p. 33.
66. Kalant, O. J., *The Amphetamines* (1966), University of Toronto Press, Toronto, pp. 71, 96, 134.
67. Glatt, M. M., In *Progress in Clinical Medicine* (1971). (Eds. R. Daley and H. Miller). 6th ed. Churchill, Livingstone, Edinburgh, London, p. 522.

After a discussion of social and biological factors which influence human fertility Dr Potts presents the currently-available methods to control procreation, together with the advantages and drawbacks of each contraceptive method.

A Guide to Modern Contraceptive Practice

The doctor's role in the nineteen-seventies

by

Malcolm Potts
Medical Director, The International Planned Parenthood Federation, London

Contraception and the clinician

Birth control is a private and individual affair but professional assistance, when properly trained and fully informed, can be of great benefit both to individual health and social advancement as well as to making an essential contribution to the well being of the community as a whole. Economic progress is virtually halted when demographic growth rates exceed 2 per cent. per year and a formidable challenge to the global resources and environment is obviously presented by rates in this order. Our present situation is difficult for anyone accurately to imagine, but the scale of the problem may partially be gained by realising that there will be an increase of more people in the next decade than those who presently live in North and South America combined or (to put it in historical terms) by a number exceeding the estimated population of the planet 200 years ago.

From the medical viewpoint family planning is made up of a limited series of well tried and relatively simple techniques. But in social and human terms the problem is more complicated and the clinician is often wise to build upon the foundations of what couples already do, rather than to try and impose a series of semi-sophisticated methods in a foreign and insensitive way. Over the past hundred years the need for family planning has become more apparent than previously, the goals set by couples in the control of their own fertility have become more exact. There has been moderate improvement in methods and an increasing involvement and interest by physicians in meeting the universal need for birth control.

But *some* degree of family limitation can be identified in most historical communities and most contemporary cultures. In fact, the artificial limitation of human fertility is so widespread among practically all known human communities that it is difficult to estimate the full potential of the human reproductive system over a fertile life time. The Huttarites, who are an eccentric religious group in the USA, are exposed on the one hand to efficient modern preventive and curative medicine but reject, on the other hand, artificial contraception and abortion. Girls marrying under 20 produce, *on average*, 10 live children before the menopause. But even in this community the rules of monogamy and of chastity before marriage ensure that fertility is less than the maximum possible. Nevertheless the Huttarites remain an exception and average family sizes in both developed and developing countries demonstrate that fertility is always curtailed by one or more man-made limiting factors.

Social factors and fertility

A very important factor influencing fertility is the age of marriage. During the twentieth century the average age of the menarche in developed countries has fallen below the teens and almost into the first decade of life. The first menses are often irregular and may be anovulatory but most girls will run through seven or eight years of fertile life and many will experience ten years or more before marriage.

The medical profession clearly has little direct influence in altering the pattern of relations that determines the age of marriage but the profession sometimes plays the role of an impassioned bystander and should always be an interested observer. Early marriage is associated with a higher divorce rate later on in life and pregnancy early in life carries higher risks to the mother and baby. Among other important social variables in the limitation of human fertility are of course the rate of divorce and remarriage, the level of celibacy (which tends to be positively correlated with late marriage, for example in Eire) and the prevalence of primary or secondary infertility due to venereal disease.

Sexual intercourse prior to marriage has been a feature of many Western communities for generations but currently three additional trends have started to emerge: the age of first intercourse has fallen; the length of time before marriage (and therefore the number of partners involved) has increased; and a proportion of young women are turning to doctors for contraceptive advice whereas previously only the male partner used contraceptives and obtained them anonymously. The events which are taking place seem to be mainly the result of economic and educational changes among young people and do not appear to be directly related to the availability or non-availability of birth control advice. For example, Japan has had a liberal abortion law for over twenty years but only 10 to 12 per cent. of those who have legal terminations are unmarried. In Britain however half those having terminations are unmarried, and similarly, the British illegitimacy rate is five times that of Japan. In other words, broad cultural influences, rather than an ability to deal with an unwanted pregnancy determine premarital sexual behaviour. The illegitimate pregnancy is, after all, something that happens to *other girls.*

Illegitimate babies have a higher neonatal death rate than those born in wedlock and the mother can also be shown to be at greater risk during pregnancy and delivery. There is therefore a great deal of scope for improvement in family planning services among the unmarried. Among a series of over 1,000 single girls seeking advice on abortions in Birmingham between 1968 and 1970 approximately half never used any form of contraception and two thirds omitted any protection on the occasion they became pregnant.

Oral contraceptives, because of their high degree of predictability and their freedom from coitally-dependent manoeuvring are first choice for single women seeking a physician's advice. Condoms, because of their fair reliability and the opportunity to obtain them without unsavoury interrogation are first choice among men. But some unmarried individuals or couples present with additional sexual or emotional problems and may be in need of wise counsel as well as reliable contraceptives.

Biological factors and fertility

The declining age of the menarche has been remarked upon. The age of cessation of periods tends to be inversely correlated with their onset. Within the fertile years primary and secondary infertility (infertility after one or more conceptions) due for example to endocrine disorders or infectious disease cuts down the number of women who run the risk of conception, a factor which must not be overlooked when considering the fertility of a society as a whole.

When a healthy woman, not using any form of contraception, begins to have regular intercourse a cycle of reproductive activity will be set in motion which has two distinct components.

(1) Regular intercourse, which on average takes place for three to six ovulatory cycles before pregnancy occurs. But this mean figure conceals a skewed distribution curve in which most women fall pregnant rapidly but a minority may go for a year or more of unprotected intercourse before conception occurs. It can be demonstrated that the frequency of intercourse is a determinant in the length of time taken to get pregnant, but it is not an outstandingly important one.

(2) Pregnancy itself, and the anovulatory interval which will succeed the end of pregnancy. In the case of term delivery followed by a stillbirth or without breast feeding this latter interval may last for two to three months, but if lactation is established it can continue for a year or more. When the pregnancy results in a spontaneous or induced abortion fertility may return within two cycles. In the absence of contraceptive protection more abortions can be fitted into a given interval of a woman's fertile life than term deliveries, and if term delivery is associated with lactation then two, or possibly three, induced abortions might be needed to avert one live birth. But the use of contraceptives greatly extends the time taken to conceive. In these circumstances even with the use of a relatively ineffective method of contraception, the interval between pregnancies may be greatly extended.

Contraceptive methods

Today, the use of reversible contraceptive methods is divided in approximately three equal ways. In the UK the sale of condoms and spermicides, through a variety of retail outlets, accounts for the largest single body of contraceptive users. Coitus interruptus remains the second most frequently used method, and together with the rhythm method, accounts in general terms for approximately one third of users. The remaining third of the population plans its families with advice from doctors and very occasionally nurses and midwives. In this group the oral contraceptives are now used by approximately one in five of the population and their use exceeds that of other methods distributed by physicians. In the rest of Europe coitus interruptus is relatively more important while in North America physicians play a larger role in contraception than is the case in Britain. It is important to remember this general division of usage in order to establish realistic perspectives by which to judge standards of clinical care for physician-medical methods and to mark out the very large area of potential improvement in family planning services. The single most important contribution of any physician to family planning is to keep the topic in mind; to use his influence to help a couple establish rational contraceptive measures; and, above all, to create opportunities when help may be sought. All women who have had a baby or an abortion, as well as a great many others (and many husbands) should be *offered* the opportunity to discuss family planning methods. The discussion should not have to be initiated by the patient herself.

(a) *User Dependent Methods*
Contraceptive methods have in the past been classified in a large number of different ways. However there is little point in over complicating what is in fact a very simple set of distinctions. It is proposed here to discuss the methods under three separate headings – methods that depend upon the user alone; methods that involve the use of some equipment which is readily and commercially available; and methods which necessitate the involvement of the physician.

(i) *Coitus interruptus.* At a world level male withdrawal before ejaculations is almost certainly the commonest form of reversible contraception. It is so widely used in the western world that it can easily be overlooked. The question 'Do you use any method of contraception?' may elicit the answer 'No', while the same patient may tell you 'My husband is always careful'. The method is known by various colloquial terms and one quoted in East Yorkshire is 'Going to Beverley and getting off at Cottingham'.

Demographically, the use of coitus interruptus is very significant and partly accounts for the fact that birth rates when Western Europe entered the historical period of industrialisation were considerably lower than those found in many contemporary developing countries.

Like many common activities whose significance is often underestimated, coitus interruptus has been the subject of myth making rather than scientific observation. It has been said to be ineffective because the pre-ejaculatory fluid is supposedly capable of fertilisation – a contention which has never been proved. The method is widely claimed by doctors to be psychologically harmful for one or both partners, a thesis which is certainly not substantiated by a review of the literature on mental illness in Britain. The unreliability of the method is also over-emphasised.

When presented with a couple who has habitually practised the method but who feels in need of advice the attitude of the helpful clinician towards withdrawal should not be to deter them from its use by unsubstantiated criticism, but to suggest, at least in suitable cases, that there are probably better ways of planning one's family.

(ii) *The rhythm method.* There are two distinct 'safe period' methods, one of which, since it requires a thermometer, might properly be placed in the 'equipment' category. Any safe period variation of course depends upon being able to predict (or at least detect) the time of ovulation and hence avoid intercourse at or around this time. The difficulties of being able to detect with certainty when a follicle has ruptured, let alone *predicting* when it will do so are sufficiently well known to require little comment here.

The least reliable of the two rhythm variants is that depending on the use of the calendar. The patient notes the length of six to twelve menstrual cycles, and on the basis of this information attempts to assess what her 'normal' cycle length might be. In so doing she makes the assumption that she *does* show some degree of menstrual regularity and also that variations in cycle length are largely due to differences in the proliferative rather than the secretory phase of the cycle.

The two sets of rules which have been adopted for determining on which days to avoid intercourse were elaborated independently by Knaus in Austria and Ogino in Japan over 30 years ago. Using the Knaus criteria, 18 days are subtracted from the duration of the shortest cycle of the twelve and 11 from the duration of the longest. This calculation gives the 'outer limits' of the safe period between for the cycle in question. For example, the limits range from days 7 to 21 for a woman whose cycle length ranges from 25 to 32 days and during this time intercourse is not permitted. It takes little mathematical skill to realise that for a woman who shows such a range of variation (and such women are by no means uncommon) intercourse must be restricted to rather less than half of the cycle if these criteria are rigorously followed.

The temperature method depends upon the fact that following ovulation in some women there is a rise in basal body temperature of some one half of one degree Fahrenheit. This effect is said to be due to the pyrogenic effects of progesterone but the statement has never been proved. Whatever the reason for the temperature shift, the woman attempts to detect it by taking daily readings of her rectal temperature immediately on waking and plotting them on an appropriate chart. Ideally, the chart should show a biphasic aspect, having a higher mean value in the second half of the cycle than in the first. Once a rise has occurred, intercourse is generally regarded as being safe. Again, if the regime is adhered to strictly the opportunities for intercourse during the cycle are very severely restricted.

The value of the rhythm method has been hotly debated in the medical literature and a number of reports exist which suggest that it shows a relatively high level of effectiveness especially when it is the temperature version that is being practised. Certainly, every clinician knows at least one couple either as patients or as friends who have used the method successfully for years. But it would be most unwise to attempt to generalise from a small sample of highly motivated individuals to a far larger group of relatively indifferent ones. Although rhythm can work effectively if all the rules are strictly observed it is unlikely to work well in the population as a whole, despite well publicised statements to the contrary. Its one advantage appears to be that it does not need the involvement of a physician.

(b) *Commercially Available Methods*

(i) *Condom*. The sheath, or French letter, has a long but uncertain history since its invention in the sixteenth century as a protection against syphilis. It is an obvious, safe and sensible method of contraception and for many it has the added appeal of not requiring the advice or involvement of a third party.

Condoms are made plain or teat-ended and are generally coated with some form of lubricant. Users tend to buy the most expensive available, although price is not necessarily the best criterion of quality. Much attention is paid to adequate standards of manufacture and it should always be remembered that rubber goods have a limited shelf life and are therefore marked with an expiry date on the packet.

The effectiveness *can* be increased by the use of a spermicide, but it should rarely be necessary to use such a material. It should be clearly stated that condoms burst extremely seldom and that defects in manufacture (pinhole flaws and similar deficiencies) very rarely occur, despite ideas which have entered the folk lore and which are based on condom surveys carried out many years ago. It therefore follows that it is not necessary to blow them up or fill them with water or cigarette smoke prior to use. Indeed, these unrolling and handling processes are likely to do more harm than good to the tough but thin latex membrane.

It also follows that pregnancies which occur amongst condom users are largely the result of misuse rather than of deficiencies in the sheath itself. Probably the greatest cause of conception in this situation is allowing the penis to become flaccid whilst it is still within the vagina. Semen can then leak past the ring at the distal end (rather than through any holes in the proximal region) and hence gain access to the cervix. An opportunity should always therefore be taken to encourage any men who enquire about the matter to withdraw from the vagina soon after orgasm and to grip the ring of the condom with their fingers whilst they are doing so.

Condoms should be available in all family planning clinics. For some couples who have sought professional advice they may still be the best single choice of method. They are useful during lactation or when intercourse is being resumed after a pregnancy; for covering the initial interval until an oral contraceptive can be relied upon, or a vasectomy becomes effective; or indeed at any time of change or uncertainty. Classically, they have the advantage of reducing the risks of infection for those men exposed to venereal diseases and there is reasonable evidence that prolonged use of the condom in a partnership reduces the woman's risk of developing cancer of the cervix.

They have the disadvantage of interrupting the sequence of play which precedes intercourse and some men object that they seriously diminish sensation. There has been a certain shyness on the part of professional family planners in trying to create an erotic image for this form of contraception. Although difficult, such an approach does not seem impossible, as the trade in coloured condoms and patterns with comic devices at the closed end testifies.

(ii) *Spermicidal preparations.* There are a number of different spermicidal preparations available on the market which are intended to be used alone rather than in combination with a diaphragm, cap or condom. At least four different physical forms exist – creams, jellies, foams and suppositories and newer methods of delivering spermicides into the vagina are currently being developed. Historically, the pessary or suppository – a solid object with a fairly large volume – was the first to make a commercial appearance and the first spermicide to be incorporated into such a formulation was a quinine derivative. Today, a good deal more investigation has been performed, both into the nature of the ideal spermicide and into the nature of the vehicle which should be used to deliver it.

Because of their large bulk, their relative messiness and the fact that they tend to produce a certain amount of leakage from the vagina, pessaries and suppositories are probably losing a certain amount of their popularity in the face of such preparations as the aerosol foam.

Nonetheless they are still bought in substantial quantities. Jellies and creams also suffer from the practical drawback that they have to be applied to the vagina through some form of applicator nozzle, which must necessarily involve a degree of premeditation on the woman's part.

It is widely believed that the use of a vaginal spermicide alone represents a particularly ineffective form of birth control. However, this is not necessarily true. Some of the published figures for creams, aerosols and jellies show that when properly used they give levels of contraceptive protection probably good as those afforded by the condom among a comparable group of users.

(c) *Physician Involved Methods*

(i) *Vaginal barriers.* Rubber or plastic barriers that cover the anterior wall of the vagina and cervix, or simply fit over the cervix itself, have been known for over a century. At one time they were almost the only reasonable option open to a woman who wanted to control her fertility and their use has played a very significant role in the evolution of the family planning movement and in the involvement of physicians, especially female, in contraceptive matters.

Today by far the commonest of the barrier methods is the diaphragm or Dutch cap, a rubber domed device varying from about 5–10 cm in diameter with a coiled or flat spring in the circumference. To some women, who are unfamiliar with the capacity of their own vaginas, the diaphragm when first seen appears more like a rubber dustbin lid than a contraceptive. However, when properly fitted both partners should be virtually unaware of its presence. A good fit is essential and to ensure it the potential user should be examined vaginally to determine the tone of the perineal muscles, whether there is any degree of prolapse and if the cervix is likely to be accessible on self examination.

The diaphragm should never be used without a spermicide and indeed there are those who would argue that its principal function is not to act as a mechanical barrier but to hold a sufficiently high concentration of spermicide close to the cervix. Because of the need to apply the spermicide to the diaphragm prior to its insertion; the need to leave it in place for eight hours after the last intercourse; and the need to apply a second quantity of spermicide to the vagina if a morning intercourse occurs, some women find the method tedious.

Certainly the diaphragm is only suitable for a minority of women engaging in premarital relationships and in this situation the failure rate, even when the method is used consistently, is high enough to cause concern. The freedom from side effects and relative simplicity of the method make it a much more attractive choice during family building. The ability unconsciously to misuse the method is said sometimes to be turned to advantage by women who emotionally want a child, but feel on rational (usually monetary) grounds that it would be wise to wait a little longer.

Observation shows that with practice the use effectiveness of the method improves and after the desired family size has been achieved some women use the method well and find it satisfactory over many years. However, where a high degree of predictability is desired the physician might, as time passes, find it wise to be increasingly sympathetic towards sterilisation of one or other partner. Perhaps even more than most methods, the use of vaginal barriers is greatly influenced by the enthusiasm of the adviser. While not often a method of choice among socially underprivileged groups, it has been well used even in those cases, when the woman has been looked after by someone (usually a nurse or midwife) who strongly favours the method and who is also a good teacher.

(ii) *Steroidal contraceptives*. The possibility of evolving a contraceptive method using exogenous ovarian hormones to inhibit ovulation was first explored by the Austrian physiologist, Ludwig Harberlant in the 1920s, but he was unable to interest the medical profession in such a possibility. When the first synthetic steroids were used, among other things, for the treatment of dysmenorrhoea it was noted that one of the side effects of therapy was an inhibition of ovulation. But still the contraceptive potential of the method was not exploited. It took the forcefulness of Margaret Sanger and the foresightedness of the Planned Parenthood Federation of the USA, which gave a small grant to Gregory Pincus at the Worcester Foundation in Massachusetts, to initiate the work which was to lead in 1956 to the first trials of what was to become known all over the world as 'the Pill'.

In developed countries oral contraceptives are now by far the commonest method of contraception used by couples who seek the advice of a physician on family planning. In the developing world they constitute a minority method, because it has been judged – some experts believe erroneously – that the supervision of a doctor is mandatory for their distribution and this assumed prerequisite has been the major rate-limiting factor in their distribution. Today over 20 million women use oral contraceptives and probably only two million of those are in the developing countries.

The pill has one singular advantage over all other contraceptive methods – its effectiveness is virtually 100 per cent. when it is properly used. It has given women a degree of freedom from the fear of pregnancy that they never previously imagined to be possible. In Western countries, sexual attitudes have been markedly changed since its introduction. Contraception has become a subject which can be discussed far more freely than before. A question like 'are you on the pill?' can be both asked and answered with relatively little embarrassment and the revolution that goes with pill taking is as much a social as a biological one.

However, there are problems which a number of clinicians have had to face when involved in prescribing oral contraception for their patients. The first problem is to some degree an ethical one because there is some evidence which has been used to suggest that the ready availability of oral contraceptives (especially amongst the young and unmarried) is leading to a degree of sexual promiscuity which has not been experienced in recent years. The evidence is conflicting, but some physicians feel a concern about the increasing spread of gonorrhoea for example, an increase which might indeed correlate with an increase in this pill-induced sexual liberation.

Their concern is justifiable in the sense that no medical man wishes to be responsible for the spread of a disease of epidemic proportions. However, the more realistic of them now realise that whatever its origins, this so-called liberation is here to stay. In that circumstance, once they accept it as a fact, they must also come to realise that their duty now lies in trying to prevent unwanted pregnancies – something that oral contraceptives do extremely well. In this sense their moral dilemma may be more apparent than real.

The second problem is biological as well as ethical. It concerns the much publicised (though extremely rare) fatalities that occur as a direct result of thrombo-embolic disorders among pill takers. Precise figures are still being computed but a fatality of some 10 women per million per year is the order of magnitude with which we are dealing.

'Am I justified in subjecting my patients to this risk?' is a question which a number of medical men must ask themselves and the answer of course will be a personal one. But the answer should certainly depend above all on an analysis of the other risks which his patient runs, particularly those risks associated with *not* using an adequate form of contraceptive protection. The simplest calculations show that the risk of pill-induced fatalities is considerably less than the risk of maternal mortality associated with gestation and labour, to say nothing of the particular problems both physical and emotional which face an unwanted child after its birth.

One school of thought maintains that the risks of pregnancy are more 'natural' and therefore by some strange implication more acceptable than those associated with the pill. It would be interesting to discover what women themselves thought about this natural argument. One imagines that few of them would find it totally convincing. Certainly no-one pretends that the pill is the ultimate contraceptive panacea, but for large numbers of women, and indeed for their medical advisers, it is looked upon as a singularly fortunate discovery and one whose potential should have been realised a good deal earlier than it actually was.

(iii) *The intrauterine device*. Just as the pill was hailed in the mid nineteen-sixties as being the answer to all our contraceptive problems, so too, after a slightly more cautious period of evaluation, was the intrauterine device. The virtual rediscovery of the IUD in 1959, after it had fallen from popularity in the nineteen-thirties, forms a fascinating chapter in medical history. Within a short time, a spate of different designs appeared, each with some hoped-for advantage over other designs, and each of them was hopefully patentable.

The results of trials with such devices as the Lippes loop and the Margulies spiral, trials carried out under strict medical supervision, were remarkably encouraging. The pregnancy rate appeared to be lower than that found with any other contraceptive method except the pill. In addition of course, a method which would give such protection after only one single application and a method which required a positive effort of will to have it removed and hence to remove its (totally reversible) contraceptive effects obviously had a great deal to be said for it.

Much debate centred around the problem of whether the introduction of a foreign body into the uterus would cause a pelvic infection or stir up a pre-existing but dormant pelvic inflammation. However, the evidence finally suggested fairly conclusively that inflammatory conditions of this type need not be a serious problem. Debate also surrounded the problem of inserting such devices into the nulliparous, and even now opinion is divided on this question. Those physicians who feel that they can do so with ease continue to do so. Others regard it as a slightly hazardous enterprise.

Ironically enough, despite very considerable research efforts which have been devoted to the problem, it is still not established precisely why such devices exert a contraceptive action at all. There have been almost as many theories as there have investigators. Most of them now agree that the device's action is exerted within the uterine cavity, perhaps by destroying the egg (or even the sperm), perhaps by altering the endometrium. Although the final explanation still eludes us we can be confident that if the device stays in place then its level of contraceptive protection will be high.

However, the results of large-scale field use of IUDs in Korea and elsewhere have shown that to ensure that the device does remain within the uterine cavity is a major problem in any population where almost continual access to the physician is not easily attained. The problem is two-fold. In the first place the difficulty is that IUDs tend to be rejected spontaneously by the uterus – a rejection that depends upon the design of the product, age, parity and so on. In addition, requests for removal of a device because its presence produces pain and bleeding during the first post-insertion cycles have started to become highly significant. For these reasons it now seems unlikely that certain IUD programmes will ever attain the goals that were originally set. The devices are tending to be lost or deliberately removed from the uterus as quickly as they can be inserted. In other words, the retention rate has started to reach a plateau.

In Western countries this is less of a problem. The continuation rate is higher simply because a woman who thinks she has lost her IUD can have its presence immediately checked by her doctor and a woman who feels that she is having trouble with the method can go to him for guidance – assuming of course that he is sufficiently knowledgeable about the topic to be able to provide it and also assuming that he himself believes in the value of intrauterine contraception.

It may well be that in the next five years the situation will improve immeasurably. New designs of device which have been intensively studied appear to be free from many of these drawbacks, and a whole new generation of IUDs containing metallic copper are currently under investigation. For some reason, the presence of this metal appears to lessen the expulsion rate, the bleeding rate and the pregnancy rate and it is possible that by 1975, the simple plastic devices with which we are familiar may be largely of historic interest only. In the meantime, although the actual fitting and removal of an IUD requires only a modicum of skill, the ability to inspire confidence in the method does demand a particular set of attitudes on the part of the doctor involved.

ABORTION AND STERILISATION

All reversible methods of contraception have a measurable failure rate. It has to be recognised that no currently available method, with the possible exception of the use of oral contraceptives over many years, is sufficiently practical to permit a population of users to achieve the fertility goals which rae common in developed countries.

Sterilisation should be available as a free choice to men and women who have the number of children they feel they want. Male sterilistion is less demanding in surgical skill, less hazardous and more open to reversibility than female sterilisation.

The need for abortion is unlikely to be eliminated even amongst those practising contraception in the immediately foreseeable future. Termination before twelve weeks is fundamentally different from termination after twelve weeks. The former procedure is simple, can be done by a relatively inexperienced surgeon, can be done as an out-patient procedure and the operation can be performed in a matter of minutes and the total contact with professional care need not extend over a few hours. Termination after twelve weeks is more hazardous, it usually requires a general anaesthetic and in-patient treatment.

The role of the physician

What specifically should be the role of the physician, as far as the spread of family planning practices, at least in Western nations, is concerned? The answer is three-fold: he must be a clinician in the obvious sense of the word but he must also be both a psychologist and a salesman if he, by his own efforts, is to make a significant contribution to the contraceptive practices of his patient population.

He must be a clinician for obvious reasons. He must be competent to deal with the medical aspects of the contraceptives which he is distributing. He must be able, for example, to detect a woman with dubious liver function or a history of migraine for whom the pill should not be prescribed, or to detect a very occasional patient presenting with abdominal symptoms due to uterine perforation by an IUD. But in general these strictly 'medical' aspects of the subject will not take up the greater part of his time. Far more of it will be spent discussing the forms of contraception (if any) that his patients are currently using and perhaps suggesting that more effective or acceptable alternatives exist.

The doctor himself must fully realise that no one method will suit any one couple for their entire reproductive lives. The newly wed pair, desperately anxious to avoid the birth of their first child until they are properly established, must have an absolute assurance that an unwanted pregnancy will not occur. For them the use of a hormonal preparation might seem ideal. After five years, however, and the birth of their first (planned) child, they may wish to *delay* the appearance of the second although they would not be unduly alarmed if it followed the first fairly quickly. For them at that stage the use of the condom or possibly a spermicide might be indicated.

After the second birth the couple may well reserve final judgement on a third. If it occurs they will be happy, but if not they will be equally pleased. By this time it may be assumed that they do not want to put a great deal of effort into their contraceptive practices although they do require a reasonably effective method of protection. Here an intra-uterine device might well be appropriate. If a decision *is* made to have a third child and thus achieve a completed family size then removal of the device will ensure that this can happen. If not, then its continued presence will make a subsequent pregnancy most unlikely.

When the family size is finally completed then again a good deal of reassurance against an unwanted pregnancy becomes important. A case can be made here for the sterilisation of one or other partner although few responsible doctors would recommend such a decision (in the absence of any disposing maternal symptoms) during the initial stages of the marriage.

Thus the couple's contraceptive needs change and thus the doctor's own attitudes have to remain flexible to accommodate them. But in one respect he has to be inflexible and that is in his role as a contraceptive salesman. Even today, distressingly few couples approach their medical advisers for help in this highly personal and sometimes embarrassing area. Even today in Britain, America and much of Western Europe a distressingly large number of unplanned pregnancies occur. It is one of the roles of the physician to take the notion of birth control to his patients rather than waiting for them to come to him. By that time it may well be too late to prevent the appearance of the fourth daughter or fifth son. He must do it tactfully and helpfully but above all he must do it. And in order to do so, he himself must believe in the message that he is broadcasting.

(*It is a pleasure to acknowledge the help of my friend Dr Clive Wood in the preparation of this chapter.*)

With the growth of aircraft travel many people are now travelling to all parts of the world for both business and pleasure. This section gives a guide to the health regulations and methods of preventing ill-health due to exposure to tropical diseases. A guide to treatment of these diseases contracted by a person who has now returned to a non-tropical country is presented.

A Guide to the Treatment of Tropical Diseases in Non-Tropical Countries

by

H. A. K. Rowland

Senior Lecturer in Clinical Tropical Medicine, London School of Hygiene and Tropical Medicine, and First Assistant, Medical Unit, Hospital for Tropical Diseases, London

Every year large numbers of people travel abroad to all parts of the world, for a variety of reasons and for varying lengths of stay. They often seek advice on what they should do to comply with health regulations and to prevent ill health while they are away. Large numbers of people also return from abroad each year after varying stays in different parts of the world; on or after entry they may seek medical advice because of symptoms; alternatively they may want to know whether they have 'picked up a bug' on their travels. This chapter is concerned with the management of such persons.

TRAVELLING OVERSEAS

Persons travelling overseas may encounter diseases which are either absent in their own country or less common there than in countries which they may visit; they will want to be protected against such infections as far as is possible. The particular infection will of course vary from country to country and will also depend on the circumstances under which the traveller lives and the duration of his stay; thus the risks are quite different in a crowded holiday resort in Europe, a rural area of West Africa, a desert area in the Middle East and a congested city in the Orient; they are different if the journey is made overland to Nepal and sleeping in a tent or by fast aircraft to an air conditioned hotel in Bangkok or Rio de Janeiro.

Protection against illness may be afforded by (i) avoidance of infection such as by the use of a mosquito net or the boiling of water for drinking, or (ii) combating infection acquired by immunisation or suppression.

Malaria

Malaria has been eradicated from large areas in which it was previously endemic but there are still many parts of the world, especially in Africa where it remains. Prophylaxis, meaning protection from infection cannot be achieved because there is no non-toxic drug capable of destroying sporozoites, the infective form of the parasite injected by the biting mosquito; protection therefore depends on causal prophylaxis and suppression. There are drugs available which destroy the pre-erythrocytic forms of *Plasmodium falciparum*, that species of parasite responsible for malignant tertian (MT) malaria, infection with which carries a mortality; they therefore destroy the source of the blood forms giving rise to the clinical attack and are referred to as 'causal prophylactics'; proguanil (paludrine) and pyrimethamine (daraprim) are such drugs. Schizonticides are those compounds having an effect on the asexual forms of the parasite developing within the red cells and regular treatment with such drugs may keep the level of infection in the blood below that at which clinical manifestations are present; they are known as 'suppressives' and include paludrine and daraprim and the more powerful schizonticides, quinine, nivaquine and chloroquine, camoquine and mepacrine.

Persons returning from malarious areas frequently give a history of malaria while on suppressive. So often a blood film was not taken at the time of the febrile attack so that the diagnosis may be in question. Even if parasites are seen in the film it is possible that the suppressive was not taken regularly; finally it may be that the parasite is truly resistant to the blood concentration of drug resulting from the particular suppressive regimen. There is no doubt that *P. falciparum* parasites in certain parts of the world are resistant to blood levels of drug produced by standard courses of treatment; this is a quantitative phenomenon rather than an all-or-nothing one so that increased dosage may be successful. Since nivaquine (or chloroquine which is merely a different salt) is the most powerful schizonticide available it is advisable to reserve this drug for the treatment of an acute attack of malaria; paludrine and daraprim therefore remain the drugs of choice for suppression. For an adult, paludrine 100 mg daily or daraprim 25 mg weekly is the standard dosage; children should be given a proportionate dose and syrup is available for very small children. Suppression should be started on arrival in a malarious area, continued for the whole of the stay without fail and for four weeks after leaving the endemic region.

Protection against mosquito bites is afforded by netting over windows and doors provided it is intact which is so often not the case and probably mosquito nets over beds is the better method; even a still night under a net in humid West Africa is not unbearable. The best repellent, which is effective for some hours against mosquitoes and other insects, is dimethylphthalate, an oily liquid which is not unpleasant to apply, is inexpensive and makes an evening on a verandah even more pleasant.

Smallpox

Control of smallpox is being actively carried out in parts of the tropics but the disease is still endemic in some African countries, Brazil, India and Indonesia where the incidence may be greater than five cases per 100,000 population per annum. Recent vaccination against smallpox gives marked protection; there are however risks associated with the procedure so that the principle should be applied intelligently and the danger of smallpox weighed against that of vaccination.

Ill-effects are especially seen in the young in whom the incidence of severe nervous system and skin complications is greater than in older persons. Encephalomyelitis occurs in about 15 of every million children vaccinated during the first year of life and carries a 40 per cent. mortality with the possibility of permanent disability in those who survive. During the second year of life the incidence falls to three per million still with high mortality; thereafter the incidence rises again but with no mortality [1].

The important skin complication is eczema vaccinatum – a vesicular eruption at the site of skin lesions in a patient with existing eczema. Although occurring at all ages it is especially important under the age of one year because of the higher mortality at that time. An unvaccinated child with infantile eczema may also develop this complication by contact with a person who has been recently vaccinated against smallpox.

These observations suggest that smallpox vaccination should be carried out during the second year of life; in healthy children travelling to areas of the world endemic for smallpox, vaccination may be carried out between the ages of 6 and 12 months. If travelling to areas where smallpox is not endemic this should be delayed and a certificate issued giving the reason. Vaccination should not be carried out under the age of 6 months; the response tends to be less good at this time.

Existing eczema especially in a small child is an absolute contra-indication; if there is a recent history of such skin lesions and vaccination is urgent, as in those in contact with the disease, it may be carried out and anti-vaccinial gamma globulin given at the same time. Vaccination is also contraindicated during pregnancy because of the risk of foetal death from generalised vaccinia; the only possible circumstance under which this might be relaxed is close contact with a smallpox patient. In those whose immune response is less good than normal, vaccination may be followed by a progressive ulceration at the site of scarification; this may be seen in persons suffering from agammaglobulinaemia and in persons on steroid therapy. Again if vaccination is thought to be essential it should be accompanied by anti-vaccinial gamma globulin.

In 1970 smallpox was reported by only 21 countries as compared with 42 countries in 1967 [2]; it is expected that this number will fall much further so that fewer and fewer travellers will need to be vaccinated against smallpox.

Enteric Fever

Typhoid fever is unusual in this country and at least half of the 200 or so cases seen each year is in persons recently arrived from warmer climates where such infections are much more common. 'Enteric fever' covers all salmonella septicaemias and may therefore be due to *Salmonella typhi*, *S. paratyphi* or one of the many salmonella organisms acquired from animals and more often giving rise to food poisoning. All salmonellae other than *S. typhi* tend to produce a diarrhoeic illness which may be associated with constitutional upset; blood culture may be positive for the particular organism in such patients.

It is therefore advisable for travellers overseas to be protected as far as is possible from such infections. Infection is via the gastrointestinal tract, water and food being the mode of transmission. Care in the boiling of water, the preparation of ice from boiled water, the proper cooking of food and the disinfection of vegetables to be eaten raw, provide considerable protection. Enthusiasm for such measures tends to wane with time even in persons in their own quarters and is often non-existent in hotels and restaurants.

The other protective measure is immunisation, first introduced by Pfeiffer and Kolle [3] and by Wright [4] in 1896. This appeared to be of benefit although it was not properly tested until comparatively recently. It is difficult to believe that typhoid immunisation was not of value under the appalling conditions in the trenches in the First World War, and the difference in incidence of enteric infections between British and Italian troops and the effect of adequate vaccination in the latter in North Africa during the Second World War, are strongly suggestive of protection conferred by inoculation (Boyd, 1943) [5].

Only during the past few years has the value of vaccine been demonstrated; well designed experiments carried out in Yugoslavia (Yugoslav Typhoid Commission, 1957, 1962, 1964) [6, 7, 8], in British Guiana (Typhoid Panel, 1964) [9] and in Poland (Polish Typhoid Committee, 1965) [10] showed that the attack rate of typhoid fever diagnosed by blood culture positive for *S. typhi* was lower in those vaccinated than in controls. Different vaccine preparations have seemed better than others in the different trials; formol-killed, phenol-preserved vaccine is probably as good as any other, two injections of 0·5 ml ($1{\cdot}0 \times 10^9$ organisms per ml) subcutaneously at a 4 week interval giving considerable protection for a period of 2 years; that protection is not complete is shown by the fact that some inoculated persons did develop culture-positive typhoid fever. There is some evidence that intradermal inoculation in which case the dose is 0·1 ml rather than 0·5 ml is followed by fewer general and local reactions (Noble, 1966) [11]; the antibody response following immunisation by this route is as good as that after subcutaneous injection. Alcoholised vaccine may not be given intradermally.

Vaccines available in this country are either monovalent (*S. typhi* only) or contain *S. typhi* ($1{\cdot}0 \times 10^9$ organisms/ml) and *S. paratyphi A* and *B* ($0{\cdot}5 \times 10^9$ organisms/ml), and may or may not be combined with tetanus toxoid. The value of including *S. paratyphi* in the vaccine has not been proven and it has been suggested that these organisms contribute to side effects. Current practice is to give 0·5 ml subcutaneously followed by 1 ml 4 weeks later, or as long afterwards as is possible; booster doses of 0·5 ml are given at yearly or 2 yearly intervals thereafter although the optimum follow-up regimen has not yet been determined by clinical trial. Using the intradermal route all doses are 0·1 ml. Enteric fever is relatively uncommon in the very young so that immunisation need not be carried out under the age of 1 year; inoculation carries no risk to the foetus but because of the possible side effects it is perhaps better avoided during pregnancy if possible.

Cholera

Since the pandemics of cholera which occurred from the early 1800s until the early part of this century, cholera remained confined to the Far East, Bengal being its home – that is until recently when it has spread to the Middle East, Africa and Europe. Originally the responsible organism was the classical *Vibrio cholerae*; during the past 10 years its biotype *V. cholerae El Tor* has steadily ousted it so that the latter organism is now primarily responsible for infections throughout the world. It was originally thought that *V. cholerae El Tor* was less pathogenic but this is now known not to be true, the clinical course being indistinguishable from that produced by the classical vibrio. In addition it seems that the *El Tor* infection perhaps affects younger children and that the carrier state may be longer.

The portal of entry is the gastrointestinal tract, water being the important mode of transmission; the source of infection is man only and the susceptible recipient is anyone not well protected. Protection may be provided by immunisation but there is some evidence that repeated contact with the organism in endemic areas provides some degree of naturally acquired immunity; this is to some extent supported by studies on vibriocidal antibody in such areas [12]. This naturally acquired immunity may have played some part in preventing a catastrophic epidemic in Calcutta and neighbouring areas during the disasters in the summer of 1971; the circumstances – refugees living under appalling conditions of sanitation and overcrowding, the presence of a substantial number of cases of cholera and the rain starting, seemed just those required to produce a devastating epidemic, but they did not.

Inoculation against cholera is not efficient, providing partial protection for perhaps 3 or 4 months; the killed vaccine currently employed in this country contains $8{\cdot}0 \times 10^9$ organisms per ml of the Inaba and Ogawa strains, doses of 0·5 and 1·0 ml being given subcutaneously at a 4 week interval. Vaccines made from the *El Tor* strain are in use in some countries and might be expected to be more effective in the face of this infection than vaccines made from the classical vibrio. Cholera vaccination is seldom followed by side effects; it need not be given to very small children.

Vaccination should not be allowed to give a false sense of security; it is no substitute for good hygiene practice – the boiling of all water, the proper cooking of vegetables and in an endemic area, probably the avoidance of raw vegetables, are of the greatest importance. One wonders too whether the time, money and effort expended in mass vaccination of a population probably partially protected by repeated natural infections, would not be better employed in the emergency provision of clean water and better excreta disposal. However, the traveller leaving this country for anywhere overseas at this time (Summer, 1971) would be advised to be inoculated whether this is required by regulation or not.

Yellow Fever

Although causing a large number of deaths in the past in the 'White Man's Grave' of West Africa and in Panama, and although there are occasional epidemics today, yellow fever would seem to be a relatively unimportant disease at the present time. How much of this reduction in incidence is attributable to man's efforts and how much for other reasons is difficult to say. The infection is transmitted by the mosquito, *Aedes aegypti* so that measures directed against these insects are important and the remarks made regarding personal protection against the bites of malaria-transmitting anopheline mosquitoes are valid here also. Man is not the only source of infection to mosquitoes, monkeys constituting an important reservoir. The susceptible recipient is anyone not protected; clearly natural immunity or naturally acquired immunity is of importance in endemic areas because subclinical infections, as gauged by the mouse protection test, are common.

Artificially induced immunity using the 17D virus is extremely efficient, giving solid protection for at least 10 years; it is given as a single dose of 0·5 ml subcutaneously, and by International Regulation is valid as from 10 days following a primary inoculation but immediately following a revaccination within 10 years of the previous immunisation. The procedure is complicated by no side effects; it should not be carried out within 3 weeks of a primary smallpox vaccination or within 4 days of a revaccination; the reverse however is not so – smallpox vaccination may follow yellow fever inoculation without such an interval and in fact the practice in some West African countries in the past was to give the two together. Yellow fever immunisation need not be carried out in children under the age of 9 months; the preparation is available only at certain centres because it must be used within 30 minutes of exposure to room temperature.

Poliomyelitis

Poliomyelitis is common in tropical countries and conforms more to 'infantile paralysis' than it has done in this country of recent years.

Most children going overseas from Britain will have been given poliomyelitis vaccine and a certain number of adults also; if required it is given orally in a dose of 3 drops at monthly intervals for 3 doses.

Tetanus

Tetanus is also much more common in warm climates than in the United Kingdom; again most children leaving this country will have been given triple vaccine (diphtheria, whooping cough, tetanus), and adults, especially those going to work in rural areas or outside modern cities might be advised to be inoculated or reinoculated with tetanus toxoid. In fact it would seem that tetanus is extremely uncommon wherever immunisation has been carried out, no matter how long ago.

Viral Hepatitis

There is evidence that the administration of gamma globulin, even in the face of an existing epidemic affords protection against a clinical attack of viral hepatitis. Its effect which is that of passive immunity, is however short lived extending for perhaps 2 months only. There is the suggestion that under cover of such passive protection, naturally acquired immunity may develop in a subclinical attack and that this is more likely if 2 doses of gamma globulin are given at a 6 month interval. Viral hepatitis is extremely common in tropical countries at the present time; gamma globulin is given at the rate of 0·2–0·4 ml/kg body weight corresponding to about 0·5 g and should be given shortly before leaving this country to those requiring it. Who such persons should be is difficult to say; often it is the traveller who requests it.

Schedule for Travel Overseas

To comply with these recommendations for vaccination is clearly a formidable procedure and if only because of the time available the schedule must often be altered. A convenient basic course is one modified from that suggested by Dr L. Roodyn, Inoculation Centre, Hospital for Tropical Diseases, London (Roodyn, 1971) [13] and is set out in the Table; it may be adjusted or supplemented by poliomyelitis or tetanus immunisation to meet the requirements of the individual which will vary depending on the time available, the region to be visited and by previous inoculations.

Table Basic immunisation schedule for overseas travel

Attendance	Immunisation	Dose
First	Monovalent typhoid vaccine	0·1 ml intradermally
	Cholera vaccine	0·5 ml subcutaneously
	Yellow fever vaccine	0·5 ml subcutaneously
Second (4 weeks after first)	Typhoid vaccine	0·1 ml intradermally
	Cholera vaccine	1·0 ml subcutaneously
	Smallpox vaccine	single scarification
Third (just before departure)	Gamma globulin	0·2–0·4 ml kg intramuscularly

Miscellaneous disorders

Persons visiting warm climates not infrequently suffer from skin disorders of which the commonest are insect bites, prickly heat and fungus infections. The majority of people experience discomfort at the site of mosquito, sandfly or other insect bites; in some however the reaction is more violent with considerable extension of the original lesion. An antihistamine cream may give some relief; the value of dimethylphthalate as an insect repellent has already been mentioned. Prickly heat is especially seen in the moist parts of the tropics and may be very uncomfortable affecting all ages including babies: it is not painful and does not itch – it 'pricks' as its name describes. Astringent lotions of which 1:1,000 mercury perchloride is a very cheap example, give some relief. Fungus infections again are especially common in the warm damp parts of the world, the lesions being found in the warm moist parts of the body – the crutch, groins, axillae and feet; the old remedy, Whitfield's ointment (Ung. ac. benz. co.) is quite as effective as the more recent preparations such as Tineafax and much cheaper. Personal hygiene and attempts to keep affected parts dry by, for example, frequent changes of socks into which talcum powder has been sprinkled, also help; no socks at all is even better.

Diarrhoea greatly troubles many persons visiting tropical countries, the reasons for this being poorly understood. Equally inexplicable is the apparent relief afforded by Enterovioform (iodochlorhydroxyquinoline) which seems to 'keep going' so many travellers on such visits. Some people go further and take with them sulphonamide preparations or a tetracycline. Enterovioform and sulphaguanidine will do no harm and are to be valued if they make a stay overseas more enjoyable but the use of tetracycline should be discouraged.

Short visits overseas

The most common complaint made by patients after a short stay overseas is undoubtedly diarrhoea; a high proportion of persons making such visits seem to suffer from some change in bowel habit, many accepting this as an inevitable accompaniment of their stay. Some may be troubled throughout the whole of their visit but surprisingly may not be greatly incapacitated or have to alter their plans. 'Travellers' diarrhoea' as this is often termed is variously attributed to 'change in food', 'change in water' or 'change in bowel flora' but it is not at all clear what actually happens. Where facilities for investigation exist which is not the rule, pathogens are isolated from only a small proportion of such diarrhoeic stools.

On return to this country the diarrhoea often improves or does not recur but in some it continues and calls for investigation; although there are some patients whose attack remains undiagnosed, in the majority a cause is found.

Some help may be obtained from the history; fellow travellers or other members of the party may have been similarly afflicted and a common time of onset might suggest a salmonella infection; it should be remembered that diarrhoea apparently due to such an organism may persist for weeks. On the other hand they may be present in the stools without producing symptoms. Salmonellae other than *S. typhi* and *S. paratyphi* are largely infections of animals in which, in this country at any rate, the prevalence has increased of recent years, as has the proportion showing drug resistance which may be transferable to other organisms. This situation which has caused some anxiety because of the possibility that resistance may be transferred to say *S. typhi*, has been attributed to intensive farming methods, the mixing of animals in markets, transport vehicles and abattoirs, the incorporation of antibiotics in feeding stuffs and the widespread and often indiscriminate use of these drugs in both veterinary and medical practice.

The diagnosis of salmonella infections depends on the isolation of the organism from the stools, or from the blood in those whose infection becomes systemic; a positive culture can rarely be obtained in less than

4 days, typing of the organism taking even longer. Serological tests are of little help in the diagnosis of salmonella infections.

Entamoeba histolytica

This parasite, especially common in the warm humid parts of the world, more commonly produces an asymptomatic than a symptomatic infection and one which is endemic rather than epidemic; in the sort of patient being considered here diarrhoea is a more common symptom than dysentery and may appear for the first time (even years) after return to this country, and be confined to a single attack. Although frank or severe dysentery is unusual in this sort of patient, liver abscess does occur so that it is important to establish the diagnosis and institute appropriate treatment. Diagnosis depends on the recognition of the parasite, either as the vegetative amoeba or as the infective cyst in the stools where it must be differentiated from the harmless *Entamoeba coli*.

Giardia lamblia

This intestinal flagellate is also common in warm climates and is a frequent cause of diarrhoea which persists after return to this country; symptoms may be intermittent and in the absence of reinfection the infection dies out spontaneously within a few months. Diarrhoea may be troublesome and associated with weight loss, malaise and steatorrhoea; the diagnosis again depends on the recognition of the parasite in the stools and treatment is effective.

Shigella infection

Infections with *Shigella* spp. occur in all parts of the world including Britain but are especially prevalent where standards of hygiene are low. As with salmonellae, shigella organisms may be present in the stools of asymptomatic persons; they may however produce diarrhoea or frank dysentery and no doubt are responsible for a proportion of bowel upsets experienced by those on a visit overseas. Since the attack even untreated lasts only up to 2 weeks or so this organism is unlikely to be the cause of diarrhoea which persists after return to this country. The carrier state is also short-lived so that a negative stool culture does not exclude a shigella organism as the cause of recent diarrhoea. In the tropics *Sh. flexneri* is the species responsible for most cases of bacillary dysentery.

Tropical sprue

Tropical sprue, that curious condition about the aetiology of which so little is still known has a strict geographical distribution; although occurring in the Caribbean it is especially in persons who have visited India and the Far East that the diagnosis is made in this country. There are however no rules regarding the period of stay in an endemic area before the disease manifests itself; symptoms may begin 2 weeks after arrival or be delayed for 20 years. Although the character of the stools and times of bowel action may suggest the diagnosis, the onset may be acute with watery diarrhoea not characteristic of sprue. Return to the temperate climate may or may not be followed by some amelioration of symptoms. Diagnosis depends on the demonstration of malabsorption and can conveniently only be made in hospital. In the sort of patient under consideration here in whom symptoms have been short-lived treatment is almost invariably followed by complete recovery. Such an attack need not preclude a further visit to an area endemic for sprue.

A few patients remain in whom no cause can be found for their diarrhoea; spontaneous remission is fortunately the rule. Persons presenting with diarrhoea after a short visit to a warm climate must have their stools examined microscopically and bacteriologically; many otherwise excellent laboratories however are inexperienced in the examination of stools for parasites, one facilitated by a concentration technique such as the formol-ether method. If the patient's symptoms persist and if laboratory investigations are negative, it is suggested that he be referred to one of the hospitals specialising in tropical disorders or that permission be sought for a stool specimen to be examined there.

With the great increase in high-speed air travel and the extension of cholera to Africa and Europe during 1971 it is inevitable that persons will arrive in this country with *V. cholerae* in their stools; they may be asymptomatic or have diarrhoea ranging from the mild to the very severe and the possibility must always be borne in mind in those with diarrhoea and recently arrived from abroad. *V. cholerae* is not a difficult organism to isolate from stools so that a diagnosis can be made quickly, provided of course that it is considered. It would be very unlikely if such introduction into this country had not already occurred; circumstances here are however such that further transmission is unlikely.

Pyrexia

Fever is a much less common complaint of short stay visitors than is diarrhoea but may appear after their return to this country. The fact that they have recently visited a warm climate does not mean that those causes of pyrexia affecting persons who have not been out of the country, should be forgotten; additional investigations should however be carried out. The patient with pyrexia but not seriously ill and without abnormal physical signs is customarily treated symptomatically and observed; should the high temperature persist investigations are carried out by the patient's doctor or the hospital to which he may have been referred – a white count is requested, the urine is examined microscopically and cultured and a radiograph of the chest obtained; later blood culture and serological reactions may be instituted.

In persons not recently returned from overseas and without an obviously treatable condition this delay is justifiable; in those arriving from abroad especially from a malarious area and particularly one endemic for *P. falciparum* infections such a delay may be important. Recently a man developed cerebral malaria and died deeply jaundiced and in renal failure 10 days after the onset of pyrexia which started a few days after return to this country following a short visit to West Africa; it is likely that malaria suppressive taken had been intermittent; the importance of continuing suppressive measures for a month after return to this country has been stressed by others [14, 15]. A blood film for malaria parasites, preferably a thick and thin film should therefore be included in the *early* investigation of a febrile patient recently arrived from overseas; these should be examined by someone experienced in the work and it helps if 'recently arrived from . . . , ?malaria' is specifically stated on the request form. They are best examined at the tropical diseases hospitals where such material is routinely handled; a telephone call followed by the slides by post is a wise precaution.

Blood culture for enteric organisms should also be instituted earlier in recently arrived febrile patients; typhoid fever is more common in warm climates than in Britain, at least half the diagnoses made in this country being in persons entering from overseas for one reason or another. It is perhaps not generally appreciated that blood, stool and urine culture increase the likelihood of making the diagnosis no matter how long the patient has been ill; those eventually found to have enteric fever are often not severely ill when first seen.

Dengue seems to be very uncommon in persons recently returned from tropical areas where it is prevalent; it may be that a diagnosis of influenza is made in this influenza-like illness, the added features of glandular enlargement and measly rash being mild or unrecognised. The diagnosis is difficult to prove but although especially the limb pains make this a most uncomfortable illness, recovery is the rule.

Pyrexia may herald viral hepatitis, a condition so common in tropical countries at the present time; its management differs in no way from that arising in this country. Liver abscess, toxoplasmosis and trypanosomiasis, although uncommon, are causes of pyrexia in persons making only a short visit overseas; expert advice is required in both diagnosis and management.

Rash

Some persons visiting especially the humid tropics are greatly troubled by prickly heat but this improves rapidly on return to a temperate climate. Similarly insect bites which in some persons may be followed by an allergic-like local reaction or complicated by secondary infection resulting from scratching, subside on return to this country. It is also in the warm humid parts of the world that fungus infections especially of the crutch and feet are especially common; they too tend to improve on return to a cooler climate and their management does not differ from that in persons who have not been out of the country. Any vesicular eruption in a person having recently entered this country must clearly be treated with the greatest suspicion; it must be remembered that previous vaccination may modify the rash of smallpox; expert opinion should be obtained without delay.

Long term visitors overseas

Those whose home is in this country and who present after tours of duty in the tropics constitute a different group from short stay visitors overseas. Their period of residence is longer and many have spent this in rural areas of the tropics; the possibilities are therefore greater. In these persons too cosmopolitan disorders must not be forgotten but in addition must be considered disorders common to tropical areas in general and those specific for the particular region where the patient has worked. These, embracing the whole of medicine in the tropics cannot be dealt with in this chapter. The remarks made concerning the management of short-term visitors are equally applicable to those who have resided for longer in the tropics; many such persons make routine visits to one of the specialised hospitals on return to this country at the end of tours of duty. Some have no complaints while others have vague symptoms such as lassitude, weight loss or looseness of the bowels; often some abnormality is detected and these routine visits are to be encouraged. Where the cause of symptoms in such patients is not apparent, the practitioner is recommended to seek advice from one of the tropical diseases hospitals.

Immigrants from Tropical Areas

Included in this group are those entering this country for the first time and those who have been home on a visit to their country of origin; long visits of this kind are common. Such persons may reach this country by air during the incubation period of some serious infective disorders of which malaria, typhoid fever and smallpox are the most common; many patients seen suffering from these disorders have recently left their country of origin.

The management of acute illness is the same as for short stay visitors for less acute illness it is advisable to obtain a further opinion from a general or specialised hospital. While it is understandable that general hospitals should like to keep an 'interesting patient' this is not always in the best interest of the individual who might be better served if expert opinion is obtained early rather than late when all other investigations have proved negative. Just as there are good and bad ways of handling a placenta praevia, an acute abdomen and a spontaneous pneumothorax, so there are good and bad ways of handling a *P. falciparum* infection and an amoebic liver abscess.

To discover that a patient has been overseas is probably the greatest hurdle to overcome, such information not always being volunteered. The management of acute illness should be as outlined here, failure to make a diagnosis calling for assistance from a specialised hospital. The investigation of less acute illness should be as for permanent residents of this country, expert opinion being obtained when a satisfactory diagnosis is not obtained; this should be sought early rather than late – by general hospitals as well as by general practitioners.

References

1. Conybeare, E. T., *Mon. Bull. Minist. Hlth* (1964), **23,** 126 and 150.
2. World Health Organisation, *Weekly Epidemiological Record* (1971), **46,** 14.
3. Pfeiffer, R., and Kolle, W., *Dtsch. med. Wschr.* (1896), **22,** 735.
4. Wright, A. E. *Lancet* (1896), **ii,** 807.
5. Boyd, J. S. K., *Brit. med. J.* (1943), **i,** 719.
6. Yugoslav Typhoid Commission, *Bull. Wld Hlth Org.* (1957), **16,** 897.
7. Yugoslav Typhoid Commission, *ibid.* (1962), **26,** 357.
8. Yugoslav Typhoid Commission, *ibid.* (1964), **30,** 623.
9. Typhoid Panel, UK Department of Technical Cooperation, *Bull. Wld Hlth Org.* (1964), **30,** 631.

10. Polish Typhoid Committee, *Bull. Wld Hlth Org.* (1965), **32,** 15.
11. Noble, J. E., *J. Roy. Army med. Corps* (1963), **109,** 178–80.
12. Joint ICMR–GWB–WHO Cholera Study Group, Calcutta, India, *Bull. Wld Hlth Org.* (1970), **43,** 389.
13. Roodyn, L., *Community Health* (1971), **2,** 291.
14. Maegraith, B. G., *Trans. Roy. Soc. trop. Med. Hyg.* (1969), **63,** 689.
15. Shute, P. G., and Maryon, M., *Brit. med. J.* (1969), **2,** 781.

It is increasingly recognised that adolescents have special medical requirements both in terms of counselling and in terms of diseases or conditions to which they are particularly susceptible. This article provides practical guidance for those who have to care for the adolescent community.

A Guide to Adolescent Care

by

Alexander D. G. Gunn

Director of Health Service,
University of Reading

The privileges of the group

Adolescence is an artificial state, created by the demands of complex modern society for further education and training in technology and apprenticeship. Those who are better intellectually endowed than others face a time of further education that may last from at least three to six years after leaving school, others face two or three years after leaving school until a trade is learnt, whilst the great majority have to learn how to become economically self-supporting before they are entitled to the full status of adulthood. As such, however, these young people are privileged by the opportunities they can enjoy – opportunities of leisure, earning power and freedom from adult responsibilities. These privileged adolescents, nevertheless, have much need of understanding, sympathy, and help through the crises of development, be they social, psychological or environmental in cause – because the adolescent of today is the investment of the community's future. Whether it be problems of academic wastage for the student, or job changing for the apprentice, or stress, depression, and adjustment to personal relationships or the demands of just simply growing up, the adolescent has a difficult time in contemporary society.

The complications of life for all developing adolescents

Intellectually the adolescent has entered a stage of life where theories of the abstract appeal, where there is a start of the passion for ideas and ideologies, and where the concept of balance between cause and effect can be appreciated. It is a new kind of thinking to that of the child, but is untempered by the experience of the adult. Authorities have claimed that from the standpoint of psychiatry the adolescent falls 'somewhere on the border between mental health and illness'. A person all of whose organs are mature and functioning may be physically healthy, but a person with all mental functions proceeding well may still be unhealthy if the relationship between them is disturbed. Thus the boy, for example, with frequent erections and consequent nocturnal or manually-produced emissions may be in all physical terms in perfect health, but obsessed by the guilt of his fantasies and neurotic as a result. Equally the girl who pretends to be of mature sexuality to keep up with her contemporaries may pass through agonizing dysmenorrhoea, or prolonged periods of amenorrhoea, and either not be prepared to admit it – or else become an obsessional physician-consultor as a result of her feelings that all below the navel is unwell. Drives, ideas and sense of reality may well be perfectly sound in adolescence, but mental health may be upset if the necessary compromise and balance between them is absent. Thus, a girl who is truly promiscuous, may be striving to achieve a feeling of wholeness that matches her physical development, and so – if her family or personal background is disturbed – she is prone to establish unfortunate personal relationships as substitutes for the stability she needs. Her relationship with a boy may not be with him as a person but with him as a source of comfort. Adults would probably be able to develop some insight into their own needs, and the dangers of their own behaviour which would cause some automatic modification, but an adolescent is subject to almost overwhelming drives that easily lead to unbalance. There is a genuine effort nevertheless by most adolescents to keep their drives, desires and fantasies under control, but there are occasional breaks punctuating the pattern of continual strain, so that one never knows where one will meet the restrictive phase, or a breakthrough of infantile behaviour.

It is extremely unfortunate that at this time of great stress the community makes greater demands on the adolescent in the academic and other fields; in many ways this could happen at no worse time. The role of aggression, in wartime, on the sportsfield, and in deprived societies, fulfils many individual adolescents. If it shows, however, in family and personal relationships, then it can lead to great distress, for it is one of the roles that modern developed society frustrates by demanding 'civilised' conformity to adult standards. Modes of dress, behaviour, language and attitudes, adopted by the adolescent – constantly reflect the desire to rebel – and yet this is the time in their lives in which we expect them to behave, to be 'a credit' to their parents, and to wait patiently for the completion of their education and the onset of apparent adult maturity. Perhaps we expect too much, forget how as youths we felt at their age, and provide too few outlets for natural adventure, enthusiasm and energy. The Battle of Britain was won by youngsters of the age who now riot in Berkeley, in Grosvenor Square, and in Tokyo – in the World Wars they gave their lives, and now all they seem to give to the adult is trouble. Conformity is not what we should expect, for adolescence is a time of irregular physical development, differing psychological maturity, and seething social torment.

The problems of physical development

Fundamentally, the health problems that arise in adolescence are less physical than they are psychological. There is a certain incidence of undescended testicle seen in late adolescence for example (approx. 1–1,000), there is a variable incidence of menstrual problems, and fibro-adenosis of the breast – and the major causes of mortality in this age group are accidents and cancer, with the leukaemias as the pre-dominant type of malignancy. The main feature of adolescent development is, however, the one that is most frequently ignored – and that is that individuals vary in the rate at which they achieve the physical and hence the psychological milestones of maturity.

This variation in rate of achievement is influenced by several factors including race, nutrition, income and sex. Not only are there sex differences in all forms of physical development, but there is a broad range of age of achievement for each sex, as wide a range in fact as 4–5 years. For some individuals there is a wide range of the speed at which developmental stages are achieved, and passed through – some boys may go through a penile growth stage in 3 years, others in 5; some girls regularly menstruate from the onset of the menarche, others have grossly irregular cycles for as long as 4 or 5 years. The significance of this is that any doctor, teacher or parent may have in the practice, class, or family, adolescents who may be of a particular age, but nevertheless are at a quite different stage of physical development from that of their contemporaries, or from that at which their siblings were, when they were that age. This is not always appreciated, and to grade adolescents by precise ages is physically and psychologically meaningless. In a class of 14-year olds some girls will be fully sexually aware and developed, others will be still pre-pubescent. With boys the physically developed will be separated at the same age in any group by their physique, attitude of mind and social behaviour, from those who are not. It must be remembered that: (1) individuals grow and develop at different rates dependent on race, nutrition, sex and family income; (2) social and cultural differences influence the rates; (3) psychological maturation is directly affected by the stage of physical development reached.

It is not surprising therefore, that the one feature predominantly met with in adolescence is narcissism. Visibly conscious of the changes occurring within their bodies, restrained often by the conventions of relationships with others who are older or younger, there is a 'we-are-alone' situation for the adolescent of today, and the problems that they have stem from such psychological difficulties rather than specific physical abnormalities.

Our knowledge of adolescent sex

Most of the attitudes towards adolescent sexual mores stem from opinion and not fact. The only reasonable survey carried out in the United Kingdom within recent years was by Schofield and that being in 1965 must already be considered to be out of date.

Age of experience of sexual intercourse*

Age	Male	Female
17	11 per cent.	6 per cent.
19	30 per cent.	16 per cent.

*Schofield, reference [4]

Some contemporary evidence may be derived from the current notification of abortion figures, which indicate that nearly 2,000 terminations a year are being carried out on girls under 16, and of these some 25 per cent. are on girls under the age of 14. More important, is the general picture that emerges from working in the care of adolescents because it is in a comprehension of their difficulties, that we are enabled to offer sympathy and offer guidance, and not, as is inevitably relied upon, our own personal experience which is irrelevant to contemporary society.

Sexual activity in the adolescent, is largely determined by group pressures, the desire to be thought 'experienced' and to prove masculinity, whilst among girls it is motivated often by the fear of losing a prized friendship. The most usual restraining influence for girls, and an important one for boys, is moral or religious training, but fear of pregnancy is also an important inhibiting factor. Fear of venereal disease seems to be of small importance. It is interesting to note that though we are in days of apparent individual freedom, with adequate and safe fertility-control becoming continually more easy of access, youth is still subject to a morality based on fear – the fear of not conforming, and the fear of pregnancy. Where these scruples have been rejected by the young people of today (e.g. 'hippy cults'), we have a new morality which the older generation cannot understand because they, in their turn were subjected to the same standard fears a generation ago and were unable to reject them.

The adolescents' knowledge about sex seems to be almost invariably acquired from friends and often through the medium of 'jokes'. Though from surveys, up to one-third of girls indicate that they receive information from their mothers, very few boys seem to have done so, and the part of fathers in giving information seems to be negligible. Middle-class children are found to be more likely to have learnt from their parents than those of a lower socio-economic group, but even so some two-thirds of sons and one-third of daughters of middle class families would seem to receive no advice about sex from their parents. At school, whilst the majority of girls (but only half the boys) receive some kind of formal sex education, this is still mainly in the form of biological information. Of equal interest is the fact that the majority of boys and girls claim to have knowledge of contraception, and yet of those with sexual experience less than half the boys, and only one girl in five always use some method of birth control. The paradox is nevertheless in keeping with the actual facts concerning experience, for in the teenage years intercourse is more often unpredictable than premeditated, and explorative rather than mutually decided. At least the 'first time' is.

Thus we have an adolescent culture that has absorbed its information, and developed its attitude to sexual relationships from a combination of sources, few of which might be regarded as unimpeachable. We have a large group in our community who although unmarried have already experimented (at least one-third of girls and half the boys) by the age of 18 with full sexual activity and we have a larger group who have many times been mutually 'on the brink' but have restricted their activities because of a morality based on either fear or their upbringing. Firstly, therefore, one would expect, medically, to see the effects of this on the birth rate and indeed illegitimacy rates have been showing an almost international increase, though it must not be forgotten that a large number of babies who are technically illegitimate are born to older women. Though we say that the rates are rising steeply (and they certainly are in the younger age groups) we find that the pre-marital conception rate in Great Britain represented 14·5 per cent. of all live births in 1938, and they are the same today, the difference being that in 1938 a higher proportion (75–80 per cent.) married than now. Secondly, we can justifiably expect to see problems emerging from the unchannelled and uneducated sexual drives of the adolescent. For example there has always been and always will be the small minority who deliberately debase the sexual act, and themselves, by promiscuous behaviour. The strongest of correlations exist between emotional instability and psychological ill-health. The more immature may not be able to accept or appreciate the feeling of responsibility that sex should and can bring and seek for gratification at a more superficial level. The need to make responsible choices concerning sexual behaviour is made particularly difficult where there is a vast area of social confusion and a pathological need to rebel. There are some who may act out their conflicts with society in a delinquent or aggressive way, frantically trying to disprove their fears of homosexuality, or trying to get their own back for frustrations suffered in childhood. Sexuality is made use of as an expression of neurosis and in terms of meaning, their activity has little effect on them emotionally. There is no satisfaction to be had from promiscuity, beyond the spinal reflexes (which in the girl's case may not be all that frequent), for real satisfaction is derived only from an emotionally stable relationship. Girls will consult a physician and complain of their promiscuity because it is something they are frightened of and do not enjoy. The boy will give a history of many shallow relationships as part of the story of his depressive illness. Genuine nymphomania is another of the myths modern society has created for itself, for promiscuity is an illness. This is not to state that any girl of 21 may not have had sexual relationships with perhaps two or three men since the age of 17 and yet been perfectly healthy emotionally, for each relationship at the time and for its duration has been one of love and affection later to be discovered as mistaken by one or other of the partners. In the context of current behavioural patterns of late adolescence this might be considered as normal, just as her mother was 'in love' with two or three 'lady-killers' before she met her husband and was kissed by them all. The girl of contemporary society can 'go further' if she wishes to, without fear of pregnancy, than her mother could. Society continually confuses promiscuity with pre-marital intercourse.

Venereal disease is one of the prices, however, of plurality in sexual contact, and whilst syphilis may be diminishing (except amongst homosexuals) gonorrhoea is increasing in its incidence. This is the pattern in contemporary society where, for example, nearly a third of all female attendances in the UK for the treatment of gonorrhoea, are made by girls under the age of 20. Similarly, most physicians concerned with the care of adolescents are seeing a considerable rise in what might be termed, 'gynaecological' complaints. The incidence of monilial and trichomonas infections is increasing annually and currently reflected in the number of new pharmaceutical preparations being introduced for their treatment.

It is interesting to note, however, that the complaint of vaginal discharge is frequently the first attendance of the girl in which she initiates a discussion of sexual activity. 'Honeymoon' cystitis is another. Both have a degree of guilt connotation and once any dam of embarrassment is breached there is a flood of eager questions and a genuine desire for open discussion. The girl will frequently have her boy-friend with her in the waiting room and enthusiastically asks if he can come in too. This genuine need for information is an expression of the paucity of agencies, reliable sources, and confidential counselling services available for adolescents in general, for who else can a young couple turn to for advice and help? There is, in general, an appalling ignorance about venereal disease and its symptoms, and an equally misplaced confidence about the 'safe' period with a widespread fear of their parents finding out. The typical pattern of a teenager's sexual relationship is one of advancing sexual exploration leading to the first act of intercourse for both, which ends prematurely, and in tears or guilt. The boy then makes some immature and half-hearted attempts to 'use something', which results in both partners hating the whole procedure. The girl, with worry more often than with conception, becomes overdue menstrually, and then – and only then – do they seek some help. The menstrual period for the fortunate ones eventually comes and they decide together that never again will they go through such agony and torment – such is a typical couple attending for contraceptive advice. The 'pill' and 'advice' have no contribution to make to increasing the numbers of adolescents who are having intercourse; they only reduce the pregnancy rate. For those who are not involved with the care of adolescents, or who are not in their intimate confidence, myths about sex have in many ways become modern fantasies of the adult world, fantasies that are quite unfounded, as facts prove, when proper investigation is undertaken.

It is admittedly exceptionally difficult for the older generation to appreciate the sexual stress and strains of a prolonged and artificial adolescence – when they were the same age they were either sublimating their desires in the desperate need to secure economic independence or else were married. Constantly, parents imagine that their unmarried daughters or sons, even at the age of 20 or 21, are either totally ignorant of sex or indulging in lustful pursuits that are in all probability more often parental imagination than adolescent fact. Communication between parent and offspring on this subject is too frequently non-existent – as indeed it is at the earlier ages in terms of sexual education. Marriage is resisted, and parental pressure is invariably brought to bear to prevent it, from the best of motives perhaps, and parents fear constantly that their daughters will turn up pregnant, or their sons be ensnared by some 'scheming girl'. Indeed the fact is that if more open discussion, confidence and trust could be found in the home, many of the adolescents' stresses and strains, and those of the adults too, could be reduced.

Misuse of drugs – the basic problems

Probably the most publicised aspect of adolescent behaviour, in recent years, has been the 'drug scene' – a distortion of the lives of a minority but taken too often, and wrongly, to reflect a pattern for the majority. It is a paradox of a divorce-prone, tobacco-smoking, alcohol-drinking and sleeping-pill-taking society that the adolescent's exploration of sensation – whether the body's senses as with sex, or the psychological perceptions as with various pharmacological substances – should receive such ferocious condemnation. That the developing youth should feel a need for 'escape' from the society he sees himself being plunged into is perhaps more a condemnation of the society than of the youth. But then the older generation has ever been prone to a judgement of its young which is tainted by the guilt of its own experience.

The misuse of drug substances by adolescents is international. In London coffee bars it may be amphetamine-type stimulants, in Scandinavia strong alcohol. In other European towns, glue-sniffing or inhaling paint-thinners are serious problems, whilst in California marijuana and LSD feature prominently in the 'hippie' cultures. The greater ease of travel to the near East and North Africa, has meant that marijuana is also a more common European feature of adolescent life, whilst in the UK particularly the misuse of 'pep' pills by adolescents seems to have followed historically, and directly, the widespread prescription of them by the medical profession for their obese, depressed and unhappy parents.

The adolescent is exceptionally vulnerable to the misuse of any drug and to dependence upon its effect for solace, comfort, confidence or escape. There is a risk of total involvement with the experience, and with the group, or the community who use drugs, for whatever purpose. There is a relief to be gained perhaps from the stress of adolescence or a sensual pleasure which gives them a feeling of daring, or of being unique, and rejecting adult standards. They will conform in being society's non-conformists. There is a danger, however, that those who are least sure of their capacity to be independent are the ones who are also most likely to take drugs for relief from their stress and so therefore the most likely to become dependent on them. Drugs may be taken in defiance of the adult community or imitation of them. The cigarette may be a symbol of adulthood, but the 'reefer' is a group experience which they alone share. Hallucinogenic substances offer the knives that cut the knots of an adolescent's feeling 'up-tight' about sex, college, thermonuclear war, Vietnam, parents and the so-called 'standards' of the adult world, just as alcohol eases the social tension of the grown-ups' situations, and the cigarette is lit by the chronic bronchitic who is permanently worried about his respiratory invalidism but cannot break the habit.

It is dependence or habituation which is the danger with any experience, from taking drugs to being superstitious, and this is, par excellence, the crux of any drug problem in adolescence. Where a personality is immature there is the greatest risk of warping its development – and even the most enthusiastic protagonists of 'legalising' marijuana would hesitate to suggest that small children should be enabled to smoke it. Thus, the adolescent must be seen as being in need of some protection from the pharmacological hazards of the world at large for three reasons. Firstly their development, emotionally and psychologically, is incomplete, secondly all persistent drug misuse carries with it inevitably crippling personality deterioration and thirdly the already unstable personality may be precipitated into permanent mental ill-health.

Marijuana

Almost invariably, 'pot' is a group experience, and is passed around at parties by the group leaders or those who wish to impress the uninitiated. The effect on the indulger is predominantly to enhance the mood that the person is, at the time, experiencing – relaxation of body and mind, with a degree of heightened perception of those things which the individual finds pleasant, colours, music, shapes, animals or sexual sensations. This latter may be particularly deceptive, for impotence under its use is a common male experience. In exactly the same way, if a person is frightened of its use because of its illegality or fear of what they may experience then marijuana may well prove unpleasant for them and they express a dislike for it. They may feel sick, vomit or sweat excessively. If they persist, again in order to conform, the hallucinogenic experiences may eventually become more pleasant, but nevertheless there are more people in the adolescent community who 'tried it once and it did nothing for me' than there are regular users. Sore and bloodshot eyes from the smoke and a persistent dry cough are signs of its regular use but a more marked sign is that the regular use distorts the individual's critical perception of their own intellectual and skilled abilities.

There is no evidence of any intellectual or physical achievement ever being better due to the influence of marijuana. With a degree of inevitability smokers of pot run the risk of becoming ever-more regular users. It may well be, however, that only the 'side-steppers', the weaker ones and those who would be prone to seek escape and not the mastery of a setback, follow this path. With regular 'escape' comes thus the first aspect of personality deterioration – just as with the adults who cannot face the stress of an important interview situation without the 'dutch' courage of a double gin. Excessive use of marijuana is rare, if only because it is expensive, but occasionally it is seen, and appetite suppression frequently occurs, along with an almost psychotic increase in fantasy. Patients who have smoked up to 20 'reefers' a day for as long as a week or more, become grossly disorientated and frequently withdraw totally from involvement with all aspects of the outside world. Vivid aggressive fantasies may be experienced, and lead to bizarre forms of self-damage – from the production of skin slashes with a palette knife 'because the blood looked pretty', to drowning because 'she said she wanted to walk on the water'. The excessive, and exclusive use of marijuana is as hazardous and as disorientating as is the excessive and exclusive use of alcohol – they both produce an acute psychosis. It is the disintegration of the critical faculties, however, that remains the danger of marijuana, which occurs, albeit temporarily, whenever it is used. Sensual pleasure is bought, at the price of critical judgement and its regular excessive use is paid for in an impairment or serious deterioration of the individual's intellect. There are many comparisons that can be made with alcohol, but unfortunately with marijuana the awareness of being drunk is not so precise or so specific as it is with alcohol, nor does it wear off so quickly. The body can vomit an excessive intake of drink, but its rejection of being 'turned-on' is much slower and less recognizable.

The Opiates

The addiction to hard drugs – opiate derivatives – are totally destructive of personality and life. The average mortality after leaving hospital for the treatment of addiction to a 'hard' drug is 20 per cent. in the first year and the average death rate within five years of addiction developing is 60 per cent. 'Hard' drug addiction is suicide by inches. But the misfortune is that those adolescents who are in contact with the illegal underworld for supplies of marijuana are highly likely to meet 'pushers' who wish to increase their own income further, in order to obtain more supplies of the 'hard' drugs they need, and this initiates the weaker ones into experience with 'hard' drugs. This initiation may even be offered free. There is a degree of social contagion to drug-taking and a malignancy that can spread; thus the maladjusted adolescent (there are approximately three male 'hard' addicts to every one female) finding solace for his disturbance in marijuana and selling it to others may become also the initiate into the 'hard' market and in turn pass the contagion on once he is addicted. All drug-taking has a certain individual price, and that of true addiction demands complete 'drop-out' from life as we know it, gross personality disintegration, and eventually death. Furthermore, the addict, who is in all probability suffering from a personality defect that antedated the addiction anyway, becomes to the community a social canker.

The major hallucinogens

The mind-bending of an acid trip is fraught with dangers – in the short term, those of a 'bad trip', which leaves the indulger suffering from an acute psychosis, marked by mental disorientation and mania, with physical lack of control, characterised either by withdrawing curled up in the corner of a room, or by running about screaming and harming themselves and others. In the long term, frequent trips produce a greater degree of psychological and social withdrawal from the world and users retreat into their own inner world of hallucination, whilst in the excessive use of 'acid' a state akin to a catatonic schizophrenic trance is produced which may last for weeks and require semi-permanent hospitalisation afterwards, the mind being truly 'blown'.

Even isolated use may be permanently harmful, for evidence is accumulating not only on the incidence of chromosomal damage, but the long lasting, psychotic after effects, which suggest that once a person has been on a 'trip' his or her personality may well be permanently impaired. The individual concerned will not appreciate that this is so, nor will the group who collectively indulge in acid-trips. Indeed, as groups, those who 'turn on' tend invariably to 'drop out' from normal society as a consequence, not necessarily as a voluntary wish. Then cults develop whose individual mystiques derive essentially from the hallucinogenic drugs they employ. There is, as in hard drug addiction, a certain latent predisposition in those who become 'acid-heads', and in a recent study conducted by the University of Southern California it was found that the primary quality in common among LSD 'trippers' was a history of unhappy family life. The 'loner' and the 'loser', with few friends and few accomplishments, is the individual particularly prone to find his or her valhalla only in the hallucinations obtained by the severe disturbance of cerebral metabolism produced by varieties of 'acid'.

The dirty youth who wants to stay in bed all day is not normal. Failure to turn up for work, persistent evidence of severe money shortage, or continual all-night parties are often suspicious signs and sooner or later drop-out will become inevitable. Psychiatric assistance at an early stage can help, given a willing attitude towards therapy. Support which is continual, no matter how trying and frustrating, is the only hope for the inadequate personality who is a potential or committed addict of drug-abuse. Punishment is irrelevant because they are punishing themselves far more than society can.

The frustrations of adolescence

Sexual and social frustrations – and their effects – are common enough in adolescence, but a particular sense of utter despair can be initiated by grief, by failure to resolve personal emotional crises over, say, homosexuality or by the broken engagement, where one or other partner blames themselves for imagined inadequacies, physically, psychologically or in an apparent inborn failure to feel sufficiently affectionate. Homesickness, creating a very real sense of isolation, is commonly experienced by those adolescents who have chosen the freedom of independence. Those who suffer worst are the ones who looked forward to leaving the parental environment and said so before they left, only to find that little satisfaction and a lot of problems can arise as a result of their new found freedom and responsibility. Eating humble pie and admitting they were wrong does not come easily in youth.

Adolescent depression

In depressive illness in the adolescent, the symptomatology is complex, but generally, though not always, obvious. A loss of interest is paramount, whether it is in work, pleasure, or the future, and there is often an allied criticism-of-self, combined with many vague physical complaints from loss of appetite to constipation, and fleeting pains to dyspepsia, all of which may classify the patient as a high 'doctor-usage' candidate, for he or she will be seen frequently in consultation. Apathy towards life is a hallmark of adolescent depression. This apathy is nevertheless a defence mechanism that protects the patient from being hurt. By living out a role of being deficient, the patient prevents himself from dealing with circumstances that might be painful – intellectually or socially – until forced to. Hostility and anger is directed inwards and expressed sometimes at this age in attacks of acute hysteria.

The apathy of adolescence may also be seen, however, as a positive physical expression, as obesity in the female compulsive over-eater, who constantly states she wants to be slim – as personal and deliberate slovenliness and the purposeful buying of second-hand clothes in order to look outrageous, despite parental gifts of money to go out and buy a new coat or suit – as sexual experimentation of the most flagrant manner where girls deliberately permit themselves to be used, or insist that their casual male partners take no contraceptive precautions and so present pregnant to their medical advisers as if it was an act of 'sexual suicide'. There is a constantly reappearing sign of self-harm in most of their actions from the obvious case where a boy drives his parents' car into a wall provoking disciplinary reaction, to the more obscure but equally deliberate case of the girl who rejects her loved fiance and becomes promiscuous with boys from town she met in a coffee-bar.

That same degree of self-harm is seen in suicide, for this is the most flagrant and instantly recognizable symptom of a depression. If an individual is depressed yet still capable enough of reacting, angry enough with himself or with others yet reduced to a particular kind of desperate aggression and frustration with everything – and sees no future before him or only ruin and disgrace – then suicide is the result. It is a cry for help from the wounded, and cornered animal, the last desperate throw of the dice.

Adolescent suicides account for about 3 per cent. of the total figure for all ages, but it has been estimated that for every teenager who succeeds in taking his own life there are 30 others who make serious suicidal attempts. At the Los Angeles Suicide Prevention Centre two psychologists carried out an investigation into the backgrounds of adolescent girls who made attempts on their own lives for a period of three years, and many common features emerged. Typically the girls came from emotionally chaotic families, 60 per cent. having been brought up in homes broken by divorce or separation. Rightly or wrongly, the girls were convinced that their parents, fathers especially had rejected them because they were social or educational failures. They felt that it was impossible to please their parents and had come to think that the parents were unconsciously conveying the message 'Everyone would be happier if you were not around'. Thirty per cent. of the girls had attempted suicide after rejection by a lover or boy friend. The mothers of the girls, it was found, had constantly expressed hostile attitudes towards men, warning their daughters that men would be insincere, untrustworthy and likely to exploit girls sexually and then abandon them. Some girls saw suicide as the most effective way of punishing their unloving parents or as a way to compel their parents to accept them and show concern. Others saw it as a form of self-punishment which would expiate their guilt or else prove their basic goodness. Because many of the girls were suspicious of all adults, then for the therapist, as there is for all of us, there was the constant danger of being viewed, as yet another rejecting 'parent'.

To be effective in a therapeutic role with adolescents, one must recognise their problems and their pressures and in the counselling role one must recall the vocational, motivational and environmental problems being acted out in the face of physical, family, group and commercial pressures.

Bibliography

1. Tanner, J. M., *Education and Physical Growth* (1961). Univ. of London Press, London.
2. Tanner, J. M., *Scientific American* (1968), **218,** 21.

3. Martin, B., *Practitioner* (1971), **206**, 256.
4. Schofield, M., *The Sexual Behaviour of Young People* (1965). Longman, London.
5. Miller, D. H., *The Age Between* (1969). Cornmarket-Hutchinson, London.
6. Gunn, A. D. G., *Roy. Soc. Health J.* (1971), **91**, 4.
7. Braceland, F. J., and Farnsworth, D. L., *Maryland Med. Journ.* (1969), 18, **4**, 67.
8. Maxwell Atkinson, *Univ. Quart.* (1969). Spring, **213**.
9. Binnie, H. L., *Vaughan Papers* (1969), **14**. Univ. of Leicester.
10. *Time* (1970), March 16, 16.

This section serves as both an introduction to electrocardiography and guide to diagnosis of coronary thrombosis by this method.

A Guide to Diagnosis by Electrocardiography with Special Reference to Coronary Thrombosis

by

D. Vérel

Regional Cardiologist, Sheffield

In planning this brief account of electrocardiography it seemed reasonable to give space in proportion to the information requested by doctors working outside hospitals who referred their patients to a hospital Outpatient Electrocardiographic Service in which electrocardiogram with report was supplied without any Consultant Medical opinion. Over 80 per cent. of requests were related to the possibility of ischaemic heart disease. Some 5 per cent. of request related to the diagnosis of cardiac arrhythmias, the remaining diagnostic needs did not reach 3 per cent. and covered a miscellaneous collection of diagnostic labels. Accordingly, in this review we shall consider the changes relating to ischaemic heart disease as the primary interest.

The electrocardiograph is a volt-meter. It provides a relatively sensitive record of changes measured in millivolts. The heart like any other muscle is a chemical machine and the voltage change which is measured by the electrocardiograph comes about as a result of the migration of positively charged ions, mainly potassium, from outside the muscle cell surface to within the muscle cell immediately before the mechanical contraction occurs. It is very crudely quantitative, larger masses of muscle producing a bigger voltage change than small ones, and clearly it is likely to be a very non-specific measurement which could be disturbed by a variety of causes. Further, with so simple a measurement it is unlikely that any change seen will be very specific for some particular phenomenon.

The conventional method of recording the electrocardiogram has grown up over the past century. Since a volt-meter has only two terminals it can only record the potential difference between two points. The heart however, is a three-dimensional body so that any electrocardiographic system must attempt to analyse a three-dimensional happening by observations made along a line or at best in a single plane. No-one today setting out to devise a system of electrocardiography would use the techniques in common use today. The very insensitive instruments which were in use thirty years ago required contact with very large skin surfaces to give any recording at all. It was conventional to make recordings by placing the subjects' hands and feet in bowls of warm saline to which the machine was attached. The very large body of knowledge relating to recordings obtained in this way has resulted in a sort of traditional usage for electrocardiography which is likely to persist despite the development of more rational systems such as that proposed by Frank.

The conventional connections used today are as follows:

Lead I — Right arm to left arm.
Lead II — Right arm to left leg.
Lead III — Left arm to left leg.
AVR — Right arm to left arm and left leg together.
AVL — Left arm to right arm and left leg together.
AVF — Left leg to right arm and left arm.
V1 — 4th right intercostal space parasternally to I, II and III.
V2 — 4th left intercostal space parasternally to I, II and III.
V3 — Halfway between V2 and the 5th space midclavicular line to I, II and III.
V4 — 5th left interspace midclavicular line to I, II and III.
V5 — Anterior axillary line at the same horizontal plane as V4 to I, II and III.
V6 — Mid-axillary line in the same plane to I, II and III.
V7 — Posterior axillary line in the same plane to I, II and III.

It will be noted in this series of chest connections there is an attempt to get a special idea of the electrical changes in the heart by connecting several leads to one pole of the volt-meter with a single lead connected to the other pole. Note the irrational numbering of the V leads where V1 and V2 straddle the sternum. When recording to the right it is conventional to correct the numbering, e.g. the point in the 4th right interspace midclavicular line is called V4R as though V1R were to the left of the sternum.

The normal electrocardiogram

The normal electrocardiogram is shown diagrammatically in Figure 1. There is an initial positive deflection called the P wave which occurs as the result of depolarisation of the atrium. Depolarisation describes the change in voltage preceding contraction. The voltage returns briefly to the iso-electric line and there then follows a rapid series of changes termed the QRS complex which is due to the depolarisation of the ventricles. After a brief return to the iso-electric line there follows the T wave which is due to the repolarisation of the ventricles and in some patients there may be seen a further lower deflection termed the U wave. Both the T wave and the U wave are positive in direction in most leads. The Q wave may not be found in some leads in all subjects. The P–R interval measured from the beginning of the P wave to the beginning of the QRS complex depends on heart rate but is not usually greater than 0·2 seconds. The QRS interval is the time measured from the beginning of the Q wave to the end of the S wave. It does not normally exceed 0·1 seconds. In some normal subjects and in many abnormal conditions the QRS complex has more oscillations than are shown in Figure 1. When there is a second R wave or second S wave the notation used is to term the first R wave R1 and the second R wave R2. Similarly the first S wave S1, the second S2. A typical 13 lead electrocardiogram is shown in Figure 2. It should be noted that because of the connections normally made to the electrocardiograph the tracing comes out 'upside down' in AVR.

The changes accompanying coronary thrombosis and cardiac ischaemia will now be considered and the possible other causes of similar changes discussed. Because the cardinal changes of cardiac infarction are seen in the ventricular complexes we begin with the QRS complex.

The most frequent and important evidence of cardiac infarction in the QRS complex is the development of a Q wave. It is usually evidence of a considerable infarct and has been interpreted as evidence of complete loss of electrical activity in the anterior or posterior wall of the heart depending upon which leads show the Q wave. In an anterior infarction it is usually seen in leads 1 and AVL, in a posterior infarction in leads 3 and AVF. It is also commonly seen in the chest leads V1 to V5 or even further in an anterior infarction. A deep Q wave (6 mm or more) rarely reverts to an R wave but it is not uncommon to find the depth of the Q wave diminishing as recovery occurs (see Figures 3 and 4).

Two fairly common conditions should be distinguished from the Q wave of cardiac infarction. The first is a Q wave found in lead III and sometimes AVL which will revert to an R wave if the subject takes a deep breath and holds it while the record is made. This is called a 'postural' Q and is due to a high diaphragm producing a very horizontal anatomical position for the heart. Taking a deep breath pulls the heart down vertically and the apparent Q wave then becomes an R wave. The second condition which can be exceedingly difficult to be sure of is the clockwise rotation of the heart which is fairly common in patients with emphysema. This can produce Q waves in the anterior chest leads (V1 to V5) indistinguishable from those resulting from cardiac infarction and only a careful history and examination enables a differentiation to be made. However, the T waves in this condition are normal.

The QRS complex may be widened by ischaemic damage to the conducting mechanism, thus producing a bundle branch block. In this situation the QRS interval is prolonged and, if the damage is acute, it is usual on an Intensive Care Unit to take the change as an indication for a prophylactic insertion of pace-making catheter in case the block should become complete. The condition has to be distinguished from bundle branch block occurring as a result of other causes, e.g. virus infections of the heart and congenital lesions, and must also be distinguished from a 'bundle branch block pattern' in which R1 S1 R2 S2 patterns occur but the total QRS interval is normal. These are not uncommon in normal subjects and are characteristic of certain congenital conditions (Figure 5).

The S–T segment is of great importance in the assessment of cardiac injury (Figure 6). Typically the S–T segment is elevated, the elevation being found in the leads appropriate to the site of the infarct, that is S1 and AVL in an anterior infarction S3 and AVF in a posterior infarction. In large infarcts the S–T changes may be found in other standard leads, and in anterior infarctions they are very characteristically encountered in the chest leads, V1 to V4 in an anterior lesion and V5 to V7 in a lateral or diaphragmatic lesion. Elevation of the S–T segment usually means the infarct is a matter of hours or days old only. Daily records will show that over 3–4 days the S–T segment elevation becomes progressively less and as it does so the T wave begins to invert. After 7–10 days in a typical example the S–T segment is once more iso-electric and the T wave has become inverted.

The changes in the S–T segment which have been described above must be distinguished from two conditions. The first is persistent S–T elevation usually in the chest leads (the V leads) which may be a permanent feature following a cardiac infarction. It has been in the past usual to regard this S–T elevation as evidence of a cardiac aneurysm. However, the methods of investigation and surgery which have become available indicate that this is not so. It is usually found that such permanent S–T elevation is associated with thinning and fibrosis in the cardiac wall but aneurysmal formation is not necessarily present. The other condition producing S–T elevation is acute pericarditis. Typically the S–T elevation here has a different form from that seen in a recent cardiac infarct but in the early stages the two conditions might be quite indistinguishable and only the progress of the condition and serial electrocardiography enable a firm distinction to be made.

While the S–T changes described may be seen in acute infarction it should be noted that S–T elevation may not be recorded, particularly in posterior infarctions. Here the only change may be the appearance of a Q wave with T wave inversion particularly if the infarct be small. Another point to note is that acute ischaemia does not usually produce S–T elevation. It is much more usual to see S–T depression below the isoelectric line as a result of acute ischaemic changes in the heart (Figure 8). Similarly acute anoxia, for example that due to obstructed breathing, will produce T wave inversion in most subjects with depression of the S–T segment. The S–T elevation as described is a particularly reliable sign of cardiac infarct.

The T wave changes associated with cardiac infarction are essentially inversion of the T wave. This can be a permanent feature and is a reliable guide to past damage. It is however, a poor indication of the time at which damage has occurred.

It was mentioned earlier that the voltage change is unlikely to provide a very specific measure of events in the heart muscle. This is well demonstrated in the part of the electrocardiogram we have now reached. Changes in the S–T segment with inversion of the T wave, although characteristic of cardiac infarction, must be distinguished from two other important conditions. The first of these is the effect of hypertrophy and strain. Over-action of either ventricle over a long period produces thickening of the wall with ultimately fibrosis among the muscle fibres. The resultant change on the electrocardiogram is important and characteristic. The voltages increase in the leads appropriate to the ventricle concerned and when 'strain' occurs the

T wave inverts. Right ventricular hypertrophy and strain are seen as increased voltage with S–T depression and T wave inversion in leads 3, AVF and the early chest leads V4R to V3 or further (Figure 9). Left ventricular hypertrophy produces increased voltage with S–T depression and T wave inversion in leads 1, AVL and V4 to V7 (Figure 10). These are sensitive indices of the progress of disease of the ventricle, for example, in aortic stenosis the spread of T wave inversion from V7 to the earlier chest leads can be observed as time passes and the ventricle becomes progressively embarrassed by its excessive load. Similarly observation of the regression of these changes after successful surgery is a sure index of success.

The other major cause of T wave changes is the administration of Digitalis. This will produce electrocardiographic changes very similar to those due to hypertrophy or to cardiac disease and not infrequently the changes are not seen evenly in every lead but occur predominantly in the standard leads mainly affected by one or other ventricle (Figure 11).

It is clear from the foregoing that in order to assess an electrocardiogram it is essential to know whether the patient's blood pressure is normal, whether or not there is evidence of valve disease, and whether or not he is taking any preparation of foxglove. It is also clearly desirable to know whether there is a history of previous cardiac infarction and, if this was documented by electrocardiography, in which lead changes were found. The changes which have been described may be exceedingly transient and it is possible to record an hour or two after an infarct clear-cut changes suggesting cardiac infarction and to repeat the recording three days later and find a normal tracing. It is also possible to encounter a patient with a clear history of cardiac infarct and find that no unequivocal evidence of disease appears for forty-eight hours after the infarction. This is not rare in posterior cardiac infarct. A number of other causes of changes in the complexes described do exist but have not been described in this account. Textbooks should be consulted for the effects of such conditions as potassium depletion and endocrine diseases.

Disturbances of rhythm

Disturbances of rhythm are common-place in ischaemic damage to the heart. They may also, of course, occur as a result of rheumatic heart disease and almost every described arrhythmia has been seen by the author in symptomless children. In considering arrhythmias, therefore,

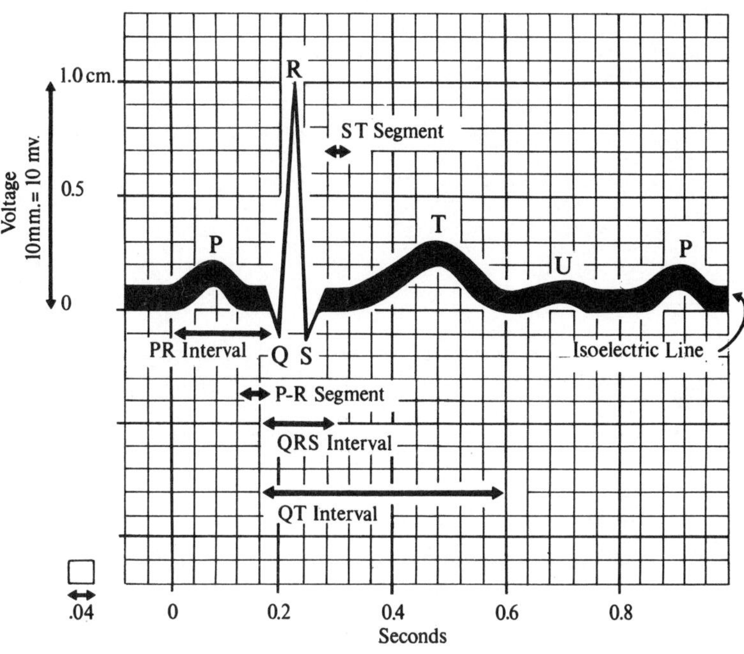

Figure 1. Diagram of the normal electrocardiogram.

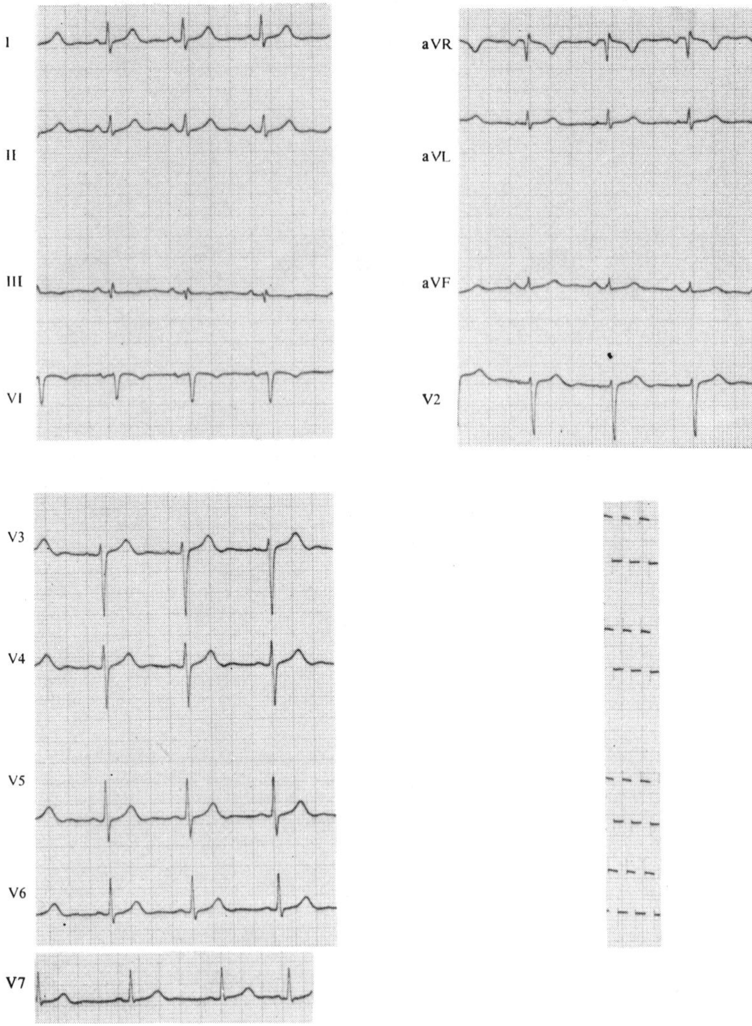

Figure 2. Normal electrocardiogram. In this example there is a very small R wave in lead 3 followed by an SR′ complex, the T wave in lead 3 being nearly flat. In AVF there is a small R wave and a normal T wave. This recording from a normal young adult shows a T wave inversion in lead V1 which is common in normal subjects.

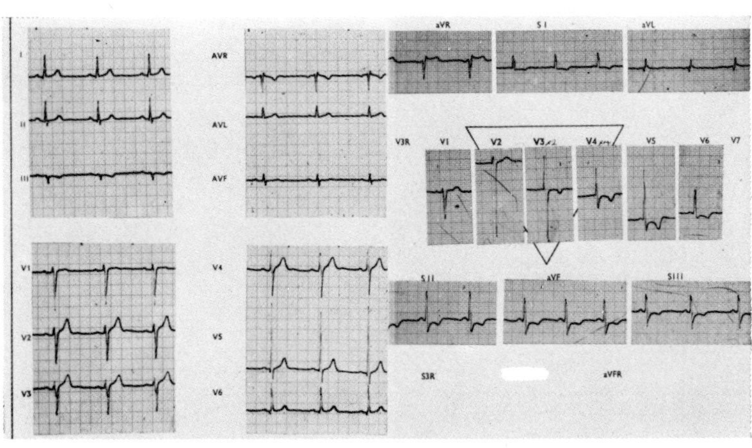

Figure 3. Cardiac infarction. Two electrocardiograms recorded at intervals of six months. That on the left was recorded two years after a cardiac infarction. The only possible abnormality is inversion of the T wave in lead S3. A further cardiac infarction occurred and the record on the right was made some 2–3 weeks after the second infarction. It now shows T wave inversion in S1, S2, AVF, and S3 and also in the chest leads V3 to V6. There is depression of the ST segments in S2, AVF, and S3. This is consistent with a small infarction mainly within the septum and posterior aspect of the heart.

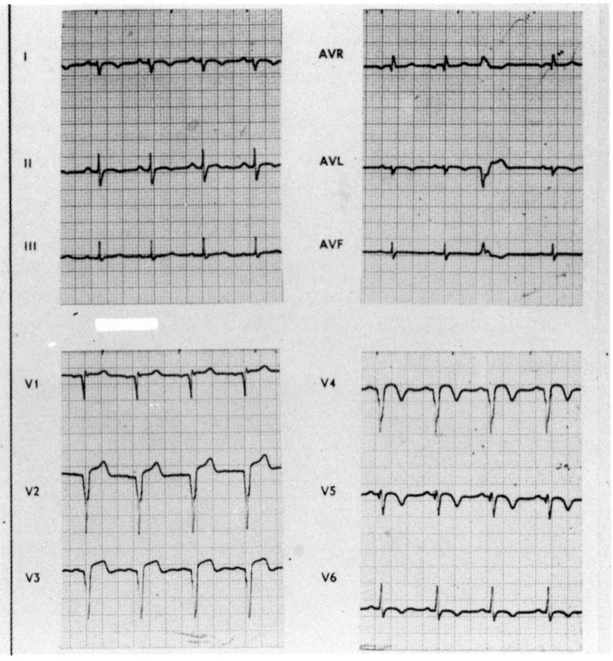

Figure 4. Electrocardiogram recorded some days after a small antero-lateral infarction. The T wave in lead 1 is inverted, there are Q waves from lead V2 to V4. The ST segments in V3 and V4 elevated, and in V4, V5 and V6 the T waves are inverted. An extra systole is seen as the 3rd beat in the block AVR, AVL, AVF. The patient recovered from this infarct and the electrocardiogram became more normal. Two years later a further episode of chest pain occurred and the electrocardiogram on the right was recorded. It shows both changes of recovery and changes of further trouble. The ST segments and T wave changes in lead 1 and the chest leads as far as V4 were much less obvious. The patient has however, developed more evident changes in V5, V6 and V7 with a deep Q wave in V5 where previously an R wave was seen. Recovery from this infarct was followed by further improvement in the electrocardiogram.

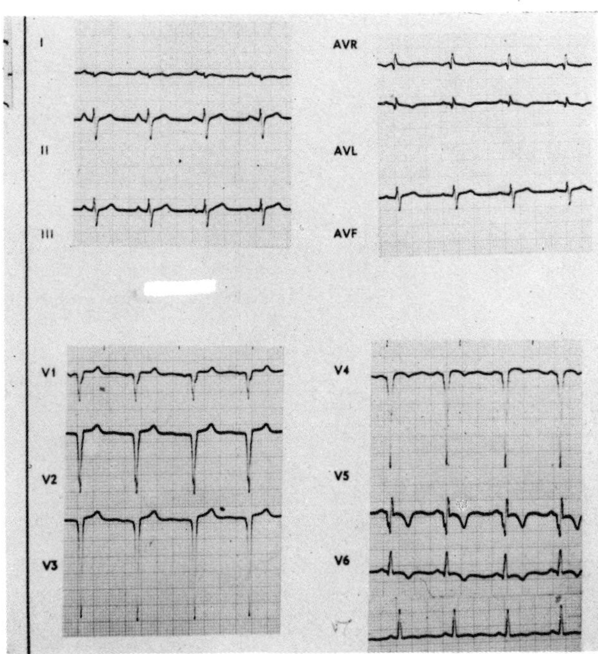
I
II
III
AVR
AVL
AVF
V1
V2
V3
V4
V5
V6

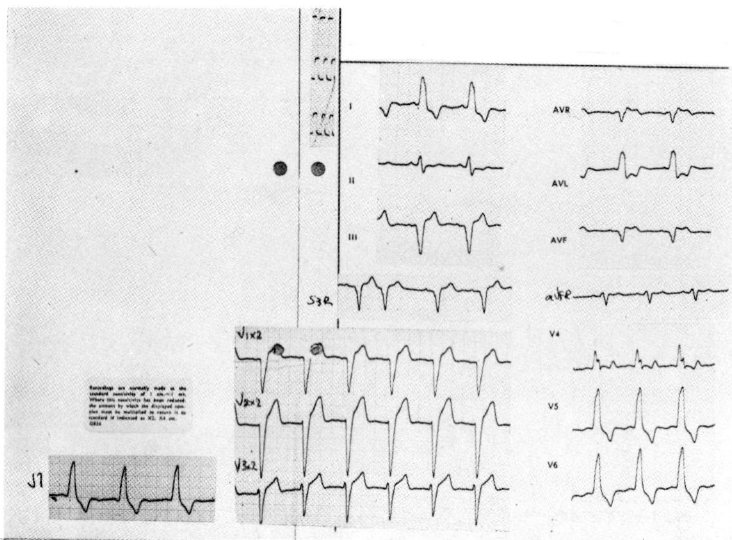

Figure 5. Bundle Branch Block. The P waves are followed by a widened QRS complex. The ST segments are displaced from the isoelectric line particularly in leads 1 and AVL. The deep Q waves in lead 3 and AVF persist after the patient takes a deep breath as shown in S3R and AVFR. However, they are the result of the abnormal conduction path and do not help to localise the ischaemic damage to the heart which has resulted in this bundle branch block. The diagnosis of cardiac infarction in the presence of bundle branch block is very difficult and can usually only be done on the basis of comparing serial electrocardiograms taken from the same patient over several days when acute changes indicate recent damage.

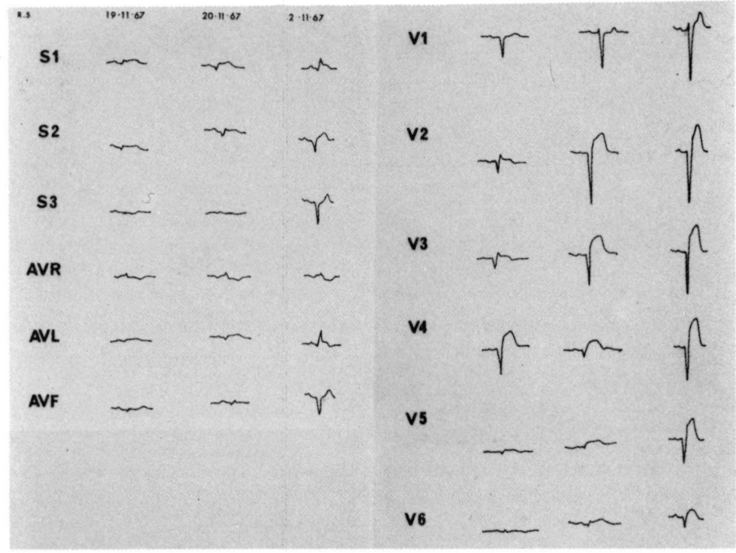

Figure 6. Electrocardiogram recorded on three successive days in a patient who died of cardiac infarction on the fourth day. Note the progressive development of a deep Q wave in lead S3 and AVF and the progressive elevation of the ST segment above the isoelectric line in the chest leads. At post-mortem a large posterior infarct was found.

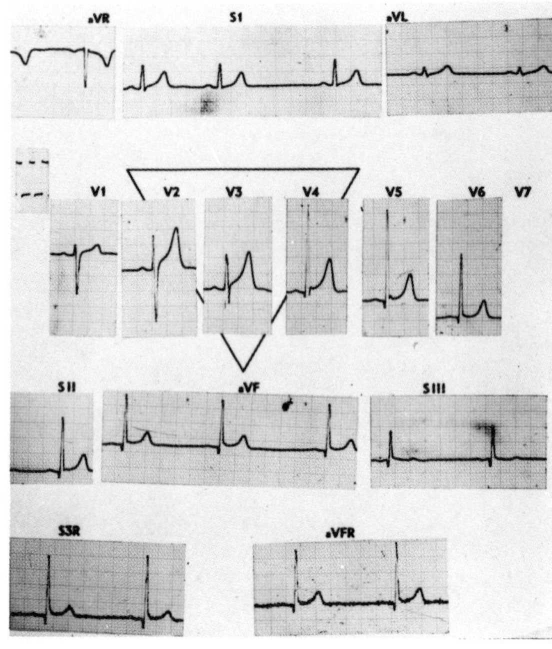

Figure 7. Acute benign pericarditis. Electrocardiogram from a patient admitted with severe precordial pain suggestive of cardiac infarction. ST elevation mainly in the chest leads. Note the typical concave upward swing of the ST segment very different from the high initial take off seen in infarction, e.g.

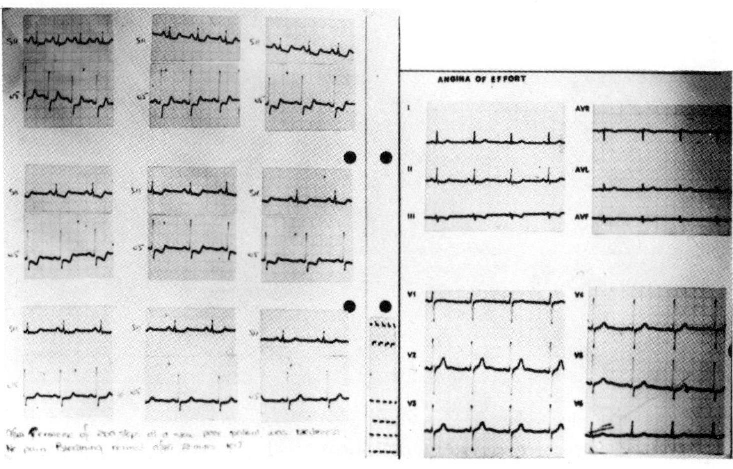

Figure 8. Ischaemic changes due to exercise. On the right is shown the standard electrocardiogram, possible ischaemic damage is indicated by T wave inversion in S3 and a biphasic T wave in AVF. On the left is shown the results of a standard exercise test. The top left recording shows S2 and V5 immediately after exercise with marked ST depression. This gradually recovers over 6–7 minutes.

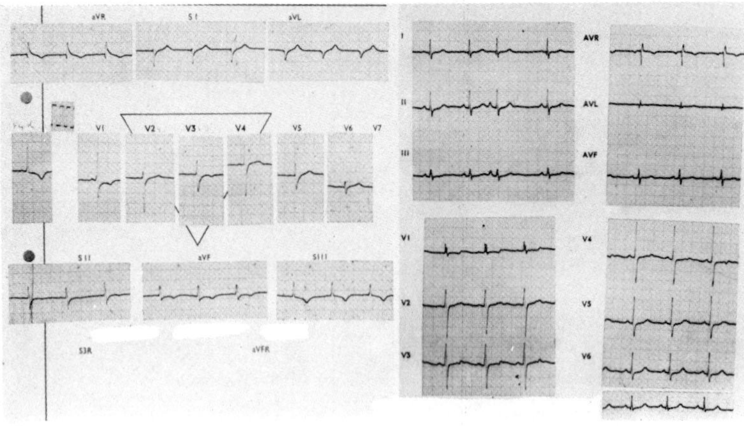

Figure 9. Electrocardiogram in pulmonary valve stenosis (right ventricular pressure 150/0). The main deflection in S1 is an S wave, in S3 an R wave. This is right axis deviation. T wave inversion is present in lead AVF, S3, V4R, and V1. One year after surgery the axis has reverted to normal with an R wave being the main deflection in lead 1 and lead 3. The T waves in lead 3 and AVF are now normal. In V1 the R wave is much smaller and there is a biphasic T wave. The patient was aged 47 at the time of operation.

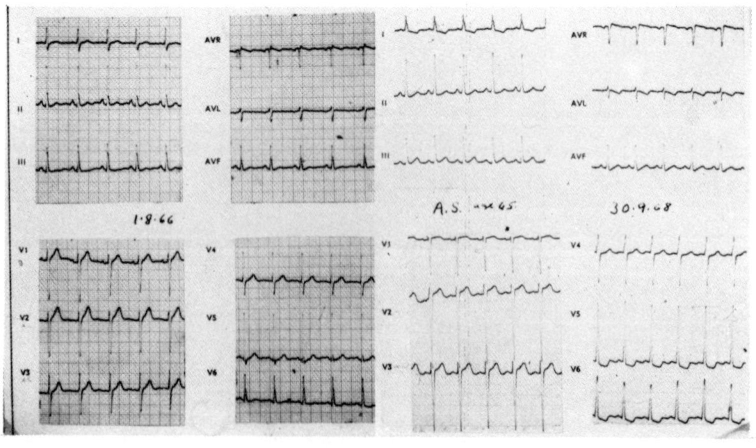

Figure 10. Progression of ST changes in aortic stenosis. On the left there is some increase in voltage but the T waves are normal. Two years later on the right the T waves are inverted in lead 1 and the S wave has been lost. The T wave has inverted in lead AVL, the voltage has increased in V5 and V6 with depression of the ST segment, and early inversion of the T wave.

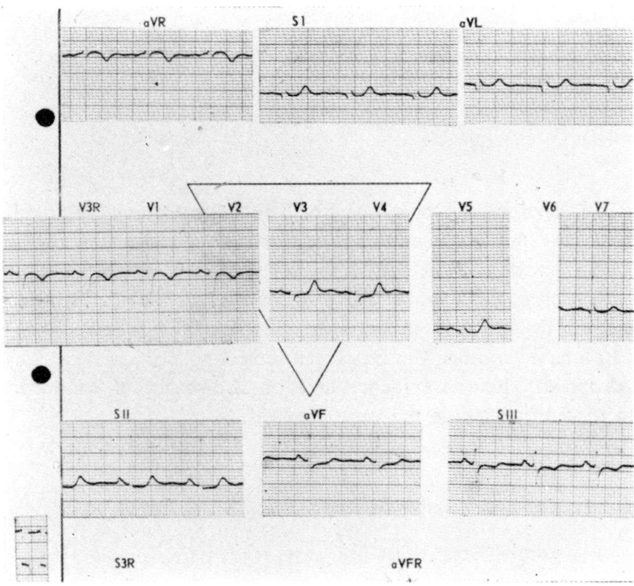

Figure 11. Electrocardiogram showing moderate changes of Digitalis therapy. There is ST depression in several leads particularly V5 and V7 and depression with some T wave inversion in lead S3. This patient was being maintained on Digitalis in sinus rhythm to prevent attacks of paroxysmal atrial tachycardia.

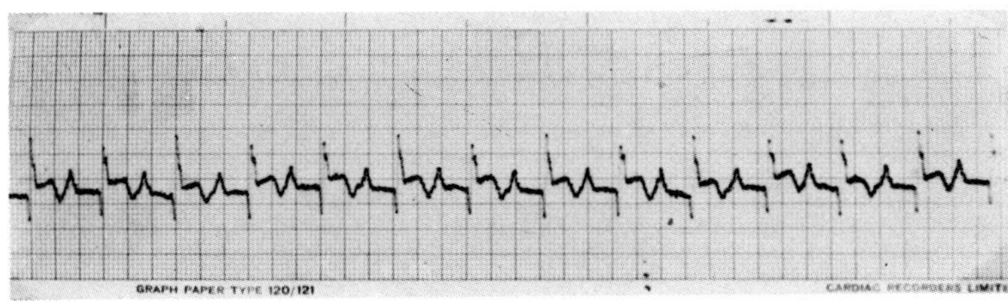

Figure 12. Electrocardiogram two days after a coronary thrombosis. On the day before this recording was made complete heart block was present. This recording shows a prolonged P–R interval followed by a Q wave. There is then a R wave with a notch in the complex suggesting some degree of bundle branch block, the ST segment is elevated and the T wave following it inverted. The patient recovered uneventfully.

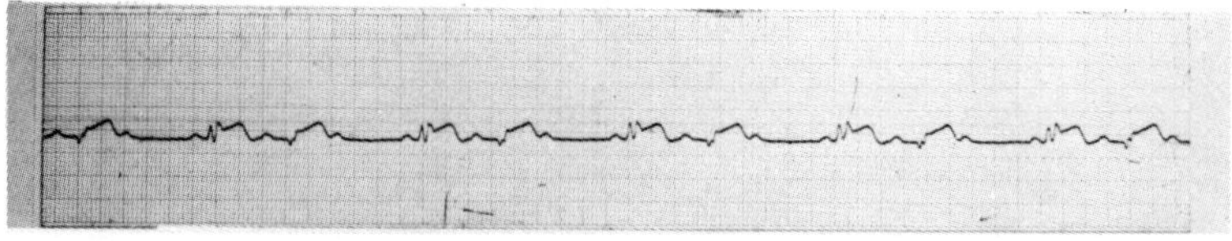

Figure 13. Wenckebach phenomenon. The tracing shows ventricular complexes in pairs (pulsus bigeminus). The first beat of each pair shows a normal P–R interval with an RSR pattern leading into an elevated ST segment and early inversion of the T wave. The P–R interval for the next ventricular beat is longer and the RSR pattern is not seen. The T wave is followed by a P wave. After an interval another P wave is seen indicating that a ventricular beat has been dropped. There is evidence here of disturbance of conduction from atrium to ventricle and in the ventricle itself.

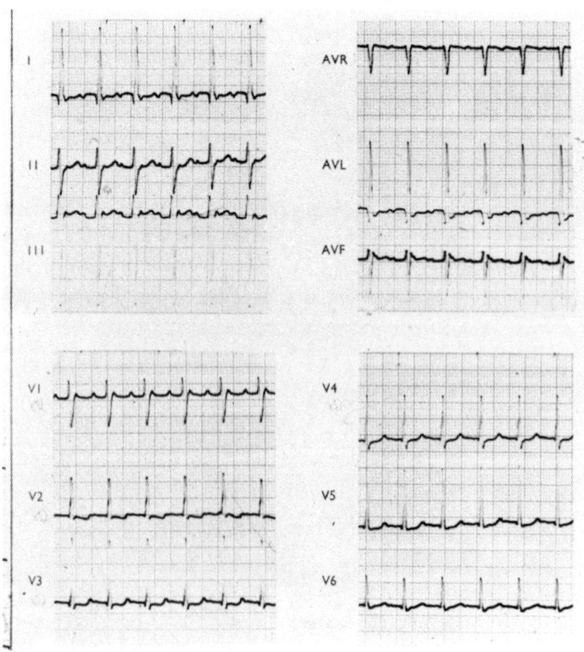

Figure 14. 2:1 heart block. The P waves are best seen in leads 2 and V1. Examination of either of these leads demonstrates that there is a P wave occurring in the QRST complex and a second P wave precedes the R wave. This is a tracing from a patient illustrated in Figure 11 showing an attack of paroxysmal tachycardia for which treatment with Digitalis was prescribed.

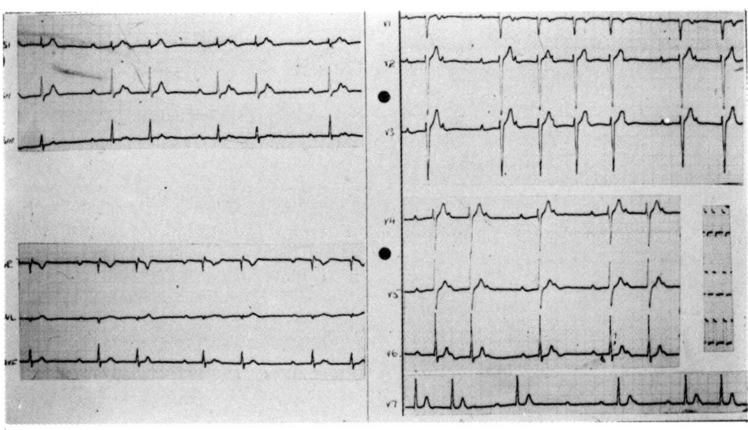

Figure 15. Complete heart block. The atrial beats are independent of the ventricular beats so in an electrocardiogram the P waves show complete dissociation from the QRS complexes.

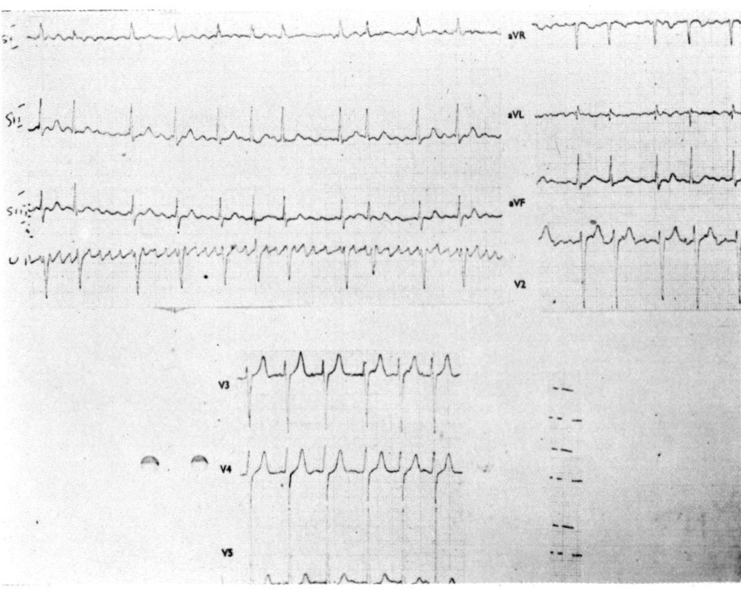

Figure 16. Uncontrolled atrial fibrillation. In this example the saw tooth appearance in V1 somewhat resembles atrial flutter but is less regular and is not regularly related to the occurrence of the QRS complex. This patient was in cardiac failure.

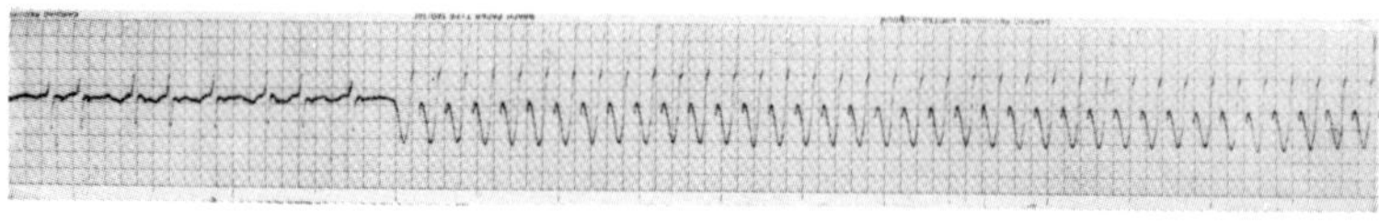

Figure 17. An attack of ventricular tachycardia terminated by injection of Practolol. This record was obtained on the coronary care ward. It shows a ventricular rate of over 200 a minute which suddenly reverts to sinus rhythm. The ventricular tachycardia had caused acute angina. Reversion to sinus rhythm relieved this in less than one minute.

one must always bear in mind that the condition may be congenital. It is also important to remember that virtually every arrhythmia can be completely asymptomatic in one patient and the cause of severe and disabling symptoms in another. This variability in the causation of symptoms is fundamentally one of rate. When the heart goes too quickly it does not get time to fill so that the output falls and the perfusion of vital tissues of the body is inadequate. When the heart goes too slowly the perfusion of the coronary vessels is inadequate since the diastolic pressure is not held at a level enough to perfuse the coronary arteries for a sufficient fraction of the cardiac cycle. This difference is well exemplified in Adams-Stokes attacks where the embarrassment is sufficient to produce syncope. Here unconsciousness may result either from gross tachycardia or from functional stand-still of the ventricles. Stand-still may be the result of either ventricular fibrillation or asystole.

Cardiac ischaemia may affect the transmission of the impulse from the atrium to the ventricle. The earliest evidence of this is prolongation of the P–R interval or first degree heart block. This is not uncommonly seen in acute coronary thrombosis and may precede a complete failure of transmission. It is, of course, found in other conditions. It may be due to rheumatic fever, to over-dosage with drugs, for example Digitalis, and it may be found as a symptomless congenital abnormality. When due to coronary artery disease it is commonly transient. Patients with this condition may be referred for electrocardiography if the atrial sound is audible so producing a gallop rhythm (Figure 12).

In more severe degrees a progressive failure of transmission may be seen. Here a normal P–R interval is followed by one longer than normal and the next beat has an even longer P–R interval or the atrial beat may be dropped. This is known as the Wenckebach phenomenon. It is rarely seen in symptomless patients (Figure 13).

Other forms of block may be seen particularly if there is an atrial tachycardia. In this condition the P–R interval is usually normal but there is failure to transmit the atrial beat which may occur regularly or irregularly. The degree of block is usually expressed numerically by giving the number of atrial beats occurring followed by the number of ventricular responses, for example, two ventricular beats for every three atrial beats is referred to as 3:2 heart block (Figure 14).

In complete heart block the atrial contractions and ventricular contractions are dissociated. The ventricle usually assumes a slow inter-ventricular rate of about 30 to 40 beats per minute. When this occurs in a heart embarrassed by cardiac infarction it may be an urgent matter to increase the heart rate by pacing the heart electrically at a more normal rate. In any acquired complete heart block the myocardial ischaemia which results from the slow rate may produce arrhythmias causing unconsciousness (Adams-Stokes attacks), or may so embarrass the heart's action that cardiac failure results. This may be treated with drugs such as Saventrine to increase the rate or if these are ineffective by permanent pacing. By contrast, congenital heart block rarely produces symptoms and is compatible with normal activity (Figure 15).

When the atrium has a very rapid rate of over 200 beats per minute, the ventricle responding regularly to these beats which have on the electrocardiogram a characteristic 'saw tooth' appearance, it is commonly referred to as atrial flutter. Atrial fibrillation may also occur in cardiac infarction and is characterised by a cessation of atrial contraction (Figure 16). Irregular fibrillary contractions occur throughout the atrium. The atrio-ventricular node is subjected to very frequent stimulation with a result that the ventricle is continually stimulated to contract. The result is a rapid irregular contraction of the ventricle usually sufficiently fast to produce cardiac failure. It is commonly seen in rheumatic heart disease and may occur as a temporary event in a wide variety of severe infections – particularly pneumonias – for example that due to Frielander's bacillus. However, slow atrial fibrillation producing no symptoms is not uncommon in elderly patients. The conventional treatment of atrial fibrillation with Digitalis slows the conduction of the impulses to the ventricle and so allows an acceptable ventricular rate. Digitalis administered to a patient with slow fibrillation may produce undue bradycardia and so cause symptoms from too slow a rate.

Extrasystoles are beats which arise in a site outside the normal sino-atrial node. They may arise in the atrium, the conducting system between the atrium and the ventricle, or in the ventricle. It has been shown that extrasystoles are universal in normal human subjects and may be found in any normal person if the electrocardiogram is recorded continuously over a sufficiently long period. They are usually asymptomatic. However, some people are conscious of the larger beat which follows an extrasystole. This larger beat is due to the long diastole causing greater filling of the heart than normal.

When extrasystoles occur in rapid succession the cardiac output is temporarily greatly reduced. When this occurs in a heart embarrassed by a cardiac infarction or other cardiac disease they can have extremely serious consequences. Even in normal hearts a prolonged run of ectopic beats as is found in paroxysmal tachycardia will produce anginal symptoms and an intense feeling that death is imminent (anguor animi). The site of the ectopic beats should be identified if possible since the treatment likely to be successful varies with the site of origin. In general, atrial tachycardia and ectopics respond best to Digitalis and similar preparations. Ventricular tachycardia responds best to a beta blocking drug. The identification of the type of ectopic beat depends upon monitoring the electrocardiograph. This usually presents no problem in cardiac infarction if the patient is on the Coronary Care Unit but in conditions like paroxysmal tachycardia may be a matter of great difficult since it is surprising how rarely the condition will manifest itself during a clinical examination (Figure 17).

This brief review has taken the form of a discourse around the text of coronary thrombosis. It is intended to serve as an introduction to a more serious study of an interesting and complex subject. The most useful way of learning to interpret electrocardiograms is to record them personally. Confidence comes with experience and repetition. Ideally it should be possible to send difficult electrocardiograms to a diagnostic centre for a further opinion providing there is a Physician in the Centre who is prepared to give an opinion on an electrocardiogram without seeing the patient. It should, however, be constantly borne in mind that an electrocardiogram is only a record of voltage change. Its meaning is usually only apparent in the context of clinical history and examination of the patient.

Section C

Useful Information

This short section contains miscellaneous items of general information often useful in daily practice.

Useful Information

Introduction

In this section items of information relevant to the everyday practice of medicine are included. For the results of laboratory tests readers are referred to an earlier section of the book. Diets suggested in the section on Therapy of Common Diseases are included here as are weight, height, obstetric and therapeutic tables. The incubation periods of some common and serious infectious diseases complete this reference section.

DIETS

Free diet

(Diet devised by Dr. D. Craddock. Reproduced with the permission of the author and publishers, Messrs. E. S. Livingstone.)

1. Eat and drink as much as you like of the following:
   LEAN MEAT, including poultry and offal.
   FISH
   EGGS
   CHEESE
   SALADS
   VEGETABLES
   FRESH FRUIT or fruit bottled without sugar, but not dried or tinned fruit.
   BUTTER, margarine and cooking fat.
   CONDIMENTS, Sour pickles, thin soups, Worcestershire sauce.
   TEA, coffee, Oxo, Bovril.
   SACCHARINE for sweetening.
2. You may have:
   (a) ½ pint of fresh milk daily (This includes all milk taken in tea, coffee, etc.).
   (b) Up to 3 oz. of reducing bread, or crisp bread, or six Energen rolls daily.
   (c) One or two small potatoes per helping.

3. You may have *nothing else whatever.*
   Note especially that this means:

   No bread (except as above), biscuits (dry or sweet), cake or pastry.
   No sausages, macaroni, spaghetti, rice, cereals, thick sauces.
   No sugar, syrup, chocolate, sweets, cocoa, honey, jam (except diabetic).
   No alcoholic drink.

   In Other Words Nothing Containing Sugar or Cereal in Any Form.
   Weigh yourself before you begin, and once a week or once a fortnight afterwards, on the *same scales*, in the *same clothes* and at the *same time of day*.
   You should eat three or four meals a day.
   On this diet, you should lose between 5 and 10 lb per month.

NOTE:

1. The weight can vary up to 2 or 3 lb in the course of a day, usually being higher in the evening.
2. A glass of beer or a short drink is equivalent in food value to 1 oz of bread, and may be substituted for it. A drink is best taken with the evening meal.

1,000 or 500 calorie diet
(Devised by Miss E. P. Skinner and Miss M. Vinnecoor, Dietetic Department, St Thomas's Hospital, London).

It is a diet containing 1,000 calories, 60 g. protein, 60 g. fat and 80 g. carbohydrate. If foods marked with an asterisk are omitted the diet will provide 500 calories, 40 g. protein, 30 g. fat and 35 g. carbohydrate a day. The 500 calorie diet should be supplemented with multi-vitamin tablets.

DAILY ALLOWANCES

*90 g. Bread	= 3 thin slices
*20 g. Butter	
300 ml Milk or up to	
600 ml Skimmed milk	
3 portions fruit	= Fresh or cooked
75 g. Meat maximum	= Cooked weight
150 g. White fish	= Cooked weight

Take four or not less than three small meals regularly daily. Avoid eating between meals, but if hungry you may have low calorie drinks or clear soup, or a cup of meat or yeast extract. An extra salad or raw carrot or stick of celery may sometimes help.

The milk may be used in drinks of tea or coffee throughout the day.

A light or main meal may be taken at midday or in the evening, whichever is most convenient.

PACKED LUNCH

Take open sandwiches using bread from daily allowance. The portion of meat, or cheese or egg can be taken separately in a polythene bag or sandwich box if preferred.

Lettuce or tomato or other suitable salad may be taken if desired.

EXCHANGES

★ 1 thin slice of bread (approx 30 g.)

- ★ or 1 Carton of plain yoghurt
- ★ or 1 Boiled potato, the size of an egg
- ★ or 2 Tablespoons cooked rice
- ★ or 2 Cream crackers
- ★ or 2 Ryvita or other crispbread
- ★ or 3 Water biscuits
- ★ or 2 Semi-sweet biscuits

SUITABLE FOODS FOR USE IN THE DIET

Cereals	Bread as daily allowance. Plain biscuits or crispbread as exchange for bread only.
Fish	White fish grilled or steamed. Herrings, mackerel or salmon occasionally only.
Meat	All fresh meat preferably lean, or offal or poultry. Can be roasted, grilled, casseroled or served cold. Lean bacon or ham. Canned meat. Sausages grilled.
Cheese	Taken as exchange for meat or fish. Cream cheeses occasionally only.
Eggs	Boiled, poached or hard boiled. Scrambled or as omelette occasionally only.
Fats	Butter or margarine or dripping, as daily allowance.

Milk	Fresh whole or skimmed as daily allowance. Plain yoghurt to replace equal amount of milk, or fruit yoghurt occasionally only.
Fruit	Fresh fruit as available, or cooked without sugar.
Vegetables	Green or root vegetables as available, frozen vegetables, salads. Canned vegetables. Potato as exchange for bread only.
Drinks	Low calorie or diabetic squashes, and other low calorie cordials. Vichy water, soda water, tea, coffee. Meat or yeast extracts, Bouillon cubes.
Miscellaneous	Artificial sweeteners in liquid or tablet form. Consommé or any clear vegetable or bone soup. Vinegar, lemon juice, mint sauce, low calorie french dressing, salt, pepper, mustard, pickled onions, gherkins, or mixed pickles in vinegar or mustard. Gelatine powder or sheets.

FOODS TO BE AVOIDED

Cereals	Flour and its products, pasta, batter, sweet biscuits, cakes, pastry. Cornflour, custard powder, arrowroot, rice. Breakfast cereals, Porridge oats.
Fish	Tinned fish in oil or sauce.
Meat	Meat pies, sausage rolls, toad in the hole. Fatty and streaky bacon, meat fritters.
Cheese	Cream cheese, Camembert, blue vein cheeses, 30 g. portion only should not be taken more than twice weekly.
Eggs	Scrambled, fried or as an omelette should not be taken more than twice weekly.
Fats	Butter, margarine or dripping not exceeding the daily allowance. Oil, lard, mayonnaise and salad cream.
Milk	Evaporated and condensed milk. Single and double cream, ice cream. Fruit yoghurt should not be taken more than twice weekly.

Fruit	Bananas, grapes, dried fruit, tinned fruit including tinned fruit for diabetics containing sorbitol. Nuts, Avocado pear, olives.
Vegetables	Beans: broad, butter, haricot, red; beans canned in tomato sauce. Lentils, dried and tinned peas. Sweet corn, yam, sweet potato, plantain. Sweet pickles, chutney. Potatoes unless in exchange for bread. Vegetables canned in sauce.
Drinks	Alcohol, including beer, sweetened fruit juices, fruit squash, all other sweetened beverages or cordials, tomato juice containing sugar. All malted milk powders, drinking chocolate, cocoa, and other beverages with milk flavouring.
Miscellaneous	Sugar, glucose, jam, marmalade, honey, golden syrup, treacle. Sweets and chocolates; all types. All artificial sweeteners containing sugar. Tinned or packet soup, home made thickened soup. Thickened sauces or gravy, gravy powders. Fried food.

SUGGESTED MEAL PATTERN

Breakfast	*1 Egg – boiled or poached, or 1 rasher grilled lean bacon or grilled fish. *1 thin slice of bread (approx. 28 g.) brown or white, plain or toasted. *Butter or margarine thinly spread. Tea or coffee with milk from daily allowance. *(1 piece of fruit in the 500 calorie diet).
Mid-morning	Tea or coffee with milk from daily allowance, or meat or yeast extract.
Lunch	Average 56 g. portion of lean meat hot or cold, or poached or grilled fish (112 g.) or 1 boiled or poached egg or 40 g. Cheddar, Dutch or other hard cheese

or 30 g. any type of cream cheese including blue vein cheeses.
Any kind of green vegetables – a good helping.
Any kind of root vegetables (excluding potatoes) average portion,
or salad with vinegar or lemon if preferred.
1 piece of fruit fresh or cooked without sugar.

Supper Meat, cheese, egg or fish as at lunch.
Vegetables green or root or salad as at lunch.
*1 thin slice of bread (28 g.) brown or white, butter thinly spread,
or 1 boiled potato the size of an egg.
Fruit fresh or cooked as at lunch.

Bed-time Drink using milk from daily allowance.
1 piece of fruit.

More restricted still is the 300 calorie diet shown below. The patient should be admitted to hospital and given vitamin supplements when this is prescribed.

300 calorie diet

(Devised by Miss E. P. Skinner and Miss M. Vinnecoor, Dietetic Department, St Thomas's Hospital, London).

Breakfast 100 g. orange or grapefruit, or equivalent unsweetened fruit.
Tea or coffee using milk from daily allowance.

Dinner 20 g. Lean meat or equivalent protein.
This can be roast or grilled, or braised, served hot or cold.
100 g. divided between 2 green vegetables or small salad with vinegar.

Tea Drink of tea, using milk from daily allowance.

Supper As at dinner – hot or cold meal.

Daily 150 ml milk – for use in drinks during the day.

This diet gives 20 g. of protein, 13 g. of fat and 26 g. of carbohydrate.

TABLE SHOWING THE NORMAL WEIGHT OF ADULTS

Expected weight above the average age of 25, and in average indoor clothing.

HEIGHT (wearing ordinary shoes)			Small build		Medium build		Large build	
ft	in	cm	lb	kg	lb	kg	lb	kg
				Men				
5	2	157·5	112–120	50·8–54·4	118–129	53·5–58·5	126–141	57·2–64·0
5	3	160·0	115–123	52·2–55·8	121–133	54·9–60·3	129–144	58·5–65·3
5	4	162·6	118–126	53·5–57·2	124–136	56·2–61·7	132–148	59·9–67·1
5	5	165·1	121–129	54·9–58·5	127–139	57·6–63·0	135–152	61·2–68·9
5	6	167·6	124–133	56·2–60·3	130–143	59·0–64·9	138–156	62·6–70·8
5	7	170·2	128–137	58·1–62·1	134–147	60·8–66·7	142–161	64·4–73·0
5	8	172·7	132–141	59·9–64·0	138–152	62·6–68·9	147–166	66·7–75·3
5	9	175·3	136–145	61·7–65·8	142–156	64·4–70·8	151–170	68·5–77·1
5	10	177·8	140–150	63·5–68·0	146–160	66·2–72·6	155–174	70·3–78·9
5	11	180·3	144–154	65·3–69·9	150–165	68·0–74·8	159–179	72·1–81·2
6	0	182·9	148–158	67·1–71·7	154–170	69·9–77·1	164–184	74·4–83·5
6	1	185·4	152–162	68·9–73·5	158–175	71·7–79·4	168–189	76·2–85·7
6	2	188·0	156–167	70·8–75·7	162–180	73·5–81·6	173–194	78·5–88·0
6	3	190·5	160–171	72·6–77·6	167–185	75·7–83·5	178–199	80·7–90·3
6	4	193·0	164–175	74·4–79·4	172–190	78·1–86·2	182–204	82·7–92·5
				Women				
4	10	147·3	92– 98	41·7–44·5	96–107	43·5–48·5	104–119	47·2–54·0
4	11	149·9	94–101	42·6–45·8	98–110	44·5–49·9	106–122	48·1–55·3
5	0	152·4	96–104	43·5–47·2	101–113	45·8–51·3	109–125	49·4–56·7
5	1	154·9	99–107	44·9–48·5	104–116	47·2–52·6	112–128	50·8–58·1
5	2	157·5	102–110	46·3–49·9	107–119	48·5–54·0	115–131	52·2–59·4
5	3	160·0	105–113	47·6–51·3	110–122	49·9–55·3	118–134	53·5–60·8
5	4	162·6	108–116	49·0–52·6	113–126	51·3–57·2	121–138	54·9–62·6
5	5	165·1	111–119	50·3–54·0	116–130	49·0–59·0	125–142	49·4–64·4
5	6	167·6	114–123	51·7–55·8	120–135	54·4–61·2	129–146	59·5–66·2
5	7	170·2	118–127	53·5–57·6	124–139	56·2–63·0	133–150	60·3–68·0
5	8	172·7	122–131	55·3–59·4	128–143	58·1–64·9	137–154	62·1–69·9
5	9	175·3	126–135	57·2–61·2	132–147	59·9–66·7	141–158	64·0–71·7
5	10	177·8	130–140	59·0–63·5	136–151	61·7–68·5	145–163	65·8–73·9
5	11	180·3	134–144	60·8–65·3	140–155	63·5–70·3	149–168	67·6–76·2
6	0	182·9	138–148	62·6–67·1	144–159	65·3–72·1	153–173	69·4–78·5

TABLE SHOWING THE NORMAL HEIGHT AND WEIGHT OF CHILDREN

	Boys				*Girls*			
Age in	Height		Weight		Height		Weight	
Years	in	cm	lb	kg	in	cm	lb	kg
1	29·6	75·2	22·2	10·1	29·2	74·2	21·5	9·8
2	34·4	87·5	27·7	12·6	34·1	86·6	27·1	12·3
3	37·9	96·2	32·2	14·6	37·7	95·7	31·8	14·4
4	40·7	103·4	36·4	16·5	40·6	103·2	36·2	16·4
5	43·8	111·3	42·8	19·4	43·2	109·7	41·4	18·8
6	46·3	117·5	48·3	21·9	45·6	115·9	46·5	21·1
7	48·9	124·1	54·1	24·5	48·1	122·3	52·2	23·7
8	51·2	130·0	60·1	27·3	50·4	128·0	58·1	26·3
9	53·3	135·5	66·0	29·9	52·3	132·9	63·8	28·9
10	55·2	140·3	71·9	32·6	54·6	138·6	70·3	31·9
11	56·8	144·2	77·6	35·2	57·0	144·7	78·8	35·7
12	58·9	149·6	84·4	38·3	59·8	151·9	87·6	39·7
13	61·0	155·0	93·0	42·2	61·9	157·1	99·1	44·9
14	64·1	162·7	107·6	48·8	62·8	159·6	108·4	49·2
15	66·1	167·8	120·1	54·5	63·4	161·1	113·5	51·5
16	67·6	171·6	129·7	58·8	63·9	162·2	117·0	53·1
17	68·4	173·7	136·2	61·8	64·0	162·5	119·1	54·0
18	68·7	174·5	139·0	63·0	64·0	162·5	119·9	54·4

TABLE SHOWING NORMAL PAEDIATRIC DOSAGES

Please note that this is based on Catzel's method (the percentage method) and it should be remembered that this method does not apply to all therapeutic agents (for example, it does *not* apply to narcotics.)

Percentage method

Age	Weight kg.	Weight lb.	Percentage of adult dose
Premature	1·1	2·5	2·5–5
Premature	1·8	4	4–8
Premature	2·5	5	5–10
Term	3·2	7	12·5
2 months	4·5	10	15
4 months	6·5	14	20
12 months	10	22	25
18 months	11	25	30
3 years	15	33	33
5 years	18	40	40
7 years	23	50	50
10 years	30	66	60
11 years	36	80	70
12 years	40	88	75
14 years	45	100	80
16 years	65	120	90

TABLE SHOWING NORMAL HEAD CIRCUMFERENCES OF INFANTS

Mean Values

	Boys (inches)	Cm	Girls (inches)	Cm.
Birth	13·9	35·3	13·7	34·8
3 months	16·1	40·9	15·7	39·9
6 months	17·3	43·9	16·9	42·9
9 months	18·1	46·0	17·6	44·7
12 months	18·6	47·2	18·0	45·7
18 months	19·2	48·8	18·5	47·0
2 years	19·6	49·8	18·9	48·0
3 years	19·8	50·3	19·4	49·3

TABLE SHOWING NORMAL FUNDUS HEIGHT

12 weeks	pelvic brim
16 weeks	mid-way pubis and umbilicus
20 weeks	just below umbilicus
24 weeks	at umbilicus
30 weeks	mid-way umbilicus and xiphisternum
36 weeks	at xiphisternum

TABLE SHOWING APPROXIMATE EQUIVALENT WEIGHTS

(Based on British Pharmacopoeia, 1963)

Apothecary – to – Metric

Grains	Milligrams	Grams
$\frac{1}{200}$ gr	0·3 mg	0·0003 g.
$\frac{1}{100}$ gr	0·6 mg	0·0006 g.
$\frac{1}{60}$ gr	1 mg	0·001 g.
$\frac{1}{30}$ gr	2 mg	0·002 g.
$\frac{1}{15}$ gr	4 mg	0·004 g.
$\frac{1}{8}$ gr	7·5 mg	0·0075 g.
$\frac{1}{4}$ gr	15 mg	0·015 g.
$\frac{1}{2}$ gr	30 mg	0·03 g.
$\frac{3}{4}$ gr	50 mg	0·05 g.
1 gr	60 mg	0·06 g.
$1\frac{1}{2}$ grs	100 mg	0·1 g.
2 grs	125 mg	0·125 g.
$2\frac{1}{2}$ grs	150 mg	0·15 g.
3 grs	200 mg	0·2 g.
5 grs	300 mg	0·3 g.
$7\frac{1}{2}$ grs	450 mg	0·45 g.
10 grs	600 mg	0·6 g.
15 grs	1,000 mg	1·0 g.

TABLE SHOWING SCALE OF FAHRENHEIT TO CENTIGRADE

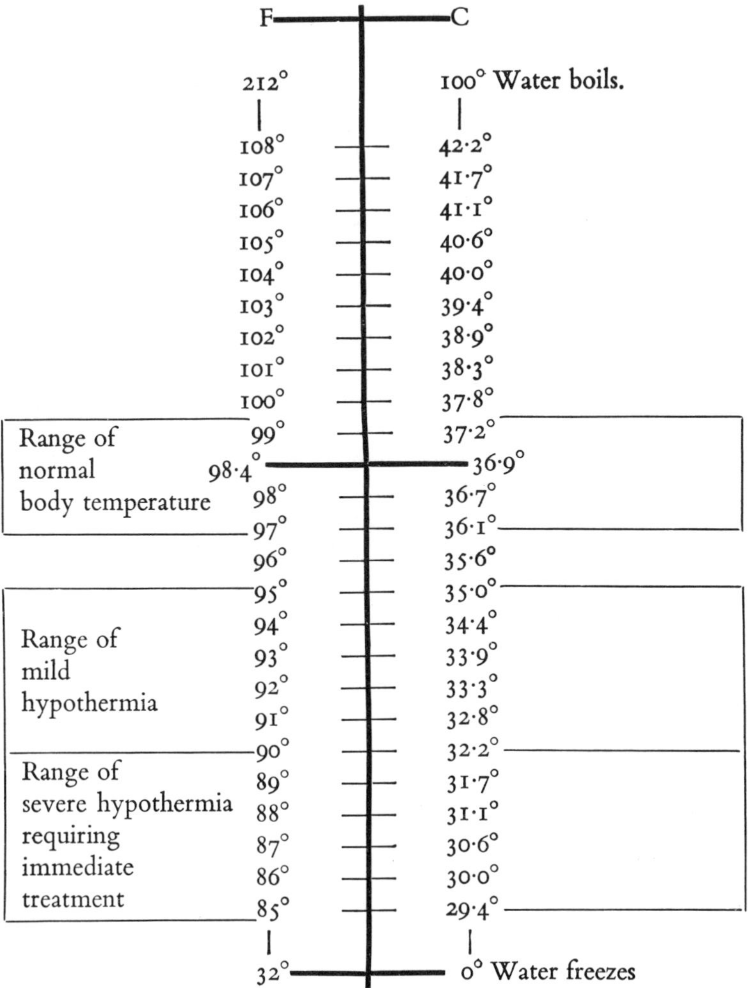

(Centigrade $\times \frac{9}{5}) + 32 =$ Fahrenheit

(Fahrenheit $- 32) \times \frac{5}{9} =$ Centigrade

OBSTETRIC DATE CALCULATION TABLE

(L.M.P. is shown in light type – E.D.C. is shown in **bold type**)

January	1	2	3	4	5	6	7	8	9	10	11	12	13	14	15	16	17	18	19	20	21	22	23	24	25	26	27	28	29	30	31	January
October	**8**	**9**	**10**	**11**	**12**	**13**	**14**	**15**	**16**	**17**	**18**	**19**	**20**	**21**	**22**	**23**	**24**	**25**	**26**	**27**	**28**	**29**	**30**	**31**	**1**	**2**	**3**	**4**	**5**	**6**	**7**	**November**
February	1	2	3	4	5	6	7	8	9	10	11	12	13	14	15	16	17	18	19	20	21	22	23	24	25	26	27	28	—	—	—	February
November	**8**	**9**	**10**	**11**	**12**	**13**	**14**	**15**	**16**	**17**	**18**	**19**	**20**	**21**	**22**	**23**	**24**	**25**	**26**	**27**	**28**	**29**	**30**	**1**	**2**	**3**	**4**	**5**	—	—	—	**December**
March	1	2	3	4	5	6	7	8	9	10	11	12	13	14	15	16	17	18	19	20	21	22	23	24	25	26	27	28	29	30	31	March
December	**6**	**7**	**8**	**9**	**10**	**11**	**12**	**13**	**14**	**15**	**16**	**17**	**18**	**19**	**20**	**21**	**22**	**23**	**24**	**25**	**26**	**27**	**28**	**29**	**30**	**31**	**1**	**2**	**3**	**4**	**5**	**January**
April	1	2	3	4	5	6	7	8	9	10	11	12	13	14	15	16	17	18	19	20	21	22	23	24	25	26	27	28	29	30	—	April
January	**6**	**7**	**8**	**9**	**10**	**11**	**12**	**13**	**14**	**15**	**16**	**17**	**18**	**19**	**20**	**21**	**22**	**23**	**24**	**25**	**26**	**27**	**28**	**29**	**30**	**31**	**1**	**2**	**3**	**4**	—	**February**
May	1	2	3	4	5	6	7	8	9	10	11	12	13	14	15	16	17	18	19	20	21	22	23	24	25	26	27	28	29	30	31	May
February	**5**	**6**	**7**	**8**	**9**	**10**	**11**	**12**	**13**	**14**	**15**	**16**	**17**	**18**	**19**	**20**	**21**	**22**	**23**	**24**	**25**	**26**	**27**	**28**	**1**	**2**	**3**	**4**	**5**	**6**	**7**	**March**
June	1	2	3	4	5	6	7	8	9	10	11	12	13	14	15	16	17	18	19	20	21	22	23	24	25	26	27	28	29	30	—	June
March	**8**	**9**	**10**	**11**	**12**	**13**	**14**	**15**	**16**	**17**	**18**	**19**	**20**	**21**	**22**	**23**	**24**	**25**	**26**	**27**	**28**	**29**	**30**	**31**	**1**	**2**	**3**	**4**	**5**	**6**	—	**April**
July	1	2	3	4	5	6	7	8	9	10	11	12	13	14	15	16	17	18	19	20	21	22	23	24	25	26	27	28	29	30	31	July
April	**7**	**8**	**9**	**10**	**11**	**12**	**13**	**14**	**15**	**16**	**17**	**18**	**19**	**20**	**21**	**22**	**23**	**24**	**25**	**26**	**27**	**28**	**29**	**30**	**1**	**2**	**3**	**4**	**5**	**6**	**7**	**May**
August	1	2	3	4	5	6	7	8	9	10	11	12	13	14	15	16	17	18	19	20	21	22	23	24	25	26	27	28	29	30	31	August
May	**8**	**9**	**10**	**11**	**12**	**13**	**14**	**15**	**16**	**17**	**18**	**19**	**20**	**21**	**22**	**23**	**24**	**25**	**26**	**27**	**28**	**29**	**30**	**31**	**1**	**2**	**3**	**4**	**5**	**6**	**7**	**June**
September	1	2	3	4	5	6	7	8	9	10	11	12	13	14	15	16	17	18	19	20	21	22	23	24	25	26	27	28	29	30	—	September
June	**8**	**9**	**10**	**11**	**12**	**13**	**14**	**15**	**16**	**17**	**18**	**19**	**20**	**21**	**22**	**23**	**24**	**25**	**26**	**27**	**28**	**29**	**30**	**1**	**2**	**3**	**4**	**5**	**6**	**7**	—	**July**
October	1	2	3	4	5	6	7	8	9	10	11	12	13	14	15	16	17	18	19	20	21	22	23	24	25	26	27	28	29	30	31	October
July	**8**	**9**	**10**	**11**	**12**	**13**	**14**	**15**	**16**	**17**	**18**	**19**	**20**	**21**	**22**	**23**	**24**	**25**	**26**	**27**	**28**	**29**	**30**	**31**	**1**	**2**	**3**	**4**	**5**	**6**	**7**	**August**
November	1	2	3	4	5	6	7	8	9	10	11	12	13	14	15	16	17	18	19	20	21	22	23	24	25	26	27	28	29	30	—	November
August	**8**	**9**	**10**	**11**	**12**	**13**	**14**	**15**	**16**	**17**	**18**	**19**	**20**	**21**	**22**	**23**	**24**	**25**	**26**	**27**	**28**	**29**	**30**	**31**	**1**	**2**	**3**	**4**	**5**	**6**	—	**September**
December	1	2	3	4	5	6	7	8	9	10	11	12	13	14	15	16	17	18	19	20	21	22	23	24	25	26	27	28	29	30	31	December
September	**7**	**8**	**9**	**10**	**11**	**12**	**13**	**14**	**15**	**16**	**17**	**18**	**19**	**20**	**21**	**22**	**23**	**24**	**25**	**26**	**27**	**28**	**29**	**30**	**1**	**2**	**3**	**4**	**5**	**6**	**7**	**October**

TABLE SHOWING THE INCUBATION PERIODS OF INFECTIOUS DISEASES

(The average expected time of development from first contact with the infecting organism – it must be remembered that individual variation is often considerable).

Within seven days from exposure:

BACILLARY DYSENTERY (SHIGELLA)
DIPHTHERIA
MENINGITIS
FOOD POISONING (Salmonella 24 hours. Staph. aureus and Cl. Welchii 4–12 hours)
GONORRHOEA
CHOLERA
STREPTOCOCCAL INFECTIONS (Scarlet Fever, Erysepelas)

From seven to fourteen days:

SMALLPOX
ENTERIC FEVER (Typhoid 12–14. Paratyphoid 10–12)
MEASLES
PERTUSSIS
PLAGUE
TETANUS (incubation periods beyond this confer good prognosis)

Within twenty-one days:

CHICKEN POX
RUBELLA
MUMPS
INFECTIOUS HEPATITIS (May extend beyond this limit)
HOMOLOGOUS SERUM HEPATITIS (May be up to 100 days or more)
BRUCELLOSIS.

Index

N.B. When the page number is shown in bold type this normally indicates a main discussion of the indexed subject (the discussion may also continue on the pages immediately following).